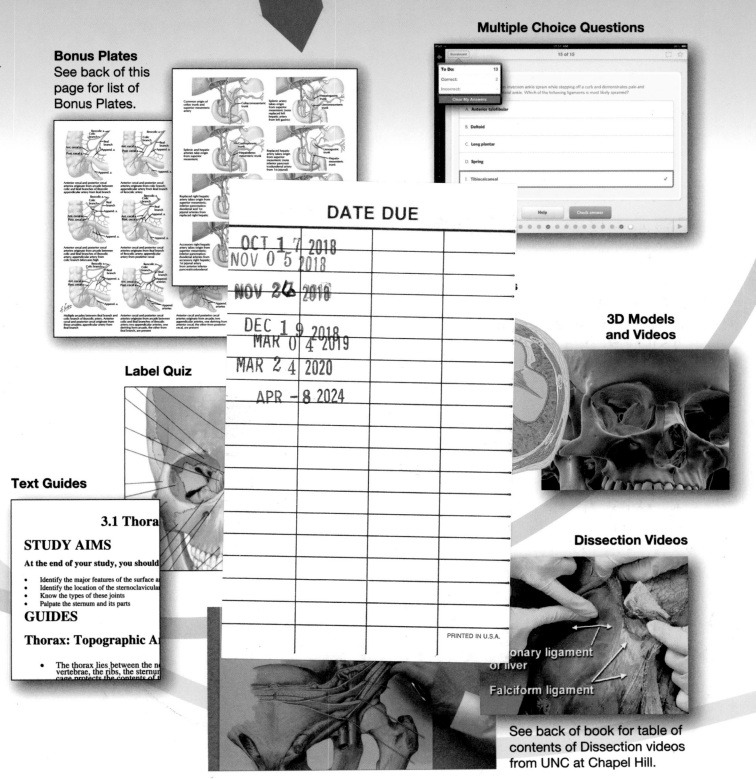

W9-AFC-574

# StudentConsult.com
## Log on now to access content beyond the book

**Bonus Plates**
See back of this page for list of Bonus Plates.

**Multiple Choice Questions**

**Label Quiz**

**Text Guides**

### 3.1 Thora

**STUDY AIMS**

At the end of your study, you should

- Identify the major features of the surface a
- Identify the location of the sternoclavicular
- Know the types of these joints
- Palpate the sternum and its parts

**GUIDES**

**Thorax: Topographic A**

- The thorax lies between the ne vertebrae, the ribs, the sternu cage protects the contents of

**3D Models and Videos**

**Dissection Videos**

...onary ligament of liver

Falciform ligament

See back of book for table of contents of Dissection videos from UNC at Chapel Hill.

**Plate Discussion Videos**

# Bonus Plates

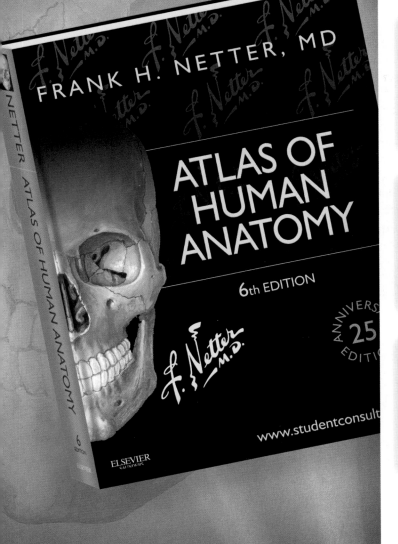
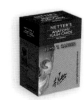
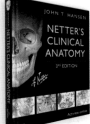
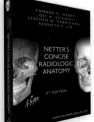
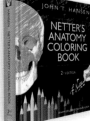

# Atlas of
# Human
# Anatomy

## Sixth Edition

Frank H. Netter, MD

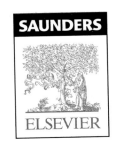

SAUNDERS

ELSEVIER

SAUNDERS
ELSEVIER

1600 John F. Kennedy Blvd.
Ste. 1800
Philadelphia, PA 19103-2899

ATLAS OF HUMAN ANATOMY
SIXTH EDITION

Standard Edition:          978-1-4557-0418-7
Professional Edition:      978-1-4557-5888-3
IE:                        978-0-8089-2451-7
Enhanced IE Edition:       978-0-323-39009-5

Previous editions copyrighted 2011, 2006, 2003, 1997, 1989

*Senior Content Strategist:* Elyse O'Grady
*Senior Content Development Specialist:* Marybeth Thiel
*Publishing Services Manager:* Patricia Tannian
*Senior Project Manager:* John Casey
*Senior Design Manager:* Lou Forgione
*Illustration Buyer:* Karen Giacomucci

Printed in the United States of America

Last digit is the print number: 9  8  7  6  5  4  3

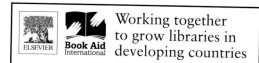

Working together
to grow libraries in
developing countries

www.elsevier.com • www.bookaid.org

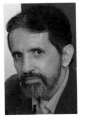

## Contributing Medical Illustrator

Carlos A. G. Machado, MD

## Consulting Editors

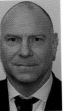

**John T. Hansen, Ph.D.**
*Lead Editor*
*Associate Dean for Admissions*
*Professor of Neurobiology and Anatomy*
*University of Rochester Medical Center*
*Rochester, New York*

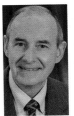

**Brion Benninger, MD, MS**
*Professor, Chair Medical Anatomical Sciences, Family Medicine,*
*and Neuromuscular Medicine College of Dental Medicine,*
*Western University of Health Sciences Lebanon, Oregon;*
*Orthopaedic and General Surgery Residency Program*
*Samaritan Hospital Corvallis, Oregon;*
*Surgery, Orthopedics & Rehabilitation,*
*and Oral Maxillofacial Surgery*
*Oregon Health & Science University*
*Portland, Oregon*

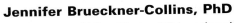

**Jennifer Brueckner-Collins, PhD**
*Professor and Vice Chair of Educational Programs*
*Anatomical Sciences and Neurobiology*
*University of Louisville School of Medicine*
*Louisville, Kentucky*

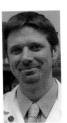

**Todd M. Hoagland, PhD**
*Associate Professor*
*Department of Cell Biology, Neurobiology, and Anatomy*
*Medical College of Wisconsin*
*Milwaukee, Wisconsin*

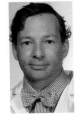

**R. Shane Tubbs, MS, PA-C, PhD**
*Pediatric Neurosurgery*
*Children's Hospital of Alabama*
*Birmingham, Alabama*
*Professor of Anatomy*
*Department of Anatomical Sciences, St. George's University,*
*Grenada Centre of Anatomy and Human Identification,*
*Dundee University, United Kingdom*

## Editors of Previous Editions

## International Advisory Board

# Netter's Atlas of Human Anatomy – Celebrating 25 Years

*"Anatomy, of course, does not change, but our understanding of anatomy and its clinical significance does."*

**– Frank H. Netter, MD**

Whether you're using this 6th edition of **Atlas of Human Anatomy** in print, as an e-Book, online, or in the Netter's Anatomy Atlas for iPad app—Dr. Netter's paintings of the intricacies of the human form remain as relevant today as at first launch. The publication of the 6th edition marks the silver anniversary of the first release of Frank H. Netter's *Atlas of Human Anatomy*—when its vibrant colors and unique clinical perspective made it a must-have companion in anatomy classes, dissection labs, and clinical professional offices worldwide—solidifying his legacy to so many as one of the world's most influential medical educators.

Anatomy remains a cornerstone of healthcare education. It is often one of the first topics taught in medical or healthcare curricula. Anatomy is also central to so much in clinical practice, from physical examination and radiologic imaging to surgery and physical rehabilitation. However, changes in anatomy education and its clinical application over these past 25 years have been significant. Medical and healthcare curricula increasingly integrate anatomy throughout and dedicated gross-anatomy hours have decreased. Some programs have discontinued full-body dissection. Advances in imaging technology have provided increasingly clearer views of living anatomy, and 3D models of anatomy continue to evolve. Likewise, the *Atlas* has evolved. Thanks to the tremendous guidance of leading clinical anatomists and expert anatomy educators, as well as the contributions of talented medical illustrators, the 6th edition features newly created illustrations and modern radiologic images that provide students with views of current clinical significance and perspectives that elucidate complex anatomic relationships. This edition also includes the illustrations from older editions of the *Atlas*, like Dr. Netter's depictions of common anatomic variations (in electronic editions and print+electronic packages) as bonus plates to help provide more comprehensive coverage that dissection lab hours may not allow. For the first time, the *Atlas* incorporates muscle tables as quick look-up appendices at the end of each section for the convenience of the clinician, student, or educator with little time. StudentConsult.com and NetterReference.com electronic resources include some 3D models extracted from Netter's 3D Interactive Anatomy, dissection video selections from Netter's Online Dissection Modules by UNC at Chapel Hill, and other supporting resources. In addition, all text throughout the Atlas has been meticulously updated to be in line with the most recent version of *Terminologia Anatomica* by the Federal International Program for Anatomical Terminology (FIPAT) of the International Federation of Associations of Anatomists (IFAA).

The unique visual perspective of Frank H. Netter is unsurpassed. Dr. Netter brought the hand of a master medical illustrator, the brain of a physician, and the soul of an artist to his depictions of the human body. This 25th anniversary edition celebrates the lasting impact of his work that continues to teach and inspire.

**We want to hear from you**—about the history and future of anatomy education and medicine and the Netter legacy and invite you to share your thoughts, inspirations, memories, tributes, and feedback with us through email: NetterAppFeedback@elsevier.com and on Facebook: www.facebook.com/NetterImages

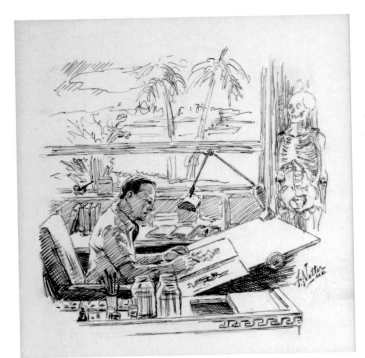

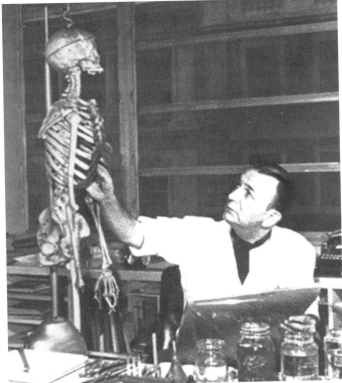

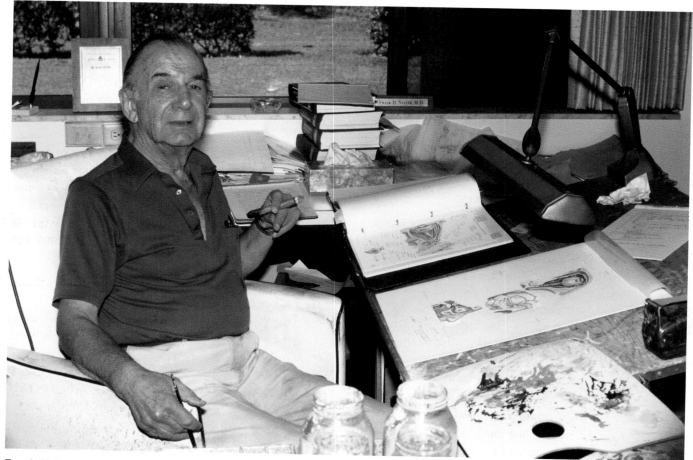

**Frank H. Netter, MD**
Photograph by James L. Clayton

**To my dear wife, Vera**

# Preface to the First Edition

I have often said that my career as a medical artist for almost 50 years has been a sort of "command performance" in the sense that it has grown in response to the desires and requests of the medical profession. Over these many years, I have produced almost 4,000 illustrations, mostly for *The CIBA* (now *Netter*) *Collection of Medical Illustrations* but also for *Clinical Symposia*. These pictures have been concerned with the varied subdivisions of medical knowledge such as gross anatomy, histology, embryology, physiology, pathology, diagnostic modalities, surgical and therapeutic techniques, and clinical manifestations of a multitude of diseases. As the years went by, however, there were more and more requests from physicians and students for me to produce an atlas purely of gross anatomy. Thus, this atlas has come about, not through any inspiration on my part but rather, like most of my previous works, as a fulfillment of the desires of the medical profession.

It involved going back over all the illustrations I had made over so many years, selecting those pertinent to gross anatomy, classifying them and organizing them by system and region, adapting them to page size and space, and arranging them in logical sequence. Anatomy of course does not change, but our understanding of anatomy and its clinical significance does change, as do anatomical terminology and

nomenclature. This therefore required much updating of many of the older pictures and even revision of a number of them in order to make them more pertinent to today's ever-expanding scope of medical and surgical practice. In addition, I found that there were gaps in the portrayal of medical knowledge as pictorialized in the illustrations I had previously done, and this necessitated my making a number of new pictures that are included in this volume.

In creating an atlas such as this, it is important to achieve a happy medium between complexity and simplification. If the pictures are too complex, they may be difficult and confusing to read; if oversimplified, they may not be adequately definitive or may even be misleading. I have therefore striven for a middle course of realism without the clutter of confusing minutiae. I hope that the students and members of the medical and allied professions will find the illustrations readily understandable, yet instructive and useful.

At one point, the publisher and I thought it might be nice to include a foreword by a truly outstanding and renowned anatomist, but there are so many in that category that we could not make a choice. We did think of men like Vesalius, Leonardo da Vinci, William Hunter, and Henry Gray, who of course are unfortunately unavailable, but I do wonder what their comments might have been about this atlas.

**Frank H. Netter, MD**
(1906–1991)

# Frank H. Netter, MD

Frank H. Netter was born in New York City in 1906. He studied art at the Art Students League and the National Academy of Design before entering medical school at New York University, where he received his Doctor of Medicine degree in 1931. During his student years, Dr. Netter's notebook sketches attracted the attention of the medical faculty and other physicians, allowing him to augment his income by illustrating articles and textbooks. He continued illustrating as a sideline after establishing a surgical practice in 1933, but he ultimately opted to give up his practice in favor of a full-time commitment to art. After service in the United States Army during World War II, Dr. Netter began his long collaboration with the CIBA Pharmaceutical Company (now Novartis Pharmaceuticals). This 45-year partnership resulted in the production of the extraordinary collection of medical art so familiar to physicians and other medical professionals worldwide.

Icon Learning Systems acquired the Netter Collection in July 2000 and continued to update Dr. Netter's original paintings and to add newly commissioned paintings by artists trained in the style of Dr. Netter. In 2005, Elsevier Inc. purchased the Netter Collection and all publications from Icon Learning Systems. There are now over 50

publications featuring the art of Dr. Netter available through Elsevier Inc.

Dr. Netter's works are among the finest examples of the use of illustration in the teaching of medical concepts. The 13-book *Netter Collection of Medical Illustrations,* which includes the greater part of the more than 20,000 paintings created by Dr. Netter, became and remains one of the most famous medical works ever published. *The Netter Atlas of Human Anatomy,* first published in 1989, presents the anatomic paintings from the Netter Collection. Now translated into 16 languages, it is the anatomy atlas of choice among medical and health professions students the world over.

The Netter illustrations are appreciated not only for their aesthetic qualities, but, more importantly, for their intellectual content. As Dr. Netter wrote in 1949 "clarification of a subject is the aim and goal of illustration. No matter how beautifully painted, how delicately and subtly rendered a subject may be, it is of little value as a *medical illustration* if it does not serve to make clear some medical point." Dr. Netter's planning, conception, point of view, and approach are what inform his paintings and what make them so intellectually valuable.

Frank H. Netter, MD, physician and artist, died in 1991.

# Acknowledgments

## Brion Benninger, MD, MS

I would like to thank my wife, Alison, and our son, Jack, for their wit, caring, and the love they provide me daily. I want to thank Elsevier, especially Marybeth Thiel, for her insight and direction, enabling John Hansen, my fellow coeditors, and Carlos Machado to work in such a rich environment. I particularly want to thank my early clinical anatomy mentors, Gerald Tressidor and Harold Ellis (Guy's Hospital); Dean P. Crone and the University Board for continuous support; all my past and future patients and students; and clinical colleagues who keep anatomy dynamic. Special thanks to Jim McDaniel and Bill Bryan and all who represent what is good in teaching. Lastly, I thank my mother for her love of education and my father for his inquisitive mind.

## Jennifer Brueckner-Collins, PhD

I am very grateful to the wonderful Elsevier team, particularly Marybeth Thiel and Elyse O'Grady, for their guidance and expertise during our preparation of the sixth edition. It is always privilege to collaborate with Carlos Machado, whose artistic talent brings our anatomical visions from concept to reality. Sincere thanks to Mark Sturgill, DO, who most generously provided us with updated images for abdominal MRCP, axial and coronal CT with contrast, as well as CT angiography. Finally, I am eternally indebted to my parents, John and Rheba, and to my husband, Kurt, for their support, encouragement, love, and inspiration; they are my raison d'etre.

## John T. Hansen, PhD

At Elsevier I would like to thank Marybeth Thiel, Senior Development Editor, Elyse O'Grady, Senior Content Strategist, John Casey, Senior Project Manager, and Madelene Hyde, Publishing Director, for their continuous support and meticulous attention to detail during the development of this sixth edition of the *Atlas of Human Anatomy*. They, along with the entire Editorial, Production, Design, and Marketing team at Elsevier have been a delight to work with and to know. I am also indebted to Carlos Machado for his superb artistic skill in producing and updating plates appearing in the *Atlas*. His renderings of human anatomy are the perfect complement to the Netter images. In addition to my fellow editors of this edition, I wish to express my thanks to my faculty colleagues at Rochester and to all my past and present students who have provided generous and constructive feedback and have enriched my life. Finally, I am indebted to my entire family for their continued support and especially to my wife, Paula. Their love and encouragement sustains me and is the source of all the happiness and joy I know.

## Todd M. Hoagland, PhD

It is a privilege to teach clinical human anatomy and I am eternally grateful to all the body donors and their families for enabling healthcare professionals to train in the dissection laboratory. It is my honor to work with outstanding medical students and colleagues at the Medical College of Wisconsin. I am grateful to John Hansen and the professionals of the Elsevier team for the opportunity to be a steward of the incomparable *Netter Atlas*. Marybeth Thiel and Elyse O'Grady were especially helpful and a pleasure to work with. It was an honor to collaborate with the brilliant Carlos Machado and all the consulting editors. I thank Joe Besharse for being an outstanding mentor. I am deeply appreciative of Stan Hillman and Jack O'Malley for inspiring me with masterful teaching and rigorous expectations. I am indebted to Richard Hoyt, Jr., for helping me become a competent anatomist, and to Rob Bouchie for his support. I am most grateful to my brother, Bill, for his unwavering optimism and gregarious nature. I thank my mother, Liz, for her dedication and love and for instilling a strong work ethic. Finally, I am humbled by my two awesome children, Ella and Caleb, for helping me redefine love, wonder, and joy.

## R. Shane Tubbs, MS, PA-C, PhD

First and foremost, I would like to thank Elsevier and in particular, Madelene Hyde, Marybeth Thiel, and Elyse O'Grady for all of their hard work in making this edition come to life. The evolution of the current atlas continues with the superb skills of Dr. Carlos Machado and his works of art. I would like to thank Dr. Satinder Singh for his kind assistance in providing radiographic images of the heart. I thank my beautiful wife, Susan, and son, Isaiah, for their patience and guidance during the editing of the sixth edition. Without the continued support of my mentor, friend, and colleague, Dr. W. Jerry Oakes, I could not fulfill all of my academic endeavors. I dedicate my efforts in this edition to my late brother-in-law, Nelson Jones, whose appetite for inquisitiveness inspires me today.

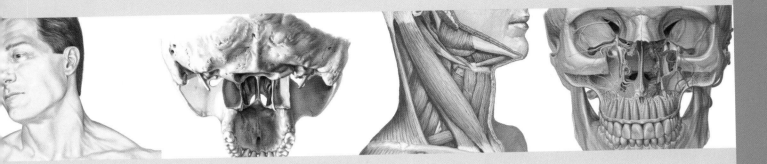

# 1 **HEAD AND NECK**

# HEAD AND NECK

## Superficial Face

**Plates 24–25**

## Neck

**Plates 26–34**

## Nasal Region

**Plates 35–55**

## Oral Region

**Plates 56–63**

## Pharynx

**Plates 64–75**

## Thyroid Gland and Larynx
**Plates 76–82**

## Orbit and Contents
**Plates 83–93**

## Ear
**Plates 94–100**

## Meninges and Brain
**Plates 101–116**

## Cranial and Cervical Nerves
**Plates 117–136**

Plate 1

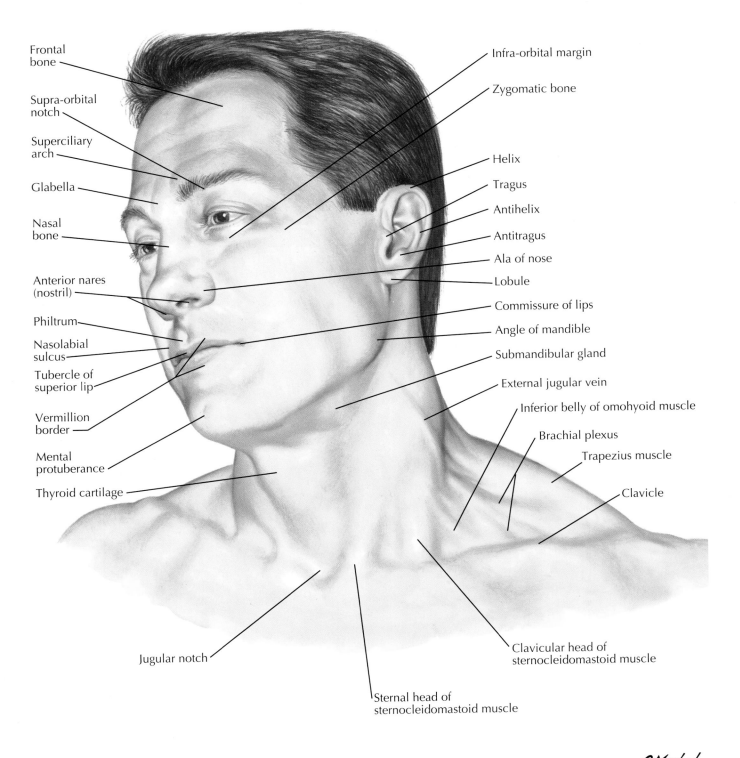

Frontal bone

Supra-orbital notch

Superciliary arch

Glabella

Nasal bone

Anterior nares (nostril)

Philtrum

Nasolabial sulcus

Tubercle of superior lip

Vermillion border

Mental protuberance

Thyroid cartilage

Jugular notch

Sternal head of sternocleidomastoid muscle

Infra-orbital margin

Zygomatic bone

Helix

Tragus

Antihelix

Antitragus

Ala of nose

Lobule

Commissure of lips

Angle of mandible

Submandibular gland

External jugular vein

Inferior belly of omohyoid muscle

Brachial plexus

Trapezius muscle

Clavicle

Clavicular head of sternocleidomastoid muscle

C. Machado
— M.D.

**Topographic Anatomy**

**Plate 1**

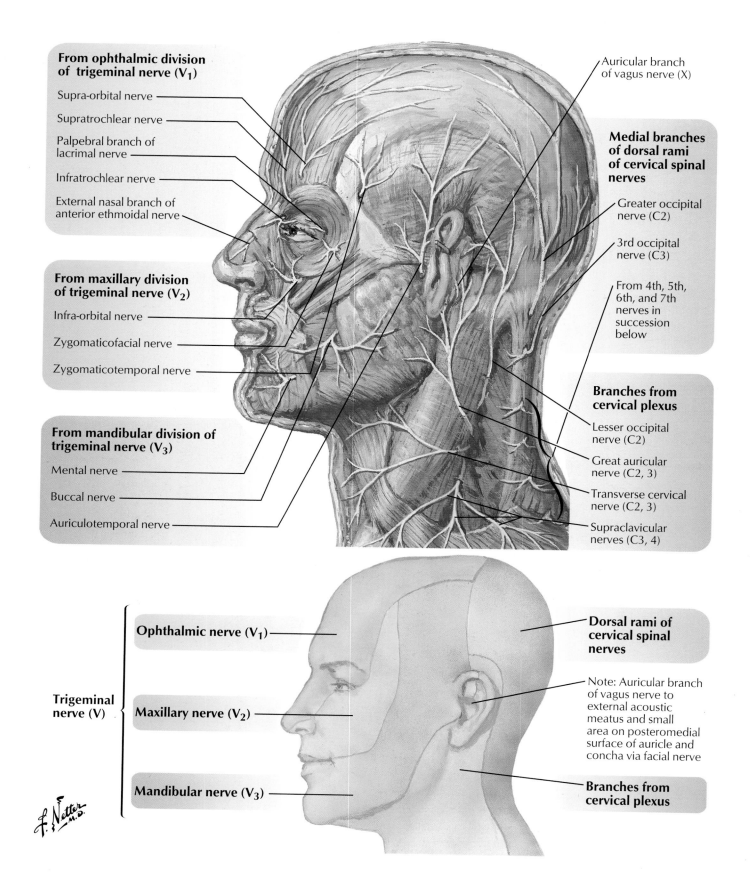

**From ophthalmic division of trigeminal nerve (V₁)**

Supra-orbital nerve

Supratrochlear nerve

Palpebral branch of lacrimal nerve

Infratrochlear nerve

External nasal branch of anterior ethmoidal nerve

**From maxillary division of trigeminal nerve (V₂)**

Infra-orbital nerve

Zygomaticofacial nerve

Zygomaticotemporal nerve

**From mandibular division of trigeminal nerve (V₃)**

Mental nerve

Buccal nerve

Auriculotemporal nerve

Auricular branch of vagus nerve (X)

**Medial branches of dorsal rami of cervical spinal nerves**

Greater occipital nerve (C2)

3rd occipital nerve (C3)

From 4th, 5th, 6th, and 7th nerves in succession below

**Branches from cervical plexus**

Lesser occipital nerve (C2)

Great auricular nerve (C2, 3)

Transverse cervical nerve (C2, 3)

Supraclavicular nerves (C3, 4)

Ophthalmic nerve (V₁)

Trigeminal nerve (V)

Maxillary nerve (V₂)

Mandibular nerve (V₃)

Dorsal rami of cervical spinal nerves

Note: Auricular branch of vagus nerve to external acoustic meatus and small area on posteromedial surface of auricle and concha via facial nerve

Branches from cervical plexus

**Plate 2**

**Superficial Head and Neck**

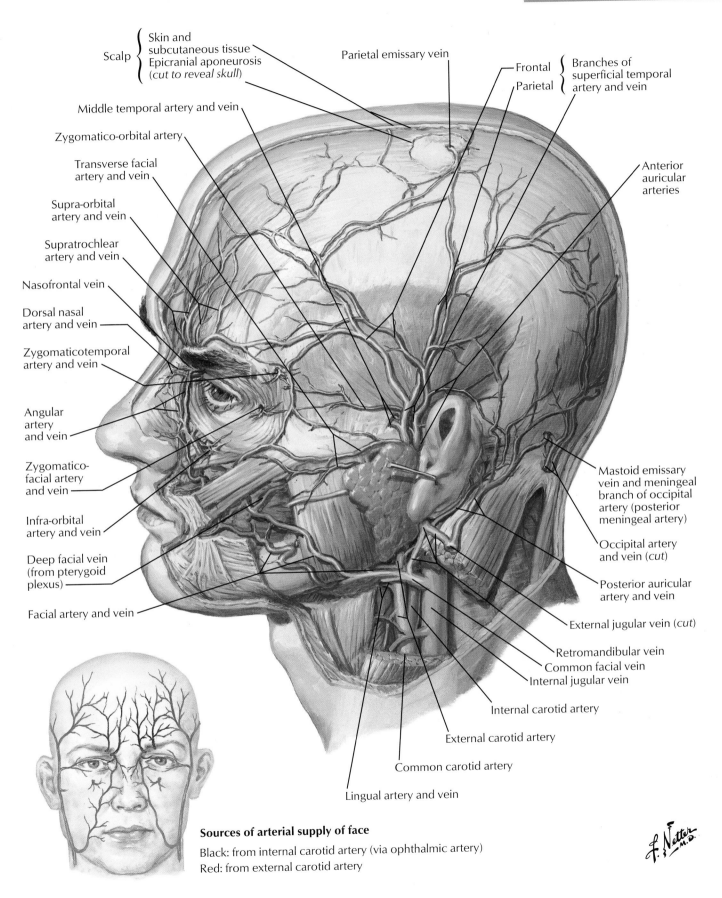

Scalp { Skin and subcutaneous tissue
Epicranial aponeurosis (*cut to reveal skull*)

Parietal emissary vein

Frontal
Parietal } Branches of superficial temporal artery and vein

Middle temporal artery and vein

Zygomatico-orbital artery

Transverse facial artery and vein

Anterior auricular arteries

Supra-orbital artery and vein

Supratrochlear artery and vein

Nasofrontal vein

Dorsal nasal artery and vein

Zygomaticotemporal artery and vein

Angular artery and vein

Zygomatico-facial artery and vein

Infra-orbital artery and vein

Deep facial vein (from pterygoid plexus)

Facial artery and vein

Mastoid emissary vein and meningeal branch of occipital artery (posterior meningeal artery)

Occipital artery and vein (*cut*)

Posterior auricular artery and vein

External jugular vein (*cut*)

Retromandibular vein

Common facial vein

Internal jugular vein

Internal carotid artery

External carotid artery

Common carotid artery

Lingual artery and vein

**Sources of arterial supply of face**

Black: from internal carotid artery (via ophthalmic artery)
Red: from external carotid artery

*f. Netter M.D.*

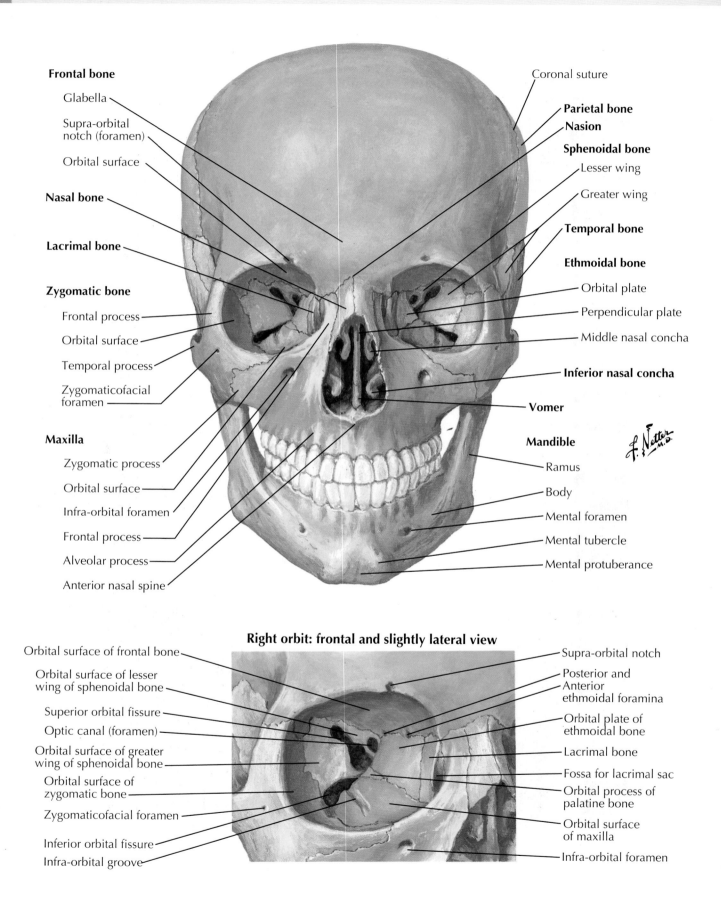

**Frontal bone**
- Glabella
- Supra-orbital notch (foramen)
- Orbital surface

**Nasal bone**

**Lacrimal bone**

**Zygomatic bone**
- Frontal process
- Orbital surface
- Temporal process
- Zygomaticofacial foramen

**Maxilla**
- Zygomatic process
- Orbital surface
- Infra-orbital foramen
- Frontal process
- Alveolar process
- Anterior nasal spine

Coronal suture

**Parietal bone**
**Nasion**
**Sphenoidal bone**
- Lesser wing
- Greater wing

**Temporal bone**

**Ethmoidal bone**
- Orbital plate
- Perpendicular plate
- Middle nasal concha

**Inferior nasal concha**

**Vomer**

**Mandible**
- Ramus
- Body
- Mental foramen
- Mental tubercle
- Mental protuberance

## Right orbit: frontal and slightly lateral view

Orbital surface of frontal bone
Orbital surface of lesser wing of sphenoidal bone
Superior orbital fissure
Optic canal (foramen)
Orbital surface of greater wing of sphenoidal bone
Orbital surface of zygomatic bone
Zygomaticofacial foramen
Inferior orbital fissure
Infra-orbital groove

Supra-orbital notch
Posterior and Anterior ethmoidal foramina
Orbital plate of ethmoidal bone
Lacrimal bone
Fossa for lacrimal sac
Orbital process of palatine bone
Orbital surface of maxilla
Infra-orbital foramen

**Plate 4**　　　　　　　　　　　　　　　**Bones and Ligaments**

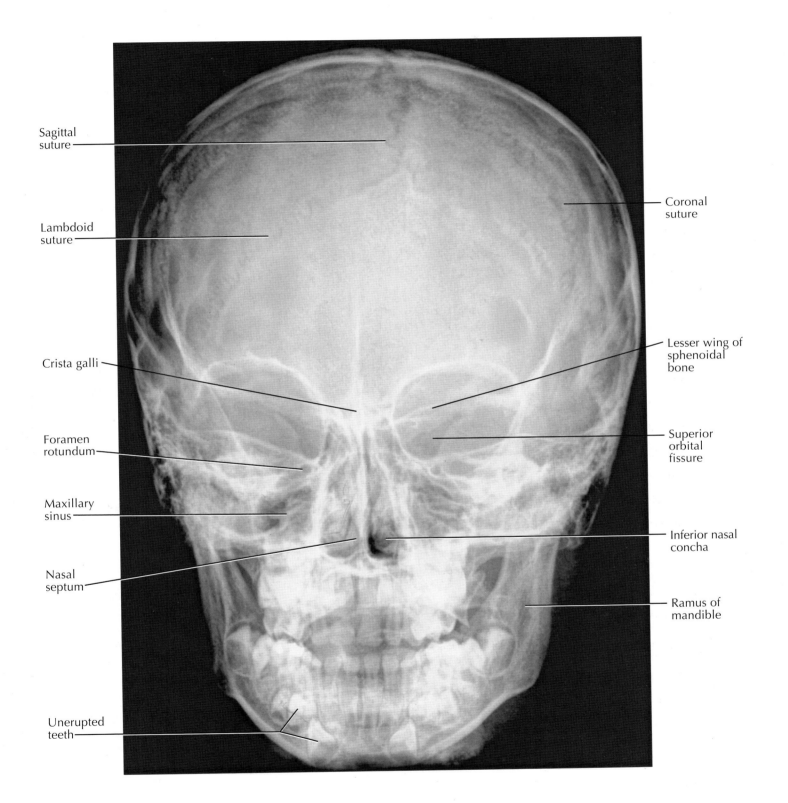

Sagittal
suture

Lambdoid
suture

Crista galli

Foramen
rotundum

Maxillary
sinus

Nasal
septum

Unerupted
teeth

Coronal
suture

Lesser wing of
sphenoidal
bone

Superior
orbital
fissure

Inferior nasal
concha

Ramus of
mandible

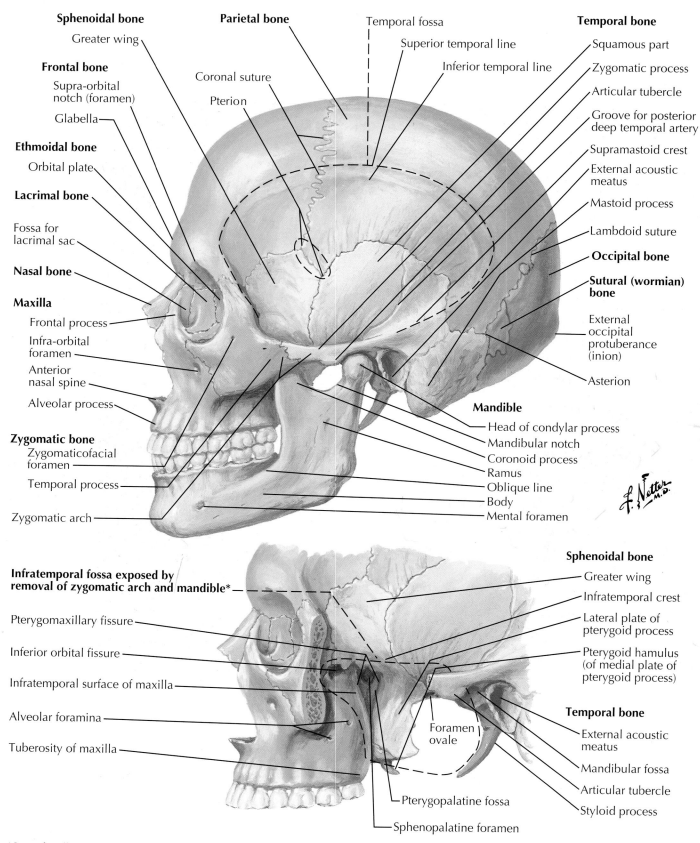

**Sphenoidal bone**
Greater wing

**Frontal bone**
Supra-orbital notch (foramen)
Glabella

**Ethmoidal bone**
Orbital plate

**Lacrimal bone**
Fossa for lacrimal sac

**Nasal bone**

**Maxilla**
Frontal process
Infra-orbital foramen
Anterior nasal spine
Alveolar process

**Zygomatic bone**
Zygomaticofacial foramen
Temporal process
Zygomatic arch

**Parietal bone**
Coronal suture
Pterion

Temporal fossa
Superior temporal line
Inferior temporal line

**Temporal bone**
Squamous part
Zygomatic process
Articular tubercle
Groove for posterior deep temporal artery
Supramastoid crest
External acoustic meatus
Mastoid process
Lambdoid suture

**Occipital bone**

**Sutural (wormian) bone**

External occipital protuberance (inion)
Asterion

**Mandible**
Head of condylar process
Mandibular notch
Coronoid process
Ramus
Oblique line
Body
Mental foramen

**Infratemporal fossa exposed by removal of zygomatic arch and mandible***

Pterygomaxillary fissure
Inferior orbital fissure
Infratemporal surface of maxilla
Alveolar foramina
Tuberosity of maxilla

Foramen ovale
Pterygopalatine fossa
Sphenopalatine foramen

**Sphenoidal bone**
Greater wing
Infratemporal crest
Lateral plate of pterygoid process
Pterygoid hamulus (of medial plate of pterygoid process)

**Temporal bone**
External acoustic meatus
Mandibular fossa
Articular tubercle
Styloid process

*Superficially, mastoid process forms posterior boundary.*

**Plate 6**

**Bones and Ligaments**

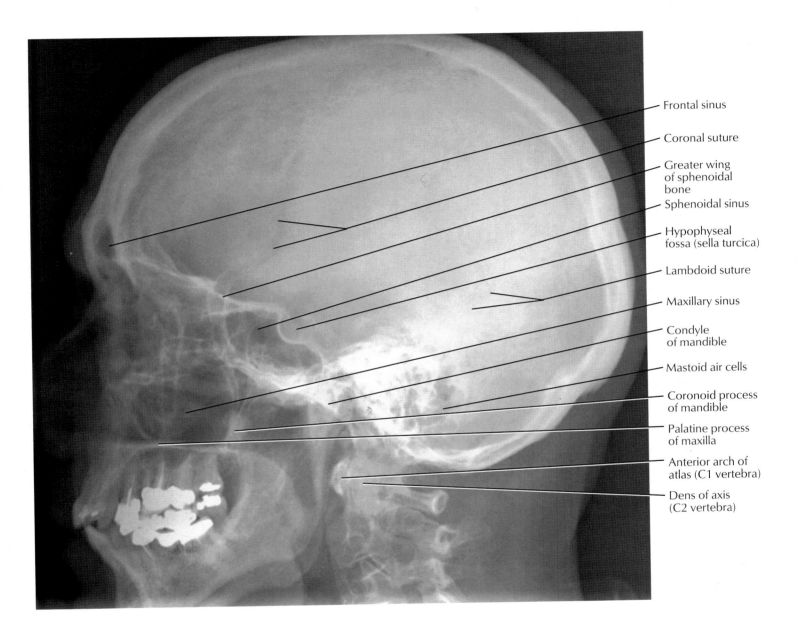

Frontal sinus

Coronal suture

Greater wing of sphenoidal bone

Sphenoidal sinus

Hypophyseal fossa (sella turcica)

Lambdoid suture

Maxillary sinus

Condyle of mandible

Mastoid air cells

Coronoid process of mandible

Palatine process of maxilla

Anterior arch of atlas (C1 vertebra)

Dens of axis (C2 vertebra)

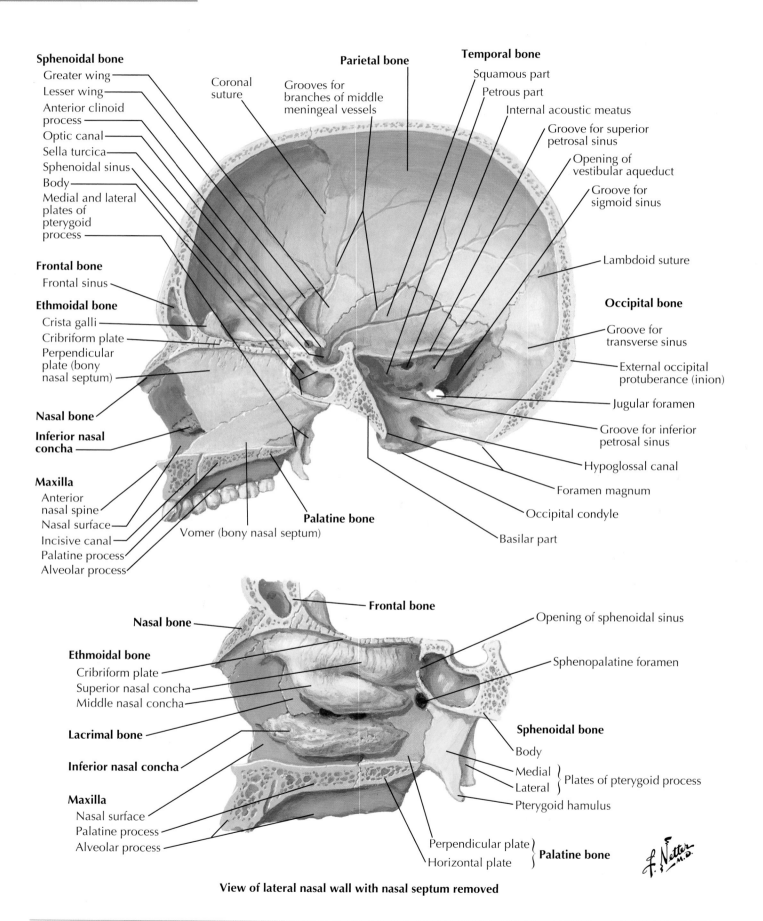

**Sphenoidal bone**
Greater wing
Lesser wing
Anterior clinoid process
Optic canal
Sella turcica
Sphenoidal sinus
Body
Medial and lateral plates of pterygoid process

**Frontal bone**
Frontal sinus

**Ethmoidal bone**
Crista galli
Cribriform plate
Perpendicular plate (bony nasal septum)

**Nasal bone**

**Inferior nasal concha**

**Maxilla**
Anterior nasal spine
Nasal surface
Incisive canal
Palatine process
Alveolar process

Coronal suture

Grooves for branches of middle meningeal vessels

**Parietal bone**

**Temporal bone**
Squamous part
Petrous part
Internal acoustic meatus
Groove for superior petrosal sinus
Opening of vestibular aqueduct
Groove for sigmoid sinus

Lambdoid suture

**Occipital bone**
Groove for transverse sinus
External occipital protuberance (inion)
Jugular foramen
Groove for inferior petrosal sinus
Hypoglossal canal
Foramen magnum
Occipital condyle
Basilar part

**Palatine bone**
Vomer (bony nasal septum)

**Nasal bone**

**Ethmoidal bone**
Cribriform plate
Superior nasal concha
Middle nasal concha

**Lacrimal bone**

**Inferior nasal concha**

**Maxilla**
Nasal surface
Palatine process
Alveolar process

**Frontal bone**

Opening of sphenoidal sinus

Sphenopalatine foramen

**Sphenoidal bone**
Body
Medial
Lateral } Plates of pterygoid process
Pterygoid hamulus

Perpendicular plate }
Horizontal plate } **Palatine bone**

**View of lateral nasal wall with nasal septum removed**

**Plate 8**

**Bones and Ligaments**

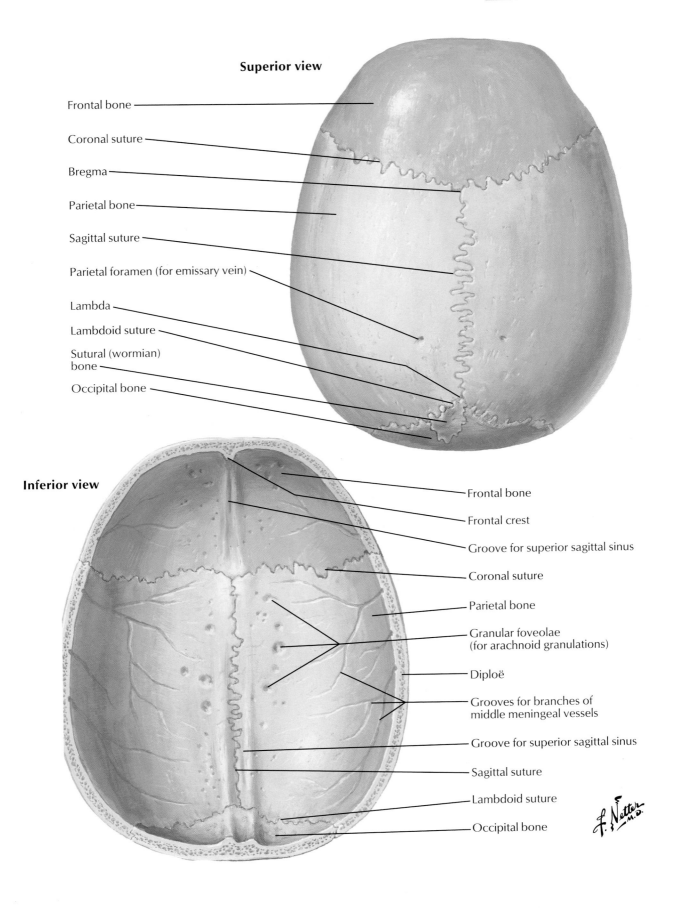

**Superior view**

Frontal bone

Coronal suture

Bregma

Parietal bone

Sagittal suture

Parietal foramen (for emissary vein)

Lambda

Lambdoid suture

Sutural (wormian) bone

Occipital bone

**Inferior view**

Frontal bone

Frontal crest

Groove for superior sagittal sinus

Coronal suture

Parietal bone

Granular foveolae (for arachnoid granulations)

Diploë

Grooves for branches of middle meningeal vessels

Groove for superior sagittal sinus

Sagittal suture

Lambdoid suture

Occipital bone

**Bones and Ligaments**

**Plate 9**

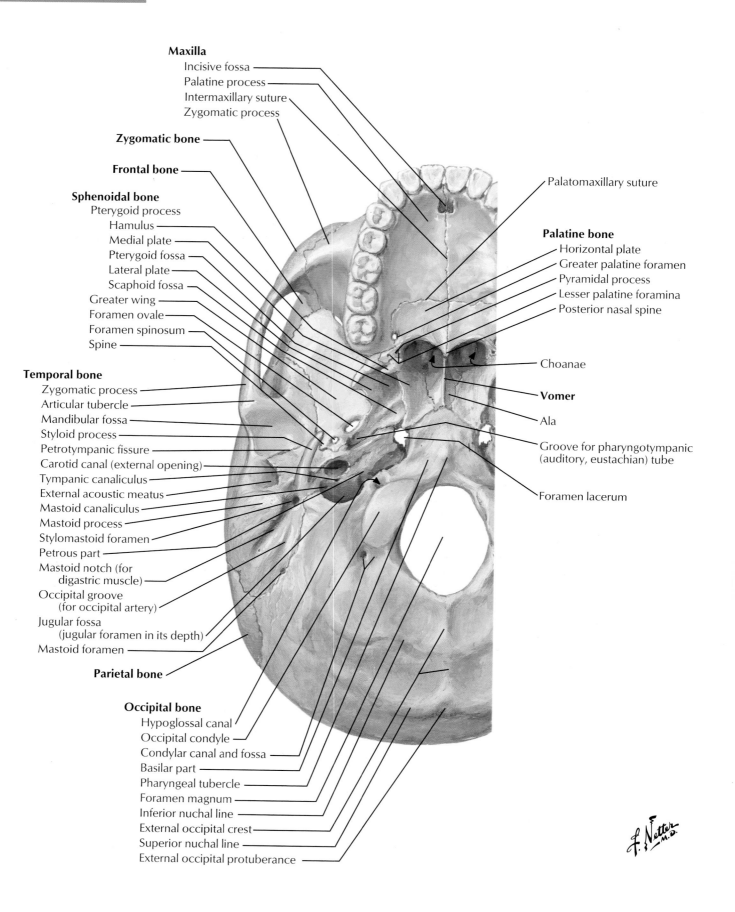

**Maxilla**
Incisive fossa
Palatine process
Intermaxillary suture
Zygomatic process

**Zygomatic bone**

**Frontal bone**

**Sphenoidal bone**
Pterygoid process
Hamulus
Medial plate
Pterygoid fossa
Lateral plate
Scaphoid fossa
Greater wing
Foramen ovale
Foramen spinosum
Spine

**Temporal bone**
Zygomatic process
Articular tubercle
Mandibular fossa
Styloid process
Petrotympanic fissure
Carotid canal (external opening)
Tympanic canaliculus
External acoustic meatus
Mastoid canaliculus
Mastoid process
Stylomastoid foramen
Petrous part
Mastoid notch (for
   digastric muscle)
Occipital groove
   (for occipital artery)
Jugular fossa
   (jugular foramen in its depth)
Mastoid foramen

**Parietal bone**

**Occipital bone**
Hypoglossal canal
Occipital condyle
Condylar canal and fossa
Basilar part
Pharyngeal tubercle
Foramen magnum
Inferior nuchal line
External occipital crest
Superior nuchal line
External occipital protuberance

Palatomaxillary suture

**Palatine bone**
Horizontal plate
Greater palatine foramen
Pyramidal process
Lesser palatine foramina
Posterior nasal spine

Choanae

**Vomer**

Ala

Groove for pharyngotympanic
(auditory, eustachian) tube

Foramen lacerum

**Plate 10**

**Bones and Ligaments**

**Frontal bone**
Groove for superior sagittal sinus
Frontal crest
Groove for anterior meningeal vessels
Foramen cecum
Superior surface of orbital part

**Ethmoidal bone**
Crista galli
Cribriform plate

**Sphenoidal bone**
Lesser wing
Anterior clinoid process
Greater wing
Groove for middle meningeal vessels (frontal branches)
Body
Jugum
Prechiasmatic groove
Sella turcica {
Tuberculum sellae
Hypophyseal fossa
Dorsum sellae
Posterior clinoid process
Carotid groove (for int. carotid a.)
Clivus

**Temporal bone**
Squamous part
Petrous part
Groove for lesser petrosal nerve
Groove for greater petrosal nerve
Arcuate eminence
Trigeminal impression
Groove for superior petrosal sinus
Groove for sigmoid sinus

**Parietal bone**
Groove for middle meningeal vessels (parietal branches)
Mastoid angle

**Occipital bone**
Clivus
Groove for inferior petrosal sinus
Basilar part
Groove for posterior meningeal vessels
Condyle
Groove for transverse sinus
Groove for occipital sinus
Internal occipital crest
Internal occipital protuberance
Groove for superior sagittal sinus

Anterior cranial fossa

Middle cranial fossa

Posterior cranial fossa

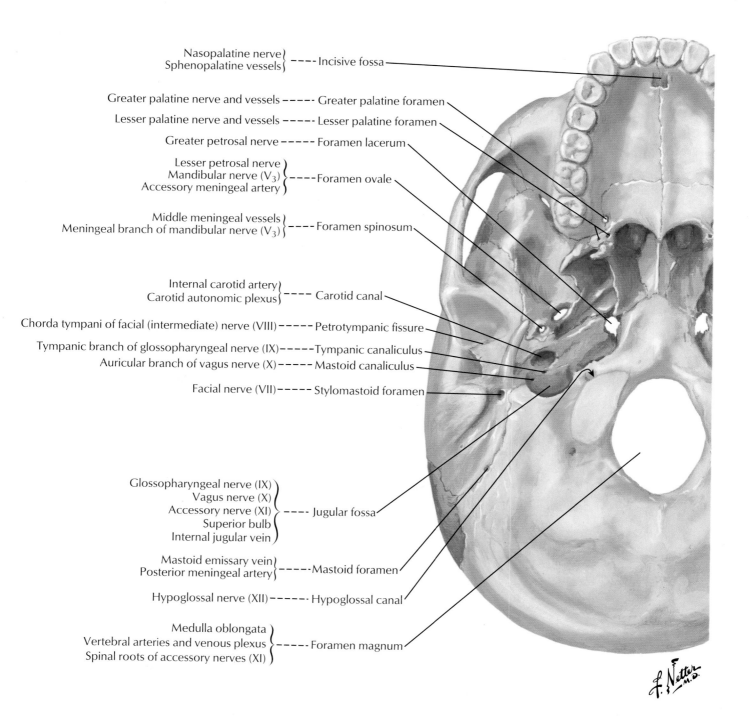

Nasopalatine nerve ⎱
Sphenopalatine vessels ⎰ ----- Incisive fossa

Greater palatine nerve and vessels ----- Greater palatine foramen

Lesser palatine nerve and vessels ----- Lesser palatine foramen

Greater petrosal nerve ----- Foramen lacerum

Lesser petrosal nerve ⎱
Mandibular nerve (V₃) ⎰ ----- Foramen ovale
Accessory meningeal artery ⎰

Middle meningeal vessels ⎱
Meningeal branch of mandibular nerve (V₃) ⎰ ----- Foramen spinosum

Internal carotid artery ⎱
Carotid autonomic plexus ⎰ ----- Carotid canal

Chorda tympani of facial (intermediate) nerve (VIII) ----- Petrotympanic fissure

Tympanic branch of glossopharyngeal nerve (IX) ----- Tympanic canaliculus

Auricular branch of vagus nerve (X) ----- Mastoid canaliculus

Facial nerve (VII) ----- Stylomastoid foramen

Glossopharyngeal nerve (IX) ⎱
Vagus nerve (X) ⎰
Accessory nerve (XI) ⎰ ----- Jugular fossa
Superior bulb ⎰
Internal jugular vein ⎰

Mastoid emissary vein ⎱
Posterior meningeal artery ⎰ ----- Mastoid foramen

Hypoglossal nerve (XII) ----- Hypoglossal canal

Medulla oblongata ⎱
Vertebral arteries and venous plexus ⎰ ----- Foramen magnum
Spinal roots of accessory nerves (XI) ⎰

**Plate 12**

**Bones and Ligaments**

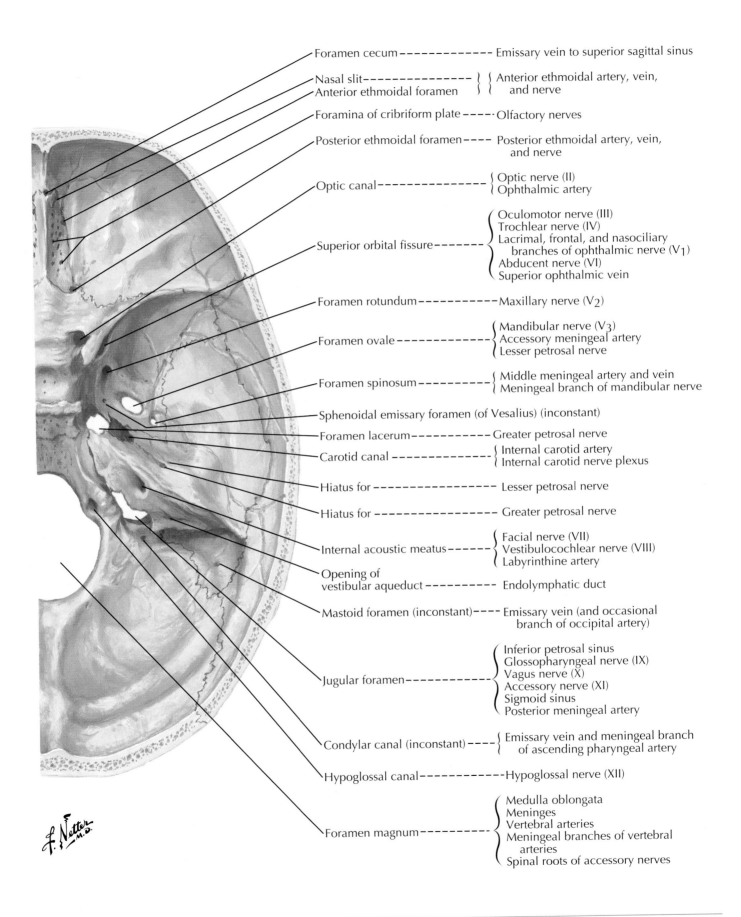

Foramen cecum – – – – – – – – – Emissary vein to superior sagittal sinus

Nasal slit – – – – – – – – – – – } } Anterior ethmoidal artery, vein,
Anterior ethmoidal foramen } } and nerve

Foramina of cribriform plate – – – · Olfactory nerves

Posterior ethmoidal foramen – – – Posterior ethmoidal artery, vein,
and nerve

Optic canal – – – – – – – – – – { Optic nerve (II)
{ Ophthalmic artery

Superior orbital fissure – – – – – { Oculomotor nerve (III)
{ Trochlear nerve (IV)
{ Lacrimal, frontal, and nasociliary
{ branches of ophthalmic nerve (V$_1$)
{ Abducent nerve (VI)
{ Superior ophthalmic vein

Foramen rotundum – – – – – – – – – Maxillary nerve (V$_2$)

Foramen ovale – – – – – – – – – { Mandibular nerve (V$_3$)
{ Accessory meningeal artery
{ Lesser petrosal nerve

Foramen spinosum – – – – – – – – { Middle meningeal artery and vein
{ Meningeal branch of mandibular nerve

Sphenoidal emissary foramen (of Vesalius) (inconstant)

Foramen lacerum – – – – – – – – – Greater petrosal nerve

Carotid canal – – – – – – – – – { Internal carotid artery
{ Internal carotid nerve plexus

Hiatus for – – – – – – – – – – – Lesser petrosal nerve

Hiatus for – – – – – – – – – – – Greater petrosal nerve

Internal acoustic meatus – – – – – { Facial nerve (VII)
{ Vestibulocochlear nerve (VIII)
{ Labyrinthine artery

Opening of
vestibular aqueduct – – – – – – – – Endolymphatic duct

Mastoid foramen (inconstant) – – – Emissary vein (and occasional
branch of occipital artery)

Jugular foramen – – – – – – – – – { Inferior petrosal sinus
{ Glossopharyngeal nerve (IX)
{ Vagus nerve (X)
{ Accessory nerve (XI)
{ Sigmoid sinus
{ Posterior meningeal artery

Condylar canal (inconstant) – – – – { Emissary vein and meningeal branch
{ of ascending pharyngeal artery

Hypoglossal canal – – – – – – – – – Hypoglossal nerve (XII)

Foramen magnum – – – – – – – – { Medulla oblongata
{ Meninges
{ Vertebral arteries
{ Meningeal branches of vertebral
{ arteries
{ Spinal roots of accessory nerves

*f. Netter, M.D.*

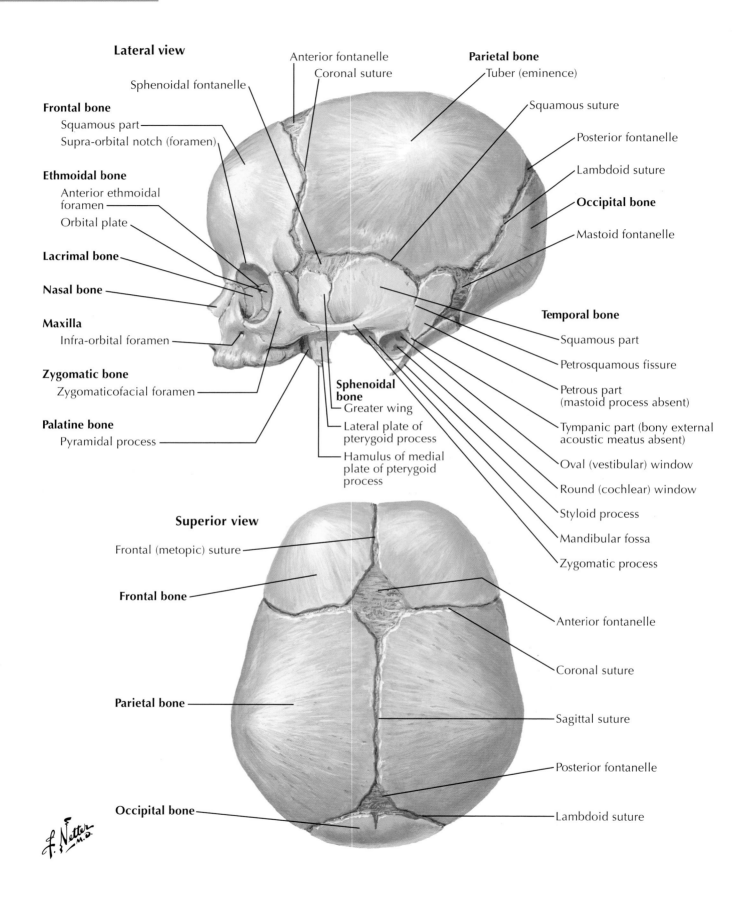

**Lateral view**

Sphenoidal fontanelle

**Frontal bone**
Squamous part
Supra-orbital notch (foramen)

**Ethmoidal bone**
Anterior ethmoidal foramen
Orbital plate

**Lacrimal bone**

**Nasal bone**

**Maxilla**
Infra-orbital foramen

**Zygomatic bone**
Zygomaticofacial foramen

**Palatine bone**
Pyramidal process

Anterior fontanelle
Coronal suture

**Parietal bone**
Tuber (eminence)
Squamous suture
Posterior fontanelle
Lambdoid suture
**Occipital bone**
Mastoid fontanelle

**Temporal bone**
Squamous part
Petrosquamous fissure
Petrous part (mastoid process absent)
Tympanic part (bony external acoustic meatus absent)
Oval (vestibular) window
Round (cochlear) window
Styloid process
Mandibular fossa
Zygomatic process

**Sphenoidal bone**
Greater wing
Lateral plate of pterygoid process
Hamulus of medial plate of pterygoid process

**Superior view**

Frontal (metopic) suture

**Frontal bone**

**Parietal bone**

**Occipital bone**

Anterior fontanelle

Coronal suture

Sagittal suture

Posterior fontanelle

Lambdoid suture

**Plate 14**                                                          **Bones and Ligaments**

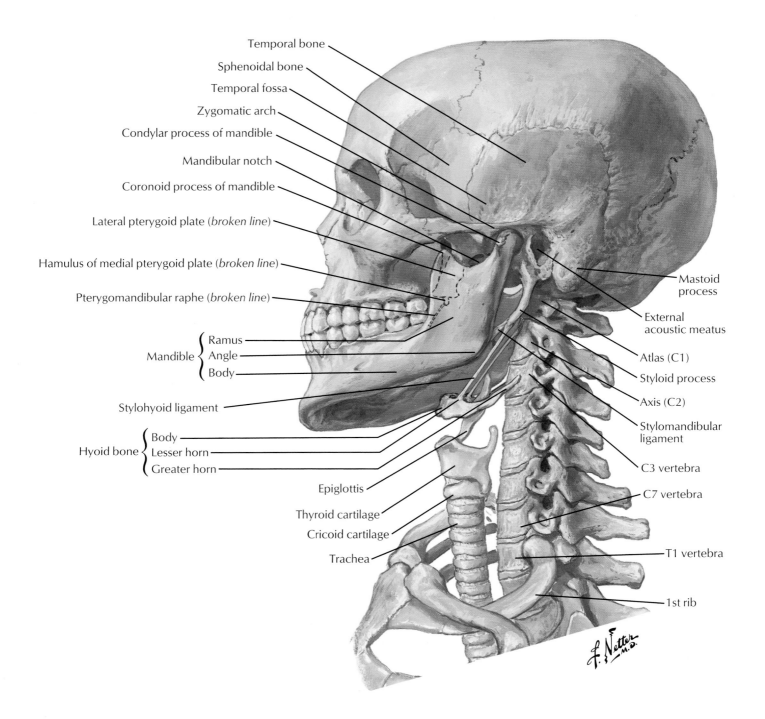

Temporal bone

Sphenoidal bone

Temporal fossa

Zygomatic arch

Condylar process of mandible

Mandibular notch

Coronoid process of mandible

Lateral pterygoid plate (*broken line*)

Hamulus of medial pterygoid plate (*broken line*)

Pterygomandibular raphe (*broken line*)

Mandible { Ramus / Angle / Body

Stylohyoid ligament

Hyoid bone { Body / Lesser horn / Greater horn

Epiglottis

Thyroid cartilage

Cricoid cartilage

Trachea

Mastoid process

External acoustic meatus

Atlas (C1)

Styloid process

Axis (C2)

Stylomandibular ligament

C3 vertebra

C7 vertebra

T1 vertebra

1st rib

**Bones and Ligaments**

**Plate 15**

**Posterior view**

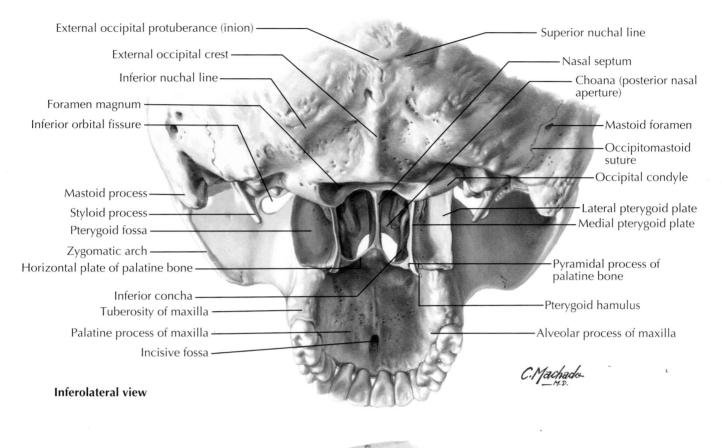

External occipital protuberance (inion)

External occipital crest

Inferior nuchal line

Foramen magnum

Inferior orbital fissure

Mastoid process

Styloid process

Pterygoid fossa

Zygomatic arch

Horizontal plate of palatine bone

Inferior concha

Tuberosity of maxilla

Palatine process of maxilla

Incisive fossa

Superior nuchal line

Nasal septum

Choana (posterior nasal aperture)

Mastoid foramen

Occipitomastoid suture

Occipital condyle

Lateral pterygoid plate

Medial pterygoid plate

Pyramidal process of palatine bone

Pterygoid hamulus

Alveolar process of maxilla

*C. Machado*
M.D.

**Inferolateral view**

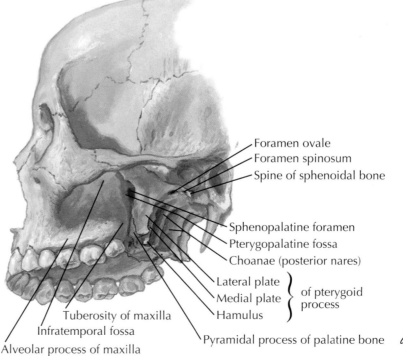

Foramen ovale

Foramen spinosum

Spine of sphenoidal bone

Sphenopalatine foramen

Pterygopalatine fossa

Choanae (posterior nares)

Lateral plate

Medial plate ⎫ of pterygoid process

Hamulus ⎭

Pyramidal process of palatine bone

Tuberosity of maxilla

Infratemporal fossa

Alveolar process of maxilla

*F. Netter*
M.D.

**Plate 16**

**Bones and Ligaments**

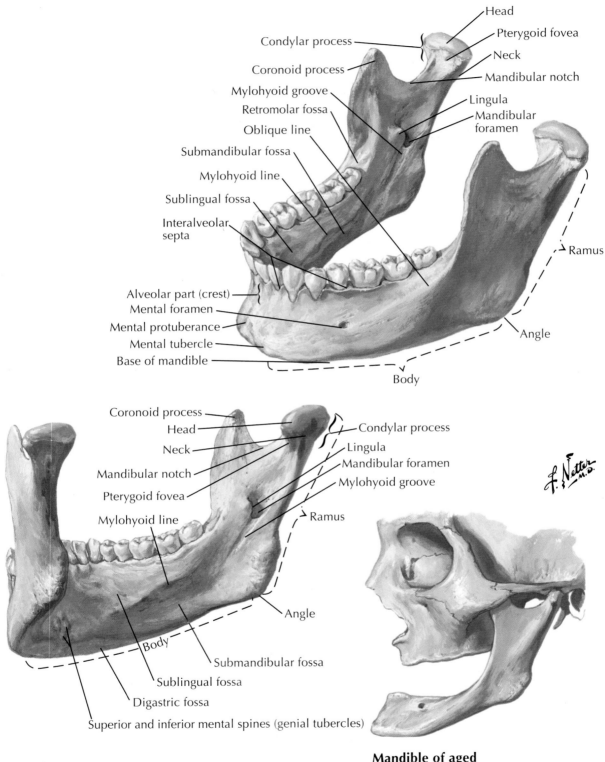

Head
Pterygoid fovea
Condylar process
Neck
Coronoid process
Mandibular notch
Mylohyoid groove
Lingula
Retromolar fossa
Mandibular foramen
Oblique line
Submandibular fossa
Mylohyoid line
Sublingual fossa
Interalveolar septa
Ramus
Alveolar part (crest)
Mental foramen
Mental protuberance
Angle
Mental tubercle
Base of mandible
Body

Coronoid process
Head
Condylar process
Neck
Lingula
Mandibular notch
Mandibular foramen
Pterygoid fovea
Mylohyoid groove
Mylohyoid line
Ramus
Angle
Body
Submandibular fossa
Sublingual fossa
Digastric fossa
Superior and inferior mental spines (genial tubercles)

**Mandible of aged person (edentulous)**

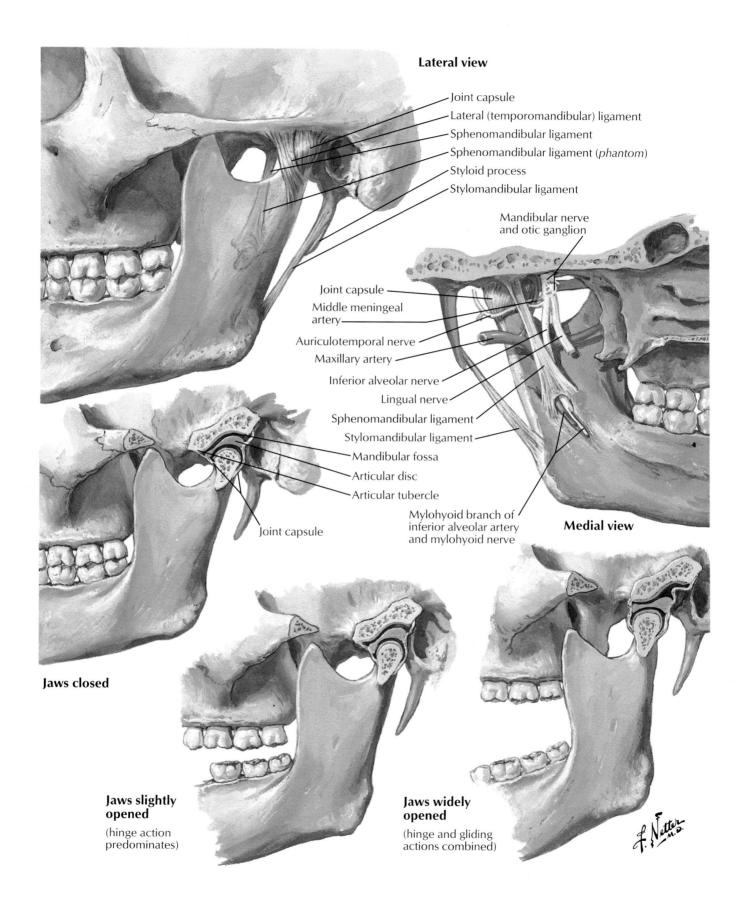

**Lateral view**

Joint capsule

Lateral (temporomandibular) ligament

Sphenomandibular ligament

Sphenomandibular ligament (*phantom*)

Styloid process

Stylomandibular ligament

Mandibular nerve and otic ganglion

Joint capsule

Middle meningeal artery

Auriculotemporal nerve

Maxillary artery

Inferior alveolar nerve

Lingual nerve

Sphenomandibular ligament

Stylomandibular ligament

Mandibular fossa

Articular disc

Articular tubercle

Mylohyoid branch of inferior alveolar artery and mylohyoid nerve

**Medial view**

Joint capsule

**Jaws closed**

**Jaws slightly opened**

(hinge action predominates)

**Jaws widely opened**

(hinge and gliding actions combined)

**Plate 18**

**Bones and Ligaments**

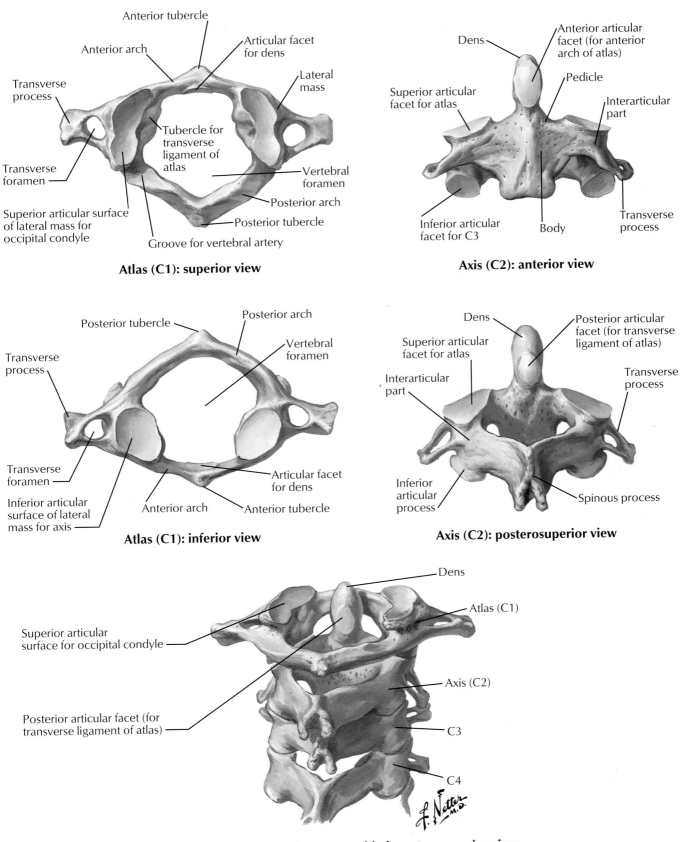

**Atlas (C1): superior view**

Anterior tubercle

Anterior arch

Articular facet for dens

Transverse process

Lateral mass

Transverse foramen

Tubercle for transverse ligament of atlas

Superior articular surface of lateral mass for occipital condyle

Vertebral foramen

Posterior arch

Posterior tubercle

Groove for vertebral artery

**Axis (C2): anterior view**

Dens

Anterior articular facet (for anterior arch of atlas)

Superior articular facet for atlas

Pedicle

Interarticular part

Inferior articular facet for C3

Body

Transverse process

**Atlas (C1): inferior view**

Posterior tubercle

Posterior arch

Vertebral foramen

Transverse process

Transverse foramen

Inferior articular surface of lateral mass for axis

Anterior arch

Articular facet for dens

Anterior tubercle

**Axis (C2): posterosuperior view**

Dens

Posterior articular facet (for transverse ligament of atlas)

Superior articular facet for atlas

Interarticular part

Transverse process

Inferior articular process

Spinous process

**Upper cervical vertebrae, assembled: posterosuperior view**

Dens

Atlas (C1)

Superior articular surface for occipital condyle

Axis (C2)

C3

Posterior articular facet (for transverse ligament of atlas)

C4

**Inferior aspect of C3 and superior aspect of C4 showing the sites of the facet and uncovertebral articulations**

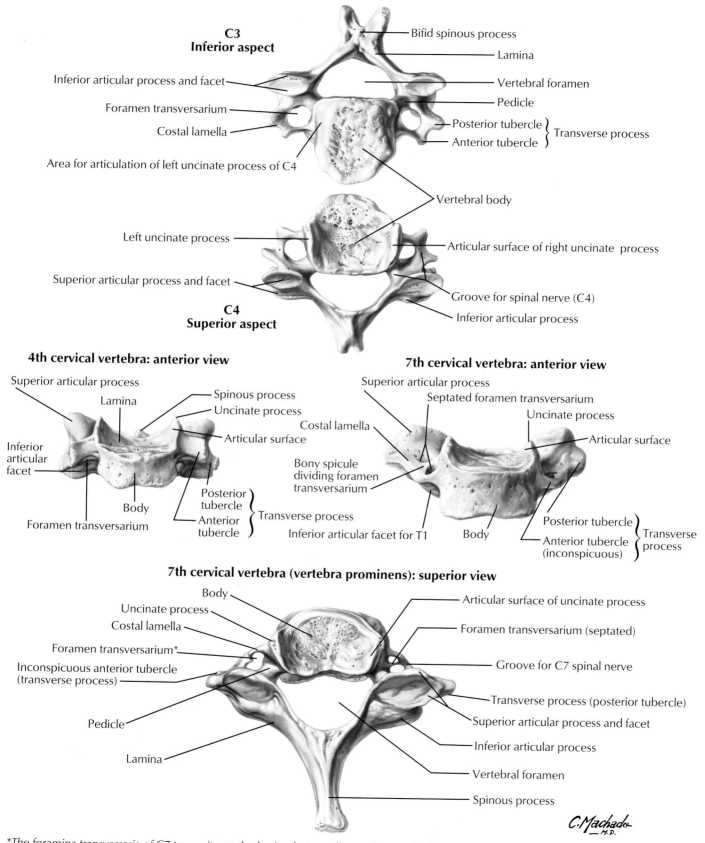

**C3
Inferior aspect**

Bifid spinous process

Lamina

Vertebral foramen

Inferior articular process and facet

Pedicle

Foramen transversarium

Posterior tubercle } Transverse process

Costal lamella

Anterior tubercle }

Area for articulation of left uncinate process of C4

Vertebral body

Left uncinate process

Articular surface of right uncinate process

Superior articular process and facet

Groove for spinal nerve (C4)

Inferior articular process

**C4
Superior aspect**

**4th cervical vertebra: anterior view**

Superior articular process

Lamina

Spinous process

Uncinate process

Articular surface

Inferior articular facet

Posterior tubercle } Transverse process

Body

Anterior tubercle }

Foramen transversarium

**7th cervical vertebra: anterior view**

Superior articular process

Septated foramen transversarium

Uncinate process

Costal lamella

Articular surface

Bony spicule dividing foramen transversarium

Posterior tubercle } Transverse process

Inferior articular facet for T1

Body

Anterior tubercle (inconspicuous) }

**7th cervical vertebra (vertebra prominens): superior view**

Body

Uncinate process

Costal lamella

Foramen transversarium*

Inconspicuous anterior tubercle (transverse process)

Pedicle

Lamina

Articular surface of uncinate process

Foramen transversarium (septated)

Groove for C7 spinal nerve

Transverse process (posterior tubercle)

Superior articular process and facet

Inferior articular process

Vertebral foramen

Spinous process

*The foramina transversaria of C7 transmit vertebral veins, but usually not the vertebral artery, and are asymmetrical in this specimen.*

**Plate 20**

**Bones and Ligaments**

**Cervical vertebrae: anterior view**

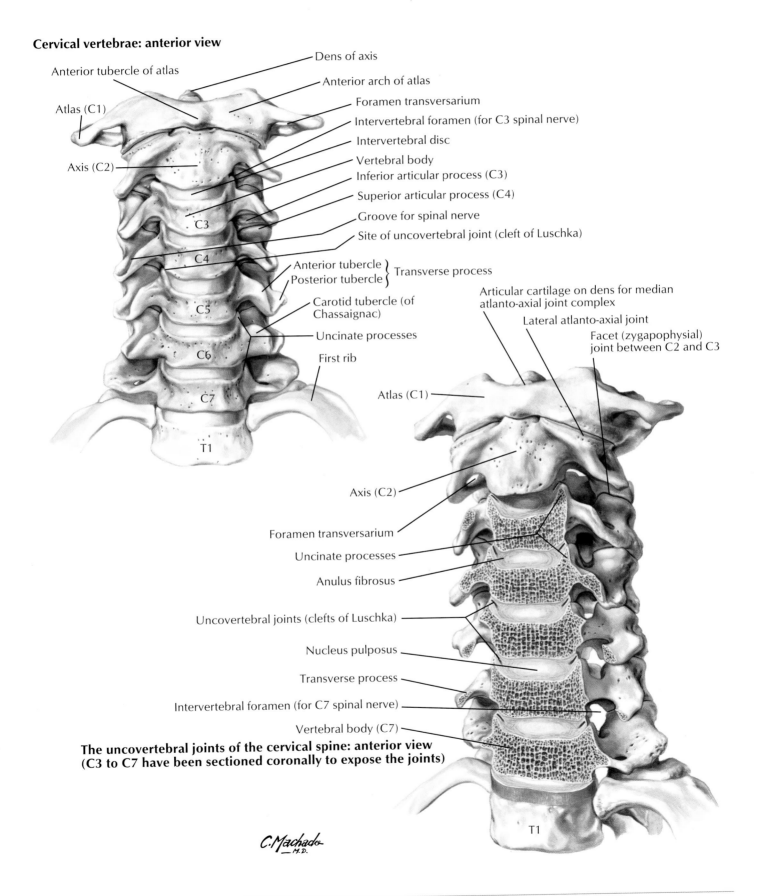

Dens of axis

Anterior tubercle of atlas

Anterior arch of atlas

Foramen transversarium

Atlas (C1)

Intervertebral foramen (for C3 spinal nerve)

Intervertebral disc

Vertebral body

Axis (C2)

Inferior articular process (C3)

Superior articular process (C4)

Groove for spinal nerve

C3

Site of uncovertebral joint (cleft of Luschka)

C4

Anterior tubercle } Transverse process
Posterior tubercle }

Articular cartilage on dens for median atlanto-axial joint complex

Lateral atlanto-axial joint

C5

Carotid tubercle (of Chassaignac)

Facet (zygapophysial) joint between C2 and C3

Uncinate processes

C6

First rib

Atlas (C1)

C7

T1

Axis (C2)

Foramen transversarium

Uncinate processes

Anulus fibrosus

Uncovertebral joints (clefts of Luschka)

Nucleus pulposus

Transverse process

Intervertebral foramen (for C7 spinal nerve)

Vertebral body (C7)

**The uncovertebral joints of the cervical spine: anterior view (C3 to C7 have been sectioned coronally to expose the joints)**

T1

C.Machado
M.D.

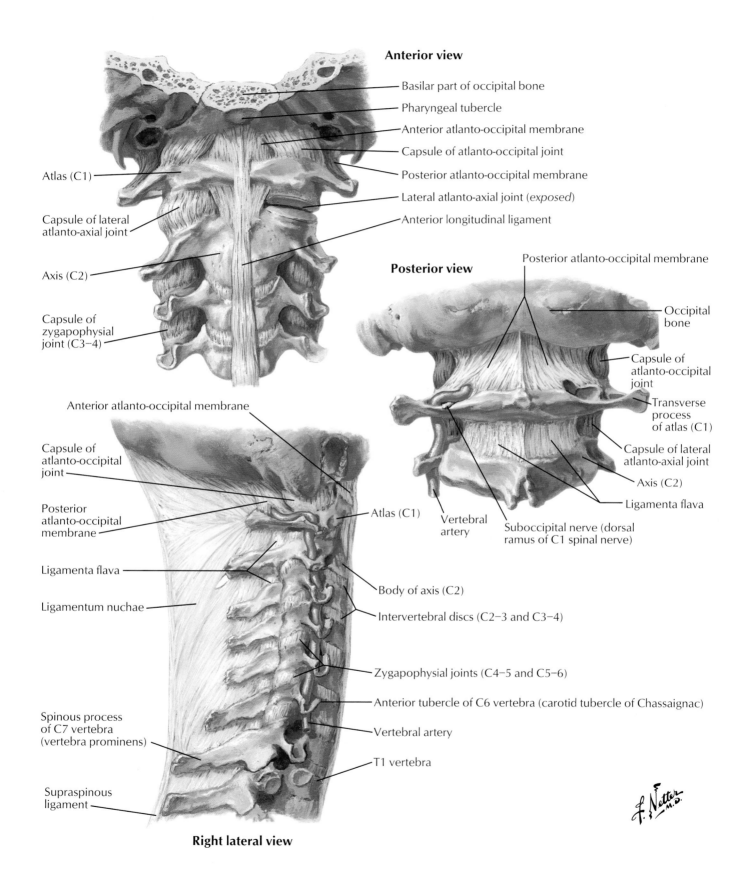

**Anterior view**

Basilar part of occipital bone

Pharyngeal tubercle

Anterior atlanto-occipital membrane

Capsule of atlanto-occipital joint

Posterior atlanto-occipital membrane

Lateral atlanto-axial joint (*exposed*)

Anterior longitudinal ligament

Atlas (C1)

Capsule of lateral atlanto-axial joint

Axis (C2)

Capsule of zygapophysial joint (C3–4)

**Posterior view**

Posterior atlanto-occipital membrane

Occipital bone

Capsule of atlanto-occipital joint

Transverse process of atlas (C1)

Capsule of lateral atlanto-axial joint

Axis (C2)

Ligamenta flava

Vertebral artery

Suboccipital nerve (dorsal ramus of C1 spinal nerve)

Anterior atlanto-occipital membrane

Capsule of atlanto-occipital joint

Posterior atlanto-occipital membrane

Ligamenta flava

Ligamentum nuchae

Atlas (C1)

Body of axis (C2)

Intervertebral discs (C2–3 and C3–4)

Zygapophysial joints (C4–5 and C5–6)

Anterior tubercle of C6 vertebra (carotid tubercle of Chassaignac)

Vertebral artery

T1 vertebra

Spinous process of C7 vertebra (vertebra prominens)

Supraspinous ligament

**Right lateral view**

**Plate 22**

**Bones and Ligaments**

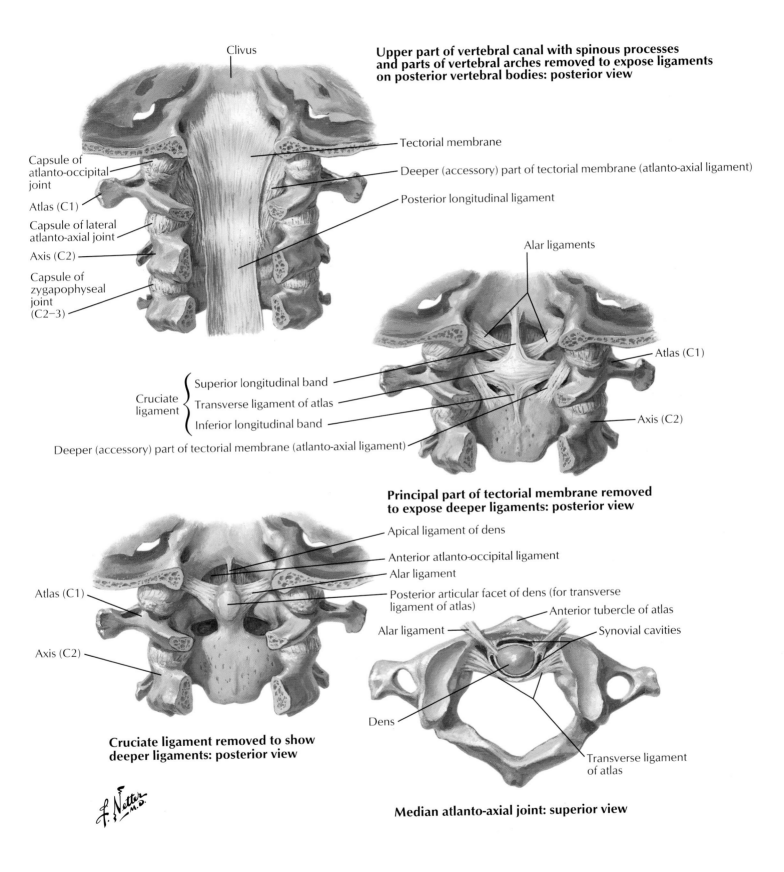

Clivus

**Upper part of vertebral canal with spinous processes and parts of vertebral arches removed to expose ligaments on posterior vertebral bodies: posterior view**

Tectorial membrane

Capsule of atlanto-occipital joint

Atlas (C1)

Deeper (accessory) part of tectorial membrane (atlanto-axial ligament)

Posterior longitudinal ligament

Capsule of lateral atlanto-axial joint

Axis (C2)

Alar ligaments

Capsule of zygapophyseal joint (C2–3)

Atlas (C1)

Cruciate ligament { Superior longitudinal band

Transverse ligament of atlas

Inferior longitudinal band

Axis (C2)

Deeper (accessory) part of tectorial membrane (atlanto-axial ligament)

**Principal part of tectorial membrane removed to expose deeper ligaments: posterior view**

Apical ligament of dens

Anterior atlanto-occipital ligament

Alar ligament

Atlas (C1)

Posterior articular facet of dens (for transverse ligament of atlas)

Anterior tubercle of atlas

Alar ligament

Synovial cavities

Axis (C2)

Dens

**Cruciate ligament removed to show deeper ligaments: posterior view**

Transverse ligament of atlas

**Median atlanto-axial joint: superior view**

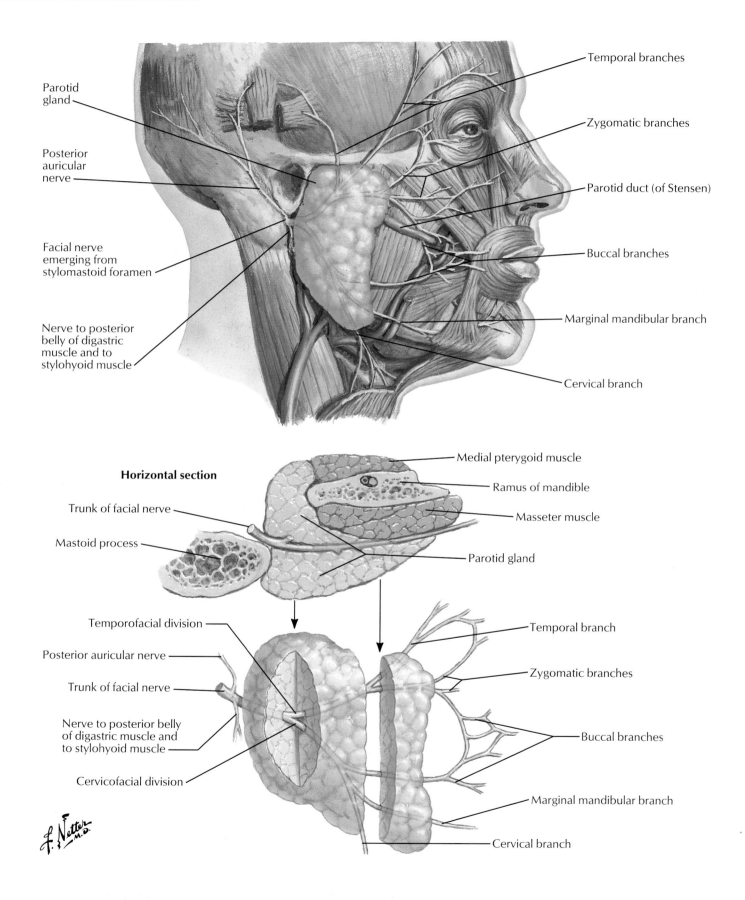

Temporal branches

Parotid gland

Zygomatic branches

Posterior auricular nerve

Parotid duct (of Stensen)

Facial nerve emerging from stylomastoid foramen

Buccal branches

Nerve to posterior belly of digastric muscle and to stylohyoid muscle

Marginal mandibular branch

Cervical branch

**Horizontal section**

Medial pterygoid muscle

Ramus of mandible

Trunk of facial nerve

Mastoid process

Masseter muscle

Parotid gland

Temporofacial division

Temporal branch

Posterior auricular nerve

Zygomatic branches

Trunk of facial nerve

Nerve to posterior belly of digastric muscle and to stylohyoid muscle

Buccal branches

Cervicofacial division

Marginal mandibular branch

Cervical branch

**Plate 24**

**Superficial Face**

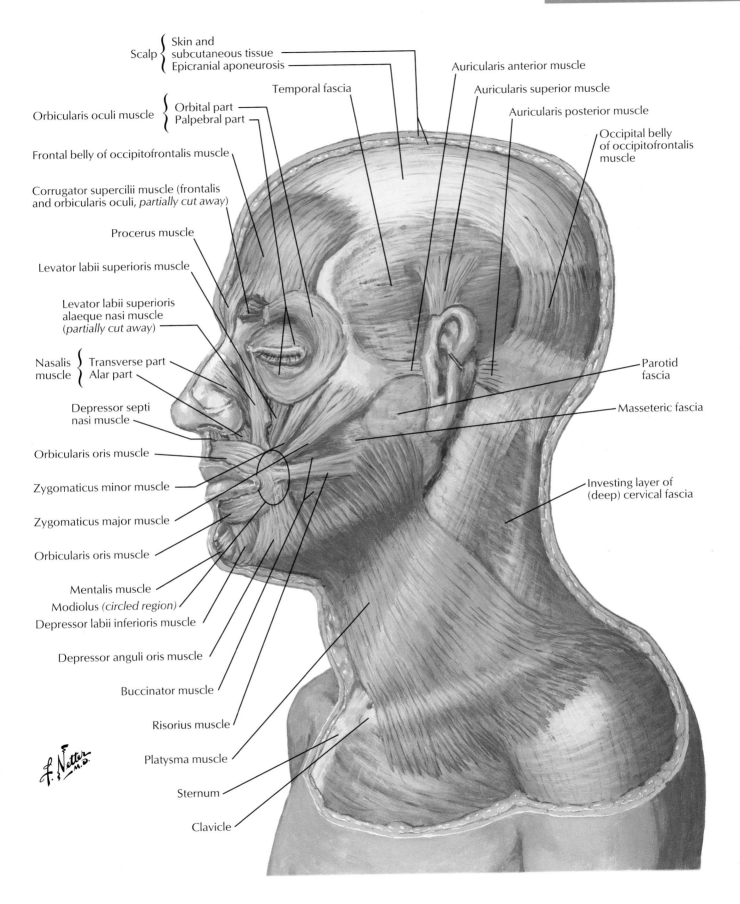

Scalp { Skin and subcutaneous tissue
Epicranial aponeurosis

Temporal fascia

Auricularis anterior muscle

Auricularis superior muscle

Auricularis posterior muscle

Occipital belly of occipitofrontalis muscle

Orbicularis oculi muscle { Orbital part
Palpebral part

Frontal belly of occipitofrontalis muscle

Corrugator supercilii muscle (frontalis and orbicularis oculi, *partially cut away*)

Procerus muscle

Levator labii superioris muscle

Levator labii superioris alaeque nasi muscle (*partially cut away*)

Nasalis muscle { Transverse part
Alar part

Depressor septi nasi muscle

Orbicularis oris muscle

Zygomaticus minor muscle

Zygomaticus major muscle

Orbicularis oris muscle

Mentalis muscle

Modiolus (*circled region*)

Depressor labii inferioris muscle

Depressor anguli oris muscle

Buccinator muscle

Risorius muscle

Platysma muscle

Sternum

Clavicle

Parotid fascia

Masseteric fascia

Investing layer of (deep) cervical fascia

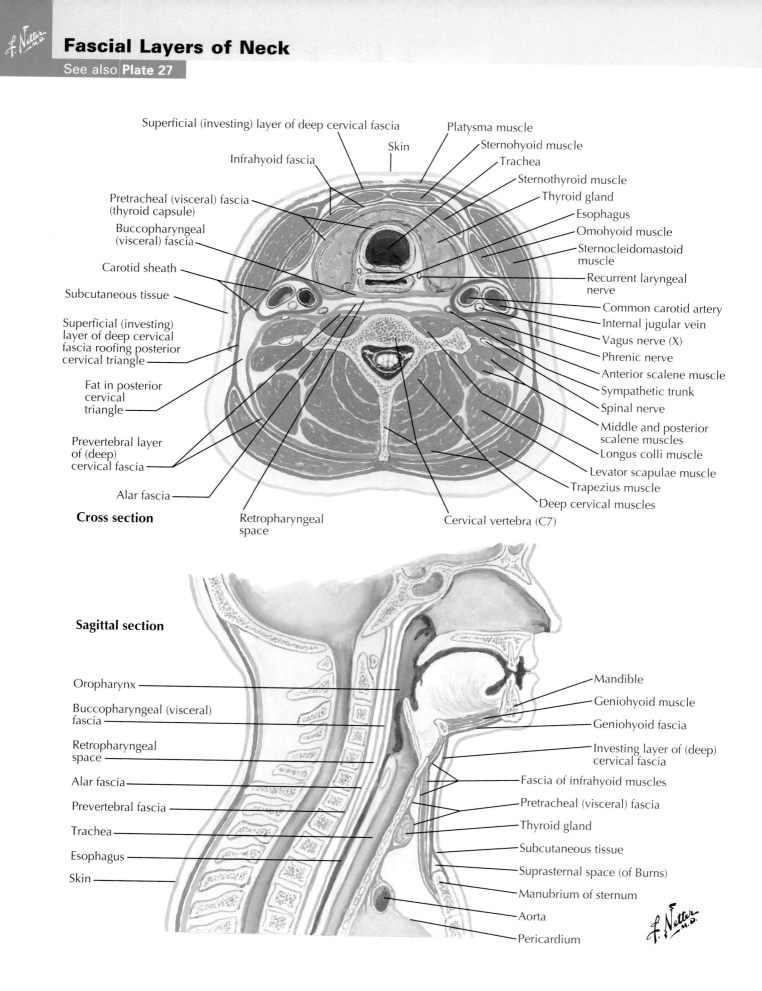

Superficial (investing) layer of deep cervical fascia

Infrahyoid fascia

Skin

Platysma muscle

Sternohyoid muscle

Trachea

Sternothyroid muscle

Thyroid gland

Pretracheal (visceral) fascia (thyroid capsule)

Buccopharyngeal (visceral) fascia

Esophagus

Omohyoid muscle

Sternocleidomastoid muscle

Carotid sheath

Subcutaneous tissue

Recurrent laryngeal nerve

Common carotid artery

Internal jugular vein

Superficial (investing) layer of deep cervical fascia roofing posterior cervical triangle

Vagus nerve (X)

Phrenic nerve

Anterior scalene muscle

Sympathetic trunk

Spinal nerve

Fat in posterior cervical triangle

Middle and posterior scalene muscles

Longus colli muscle

Prevertebral layer of (deep) cervical fascia

Levator scapulae muscle

Trapezius muscle

Deep cervical muscles

Alar fascia

**Cross section**

Retropharyngeal space

Cervical vertebra (C7)

**Sagittal section**

Oropharynx

Mandible

Buccopharyngeal (visceral) fascia

Geniohyoid muscle

Geniohyoid fascia

Retropharyngeal space

Investing layer of (deep) cervical fascia

Alar fascia

Fascia of infrahyoid muscles

Prevertebral fascia

Pretracheal (visceral) fascia

Trachea

Thyroid gland

Esophagus

Subcutaneous tissue

Skin

Suprasternal space (of Burns)

Manubrium of sternum

Aorta

Pericardium

**Plate 26**

**Neck**

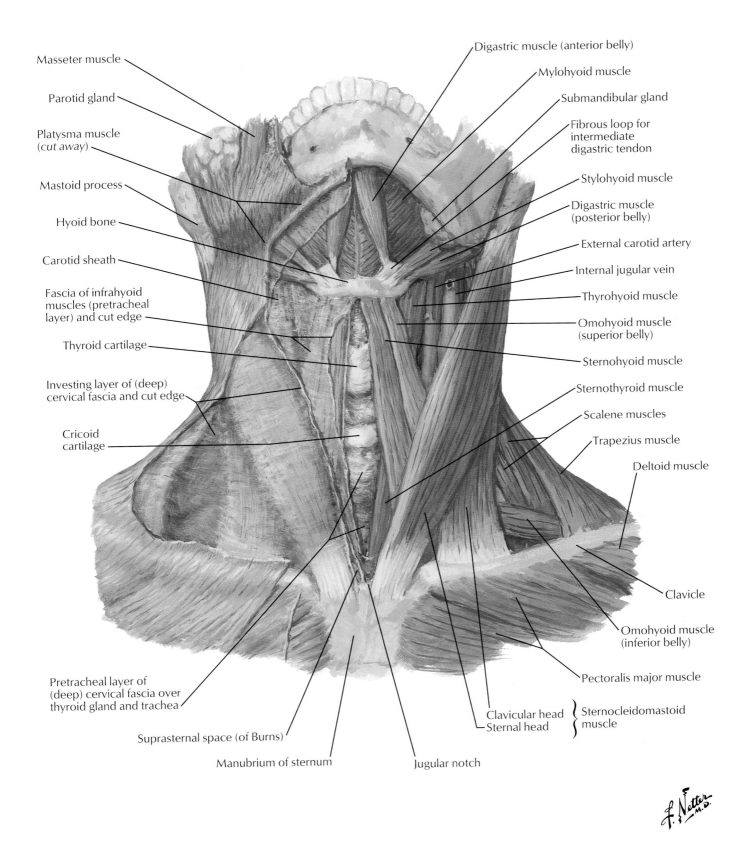

Masseter muscle

Parotid gland

Platysma muscle (*cut away*)

Mastoid process

Hyoid bone

Carotid sheath

Fascia of infrahyoid muscles (pretracheal layer) and cut edge

Thyroid cartilage

Investing layer of (deep) cervical fascia and cut edge

Cricoid cartilage

Pretracheal layer of (deep) cervical fascia over thyroid gland and trachea

Suprasternal space (of Burns)

Manubrium of sternum

Digastric muscle (anterior belly)

Mylohyoid muscle

Submandibular gland

Fibrous loop for intermediate digastric tendon

Stylohyoid muscle

Digastric muscle (posterior belly)

External carotid artery

Internal jugular vein

Thyrohyoid muscle

Omohyoid muscle (superior belly)

Sternohyoid muscle

Sternothyroid muscle

Scalene muscles

Trapezius muscle

Deltoid muscle

Clavicle

Omohyoid muscle (inferior belly)

Pectoralis major muscle

Clavicular head
Sternal head
} Sternocleidomastoid muscle

Jugular notch

**Neck**

**Plate 27**

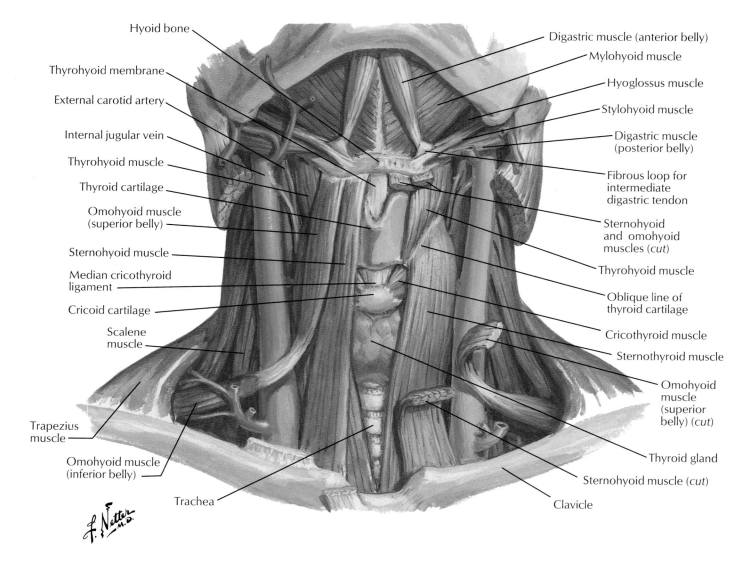

Hyoid bone

Thyrohyoid membrane

External carotid artery

Internal jugular vein

Thyrohyoid muscle

Thyroid cartilage

Omohyoid muscle (superior belly)

Sternohyoid muscle

Median cricothyroid ligament

Cricoid cartilage

Scalene muscle

Trapezius muscle

Omohyoid muscle (inferior belly)

Trachea

Digastric muscle (anterior belly)

Mylohyoid muscle

Hyoglossus muscle

Stylohyoid muscle

Digastric muscle (posterior belly)

Fibrous loop for intermediate digastric tendon

Sternohyoid and omohyoid muscles (cut)

Thyrohyoid muscle

Oblique line of thyroid cartilage

Cricothyroid muscle

Sternothyroid muscle

Omohyoid muscle (superior belly) (cut)

Thyroid gland

Sternohyoid muscle (cut)

Clavicle

**Plate 28**

**Neck**

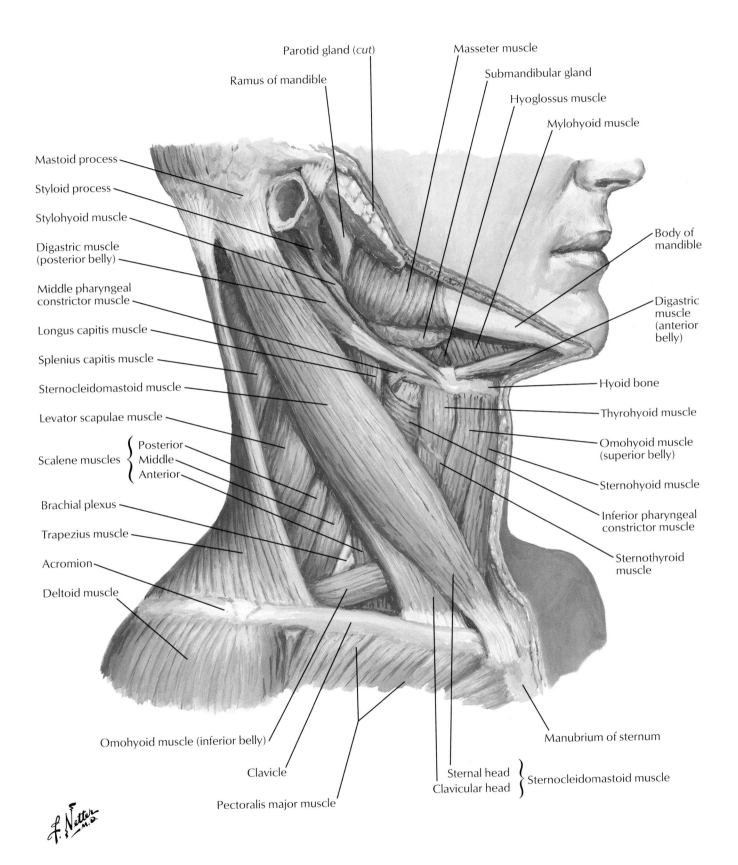

Parotid gland (*cut*)

Masseter muscle

Ramus of mandible

Submandibular gland

Hyoglossus muscle

Mylohyoid muscle

Mastoid process

Styloid process

Stylohyoid muscle

Digastric muscle (posterior belly)

Middle pharyngeal constrictor muscle

Longus capitis muscle

Splenius capitis muscle

Sternocleidomastoid muscle

Levator scapulae muscle

Scalene muscles { Posterior / Middle / Anterior

Brachial plexus

Trapezius muscle

Acromion

Deltoid muscle

Body of mandible

Digastric muscle (anterior belly)

Hyoid bone

Thyrohyoid muscle

Omohyoid muscle (superior belly)

Sternohyoid muscle

Inferior pharyngeal constrictor muscle

Sternothyroid muscle

Omohyoid muscle (inferior belly)

Clavicle

Pectoralis major muscle

Sternal head / Clavicular head } Sternocleidomastoid muscle

Manubrium of sternum

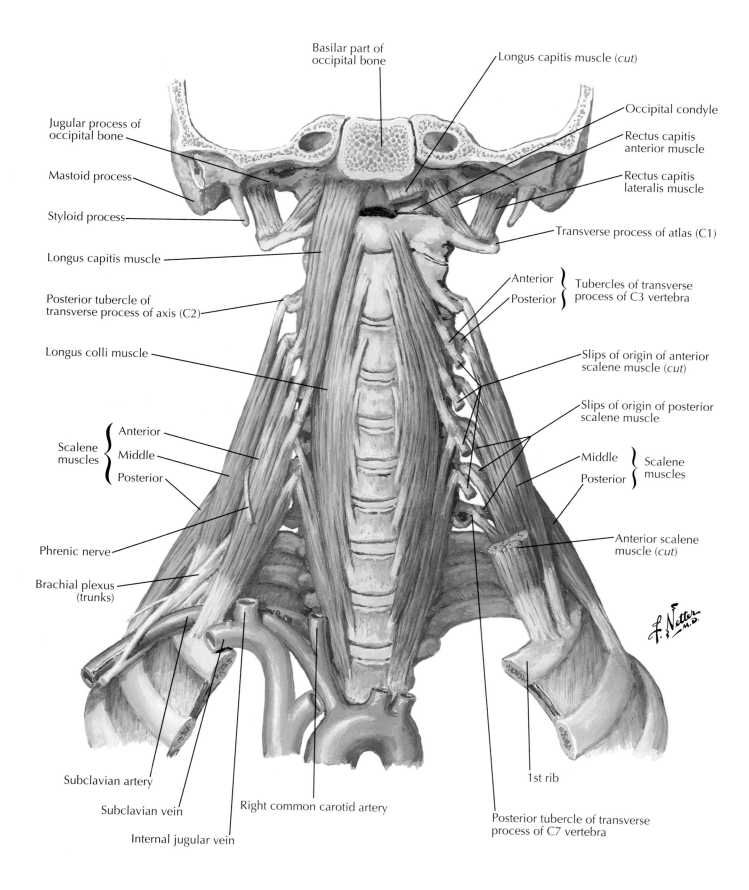

Basilar part of
occipital bone

Longus capitis muscle (*cut*)

Occipital condyle

Rectus capitis
anterior muscle

Rectus capitis
lateralis muscle

Jugular process of
occipital bone

Mastoid process

Styloid process

Transverse process of atlas (C1)

Longus capitis muscle

Posterior tubercle of
transverse process of axis (C2)

Longus colli muscle

Anterior
Posterior } Tubercles of transverse
process of C3 vertebra

Slips of origin of anterior
scalene muscle (*cut*)

Slips of origin of posterior
scalene muscle

Scalene
muscles { Anterior
Middle
Posterior

Middle
Posterior } Scalene
muscles

Phrenic nerve

Anterior scalene
muscle (*cut*)

Brachial plexus
(trunks)

1st rib

Subclavian artery

Subclavian vein

Right common carotid artery

Internal jugular vein

Posterior tubercle of transverse
process of C7 vertebra

**Plate 30**

**Neck**

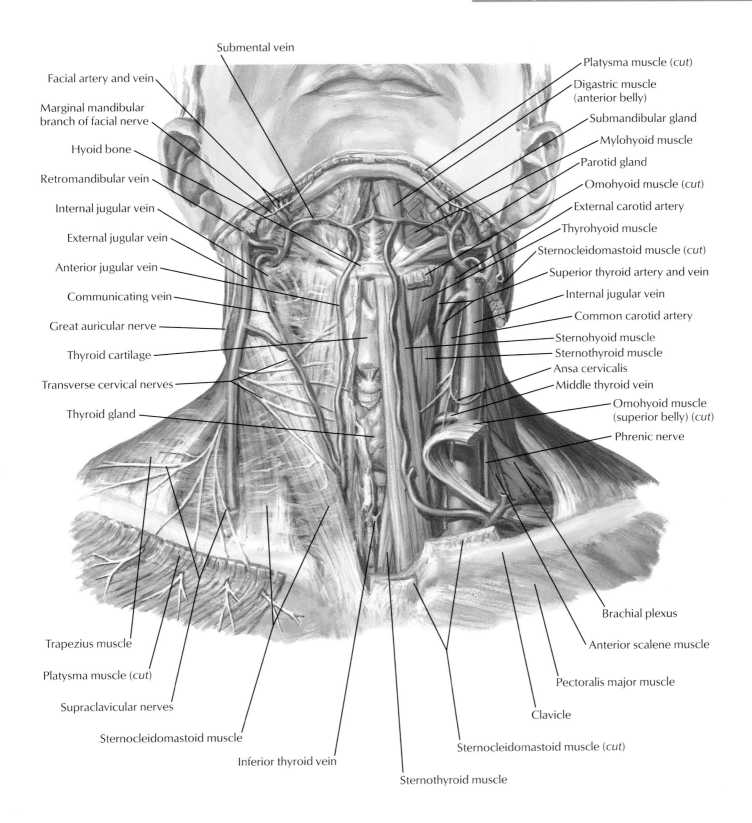

Submental vein

Facial artery and vein

Marginal mandibular branch of facial nerve

Hyoid bone

Retromandibular vein

Internal jugular vein

External jugular vein

Anterior jugular vein

Communicating vein

Great auricular nerve

Thyroid cartilage

Transverse cervical nerves

Thyroid gland

Trapezius muscle

Platysma muscle (*cut*)

Supraclavicular nerves

Sternocleidomastoid muscle

Inferior thyroid vein

Sternothyroid muscle

Platysma muscle (*cut*)

Digastric muscle (anterior belly)

Submandibular gland

Mylohyoid muscle

Parotid gland

Omohyoid muscle (*cut*)

External carotid artery

Thyrohyoid muscle

Sternocleidomastoid muscle (*cut*)

Superior thyroid artery and vein

Internal jugular vein

Common carotid artery

Sternohyoid muscle

Sternothyroid muscle

Ansa cervicalis

Middle thyroid vein

Omohyoid muscle (superior belly) (*cut*)

Phrenic nerve

Brachial plexus

Anterior scalene muscle

Pectoralis major muscle

Clavicle

Sternocleidomastoid muscle (*cut*)

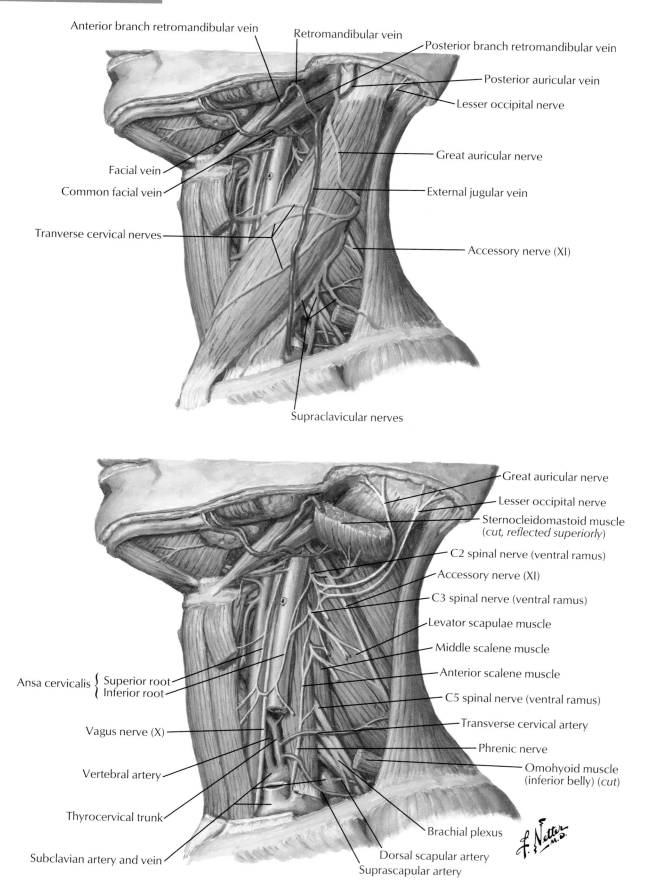

Anterior branch retromandibular vein

Retromandibular vein

Posterior branch retromandibular vein

Posterior auricular vein

Lesser occipital nerve

Great auricular nerve

Facial vein

Common facial vein

External jugular vein

Tranverse cervical nerves

Accessory nerve (XI)

Supraclavicular nerves

Great auricular nerve

Lesser occipital nerve

Sternocleidomastoid muscle *(cut, reflected superiorly)*

C2 spinal nerve (ventral ramus)

Accessory nerve (XI)

C3 spinal nerve (ventral ramus)

Levator scapulae muscle

Middle scalene muscle

Anterior scalene muscle

Ansa cervicalis { Superior root / Inferior root

C5 spinal nerve (ventral ramus)

Transverse cervical artery

Vagus nerve (X)

Phrenic nerve

Vertebral artery

Omohyoid muscle *(inferior belly) (cut)*

Thyrocervical trunk

Brachial plexus

Subclavian artery and vein

Dorsal scapular artery

Suprascapular artery

**Plate 32**

**Neck**

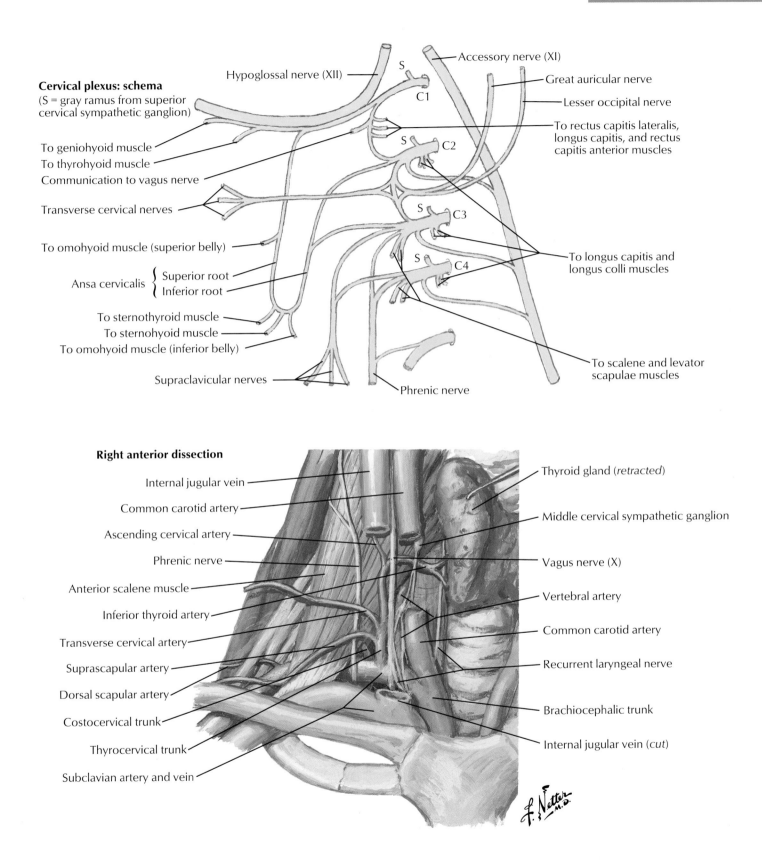

**Cervical plexus: schema**
(S = gray ramus from superior cervical sympathetic ganglion)

Hypoglossal nerve (XII)

S

Accessory nerve (XI)

C1

Great auricular nerve

Lesser occipital nerve

To geniohyoid muscle
To thyrohyoid muscle
Communication to vagus nerve

To rectus capitis lateralis, longus capitis, and rectus capitis anterior muscles

S      C2

Transverse cervical nerves

S      C3

To omohyoid muscle (superior belly)

Ansa cervicalis { Superior root
                { Inferior root

S      C4

To longus capitis and longus colli muscles

To sternothyroid muscle
To sternohyoid muscle
To omohyoid muscle (inferior belly)

To scalene and levator scapulae muscles

Supraclavicular nerves

Phrenic nerve

**Right anterior dissection**

Internal jugular vein

Common carotid artery

Ascending cervical artery

Phrenic nerve

Anterior scalene muscle

Inferior thyroid artery

Transverse cervical artery

Suprascapular artery

Dorsal scapular artery

Costocervical trunk

Thyrocervical trunk

Subclavian artery and vein

Thyroid gland (*retracted*)

Middle cervical sympathetic ganglion

Vagus nerve (X)

Vertebral artery

Common carotid artery

Recurrent laryngeal nerve

Brachiocephalic trunk

Internal jugular vein (*cut*)

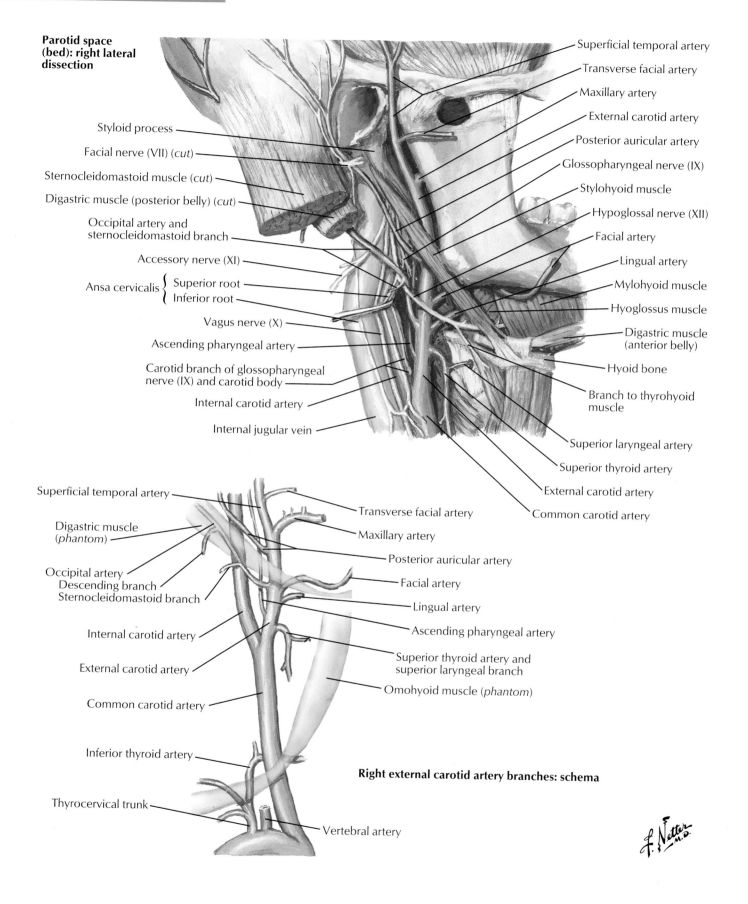

**Parotid space (bed): right lateral dissection**

Superficial temporal artery

Transverse facial artery

Maxillary artery

External carotid artery

Posterior auricular artery

Glossopharyngeal nerve (IX)

Stylohyoid muscle

Hypoglossal nerve (XII)

Facial artery

Lingual artery

Mylohyoid muscle

Hyoglossus muscle

Digastric muscle (anterior belly)

Hyoid bone

Branch to thyrohyoid muscle

Superior laryngeal artery

Superior thyroid artery

External carotid artery

Common carotid artery

Styloid process

Facial nerve (VII) (cut)

Sternocleidomastoid muscle (cut)

Digastric muscle (posterior belly) (cut)

Occipital artery and sternocleidomastoid branch

Accessory nerve (XI)

Ansa cervicalis { Superior root / Inferior root }

Vagus nerve (X)

Ascending pharyngeal artery

Carotid branch of glossopharyngeal nerve (IX) and carotid body

Internal carotid artery

Internal jugular vein

**Right external carotid artery branches: schema**

Superficial temporal artery

Digastric muscle (phantom)

Occipital artery

Descending branch

Sternocleidomastoid branch

Internal carotid artery

External carotid artery

Common carotid artery

Inferior thyroid artery

Thyrocervical trunk

Transverse facial artery

Maxillary artery

Posterior auricular artery

Facial artery

Lingual artery

Ascending pharyngeal artery

Superior thyroid artery and superior laryngeal branch

Omohyoid muscle (phantom)

Vertebral artery

**Plate 34**

**Neck**

**Anterolateral view**

Frontal bone

Nasal bones

Frontal process of maxilla

Lateral process of septal nasal cartilages

Septal cartilage

Minor alar cartilage

Accessory nasal cartilage

Major alar cartilage { Lateral crus

Medial crus

Nasal septal cartilage

Anterior nasal spine of maxilla

Alar fibrofatty tissue

Infra-orbital foramen

**Inferior view**

Major alar cartilage

Lateral crus

Medial crus

Alar fibrofatty tissue

Nasal septal cartilage

Anterior nasal spine of maxilla

Intermaxillary suture

Superficial temporal artery

Frontal belly of occipitofrontalis muscle

Supra-orbital artery and nerve

Supratrochlear artery and nerve

Procerus muscle

Corrugator supercilii muscle

Dorsal nasal artery

Infratrochlear nerve

Angular artery

External nasal artery and nerve

Nasalis muscle (transverse part)

Infra-orbital artery and nerve

Lateral nasal artery

Transverse facial artery

Nasalis muscle (alar part)

Depressor septi nasi muscle

Orbicularis oris muscle

Facial artery

Superior and inferior labial arteries

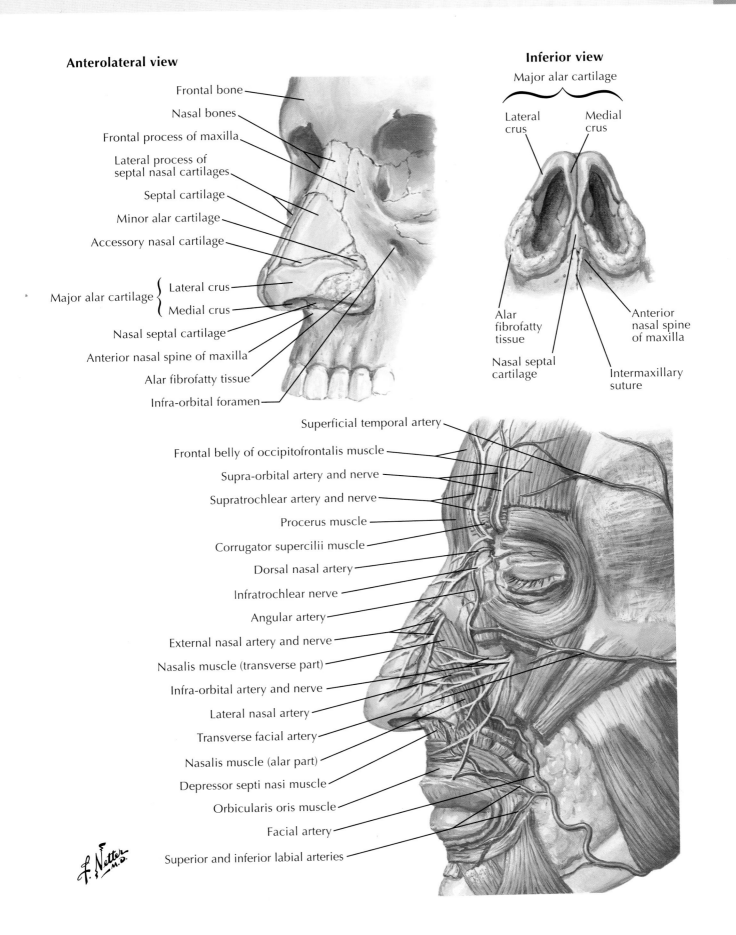

**Nasal Region**

**Plate 35**

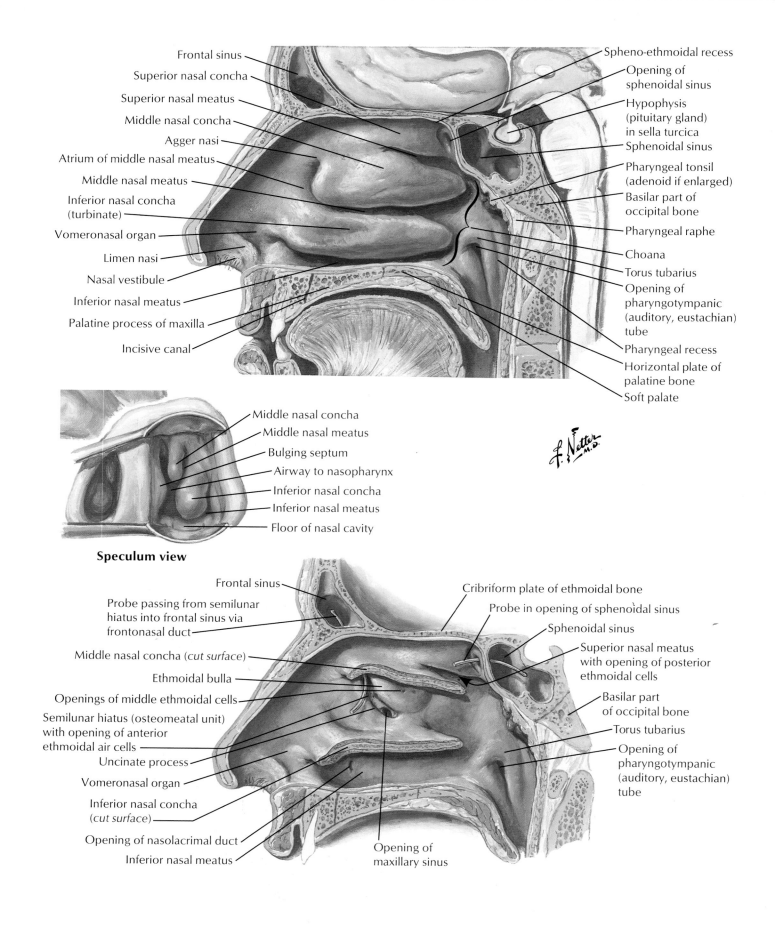

Frontal sinus

Superior nasal concha

Superior nasal meatus

Middle nasal concha

Agger nasi

Atrium of middle nasal meatus

Middle nasal meatus

Inferior nasal concha (turbinate)

Vomeronasal organ

Limen nasi

Nasal vestibule

Inferior nasal meatus

Palatine process of maxilla

Incisive canal

Spheno-ethmoidal recess

Opening of sphenoidal sinus

Hypophysis (pituitary gland) in sella turcica

Sphenoidal sinus

Pharyngeal tonsil (adenoid if enlarged)

Basilar part of occipital bone

Pharyngeal raphe

Choana

Torus tubarius

Opening of pharyngotympanic (auditory, eustachian) tube

Pharyngeal recess

Horizontal plate of palatine bone

Soft palate

Middle nasal concha

Middle nasal meatus

Bulging septum

Airway to nasopharynx

Inferior nasal concha

Inferior nasal meatus

Floor of nasal cavity

**Speculum view**

Frontal sinus

Probe passing from semilunar hiatus into frontal sinus via frontonasal duct

Middle nasal concha (*cut surface*)

Ethmoidal bulla

Openings of middle ethmoidal cells

Semilunar hiatus (osteomeatal unit) with opening of anterior ethmoidal air cells

Uncinate process

Vomeronasal organ

Inferior nasal concha (*cut surface*)

Opening of nasolacrimal duct

Inferior nasal meatus

Cribriform plate of ethmoidal bone

Probe in opening of sphenoidal sinus

Sphenoidal sinus

Superior nasal meatus with opening of posterior ethmoidal cells

Basilar part of occipital bone

Torus tubarius

Opening of pharyngotympanic (auditory, eustachian) tube

Opening of maxillary sinus

**Plate 36**

**Nasal Region**

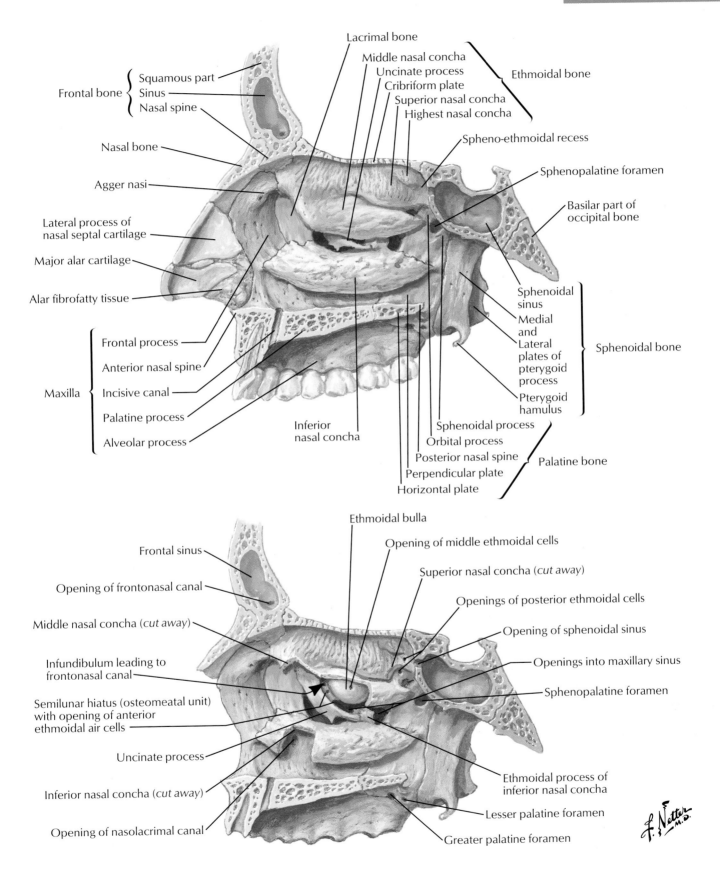

Lacrimal bone
Middle nasal concha
Uncinate process
Cribriform plate
Superior nasal concha
Highest nasal concha

Ethmoidal bone

Frontal bone
Squamous part
Sinus
Nasal spine

Nasal bone

Agger nasi

Lateral process of nasal septal cartilage

Major alar cartilage

Alar fibrofatty tissue

Spheno-ethmoidal recess

Sphenopalatine foramen

Basilar part of occipital bone

Maxilla
Frontal process
Anterior nasal spine
Incisive canal
Palatine process
Alveolar process

Sphenoidal sinus
Medial and Lateral plates of pterygoid process

Sphenoidal bone

Pterygoid hamulus

Inferior nasal concha

Sphenoidal process
Orbital process
Posterior nasal spine
Perpendicular plate
Horizontal plate

Palatine bone

Ethmoidal bulla
Opening of middle ethmoidal cells

Frontal sinus

Opening of frontonasal canal

Middle nasal concha (*cut away*)

Infundibulum leading to frontonasal canal

Semilunar hiatus (osteomeatal unit) with opening of anterior ethmoidal air cells

Uncinate process

Inferior nasal concha (*cut away*)

Opening of nasolacrimal canal

Superior nasal concha (*cut away*)

Openings of posterior ethmoidal cells

Opening of sphenoidal sinus

Openings into maxillary sinus

Sphenopalatine foramen

Ethmoidal process of inferior nasal concha

Lesser palatine foramen

Greater palatine foramen

*F. Netter M.D.*

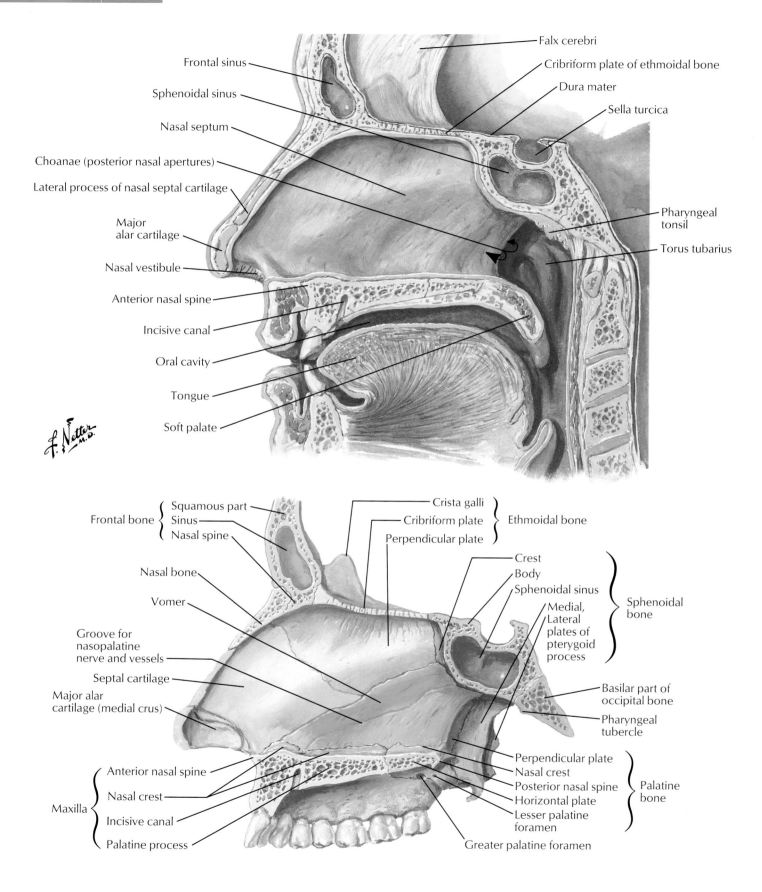

Falx cerebri

Frontal sinus

Cribriform plate of ethmoidal bone

Sphenoidal sinus

Dura mater

Nasal septum

Sella turcica

Choanae (posterior nasal apertures)

Lateral process of nasal septal cartilage

Pharyngeal tonsil

Major alar cartilage

Torus tubarius

Nasal vestibule

Anterior nasal spine

Incisive canal

Oral cavity

Tongue

Soft palate

Frontal bone
  { Squamous part
  { Sinus
  { Nasal spine

Crista galli

Cribriform plate

Ethmoidal bone

Perpendicular plate

Nasal bone

Crest

Body

Vomer

Sphenoidal sinus

Groove for nasopalatine nerve and vessels

Medial, Lateral plates of pterygoid process

Sphenoidal bone

Septal cartilage

Major alar cartilage (medial crus)

Basilar part of occipital bone

Pharyngeal tubercle

Anterior nasal spine

Perpendicular plate

Nasal crest

Nasal crest

Posterior nasal spine

Horizontal plate

Palatine bone

Maxilla

Incisive canal

Lesser palatine foramen

Palatine process

Greater palatine foramen

**Plate 38**

**Nasal Region**

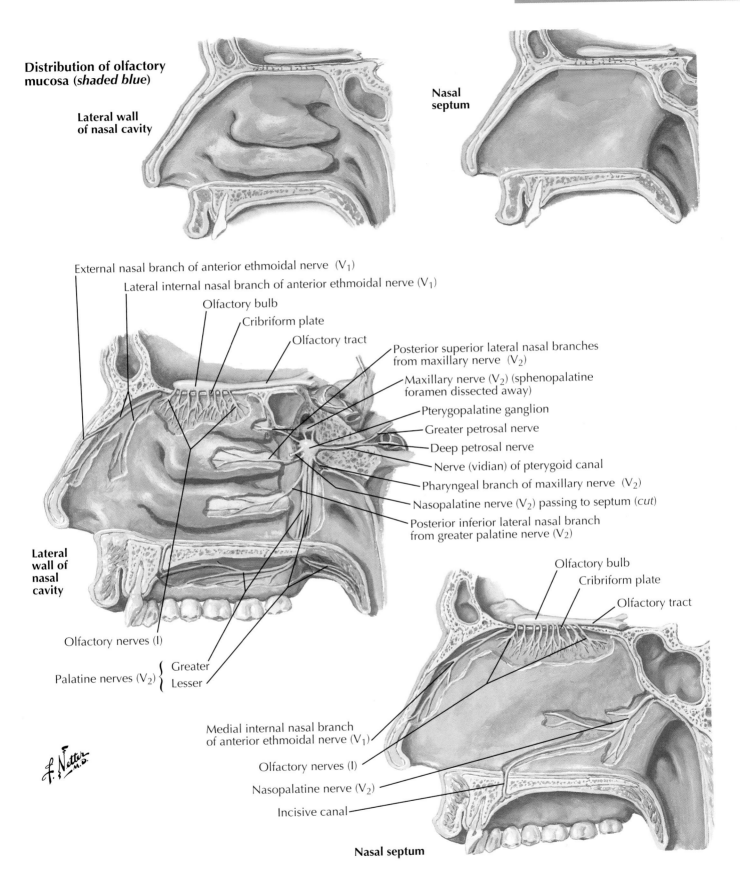

**Distribution of olfactory mucosa (*shaded blue*)**

**Lateral wall of nasal cavity**

**Nasal septum**

External nasal branch of anterior ethmoidal nerve (V$_1$)

Lateral internal nasal branch of anterior ethmoidal nerve (V$_1$)

Olfactory bulb

Cribriform plate

Olfactory tract

Posterior superior lateral nasal branches from maxillary nerve (V$_2$)

Maxillary nerve (V$_2$) (sphenopalatine foramen dissected away)

Pterygopalatine ganglion

Greater petrosal nerve

Deep petrosal nerve

Nerve (vidian) of pterygoid canal

Pharyngeal branch of maxillary nerve (V$_2$)

Nasopalatine nerve (V$_2$) passing to septum (*cut*)

Posterior inferior lateral nasal branch from greater palatine nerve (V$_2$)

**Lateral wall of nasal cavity**

Olfactory nerves (I)

Palatine nerves (V$_2$) { Greater / Lesser

Olfactory bulb

Cribriform plate

Olfactory tract

Medial internal nasal branch of anterior ethmoidal nerve (V$_1$)

Olfactory nerves (I)

Nasopalatine nerve (V$_2$)

Incisive canal

**Nasal septum**

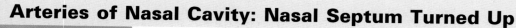

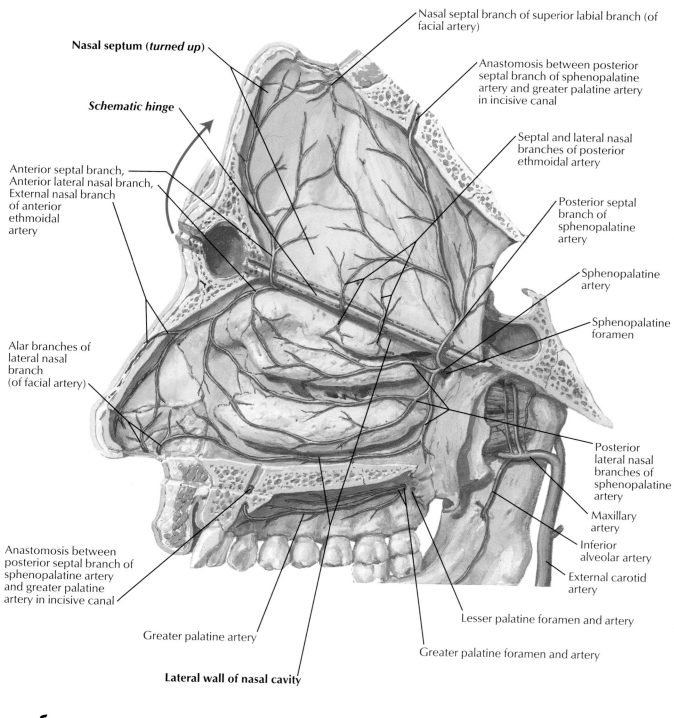

Nasal septal branch of superior labial branch (of facial artery)

**Nasal septum** (*turned up*)

Anastomosis between posterior septal branch of sphenopalatine artery and greater palatine artery in incisive canal

***Schematic hinge***

Septal and lateral nasal branches of posterior ethmoidal artery

Anterior septal branch, Anterior lateral nasal branch, External nasal branch of anterior ethmoidal artery

Posterior septal branch of sphenopalatine artery

Sphenopalatine artery

Sphenopalatine foramen

Alar branches of lateral nasal branch (of facial artery)

Posterior lateral nasal branches of sphenopalatine artery

Maxillary artery

Inferior alveolar artery

External carotid artery

Anastomosis between posterior septal branch of sphenopalatine artery and greater palatine artery in incisive canal

Lesser palatine foramen and artery

Greater palatine artery

Greater palatine foramen and artery

**Lateral wall of nasal cavity**

**Plate 40**

**Nasal Region**

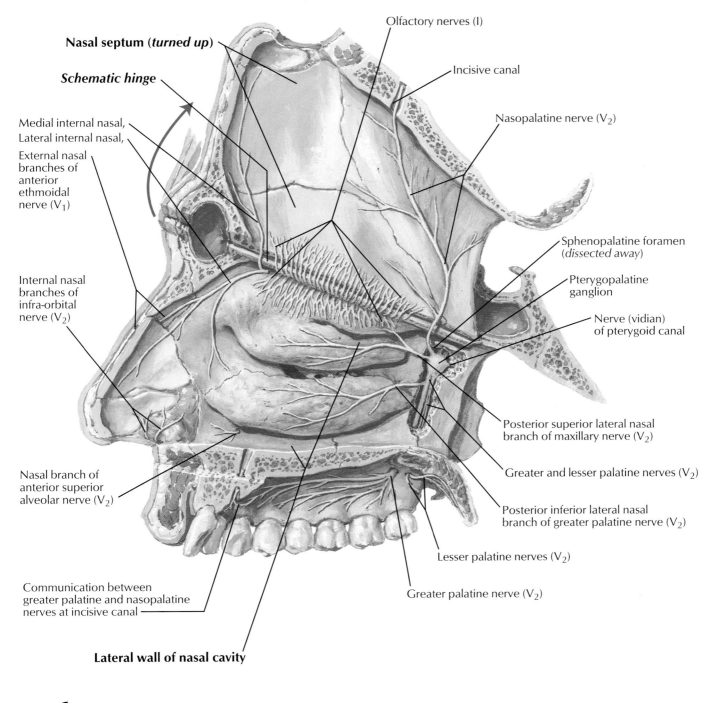

Nasal septum (*turned up*)

Schematic hinge

Medial internal nasal,
Lateral internal nasal,
External nasal branches of anterior ethmoidal nerve (V₁)

Internal nasal branches of infra-orbital nerve (V₂)

Nasal branch of anterior superior alveolar nerve (V₂)

Communication between greater palatine and nasopalatine nerves at incisive canal

**Lateral wall of nasal cavity**

Olfactory nerves (I)

Incisive canal

Nasopalatine nerve (V₂)

Sphenopalatine foramen (*dissected away*)

Pterygopalatine ganglion

Nerve (vidian) of pterygoid canal

Posterior superior lateral nasal branch of maxillary nerve (V₂)

Greater and lesser palatine nerves (V₂)

Posterior inferior lateral nasal branch of greater palatine nerve (V₂)

Lesser palatine nerves (V₂)

Greater palatine nerve (V₂)

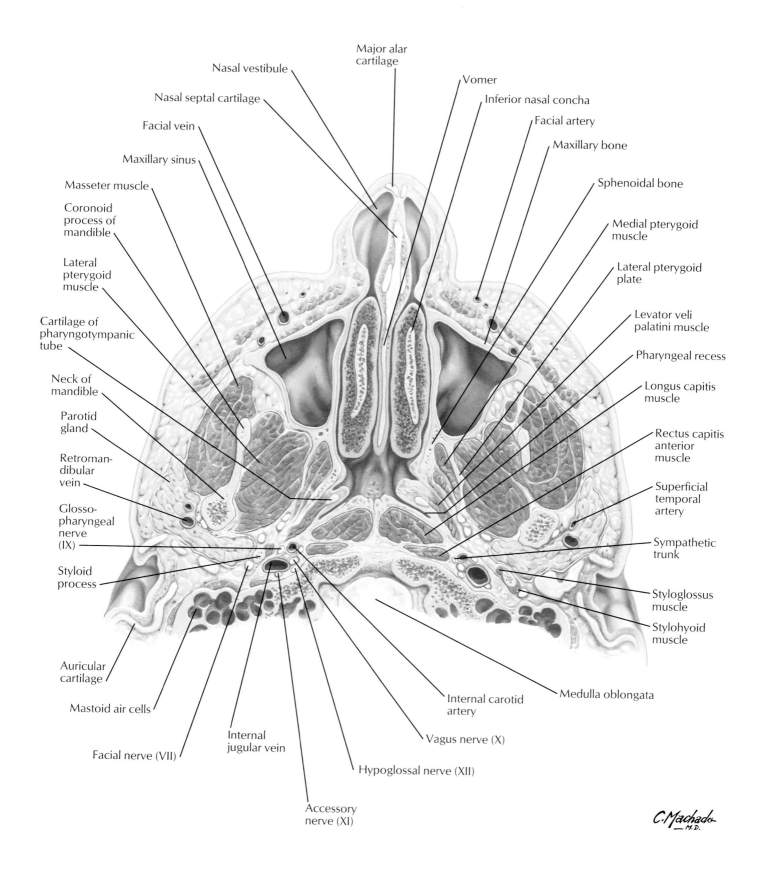

Major alar cartilage

Nasal vestibule

Vomer

Nasal septal cartilage

Inferior nasal concha

Facial vein

Facial artery

Maxillary sinus

Maxillary bone

Masseter muscle

Sphenoidal bone

Coronoid process of mandible

Medial pterygoid muscle

Lateral pterygoid muscle

Lateral pterygoid plate

Cartilage of pharyngotympanic tube

Levator veli palatini muscle

Pharyngeal recess

Neck of mandible

Longus capitis muscle

Parotid gland

Rectus capitis anterior muscle

Retromandibular vein

Superficial temporal artery

Glossopharyngeal nerve (IX)

Sympathetic trunk

Styloid process

Styloglossus muscle

Auricular cartilage

Stylohyoid muscle

Mastoid air cells

Medulla oblongata

Facial nerve (VII)

Internal carotid artery

Internal jugular vein

Vagus nerve (X)

Hypoglossal nerve (XII)

Accessory nerve (XI)

C. Machado —M.D.

**Plate 42**

**Nasal Region**

**Coronal section**

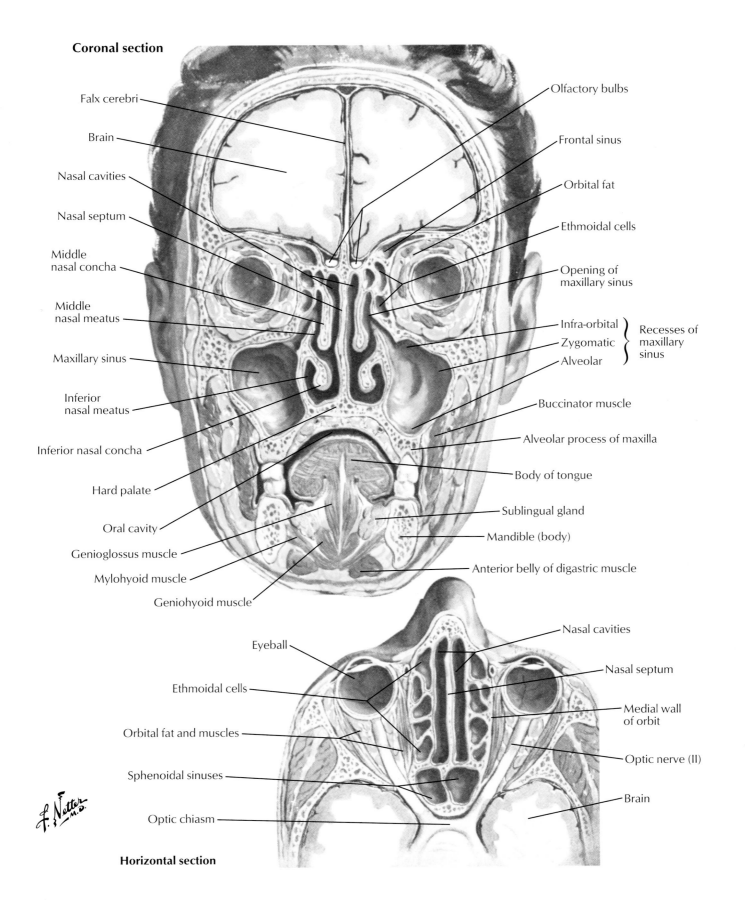

Falx cerebri

Brain

Nasal cavities

Nasal septum

Middle nasal concha

Middle nasal meatus

Maxillary sinus

Inferior nasal meatus

Inferior nasal concha

Hard palate

Oral cavity

Genioglossus muscle

Mylohyoid muscle

Geniohyoid muscle

Olfactory bulbs

Frontal sinus

Orbital fat

Ethmoidal cells

Opening of maxillary sinus

Infra-orbital }
Zygomatic    } Recesses of maxillary sinus
Alveolar     }

Buccinator muscle

Alveolar process of maxilla

Body of tongue

Sublingual gland

Mandible (body)

Anterior belly of digastric muscle

Eyeball

Ethmoidal cells

Orbital fat and muscles

Sphenoidal sinuses

Optic chiasm

Nasal cavities

Nasal septum

Medial wall of orbit

Optic nerve (II)

Brain

**Horizontal section**

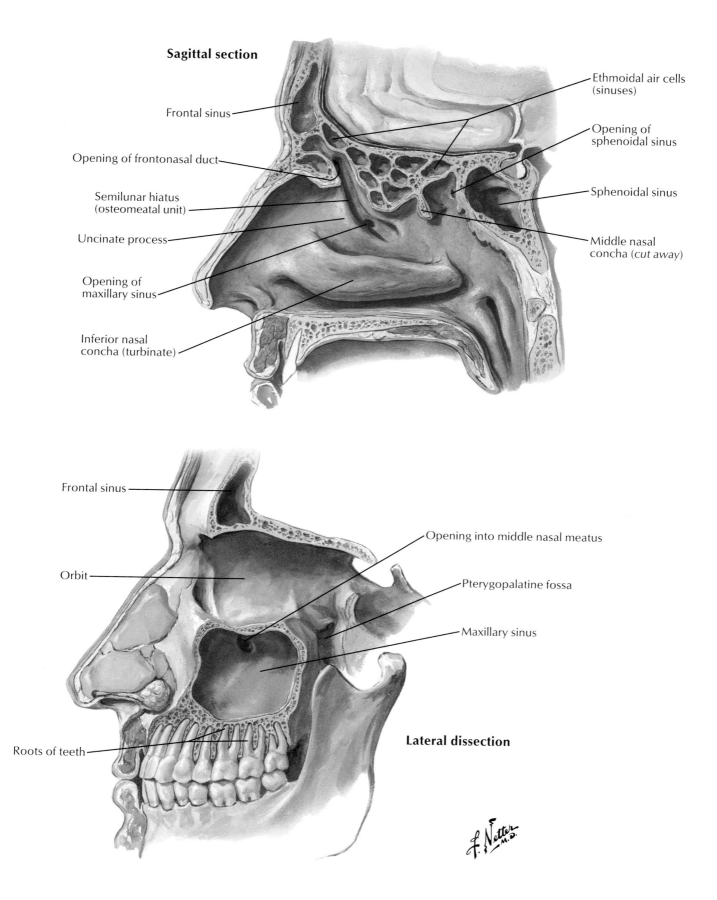

**Sagittal section**

Frontal sinus

Ethmoidal air cells (sinuses)

Opening of frontonasal duct

Opening of sphenoidal sinus

Semilunar hiatus (osteomeatal unit)

Sphenoidal sinus

Uncinate process

Middle nasal concha (cut away)

Opening of maxillary sinus

Inferior nasal concha (turbinate)

Frontal sinus

Opening into middle nasal meatus

Orbit

Pterygopalatine fossa

Maxillary sinus

Roots of teeth

**Lateral dissection**

**Plate 44**

**Nasal Region**

**Bones of nasal cavity
and paranasal sinuses
at birth**

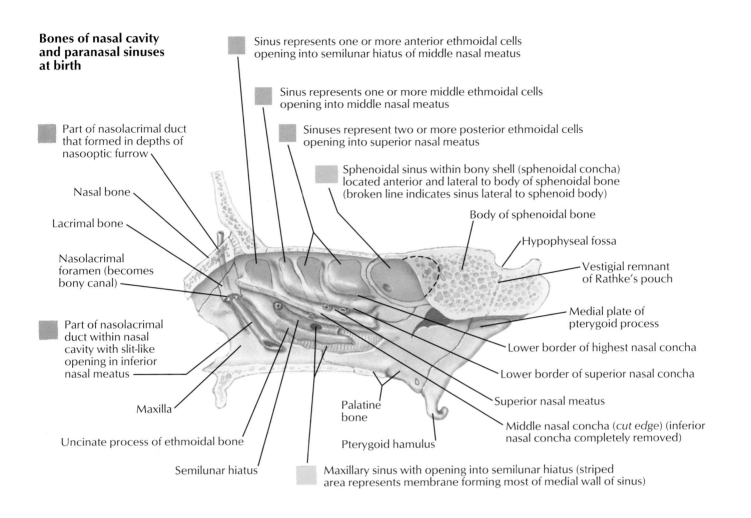

Sinus represents one or more anterior ethmoidal cells opening into semilunar hiatus of middle nasal meatus

Sinus represents one or more middle ethmoidal cells opening into middle nasal meatus

Sinuses represent two or more posterior ethmoidal cells opening into superior nasal meatus

Sphenoidal sinus within bony shell (sphenoidal concha) located anterior and lateral to body of sphenoidal bone (broken line indicates sinus lateral to sphenoid body)

Part of nasolacrimal duct that formed in depths of nasooptic furrow

Nasal bone

Lacrimal bone

Nasolacrimal foramen (becomes bony canal)

Part of nasolacrimal duct within nasal cavity with slit-like opening in inferior nasal meatus

Maxilla

Uncinate process of ethmoidal bone

Semilunar hiatus

Palatine bone

Pterygoid hamulus

Body of sphenoidal bone

Hypophyseal fossa

Vestigial remnant of Rathke's pouch

Medial plate of pterygoid process

Lower border of highest nasal concha

Lower border of superior nasal concha

Superior nasal meatus

Middle nasal concha (*cut edge*) (inferior nasal concha completely removed)

Maxillary sinus with opening into semilunar hiatus (striped area represents membrane forming most of medial wall of sinus)

**Growth of frontal and maxillary
sinuses throughout life**

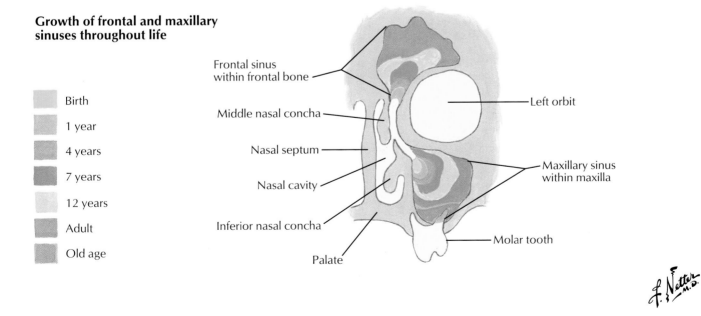

Birth

1 year

4 years

7 years

12 years

Adult

Old age

Frontal sinus within frontal bone

Middle nasal concha

Nasal septum

Nasal cavity

Inferior nasal concha

Palate

Left orbit

Maxillary sinus within maxilla

Molar tooth

Temporalis tendon

Superficial temporal artery and vein and auriculotemporal nerve

Branches of facial nerve (VII)

Transverse facial artery

Accessory parotid gland

Parotid duct

Buccinator muscle (*cut*)

Masseter muscle

Lingual nerve

Submandibular ganglion

Tongue

Frenulum of tongue

Sublingual fold with openings of sublingual ducts (of Rivinus)

Sublingual caruncle with opening of submandibular duct

Sublingual gland

Submandibular duct

Sublingual artery and vein

Mylohyoid muscle (*cut*)

Digastric muscle (anterior belly)

Submandibular gland

Facial artery and vein

Hyoid bone

Parotid gland

Retromandibular vein (anterior and posterior divisions)

Digastric muscle (posterior belly)

Stylohyoid muscle

External jugular vein

Sternocleidomastoid muscle

Common trunk receiving facial, anterior branch of retromandibular, and lingual veins (common facial vein)

Internal jugular vein

External carotid artery

**Plate 46**

**Nasal Region**

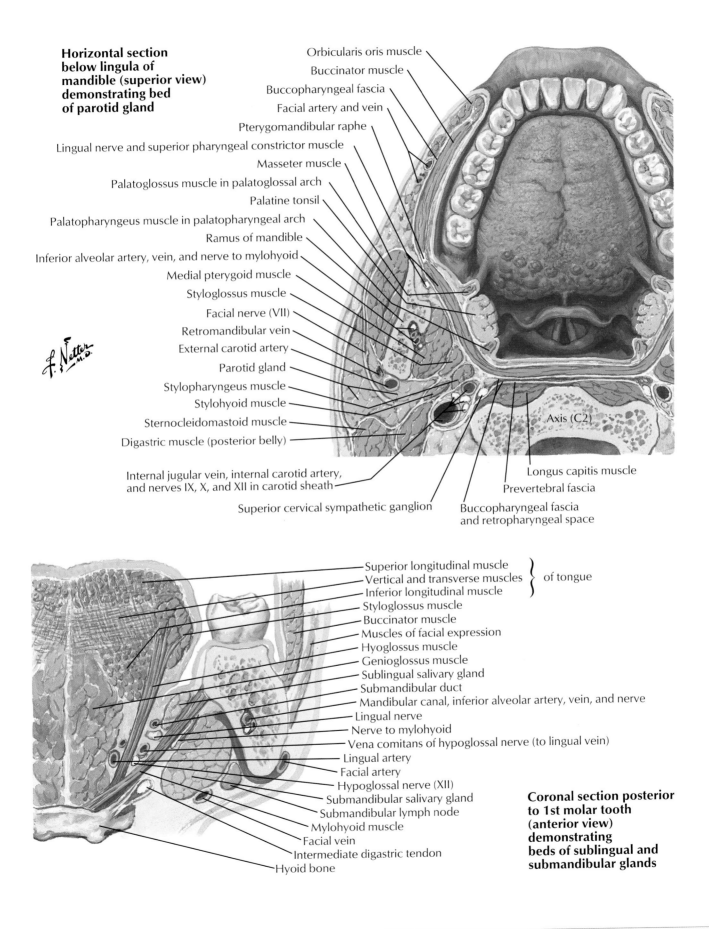

**Horizontal section below lingula of mandible (superior view) demonstrating bed of parotid gland**

Orbicularis oris muscle

Buccinator muscle

Buccopharyngeal fascia

Facial artery and vein

Pterygomandibular raphe

Lingual nerve and superior pharyngeal constrictor muscle

Masseter muscle

Palatoglossus muscle in palatoglossal arch

Palatine tonsil

Palatopharyngeus muscle in palatopharyngeal arch

Ramus of mandible

Inferior alveolar artery, vein, and nerve to mylohyoid

Medial pterygoid muscle

Styloglossus muscle

Facial nerve (VII)

Retromandibular vein

External carotid artery

Parotid gland

Stylopharyngeus muscle

Stylohyoid muscle

Sternocleidomastoid muscle

Digastric muscle (posterior belly)

Internal jugular vein, internal carotid artery, and nerves IX, X, and XII in carotid sheath

Superior cervical sympathetic ganglion

Axis (C2)

Longus capitis muscle

Prevertebral fascia

Buccopharyngeal fascia and retropharyngeal space

Superior longitudinal muscle
Vertical and transverse muscles } of tongue
Inferior longitudinal muscle

Styloglossus muscle

Buccinator muscle

Muscles of facial expression

Hyoglossus muscle

Genioglossus muscle

Sublingual salivary gland

Submandibular duct

Mandibular canal, inferior alveolar artery, vein, and nerve

Lingual nerve

Nerve to mylohyoid

Vena comitans of hypoglossal nerve (to lingual vein)

Lingual artery

Facial artery

Hypoglossal nerve (XII)

Submandibular salivary gland

Submandibular lymph node

Mylohyoid muscle

Facial vein

Intermediate digastric tendon

Hyoid bone

**Coronal section posterior to 1st molar tooth (anterior view) demonstrating beds of sublingual and submandibular glands**

**Nasal Region**

**Plate 47**

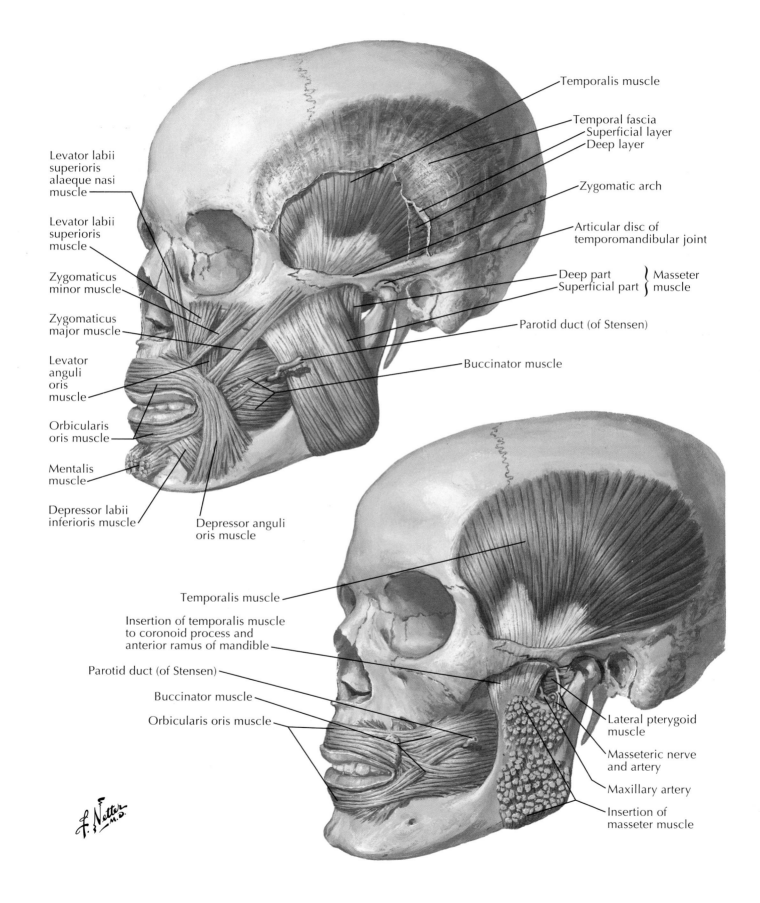

Levator labii superioris alaeque nasi muscle

Levator labii superioris muscle

Zygomaticus minor muscle

Zygomaticus major muscle

Levator anguli oris muscle

Orbicularis oris muscle

Mentalis muscle

Depressor labii inferioris muscle

Depressor anguli oris muscle

Temporalis muscle

Temporal fascia
Superficial layer
Deep layer

Zygomatic arch

Articular disc of temporomandibular joint

Deep part
Superficial part } Masseter muscle

Parotid duct (of Stensen)

Buccinator muscle

Temporalis muscle

Insertion of temporalis muscle to coronoid process and anterior ramus of mandible

Parotid duct (of Stensen)

Buccinator muscle

Orbicularis oris muscle

Lateral pterygoid muscle

Masseteric nerve and artery

Maxillary artery

Insertion of masseter muscle

**Plate 48**

**Nasal Region**

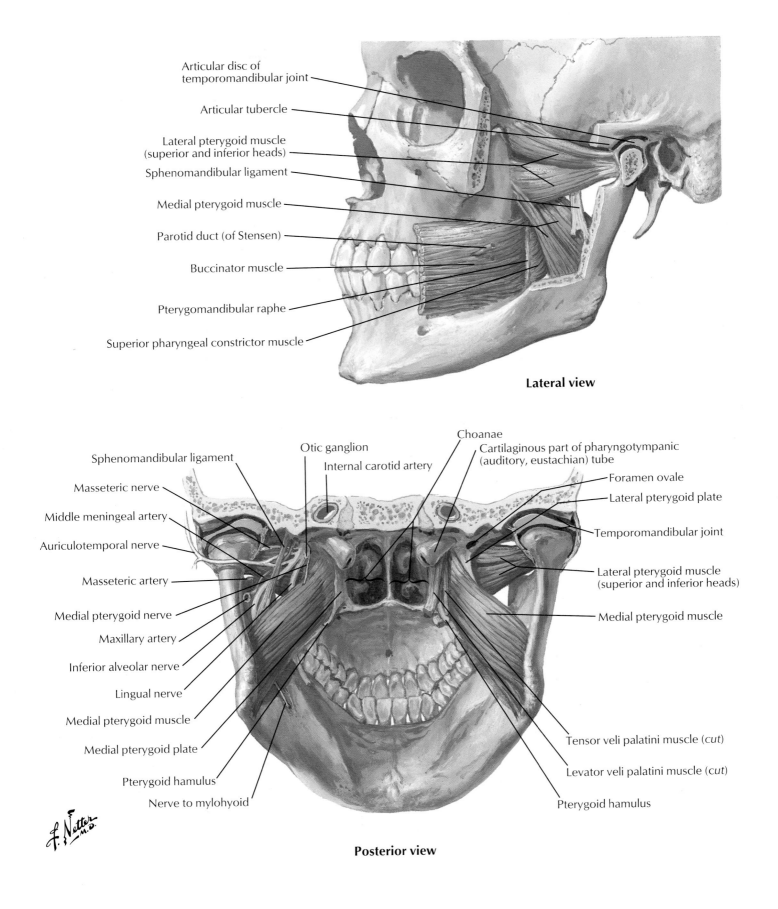

Articular disc of
temporomandibular joint

Articular tubercle

Lateral pterygoid muscle
(superior and inferior heads)

Sphenomandibular ligament

Medial pterygoid muscle

Parotid duct (of Stensen)

Buccinator muscle

Pterygomandibular raphe

Superior pharyngeal constrictor muscle

**Lateral view**

Sphenomandibular ligament

Masseteric nerve

Middle meningeal artery

Auriculotemporal nerve

Masseteric artery

Medial pterygoid nerve

Maxillary artery

Inferior alveolar nerve

Lingual nerve

Medial pterygoid muscle

Medial pterygoid plate

Pterygoid hamulus

Nerve to mylohyoid

Otic ganglion

Internal carotid artery

Choanae

Cartilaginous part of pharyngotympanic
(auditory, eustachian) tube

Foramen ovale

Lateral pterygoid plate

Temporomandibular joint

Lateral pterygoid muscle
(superior and inferior heads)

Medial pterygoid muscle

Tensor veli palatini muscle (*cut*)

Levator veli palatini muscle (*cut*)

Pterygoid hamulus

**Posterior view**

**Lateral view**

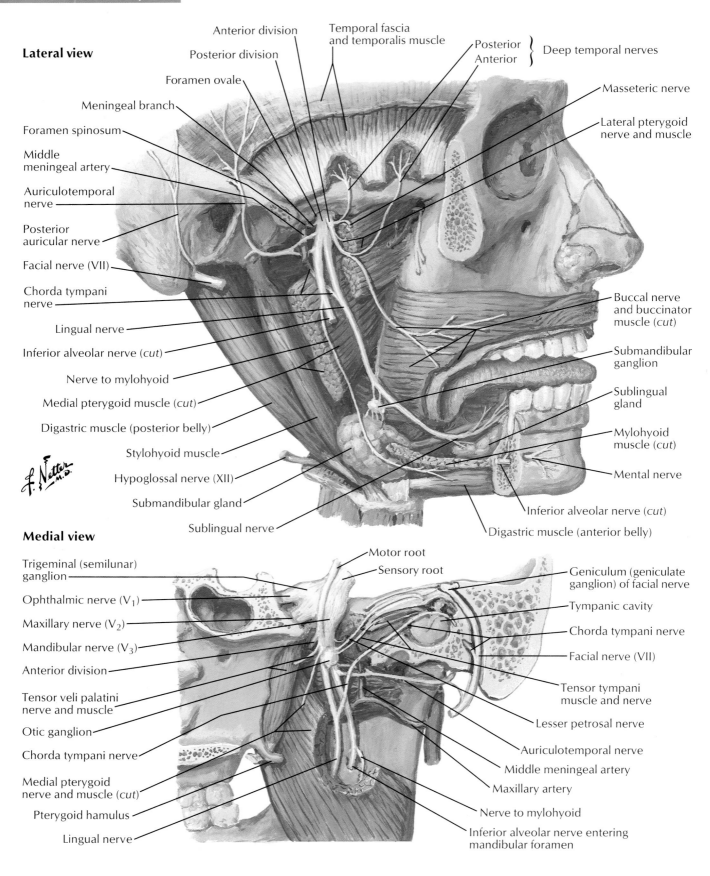

Anterior division

Posterior division

Foramen ovale

Meningeal branch

Foramen spinosum

Middle
meningeal artery

Auriculotemporal
nerve

Posterior
auricular nerve

Facial nerve (VII)

Chorda tympani
nerve

Lingual nerve

Inferior alveolar nerve (*cut*)

Nerve to mylohyoid

Medial pterygoid muscle (*cut*)

Digastric muscle (posterior belly)

Stylohyoid muscle

Hypoglossal nerve (XII)

Submandibular gland

Sublingual nerve

Temporal fascia
and temporalis muscle

Posterior } Deep temporal nerves
Anterior

Masseteric nerve

Lateral pterygoid
nerve and muscle

Buccal nerve
and buccinator
muscle (*cut*)

Submandibular
ganglion

Sublingual
gland

Mylohyoid
muscle (*cut*)

Mental nerve

Inferior alveolar nerve (*cut*)

Digastric muscle (anterior belly)

**Medial view**

Trigeminal (semilunar)
ganglion

Ophthalmic nerve (V₁)

Maxillary nerve (V₂)

Mandibular nerve (V₃)

Anterior division

Tensor veli palatini
nerve and muscle

Otic ganglion

Chorda tympani nerve

Medial pterygoid
nerve and muscle (*cut*)

Pterygoid hamulus

Lingual nerve

Motor root

Sensory root

Geniculum (geniculate
ganglion) of facial nerve

Tympanic cavity

Chorda tympani nerve

Facial nerve (VII)

Tensor tympani
muscle and nerve

Lesser petrosal nerve

Auriculotemporal nerve

Middle meningeal artery

Maxillary artery

Nerve to mylohyoid

Inferior alveolar nerve entering
mandibular foramen

**Plate 50**

**Nasal Region**

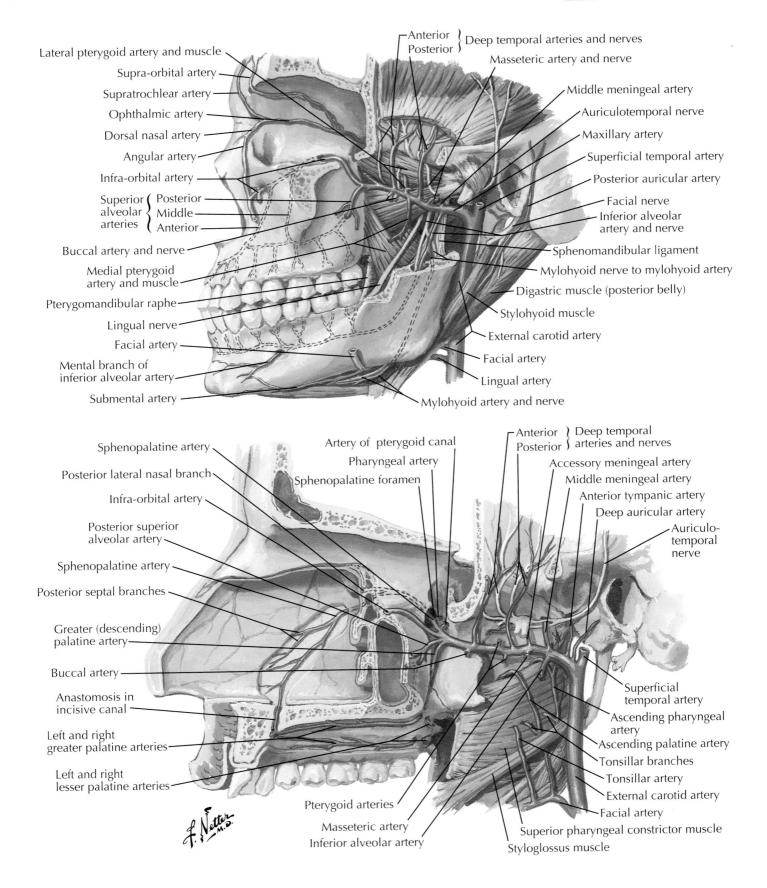

Anterior } Deep temporal arteries and nerves
Posterior

Lateral pterygoid artery and muscle

Supra-orbital artery

Supratrochlear artery

Ophthalmic artery

Dorsal nasal artery

Angular artery

Infra-orbital artery

Superior { Posterior
alveolar   Middle
arteries   Anterior

Buccal artery and nerve

Medial pterygoid artery and muscle

Pterygomandibular raphe

Lingual nerve

Facial artery

Mental branch of inferior alveolar artery

Submental artery

Masseteric artery and nerve

Middle meningeal artery

Auriculotemporal nerve

Maxillary artery

Superficial temporal artery

Posterior auricular artery

Facial nerve

Inferior alveolar artery and nerve

Sphenomandibular ligament

Mylohyoid nerve to mylohyoid artery

Digastric muscle (posterior belly)

Stylohyoid muscle

External carotid artery

Facial artery

Lingual artery

Mylohyoid artery and nerve

Sphenopalatine artery

Posterior lateral nasal branch

Infra-orbital artery

Posterior superior alveolar artery

Sphenopalatine artery

Posterior septal branches

Greater (descending) palatine artery

Buccal artery

Anastomosis in incisive canal

Left and right greater palatine arteries

Left and right lesser palatine arteries

Artery of pterygoid canal

Pharyngeal artery

Sphenopalatine foramen

Anterior } Deep temporal
Posterior   arteries and nerves

Accessory meningeal artery

Middle meningeal artery

Anterior tympanic artery

Deep auricular artery

Auriculo-temporal nerve

Superficial temporal artery

Ascending pharyngeal artery

Ascending palatine artery

Tonsillar branches

Tonsillar artery

External carotid artery

Facial artery

Superior pharyngeal constrictor muscle

Pterygoid arteries

Masseteric artery

Inferior alveolar artery

Styloglossus muscle

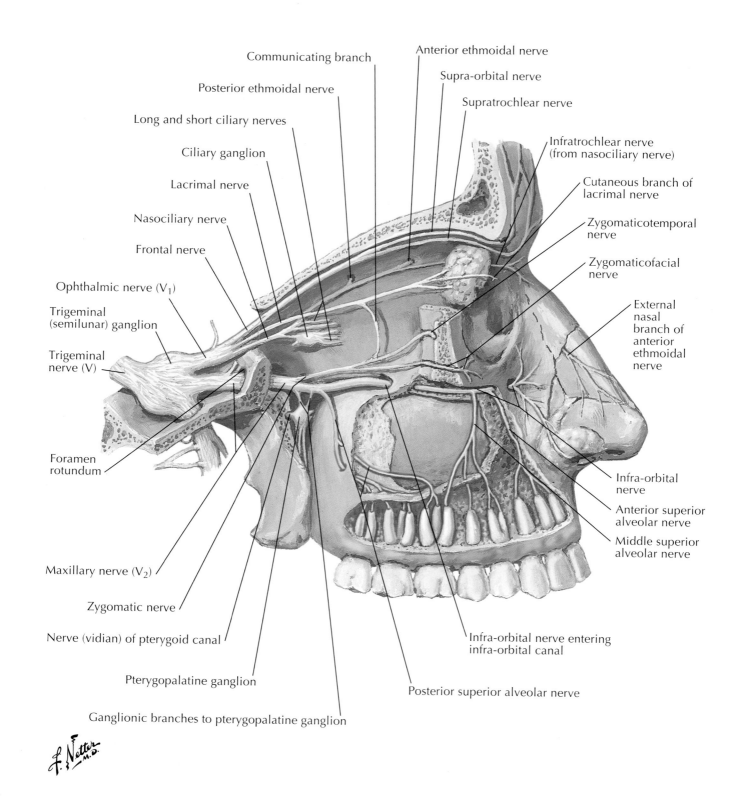

Communicating branch

Posterior ethmoidal nerve

Long and short ciliary nerves

Ciliary ganglion

Lacrimal nerve

Nasociliary nerve

Frontal nerve

Ophthalmic nerve (V₁)

Trigeminal (semilunar) ganglion

Trigeminal nerve (V)

Foramen rotundum

Maxillary nerve (V₂)

Zygomatic nerve

Nerve (vidian) of pterygoid canal

Pterygopalatine ganglion

Ganglionic branches to pterygopalatine ganglion

Anterior ethmoidal nerve

Supra-orbital nerve

Supratrochlear nerve

Infratrochlear nerve (from nasociliary nerve)

Cutaneous branch of lacrimal nerve

Zygomaticotemporal nerve

Zygomaticofacial nerve

External nasal branch of anterior ethmoidal nerve

Infra-orbital nerve

Anterior superior alveolar nerve

Middle superior alveolar nerve

Infra-orbital nerve entering infra-orbital canal

Posterior superior alveolar nerve

**Plate 52**

**Nasal Region**

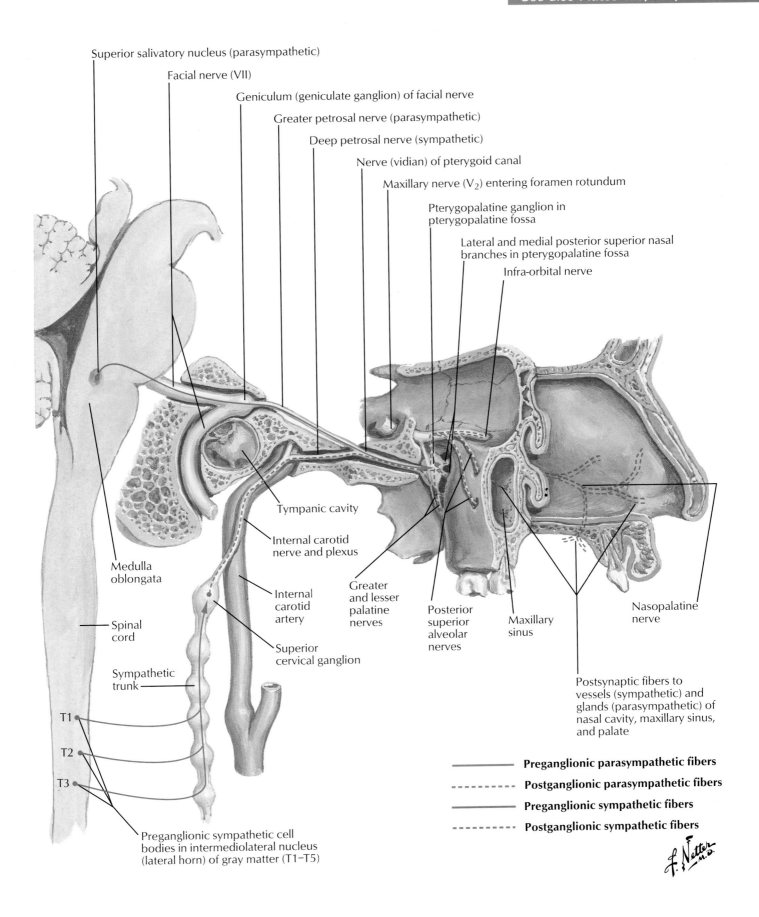

Superior salivatory nucleus (parasympathetic)

Facial nerve (VII)

Geniculum (geniculate ganglion) of facial nerve

Greater petrosal nerve (parasympathetic)

Deep petrosal nerve (sympathetic)

Nerve (vidian) of pterygoid canal

Maxillary nerve (V₂) entering foramen rotundum

Pterygopalatine ganglion in pterygopalatine fossa

Lateral and medial posterior superior nasal branches in pterygopalatine fossa

Infra-orbital nerve

Tympanic cavity

Internal carotid nerve and plexus

Medulla oblongata

Internal carotid artery

Greater and lesser palatine nerves

Posterior superior alveolar nerves

Maxillary sinus

Nasopalatine nerve

Spinal cord

Superior cervical ganglion

Sympathetic trunk

T1

T2

T3

Postsynaptic fibers to vessels (sympathetic) and glands (parasympathetic) of nasal cavity, maxillary sinus, and palate

Preganglionic sympathetic cell bodies in intermediolateral nucleus (lateral horn) of gray matter (T1–T5)

——————— **Preganglionic parasympathetic fibers**

- - - - - - - **Postganglionic parasympathetic fibers**

——————— **Preganglionic sympathetic fibers**

- - - - - - - **Postganglionic sympathetic fibers**

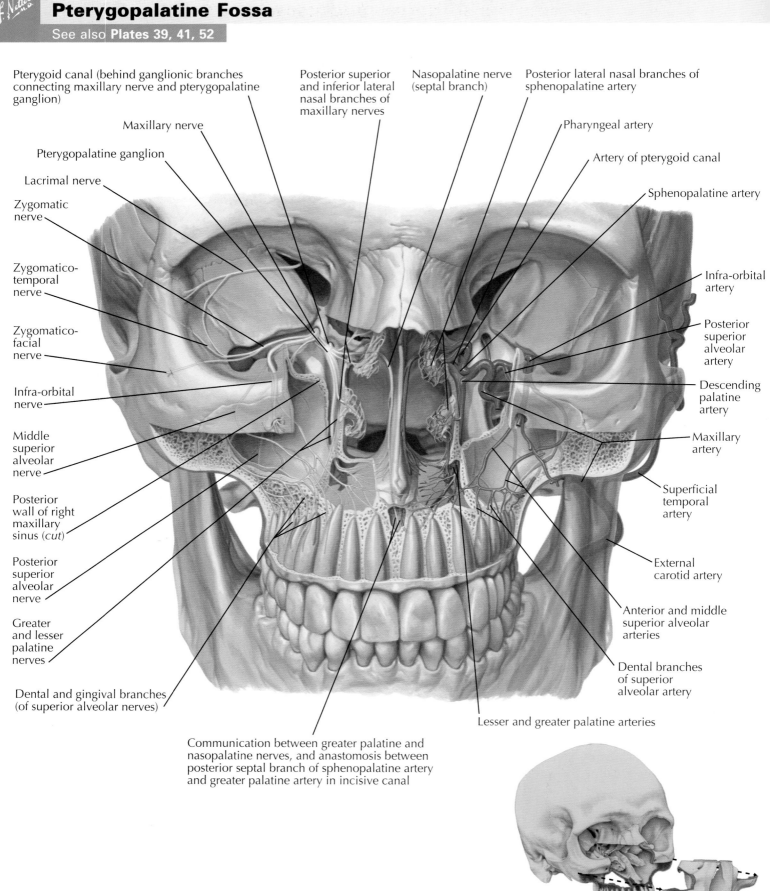

Pterygoid canal (behind ganglionic branches connecting maxillary nerve and pterygopalatine ganglion)

Maxillary nerve

Pterygopalatine ganglion

Lacrimal nerve

Zygomatic nerve

Zygomatico-temporal nerve

Zygomatico-facial nerve

Infra-orbital nerve

Middle superior alveolar nerve

Posterior wall of right maxillary sinus (cut)

Posterior superior alveolar nerve

Greater and lesser palatine nerves

Dental and gingival branches (of superior alveolar nerves)

Posterior superior and inferior lateral nasal branches of maxillary nerves

Nasopalatine nerve (septal branch)

Posterior lateral nasal branches of sphenopalatine artery

Pharyngeal artery

Artery of pterygoid canal

Sphenopalatine artery

Infra-orbital artery

Posterior superior alveolar artery

Descending palatine artery

Maxillary artery

Superficial temporal artery

External carotid artery

Anterior and middle superior alveolar arteries

Dental branches of superior alveolar artery

Lesser and greater palatine arteries

Communication between greater palatine and nasopalatine nerves, and anastomosis between posterior septal branch of sphenopalatine artery and greater palatine artery in incisive canal

Anterior perspective of fossa with lower facial skeleton removed

**Plate 54**

**Nasal Region**

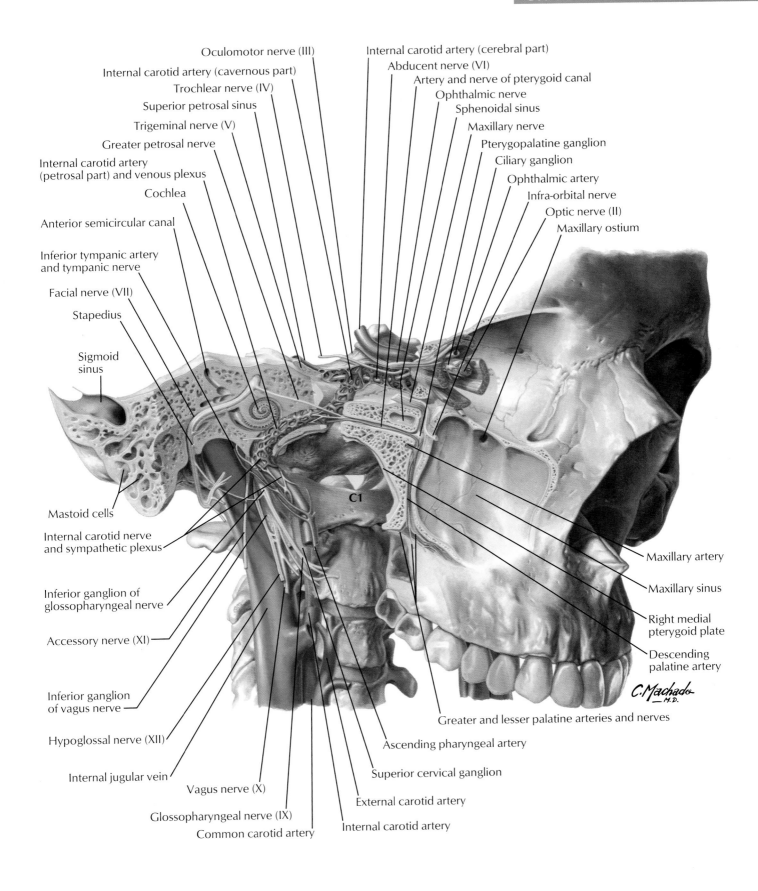

Oculomotor nerve (III)

Internal carotid artery (cavernous part)

Trochlear nerve (IV)

Superior petrosal sinus

Trigeminal nerve (V)

Greater petrosal nerve

Internal carotid artery
(petrosal part) and venous plexus

Cochlea

Anterior semicircular canal

Inferior tympanic artery
and tympanic nerve

Facial nerve (VII)

Stapedius

Sigmoid
sinus

Mastoid cells

Internal carotid nerve
and sympathetic plexus

Inferior ganglion of
glossopharyngeal nerve

Accessory nerve (XI)

Inferior ganglion
of vagus nerve

Hypoglossal nerve (XII)

Internal jugular vein

Vagus nerve (X)

Glossopharyngeal nerve (IX)

Common carotid artery

Internal carotid artery (cerebral part)

Abducent nerve (VI)

Artery and nerve of pterygoid canal

Ophthalmic nerve

Sphenoidal sinus

Maxillary nerve

Pterygopalatine ganglion

Ciliary ganglion

Ophthalmic artery

Infra-orbital nerve

Optic nerve (II)

Maxillary ostium

C1

Maxillary artery

Maxillary sinus

Right medial
pterygoid plate

Descending
palatine artery

C. Machado
_M.D._

Greater and lesser palatine arteries and nerves

Ascending pharyngeal artery

Superior cervical ganglion

External carotid artery

Internal carotid artery

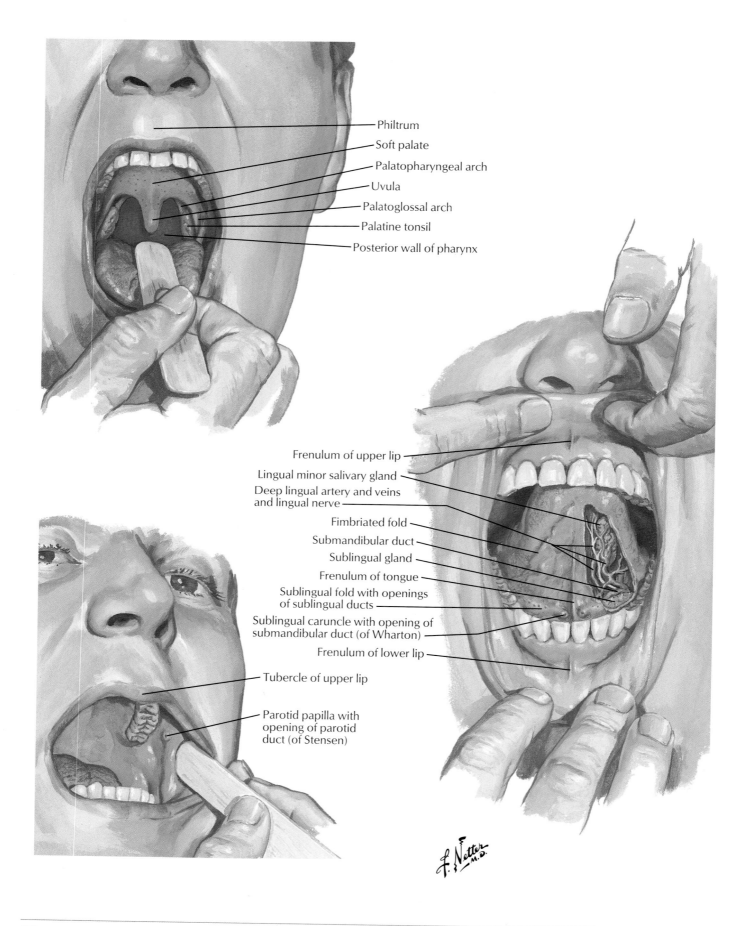

Philtrum

Soft palate

Palatopharyngeal arch

Uvula

Palatoglossal arch

Palatine tonsil

Posterior wall of pharynx

Frenulum of upper lip

Lingual minor salivary gland

Deep lingual artery and veins and lingual nerve

Fimbriated fold

Submandibular duct

Sublingual gland

Frenulum of tongue

Sublingual fold with openings of sublingual ducts

Sublingual caruncle with opening of submandibular duct (of Wharton)

Frenulum of lower lip

Tubercle of upper lip

Parotid papilla with opening of parotid duct (of Stensen)

**Plate 56**

**Oral Region**

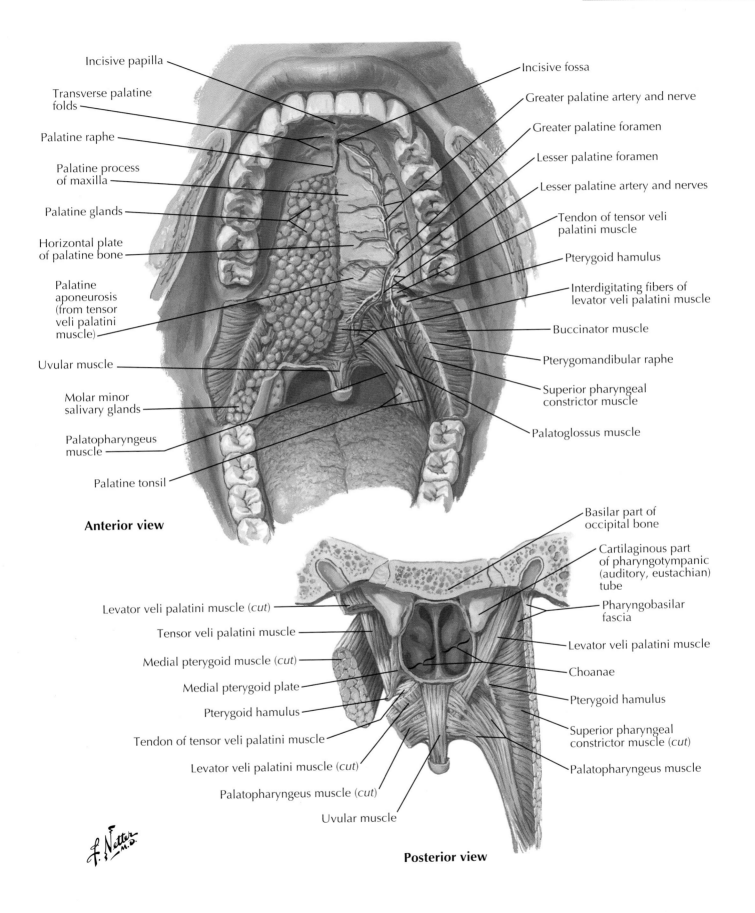

Incisive papilla

Transverse palatine folds

Palatine raphe

Palatine process of maxilla

Palatine glands

Horizontal plate of palatine bone

Palatine aponeurosis (from tensor veli palatini muscle)

Uvular muscle

Molar minor salivary glands

Palatopharyngeus muscle

Palatine tonsil

**Anterior view**

Incisive fossa

Greater palatine artery and nerve

Greater palatine foramen

Lesser palatine foramen

Lesser palatine artery and nerves

Tendon of tensor veli palatini muscle

Pterygoid hamulus

Interdigitating fibers of levator veli palatini muscle

Buccinator muscle

Pterygomandibular raphe

Superior pharyngeal constrictor muscle

Palatoglossus muscle

Levator veli palatini muscle (*cut*)

Tensor veli palatini muscle

Medial pterygoid muscle (*cut*)

Medial pterygoid plate

Pterygoid hamulus

Tendon of tensor veli palatini muscle

Levator veli palatini muscle (*cut*)

Palatopharyngeus muscle (*cut*)

Uvular muscle

Basilar part of occipital bone

Cartilaginous part of pharyngotympanic (auditory, eustachian) tube

Pharyngobasilar fascia

Levator veli palatini muscle

Choanae

Pterygoid hamulus

Superior pharyngeal constrictor muscle (*cut*)

Palatopharyngeus muscle

**Posterior view**

**Oral Region**

**Plate 57**

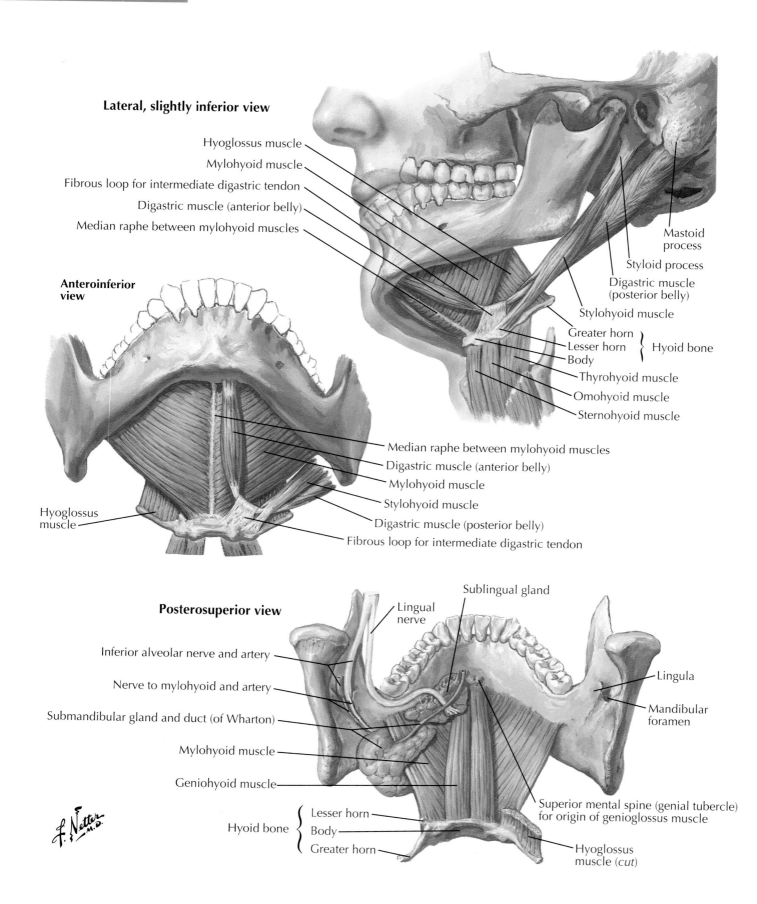

**Lateral, slightly inferior view**

Hyoglossus muscle

Mylohyoid muscle

Fibrous loop for intermediate digastric tendon

Digastric muscle (anterior belly)

Median raphe between mylohyoid muscles

Mastoid process

Styloid process

Digastric muscle (posterior belly)

Stylohyoid muscle

Greater horn

Lesser horn } Hyoid bone

Body

Thyrohyoid muscle

Omohyoid muscle

Sternohyoid muscle

**Anteroinferior view**

Median raphe between mylohyoid muscles

Digastric muscle (anterior belly)

Mylohyoid muscle

Stylohyoid muscle

Digastric muscle (posterior belly)

Hyoglossus muscle

Fibrous loop for intermediate digastric tendon

**Posterosuperior view**

Sublingual gland

Lingual nerve

Inferior alveolar nerve and artery

Nerve to mylohyoid and artery

Submandibular gland and duct (of Wharton)

Mylohyoid muscle

Geniohyoid muscle

Lingula

Mandibular foramen

Superior mental spine (genial tubercle) for origin of genioglossus muscle

Hyoglossus muscle (cut)

Hyoid bone { Lesser horn

Body

Greater horn

**Plate 58**

**Oral Region**

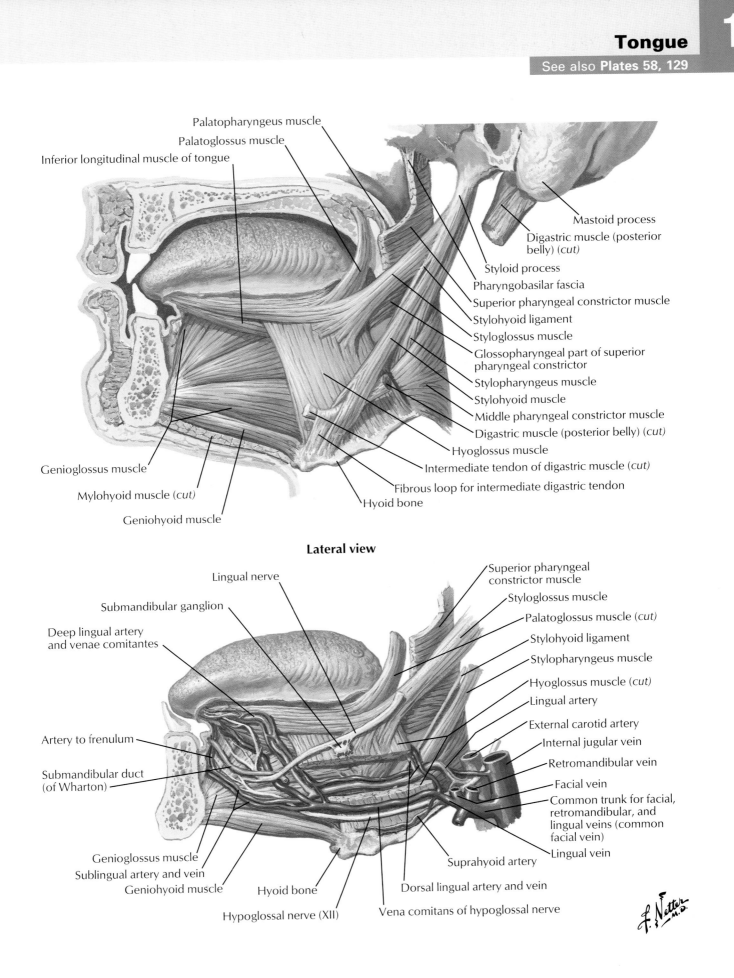

Palatopharyngeus muscle

Palatoglossus muscle

Inferior longitudinal muscle of tongue

Mastoid process

Digastric muscle (posterior belly) (*cut*)

Styloid process

Pharyngobasilar fascia

Superior pharyngeal constrictor muscle

Stylohyoid ligament

Styloglossus muscle

Glossopharyngeal part of superior pharyngeal constrictor

Stylopharyngeus muscle

Stylohyoid muscle

Middle pharyngeal constrictor muscle

Digastric muscle (posterior belly) (*cut*)

Hyoglossus muscle

Intermediate tendon of digastric muscle (*cut*)

Fibrous loop for intermediate digastric tendon

Hyoid bone

Genioglossus muscle

Mylohyoid muscle (*cut*)

Geniohyoid muscle

**Lateral view**

Lingual nerve

Submandibular ganglion

Deep lingual artery and venae comitantes

Superior pharyngeal constrictor muscle

Styloglossus muscle

Palatoglossus muscle (*cut*)

Stylohyoid ligament

Stylopharyngeus muscle

Hyoglossus muscle (*cut*)

Lingual artery

External carotid artery

Internal jugular vein

Retromandibular vein

Facial vein

Common trunk for facial, retromandibular, and lingual veins (common facial vein)

Lingual vein

Artery to frenulum

Submandibular duct (of Wharton)

Genioglossus muscle

Sublingual artery and vein

Geniohyoid muscle

Hyoid bone

Hypoglossal nerve (XII)

Vena comitans of hypoglossal nerve

Dorsal lingual artery and vein

Suprahyoid artery

**Oral Region**

**Plate 59**

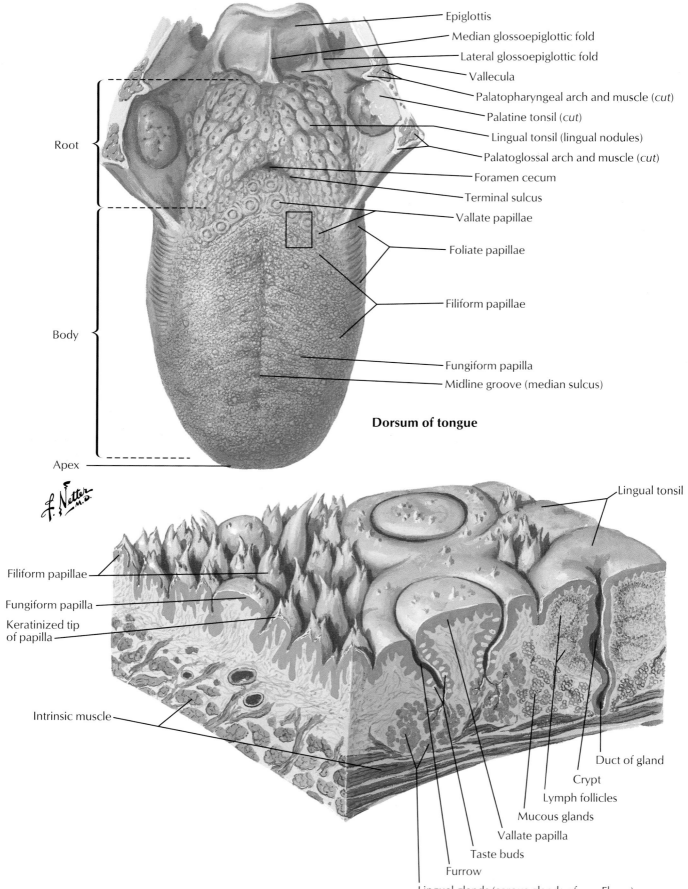

Epiglottis

Median glossoepiglottic fold

Lateral glossoepiglottic fold

Vallecula

Palatopharyngeal arch and muscle (*cut*)

Palatine tonsil (*cut*)

Lingual tonsil (lingual nodules)

Palatoglossal arch and muscle (*cut*)

Foramen cecum

Terminal sulcus

Vallate papillae

Foliate papillae

Filiform papillae

Fungiform papilla

Midline groove (median sulcus)

Root

Body

Apex

**Dorsum of tongue**

Lingual tonsil

Filiform papillae

Fungiform papilla

Keratinized tip of papilla

Intrinsic muscle

Duct of gland

Crypt

Lymph follicles

Mucous glands

Vallate papilla

Taste buds

Furrow

Lingual glands (serous glands of von Ebner)

**Schematic stereogram: area indicated above**

**Plate 60**

**Oral Region**

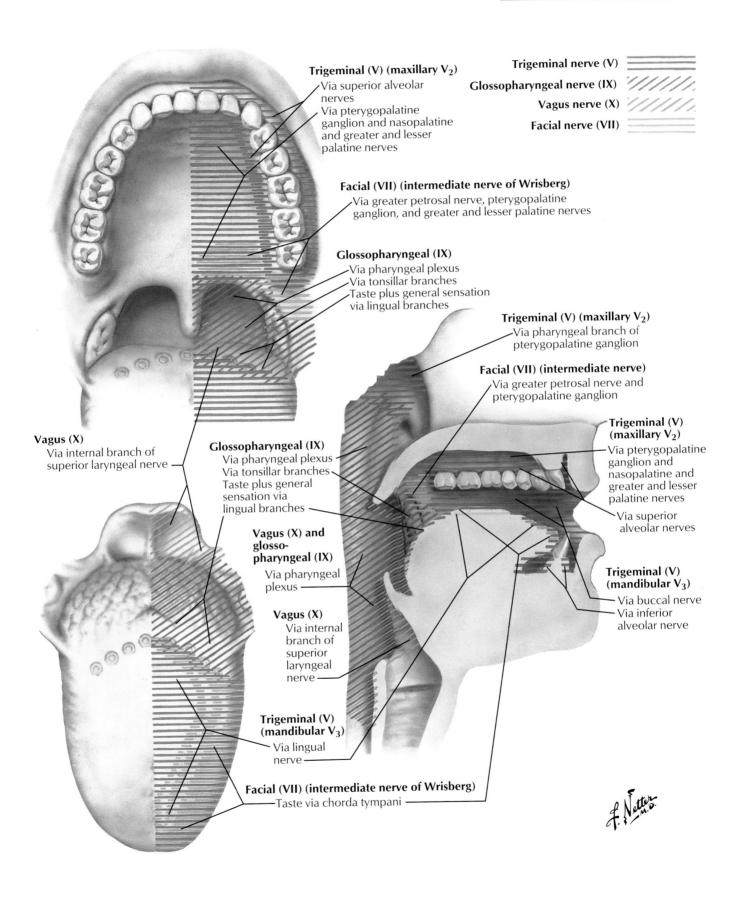

**Trigeminal (V) (maxillary V₂)**
Via superior alveolar nerves
Via pterygopalatine ganglion and nasopalatine and greater and lesser palatine nerves

Trigeminal nerve (V)
Glossopharyngeal nerve (IX)
Vagus nerve (X)
Facial nerve (VII)

**Facial (VII) (intermediate nerve of Wrisberg)**
Via greater petrosal nerve, pterygopalatine ganglion, and greater and lesser palatine nerves

**Glossopharyngeal (IX)**
Via pharyngeal plexus
Via tonsillar branches
Taste plus general sensation via lingual branches

**Trigeminal (V) (maxillary V₂)**
Via pharyngeal branch of pterygopalatine ganglion

**Facial (VII) (intermediate nerve)**
Via greater petrosal nerve and pterygopalatine ganglion

**Trigeminal (V) (maxillary V₂)**
Via pterygopalatine ganglion and nasopalatine and greater and lesser palatine nerves
Via superior alveolar nerves

**Vagus (X)**
Via internal branch of superior laryngeal nerve

**Glossopharyngeal (IX)**
Via pharyngeal plexus
Via tonsillar branches
Taste plus general sensation via lingual branches

**Vagus (X) and glosso-pharyngeal (IX)**
Via pharyngeal plexus

**Vagus (X)**
Via internal branch of superior laryngeal nerve

**Trigeminal (V) (mandibular V₃)**
Via lingual nerve

**Facial (VII) (intermediate nerve of Wrisberg)**
Taste via chorda tympani

**Trigeminal (V) (mandibular V₃)**
Via buccal nerve
Via inferior alveolar nerve

*f. Netter*

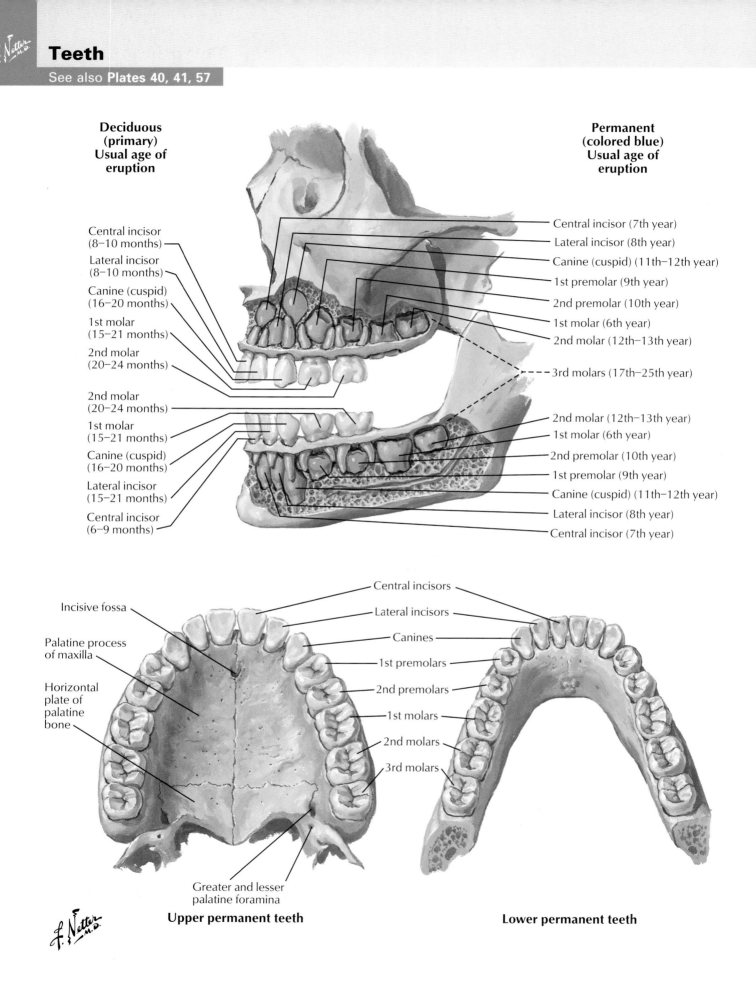

**Deciduous (primary) Usual age of eruption**

Central incisor (8–10 months)
Lateral incisor (8–10 months)
Canine (cuspid) (16–20 months)
1st molar (15–21 months)
2nd molar (20–24 months)

2nd molar (20–24 months)
1st molar (15–21 months)
Canine (cuspid) (16–20 months)
Lateral incisor (15–21 months)
Central incisor (6–9 months)

**Permanent (colored blue) Usual age of eruption**

Central incisor (7th year)
Lateral incisor (8th year)
Canine (cuspid) (11th–12th year)
1st premolar (9th year)
2nd premolar (10th year)
1st molar (6th year)
2nd molar (12th–13th year)

3rd molars (17th–25th year)

2nd molar (12th–13th year)
1st molar (6th year)
2nd premolar (10th year)
1st premolar (9th year)
Canine (cuspid) (11th–12th year)
Lateral incisor (8th year)
Central incisor (7th year)

Central incisors
Lateral incisors
Canines
1st premolars
2nd premolars
1st molars
2nd molars
3rd molars

Incisive fossa
Palatine process of maxilla
Horizontal plate of palatine bone

Greater and lesser palatine foramina

**Upper permanent teeth**

**Lower permanent teeth**

**Plate 62**

**Oral Region**

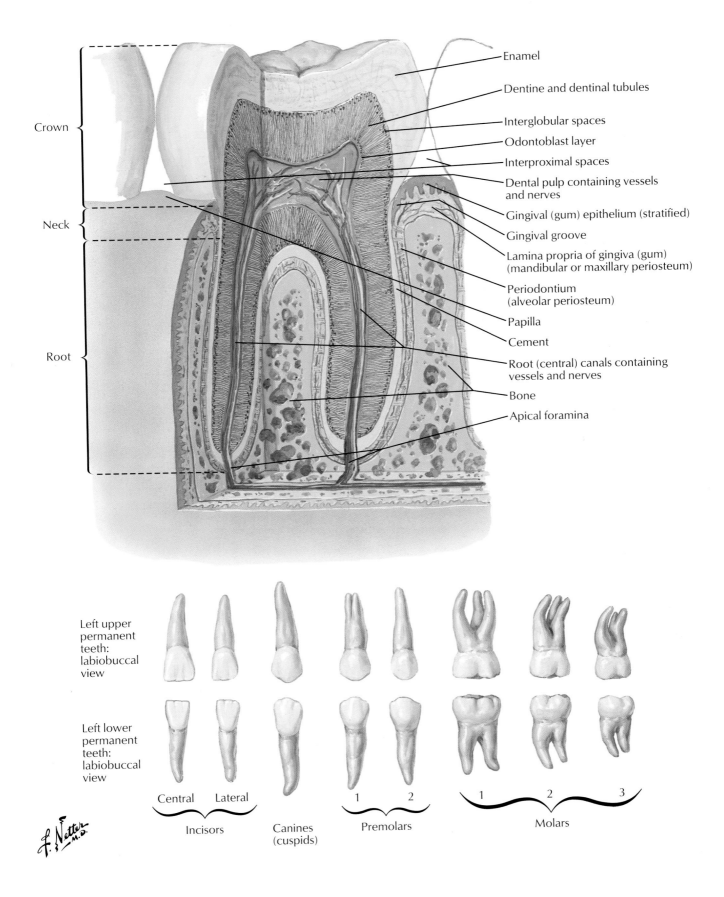

Crown

Neck

Root

Enamel

Dentine and dentinal tubules

Interglobular spaces

Odontoblast layer

Interproximal spaces

Dental pulp containing vessels and nerves

Gingival (gum) epithelium (stratified)

Gingival groove

Lamina propria of gingiva (gum) (mandibular or maxillary periosteum)

Periodontium (alveolar periosteum)

Papilla

Cement

Root (central) canals containing vessels and nerves

Bone

Apical foramina

Left upper permanent teeth: labiobuccal view

Left lower permanent teeth: labiobuccal view

Central    Lateral

Incisors

Canines (cuspids)

1    2

Premolars

1    2    3

Molars

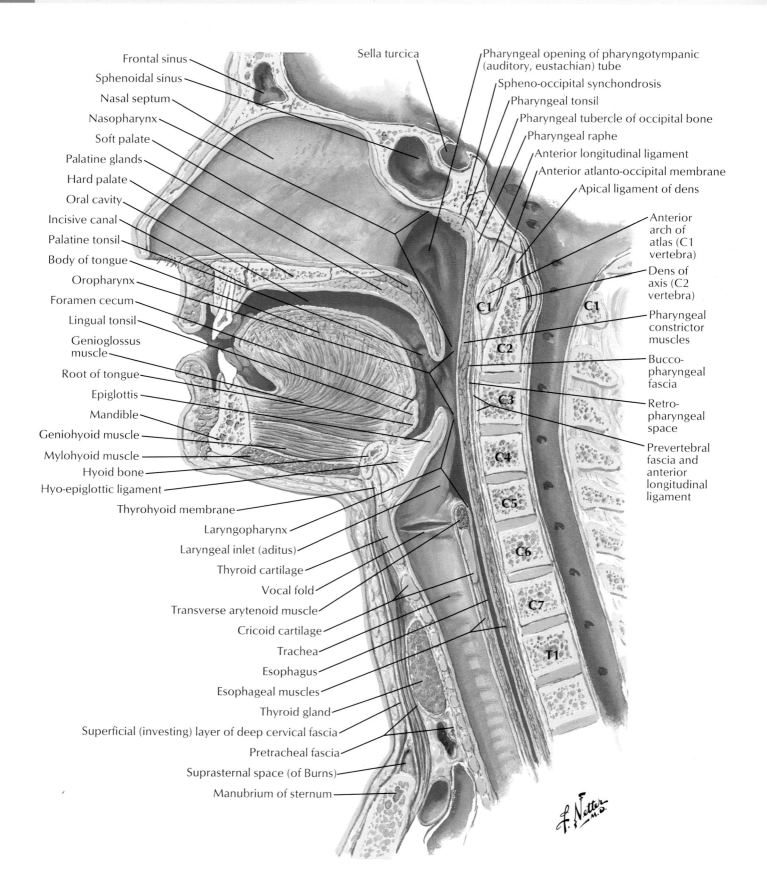

Frontal sinus
Sphenoidal sinus
Nasal septum
Nasopharynx
Soft palate
Palatine glands
Hard palate
Oral cavity
Incisive canal
Palatine tonsil
Body of tongue
Oropharynx
Foramen cecum
Lingual tonsil
Genioglossus muscle
Root of tongue
Epiglottis
Mandible
Geniohyoid muscle
Mylohyoid muscle
Hyoid bone
Hyo-epiglottic ligament
Thyrohyoid membrane
Laryngopharynx
Laryngeal inlet (aditus)
Thyroid cartilage
Vocal fold
Transverse arytenoid muscle
Cricoid cartilage
Trachea
Esophagus
Esophageal muscles
Thyroid gland
Superficial (investing) layer of deep cervical fascia
Pretracheal fascia
Suprasternal space (of Burns)
Manubrium of sternum

Sella turcica

Pharyngeal opening of pharyngotympanic (auditory, eustachian) tube
Spheno-occipital synchondrosis
Pharyngeal tonsil
Pharyngeal tubercle of occipital bone
Pharyngeal raphe
Anterior longitudinal ligament
Anterior atlanto-occipital membrane
Apical ligament of dens
Anterior arch of atlas (C1 vertebra)
Dens of axis (C2 vertebra)
Pharyngeal constrictor muscles
Bucco-pharyngeal fascia
Retro-pharyngeal space
Prevertebral fascia and anterior longitudinal ligament

C1
C2
C3
C4
C5
C6
C7
T1

C1
C1

**Plate 64**

**Pharynx**

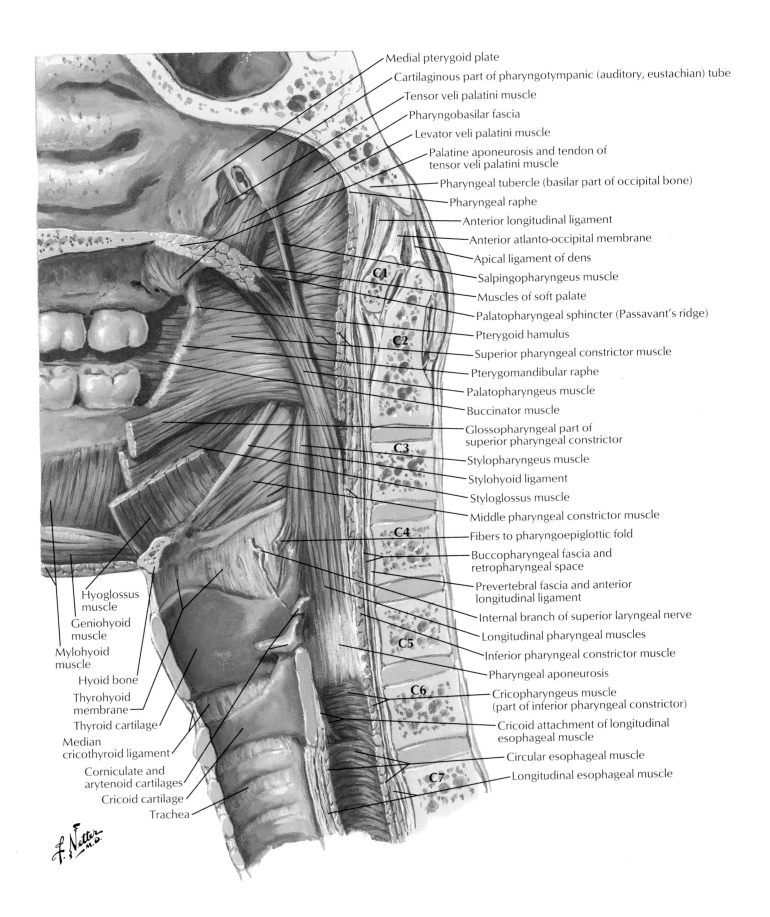

Medial pterygoid plate

Cartilaginous part of pharyngotympanic (auditory, eustachian) tube

Tensor veli palatini muscle

Pharyngobasilar fascia

Levator veli palatini muscle

Palatine aponeurosis and tendon of tensor veli palatini muscle

Pharyngeal tubercle (basilar part of occipital bone)

Pharyngeal raphe

Anterior longitudinal ligament

Anterior atlanto-occipital membrane

Apical ligament of dens

Salpingopharyngeus muscle

Muscles of soft palate

Palatopharyngeal sphincter (Passavant's ridge)

Pterygoid hamulus

Superior pharyngeal constrictor muscle

Pterygomandibular raphe

Palatopharyngeus muscle

Buccinator muscle

Glossopharyngeal part of superior pharyngeal constrictor

Stylopharyngeus muscle

Stylohyoid ligament

Styloglossus muscle

Middle pharyngeal constrictor muscle

Fibers to pharyngoepiglottic fold

Buccopharyngeal fascia and retropharyngeal space

Prevertebral fascia and anterior longitudinal ligament

Internal branch of superior laryngeal nerve

Longitudinal pharyngeal muscles

Inferior pharyngeal constrictor muscle

Pharyngeal aponeurosis

Cricopharyngeus muscle (part of inferior pharyngeal constrictor)

Cricoid attachment of longitudinal esophageal muscle

Circular esophageal muscle

Longitudinal esophageal muscle

C1
C2
C3
C4
C5
C6
C7

Hyoglossus muscle

Geniohyoid muscle

Mylohyoid muscle

Hyoid bone

Thyrohyoid membrane

Thyroid cartilage

Median cricothyroid ligament

Corniculate and arytenoid cartilages

Cricoid cartilage

Trachea

*F. Netter, M.D.*

**Pharynx**

**Plate 65**

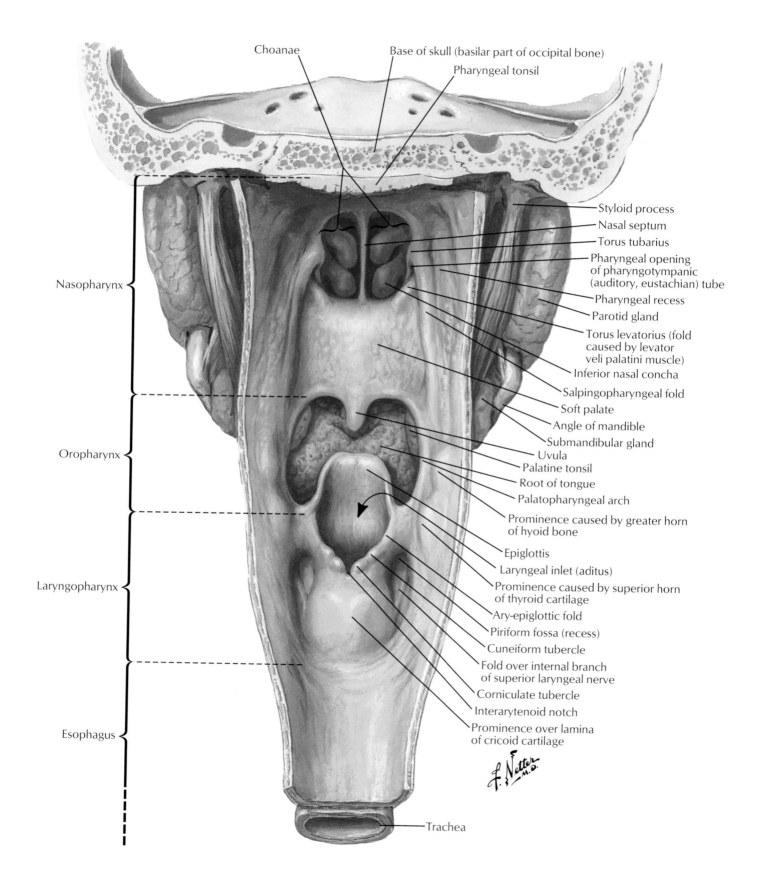

Choanae

Base of skull (basilar part of occipital bone)

Pharyngeal tonsil

Styloid process

Nasal septum

Torus tubarius

Pharyngeal opening of pharyngotympanic (auditory, eustachian) tube

Pharyngeal recess

Parotid gland

Torus levatorius (fold caused by levator veli palatini muscle)

Inferior nasal concha

Salpingopharyngeal fold

Soft palate

Angle of mandible

Submandibular gland

Uvula

Palatine tonsil

Root of tongue

Palatopharyngeal arch

Prominence caused by greater horn of hyoid bone

Epiglottis

Laryngeal inlet (aditus)

Prominence caused by superior horn of thyroid cartilage

Ary-epiglottic fold

Piriform fossa (recess)

Cuneiform tubercle

Fold over internal branch of superior laryngeal nerve

Corniculate tubercle

Interarytenoid notch

Prominence over lamina of cricoid cartilage

Nasopharynx

Oropharynx

Laryngopharynx

Esophagus

Trachea

**Plate 66**

**Pharynx**

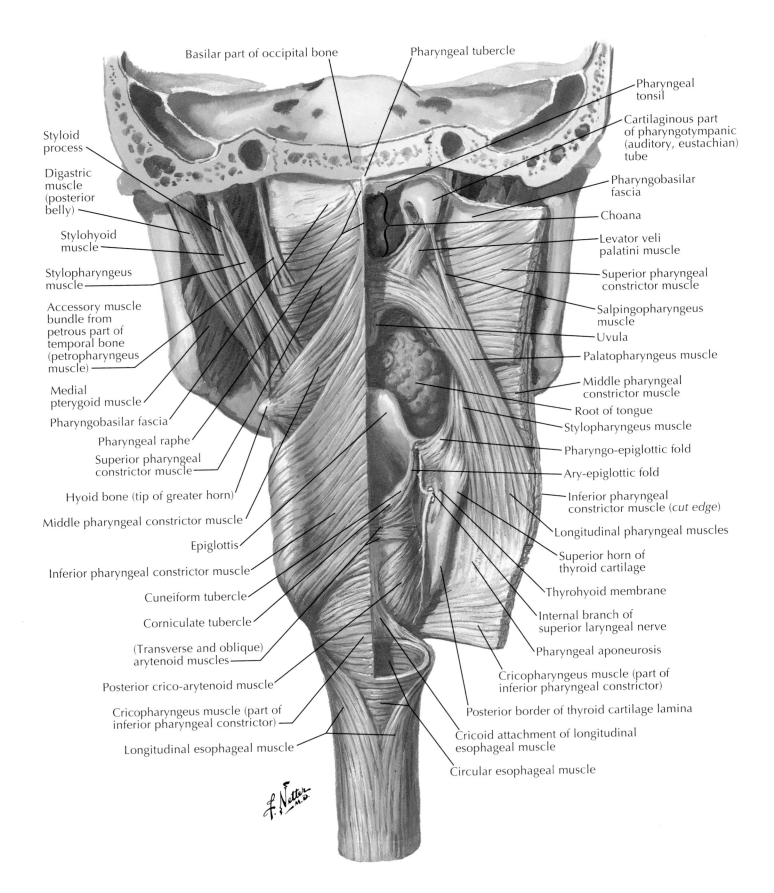

Basilar part of occipital bone

Pharyngeal tubercle

Styloid process

Digastric muscle (posterior belly)

Stylohyoid muscle

Stylopharyngeus muscle

Accessory muscle bundle from petrous part of temporal bone (petropharyngeus muscle)

Medial pterygoid muscle

Pharyngobasilar fascia

Pharyngeal raphe

Superior pharyngeal constrictor muscle

Hyoid bone (tip of greater horn)

Middle pharyngeal constrictor muscle

Epiglottis

Inferior pharyngeal constrictor muscle

Cuneiform tubercle

Corniculate tubercle

(Transverse and oblique) arytenoid muscles

Posterior crico-arytenoid muscle

Cricopharyngeus muscle (part of inferior pharyngeal constrictor)

Longitudinal esophageal muscle

Pharyngeal tonsil

Cartilaginous part of pharyngotympanic (auditory, eustachian) tube

Pharyngobasilar fascia

Choana

Levator veli palatini muscle

Superior pharyngeal constrictor muscle

Salpingopharyngeus muscle

Uvula

Palatopharyngeus muscle

Middle pharyngeal constrictor muscle

Root of tongue

Stylopharyngeus muscle

Pharyngo-epiglottic fold

Ary-epiglottic fold

Inferior pharyngeal constrictor muscle (*cut edge*)

Longitudinal pharyngeal muscles

Superior horn of thyroid cartilage

Thyrohyoid membrane

Internal branch of superior laryngeal nerve

Pharyngeal aponeurosis

Cricopharyngeus muscle (part of inferior pharyngeal constrictor)

Posterior border of thyroid cartilage lamina

Cricoid attachment of longitudinal esophageal muscle

Circular esophageal muscle

**Medial view
sagittal section**

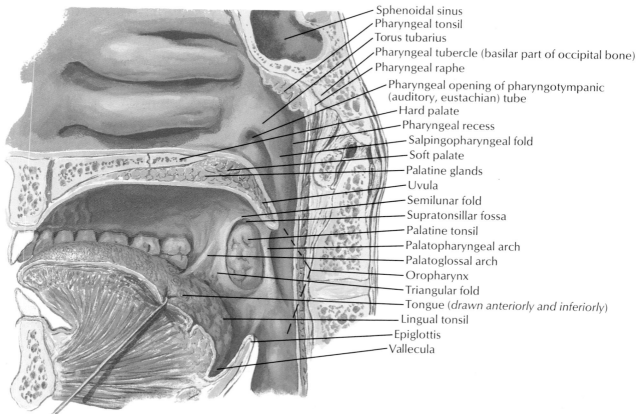

Sphenoidal sinus
Pharyngeal tonsil
Torus tubarius
Pharyngeal tubercle (basilar part of occipital bone)
Pharyngeal raphe
Pharyngeal opening of pharyngotympanic (auditory, eustachian) tube
Hard palate
Pharyngeal recess
Salpingopharyngeal fold
Soft palate
Palatine glands
Uvula
Semilunar fold
Supratonsillar fossa
Palatine tonsil
Palatopharyngeal arch
Palatoglossal arch
Oropharynx
Triangular fold
Tongue (*drawn anteriorly and inferiorly*)
Lingual tonsil
Epiglottis
Vallecula

**Pharyngeal mucosa removed**

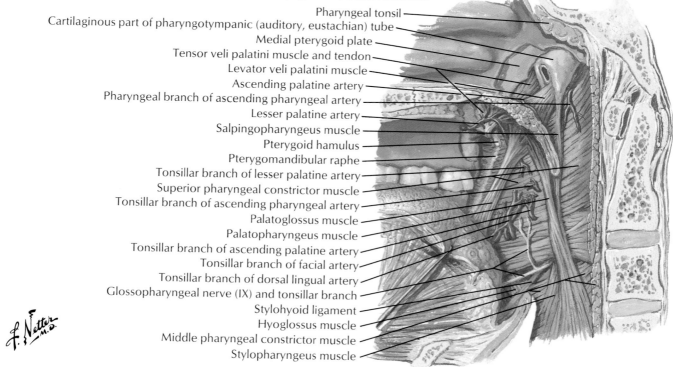

Pharyngeal tonsil
Cartilaginous part of pharyngotympanic (auditory, eustachian) tube
Medial pterygoid plate
Tensor veli palatini muscle and tendon
Levator veli palatini muscle
Ascending palatine artery
Pharyngeal branch of ascending pharyngeal artery
Lesser palatine artery
Salpingopharyngeus muscle
Pterygoid hamulus
Pterygomandibular raphe
Tonsillar branch of lesser palatine artery
Superior pharyngeal constrictor muscle
Tonsillar branch of ascending pharyngeal artery
Palatoglossus muscle
Palatopharyngeus muscle
Tonsillar branch of ascending palatine artery
Tonsillar branch of facial artery
Tonsillar branch of dorsal lingual artery
Glossopharyngeal nerve (IX) and tonsillar branch
Stylohyoid ligament
Hyoglossus muscle
Middle pharyngeal constrictor muscle
Stylopharyngeus muscle

**Plate 68**

**Pharynx**

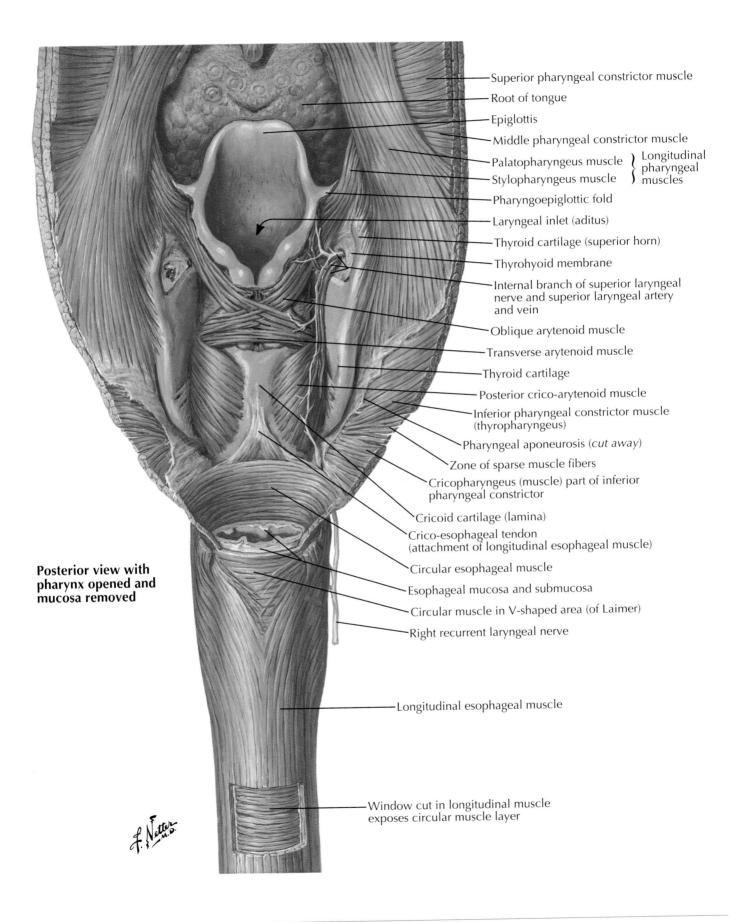

Superior pharyngeal constrictor muscle

Root of tongue

Epiglottis

Middle pharyngeal constrictor muscle

Palatopharyngeus muscle ⎱ Longitudinal
Stylopharyngeus muscle ⎰ pharyngeal muscles

Pharyngoepiglottic fold

Laryngeal inlet (aditus)

Thyroid cartilage (superior horn)

Thyrohyoid membrane

Internal branch of superior laryngeal nerve and superior laryngeal artery and vein

Oblique arytenoid muscle

Transverse arytenoid muscle

Thyroid cartilage

Posterior crico-arytenoid muscle

Inferior pharyngeal constrictor muscle (thyropharyngeus)

Pharyngeal aponeurosis (*cut away*)

Zone of sparse muscle fibers

Cricopharyngeus (muscle) part of inferior pharyngeal constrictor

Cricoid cartilage (lamina)

Crico-esophageal tendon (attachment of longitudinal esophageal muscle)

Circular esophageal muscle

Esophageal mucosa and submucosa

Circular muscle in V-shaped area (of Laimer)

Right recurrent laryngeal nerve

Longitudinal esophageal muscle

Window cut in longitudinal muscle exposes circular muscle layer

**Posterior view with pharynx opened and mucosa removed**

*F. Netter M.D.*

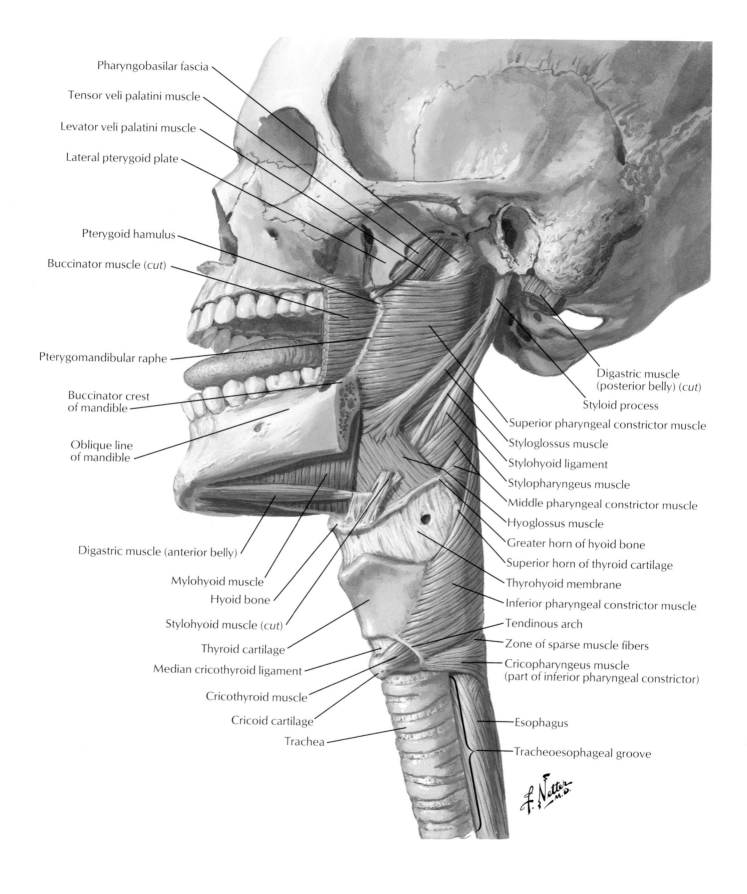

Pharyngobasilar fascia

Tensor veli palatini muscle

Levator veli palatini muscle

Lateral pterygoid plate

Pterygoid hamulus

Buccinator muscle (*cut*)

Pterygomandibular raphe

Buccinator crest
of mandible

Oblique line
of mandible

Digastric muscle (anterior belly)

Mylohyoid muscle

Hyoid bone

Stylohyoid muscle (*cut*)

Thyroid cartilage

Median cricothyroid ligament

Cricothyroid muscle

Cricoid cartilage

Trachea

Digastric muscle
(posterior belly) (*cut*)

Styloid process

Superior pharyngeal constrictor muscle

Styloglossus muscle

Stylohyoid ligament

Stylopharyngeus muscle

Middle pharyngeal constrictor muscle

Hyoglossus muscle

Greater horn of hyoid bone

Superior horn of thyroid cartilage

Thyrohyoid membrane

Inferior pharyngeal constrictor muscle

Tendinous arch

Zone of sparse muscle fibers

Cricopharyngeus muscle
(part of inferior pharyngeal constrictor)

Esophagus

Tracheoesophageal groove

**Plate 70**

**Pharynx**

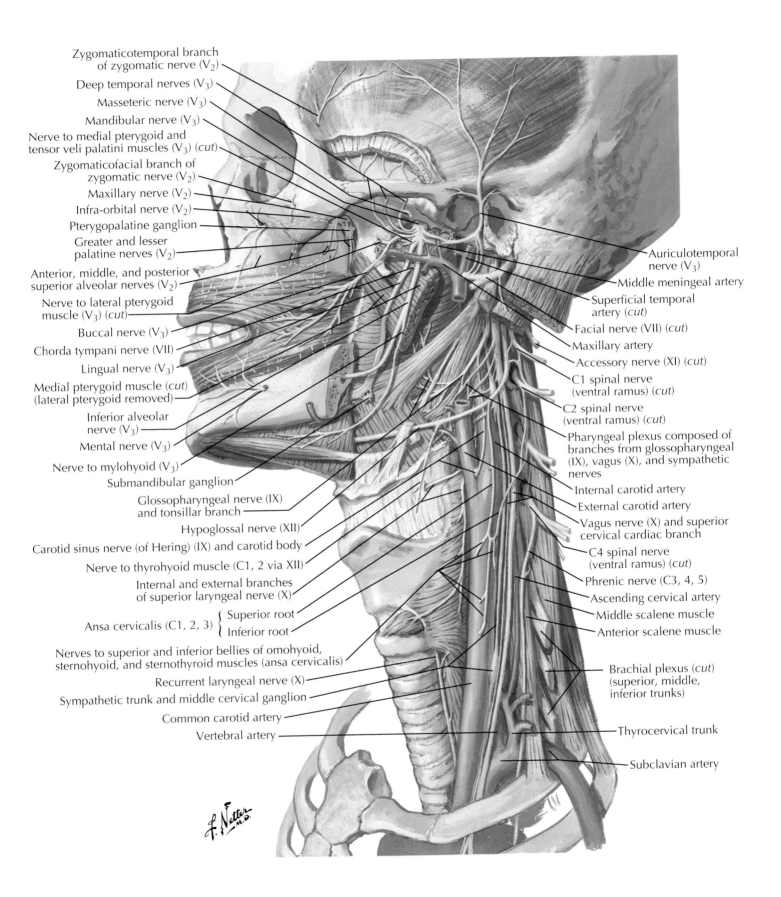

Zygomaticotemporal branch of zygomatic nerve ($V_2$)

Deep temporal nerves ($V_3$)

Masseteric nerve ($V_3$)

Mandibular nerve ($V_3$)

Nerve to medial pterygoid and tensor veli palatini muscles ($V_3$) (*cut*)

Zygomaticofacial branch of zygomatic nerve ($V_2$)

Maxillary nerve ($V_2$)

Infra-orbital nerve ($V_2$)

Pterygopalatine ganglion

Greater and lesser palatine nerves ($V_2$)

Anterior, middle, and posterior superior alveolar nerves ($V_2$)

Nerve to lateral pterygoid muscle ($V_3$) (*cut*)

Buccal nerve ($V_3$)

Chorda tympani nerve (VII)

Lingual nerve ($V_3$)

Medial pterygoid muscle (*cut*) (lateral pterygoid removed)

Inferior alveolar nerve ($V_3$)

Mental nerve ($V_3$)

Nerve to mylohyoid ($V_3$)

Submandibular ganglion

Glossopharyngeal nerve (IX) and tonsillar branch

Hypoglossal nerve (XII)

Carotid sinus nerve (of Hering) (IX) and carotid body

Nerve to thyrohyoid muscle (C1, 2 via XII)

Internal and external branches of superior laryngeal nerve (X)

Ansa cervicalis (C1, 2, 3) { Superior root / Inferior root

Nerves to superior and inferior bellies of omohyoid, sternohyoid, and sternothyroid muscles (ansa cervicalis)

Recurrent laryngeal nerve (X)

Sympathetic trunk and middle cervical ganglion

Common carotid artery

Vertebral artery

Auriculotemporal nerve ($V_3$)

Middle meningeal artery

Superficial temporal artery (*cut*)

Facial nerve (VII) (*cut*)

Maxillary artery

Accessory nerve (XI) (*cut*)

C1 spinal nerve (ventral ramus) (*cut*)

C2 spinal nerve (ventral ramus) (*cut*)

Pharyngeal plexus composed of branches from glossopharyngeal (IX), vagus (X), and sympathetic nerves

Internal carotid artery

External carotid artery

Vagus nerve (X) and superior cervical cardiac branch

C4 spinal nerve (ventral ramus) (*cut*)

Phrenic nerve (C3, 4, 5)

Ascending cervical artery

Middle scalene muscle

Anterior scalene muscle

Brachial plexus (*cut*) (superior, middle, inferior trunks)

Thyrocervical trunk

Subclavian artery

**Pharynx**

**Plate 71**

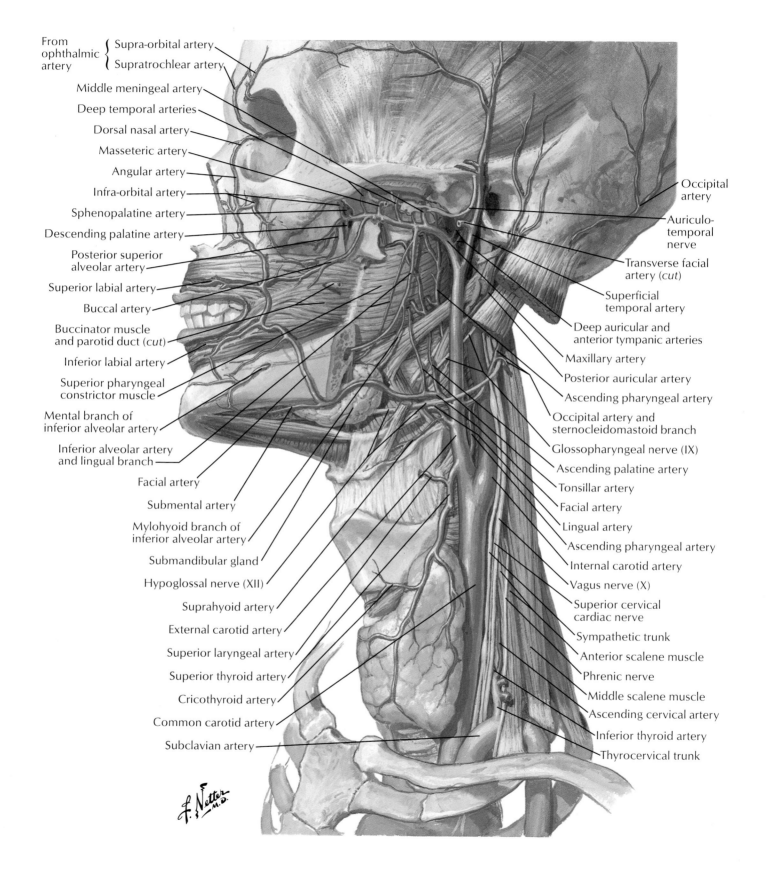

From
ophthalmic { Supra-orbital artery
artery { Supratrochlear artery

Middle meningeal artery

Deep temporal arteries

Dorsal nasal artery

Masseteric artery

Angular artery

Infra-orbital artery

Sphenopalatine artery

Descending palatine artery

Posterior superior
alveolar artery

Superior labial artery

Buccal artery

Buccinator muscle
and parotid duct (cut)

Inferior labial artery

Superior pharyngeal
constrictor muscle

Mental branch of
inferior alveolar artery

Inferior alveolar artery
and lingual branch

Facial artery

Submental artery

Mylohyoid branch of
inferior alveolar artery

Submandibular gland

Hypoglossal nerve (XII)

Suprahyoid artery

External carotid artery

Superior laryngeal artery

Superior thyroid artery

Cricothyroid artery

Common carotid artery

Subclavian artery

Occipital
artery

Auriculo-
temporal
nerve

Transverse facial
artery (cut)

Superficial
temporal artery

Deep auricular and
anterior tympanic arteries

Maxillary artery

Posterior auricular artery

Ascending pharyngeal artery

Occipital artery and
sternocleidomastoid branch

Glossopharyngeal nerve (IX)

Ascending palatine artery

Tonsillar artery

Facial artery

Lingual artery

Ascending pharyngeal artery

Internal carotid artery

Vagus nerve (X)

Superior cervical
cardiac nerve

Sympathetic trunk

Anterior scalene muscle

Phrenic nerve

Middle scalene muscle

Ascending cervical artery

Inferior thyroid artery

Thyrocervical trunk

**Plate 72**

**Pharynx**

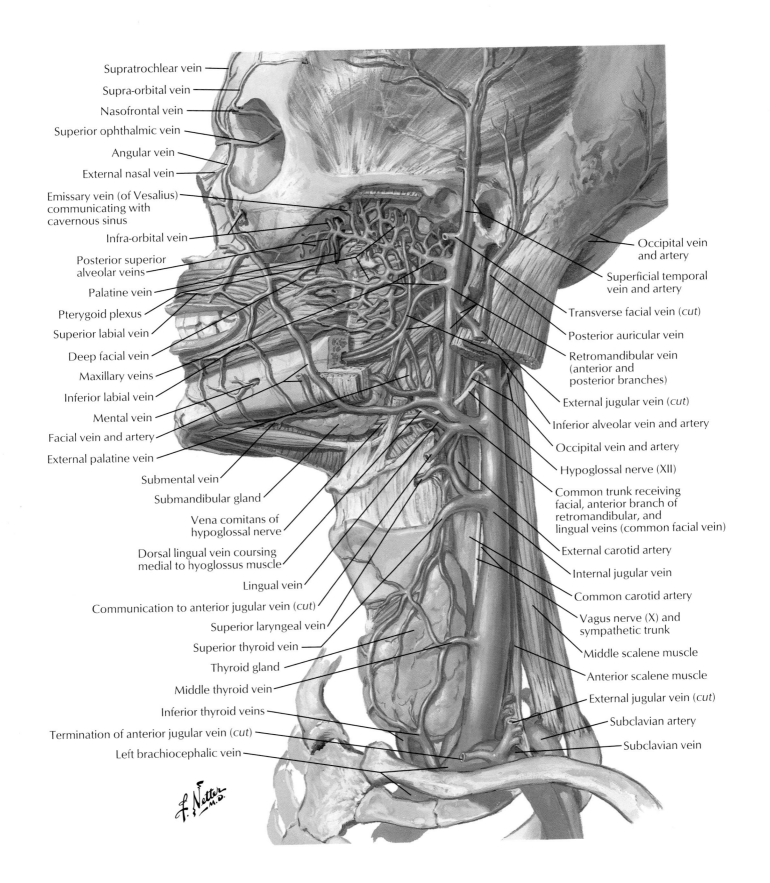

Supratrochlear vein

Supra-orbital vein

Nasofrontal vein

Superior ophthalmic vein

Angular vein

External nasal vein

Emissary vein (of Vesalius) communicating with cavernous sinus

Infra-orbital vein

Posterior superior alveolar veins

Palatine vein

Pterygoid plexus

Superior labial vein

Deep facial vein

Maxillary veins

Inferior labial vein

Mental vein

Facial vein and artery

External palatine vein

Submental vein

Submandibular gland

Vena comitans of hypoglossal nerve

Dorsal lingual vein coursing medial to hyoglossus muscle

Lingual vein

Communication to anterior jugular vein (cut)

Superior laryngeal vein

Superior thyroid vein

Thyroid gland

Middle thyroid vein

Inferior thyroid veins

Termination of anterior jugular vein (cut)

Left brachiocephalic vein

Occipital vein and artery

Superficial temporal vein and artery

Transverse facial vein (cut)

Posterior auricular vein

Retromandibular vein (anterior and posterior branches)

External jugular vein (cut)

Inferior alveolar vein and artery

Occipital vein and artery

Hypoglossal nerve (XII)

Common trunk receiving facial, anterior branch of retromandibular, and lingual veins (common facial vein)

External carotid artery

Internal jugular vein

Common carotid artery

Vagus nerve (X) and sympathetic trunk

Middle scalene muscle

Anterior scalene muscle

External jugular vein (cut)

Subclavian artery

Subclavian vein

**Pharynx**

**Plate 73**

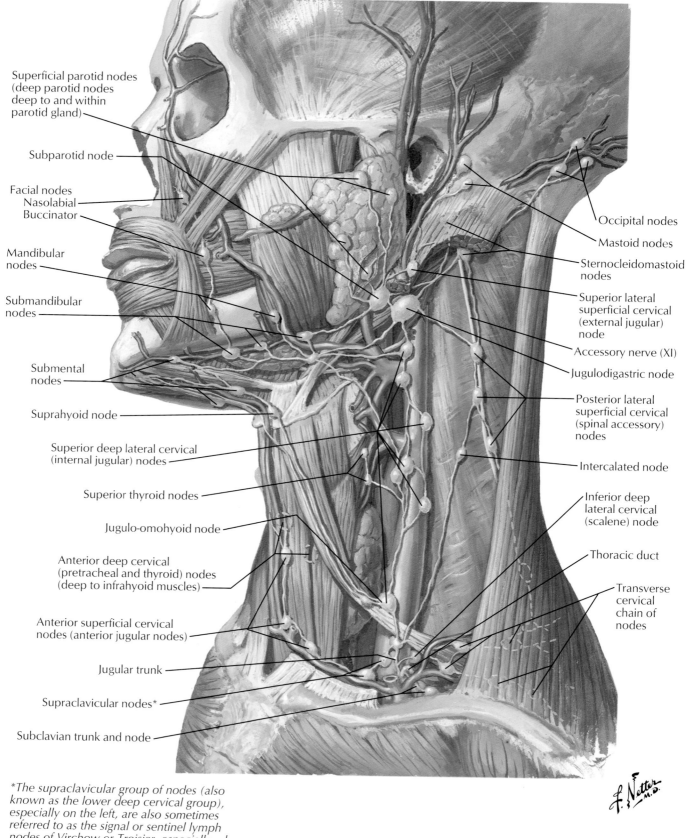

Superficial parotid nodes
(deep parotid nodes
deep to and within
parotid gland)

Subparotid node

Facial nodes
Nasolabial
Buccinator

Mandibular
nodes

Submandibular
nodes

Submental
nodes

Suprahyoid node

Superior deep lateral cervical
(internal jugular) nodes

Superior thyroid nodes

Jugulo-omohyoid node

Anterior deep cervical
(pretracheal and thyroid) nodes
(deep to infrahyoid muscles)

Anterior superficial cervical
nodes (anterior jugular nodes)

Jugular trunk

Supraclavicular nodes*

Subclavian trunk and node

Occipital nodes

Mastoid nodes

Sternocleidomastoid
nodes

Superior lateral
superficial cervical
(external jugular)
node

Accessory nerve (XI)

Jugulodigastric node

Posterior lateral
superficial cervical
(spinal accessory)
nodes

Intercalated node

Inferior deep
lateral cervical
(scalene) node

Thoracic duct

Transverse
cervical
chain of
nodes

*The supraclavicular group of nodes (also
known as the lower deep cervical group),
especially on the left, are also sometimes
referred to as the signal or sentinel lymph
nodes of Virchow or Troisier, especially when
sufficiently enlarged and palpable. These
nodes (or a single node) are so termed because
they may be the first recognized presumptive
evidence of malignant disease in the viscera.

**Plate 74**

**Pharynx**

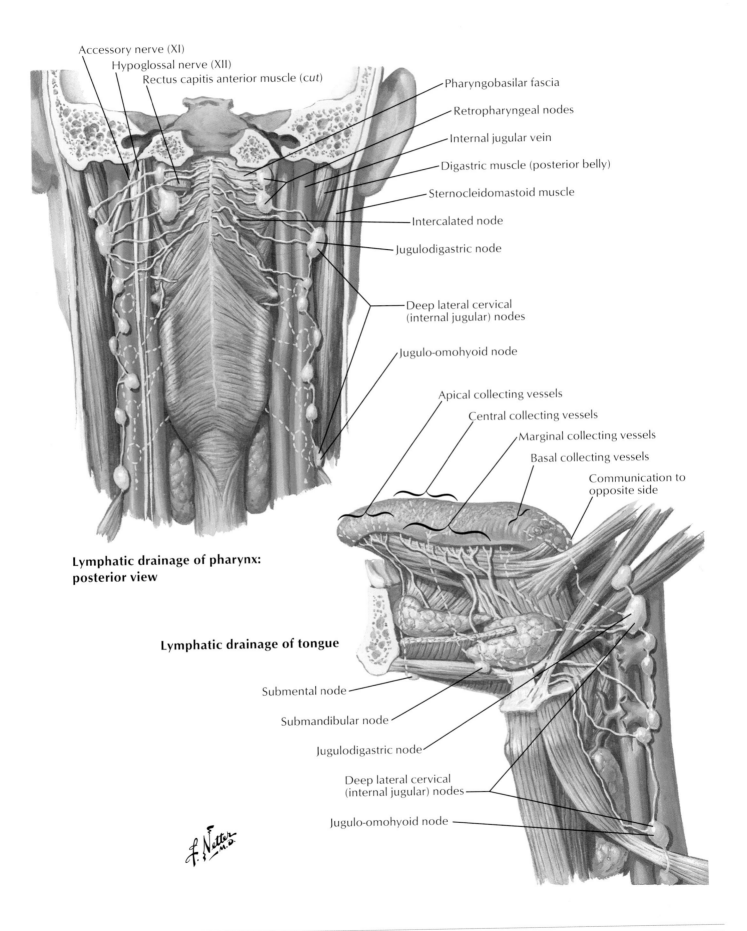

Lymphatic drainage of pharynx: posterior view

**Accessory nerve (XI)**
**Hypoglossal nerve (XII)**
**Rectus capitis anterior muscle (cut)**
Pharyngobasilar fascia
Retropharyngeal nodes
Internal jugular vein
Digastric muscle (posterior belly)
Sternocleidomastoid muscle
Intercalated node
Jugulodigastric node
Deep lateral cervical (internal jugular) nodes
Jugulo-omohyoid node

**Lymphatic drainage of pharynx: posterior view**

Apical collecting vessels
Central collecting vessels
Marginal collecting vessels
Basal collecting vessels
Communication to opposite side

**Lymphatic drainage of tongue**

Submental node
Submandibular node
Jugulodigastric node
Deep lateral cervical (internal jugular) nodes
Jugulo-omohyoid node

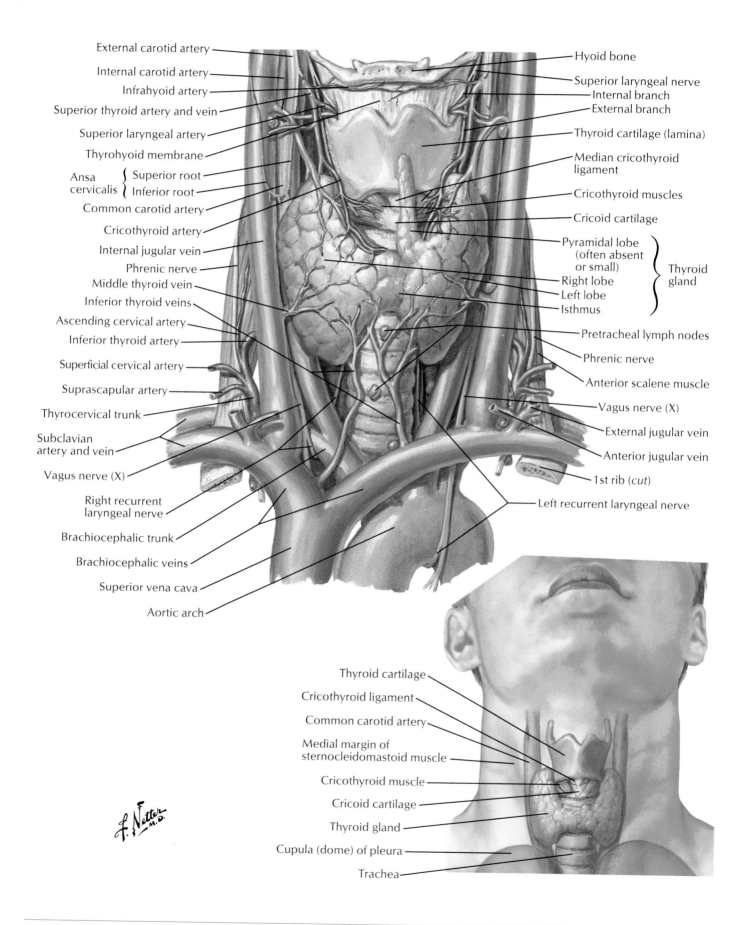

External carotid artery

Internal carotid artery

Infrahyoid artery

Superior thyroid artery and vein

Superior laryngeal artery

Thyrohyoid membrane

Ansa cervicalis { Superior root / Inferior root }

Common carotid artery

Cricothyroid artery

Internal jugular vein

Phrenic nerve

Middle thyroid vein

Inferior thyroid veins

Ascending cervical artery

Inferior thyroid artery

Superficial cervical artery

Suprascapular artery

Thyrocervical trunk

Subclavian artery and vein

Vagus nerve (X)

Right recurrent laryngeal nerve

Brachiocephalic trunk

Brachiocephalic veins

Superior vena cava

Aortic arch

Hyoid bone

Superior laryngeal nerve

Internal branch

External branch

Thyroid cartilage (lamina)

Median cricothyroid ligament

Cricothyroid muscles

Cricoid cartilage

Pyramidal lobe (often absent or small)

Right lobe

Left lobe } Thyroid gland

Isthmus

Pretracheal lymph nodes

Phrenic nerve

Anterior scalene muscle

Vagus nerve (X)

External jugular vein

Anterior jugular vein

1st rib (cut)

Left recurrent laryngeal nerve

Thyroid cartilage

Cricothyroid ligament

Common carotid artery

Medial margin of sternocleidomastoid muscle

Cricothyroid muscle

Cricoid cartilage

Thyroid gland

Cupula (dome) of pleura

Trachea

**Plate 76**

**Thyroid Gland and Larynx**

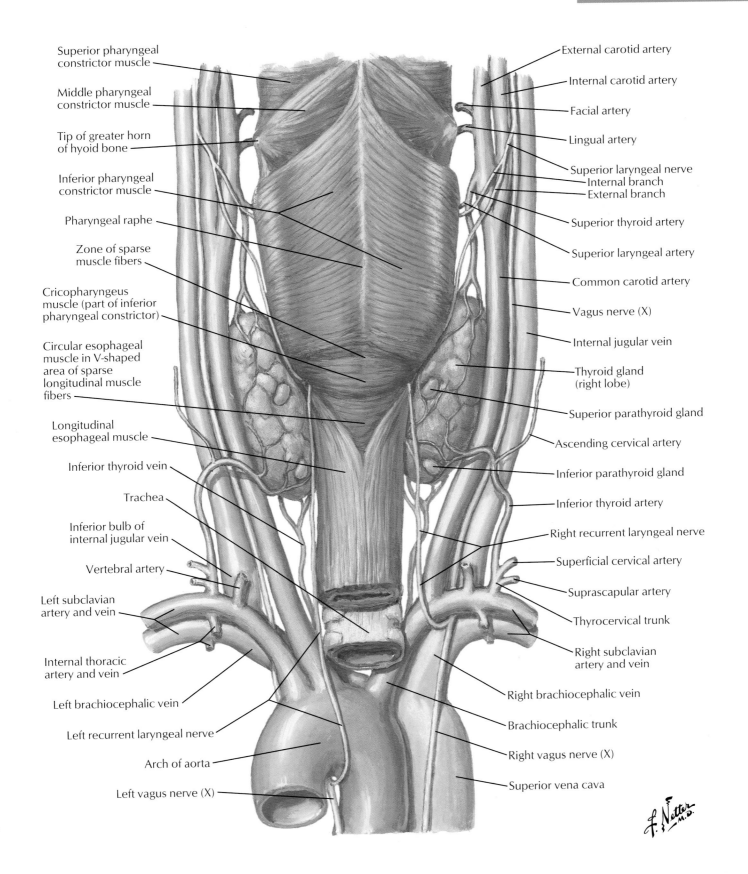

Superior pharyngeal constrictor muscle

Middle pharyngeal constrictor muscle

Tip of greater horn of hyoid bone

Inferior pharyngeal constrictor muscle

Pharyngeal raphe

Zone of sparse muscle fibers

Cricopharyngeus muscle (part of inferior pharyngeal constrictor)

Circular esophageal muscle in V-shaped area of sparse longitudinal muscle fibers

Longitudinal esophageal muscle

Inferior thyroid vein

Trachea

Inferior bulb of internal jugular vein

Vertebral artery

Left subclavian artery and vein

Internal thoracic artery and vein

Left brachiocephalic vein

Left recurrent laryngeal nerve

Arch of aorta

Left vagus nerve (X)

External carotid artery

Internal carotid artery

Facial artery

Lingual artery

Superior laryngeal nerve
Internal branch
External branch

Superior thyroid artery

Superior laryngeal artery

Common carotid artery

Vagus nerve (X)

Internal jugular vein

Thyroid gland (right lobe)

Superior parathyroid gland

Ascending cervical artery

Inferior parathyroid gland

Inferior thyroid artery

Right recurrent laryngeal nerve

Superficial cervical artery

Suprascapular artery

Thyrocervical trunk

Right subclavian artery and vein

Right brachiocephalic vein

Brachiocephalic trunk

Right vagus nerve (X)

Superior vena cava

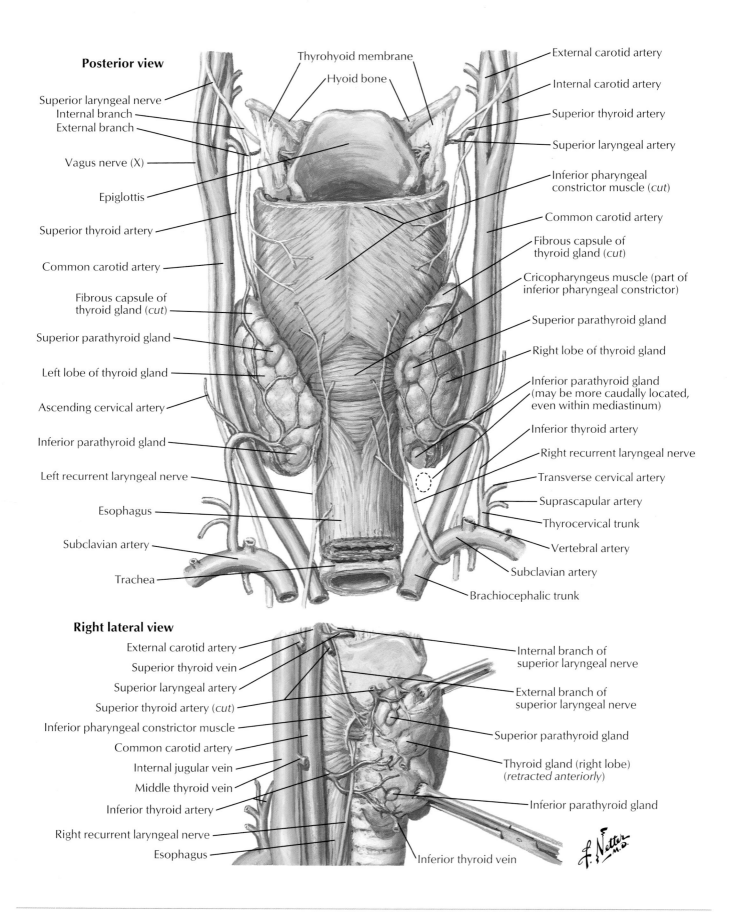

**Posterior view**

Thyrohyoid membrane

Hyoid bone

External carotid artery

Internal carotid artery

Superior thyroid artery

Superior laryngeal artery

Superior laryngeal nerve
Internal branch
External branch

Vagus nerve (X)

Epiglottis

Inferior pharyngeal
constrictor muscle (*cut*)

Common carotid artery

Fibrous capsule of
thyroid gland (*cut*)

Superior thyroid artery

Common carotid artery

Cricopharyngeus muscle (part of
inferior pharyngeal constrictor)

Superior parathyroid gland

Right lobe of thyroid gland

Fibrous capsule of
thyroid gland (*cut*)

Superior parathyroid gland

Left lobe of thyroid gland

Ascending cervical artery

Inferior parathyroid gland
(may be more caudally located,
even within mediastinum)

Inferior thyroid artery

Right recurrent laryngeal nerve

Inferior parathyroid gland

Left recurrent laryngeal nerve

Transverse cervical artery

Esophagus

Suprascapular artery

Thyrocervical trunk

Subclavian artery

Vertebral artery

Trachea

Subclavian artery

Brachiocephalic trunk

**Right lateral view**

External carotid artery

Superior thyroid vein

Superior laryngeal artery

Superior thyroid artery (*cut*)

Inferior pharyngeal constrictor muscle

Common carotid artery

Internal jugular vein

Middle thyroid vein

Inferior thyroid artery

Right recurrent laryngeal nerve

Esophagus

Internal branch of
superior laryngeal nerve

External branch of
superior laryngeal nerve

Superior parathyroid gland

Thyroid gland (right lobe)
(*retracted anteriorly*)

Inferior parathyroid gland

Inferior thyroid vein

**Plate 78**

**Thyroid Gland and Larynx**

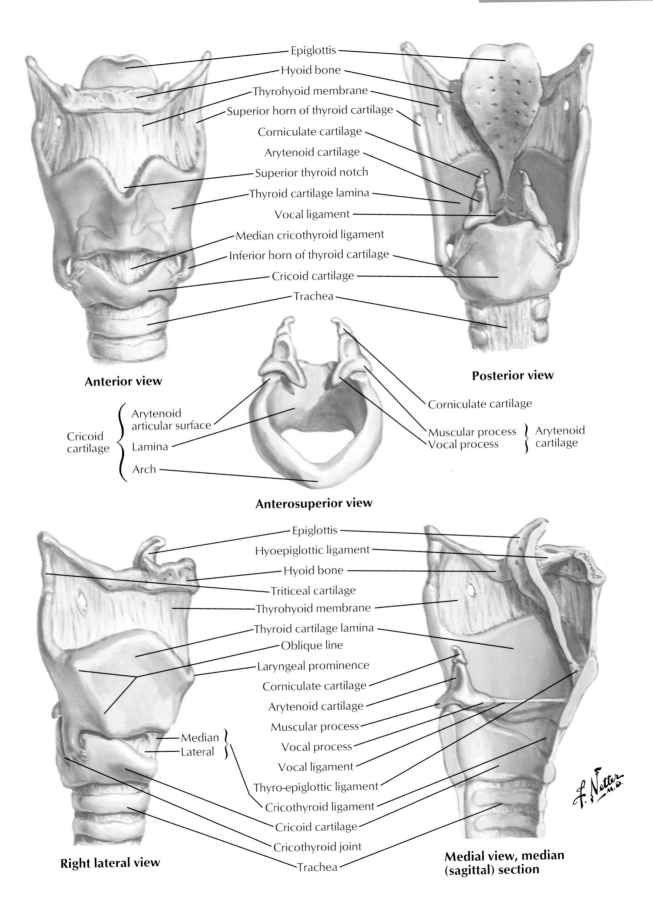

Epiglottis

Hyoid bone

Thyrohyoid membrane

Superior horn of thyroid cartilage

Corniculate cartilage

Arytenoid cartilage

Superior thyroid notch

Thyroid cartilage lamina

Vocal ligament

Median cricothyroid ligament

Inferior horn of thyroid cartilage

Cricoid cartilage

Trachea

**Anterior view**

**Posterior view**

Cricoid cartilage { Arytenoid articular surface, Lamina, Arch }

Corniculate cartilage

Muscular process, Vocal process } Arytenoid cartilage

**Anterosuperior view**

Epiglottis

Hyoepiglottic ligament

Hyoid bone

Triticeal cartilage

Thyrohyoid membrane

Thyroid cartilage lamina

Oblique line

Laryngeal prominence

Corniculate cartilage

Arytenoid cartilage

Muscular process

Vocal process

Vocal ligament

Thyro-epiglottic ligament

Cricothyroid ligament

Cricoid cartilage

Cricothyroid joint

Trachea

Median }
Lateral }

**Right lateral view**

**Medial view, median (sagittal) section**

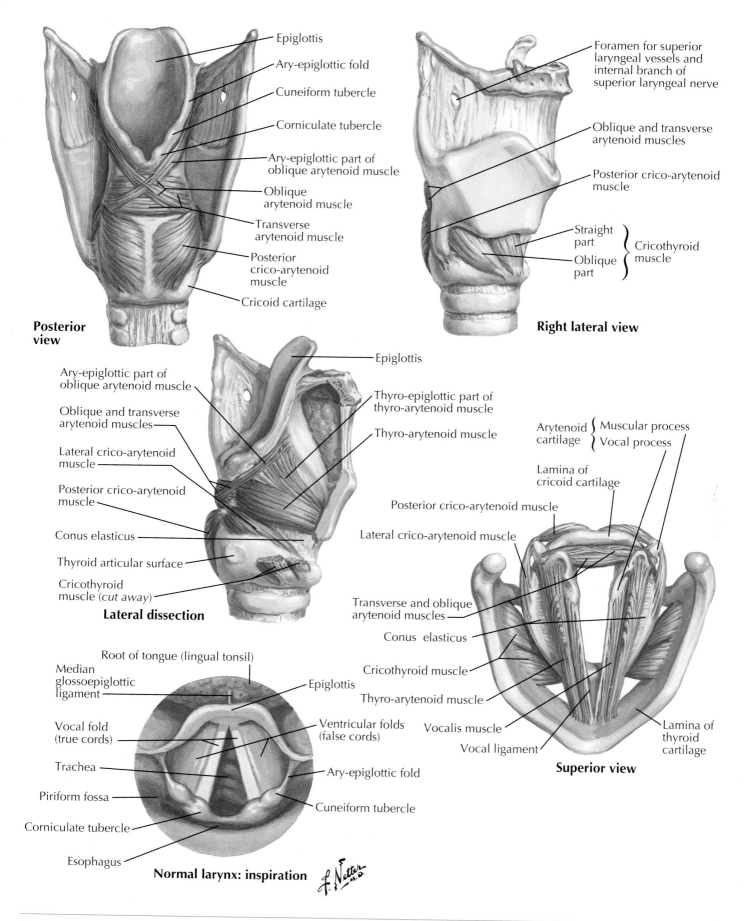

Epiglottis

Ary-epiglottic fold

Cuneiform tubercle

Corniculate tubercle

Ary-epiglottic part of oblique arytenoid muscle

Oblique arytenoid muscle

Transverse arytenoid muscle

Posterior crico-arytenoid muscle

Cricoid cartilage

**Posterior view**

Foramen for superior laryngeal vessels and internal branch of superior laryngeal nerve

Oblique and transverse arytenoid muscles

Posterior crico-arytenoid muscle

Straight part
Oblique part } Cricothyroid muscle

**Right lateral view**

Ary-epiglottic part of oblique arytenoid muscle

Oblique and transverse arytenoid muscles

Lateral crico-arytenoid muscle

Posterior crico-arytenoid muscle

Conus elasticus

Thyroid articular surface

Cricothyroid muscle (*cut away*)

**Lateral dissection**

Epiglottis

Thyro-epiglottic part of thyro-arytenoid muscle

Thyro-arytenoid muscle

Arytenoid cartilage { Muscular process
Vocal process

Lamina of cricoid cartilage

Posterior crico-arytenoid muscle

Lateral crico-arytenoid muscle

Transverse and oblique arytenoid muscles

Conus elasticus

Cricothyroid muscle

Thyro-arytenoid muscle

Vocalis muscle

Vocal ligament

Lamina of thyroid cartilage

**Superior view**

Root of tongue (lingual tonsil)

Median glossoepiglottic ligament

Vocal fold (true cords)

Trachea

Piriform fossa

Corniculate tubercle

Esophagus

Epiglottis

Ventricular folds (false cords)

Ary-epiglottic fold

Cuneiform tubercle

**Normal larynx: inspiration**

**Plate 80**

**Thyroid Gland and Larynx**

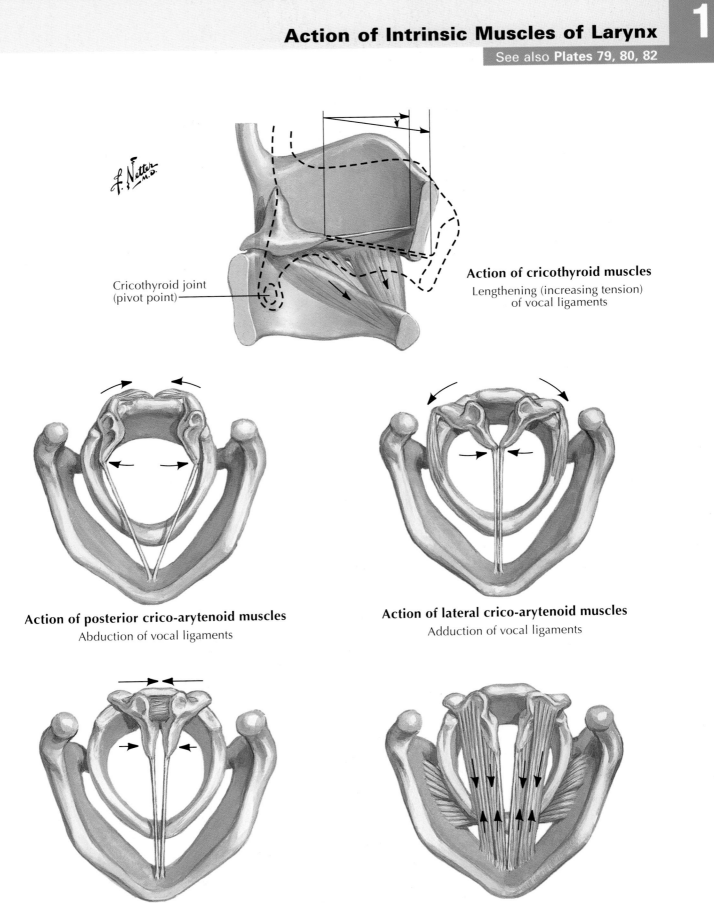

Cricothyroid joint
(pivot point)

**Action of cricothyroid muscles**
Lengthening (increasing tension)
of vocal ligaments

**Action of posterior crico-arytenoid muscles**
Abduction of vocal ligaments

**Action of lateral crico-arytenoid muscles**
Adduction of vocal ligaments

**Action of transverse and oblique arytenoid muscles**
Adduction of vocal ligaments

**Action of vocalis and thyro-arytenoid muscles**
Shortening (relaxation) of vocal ligaments

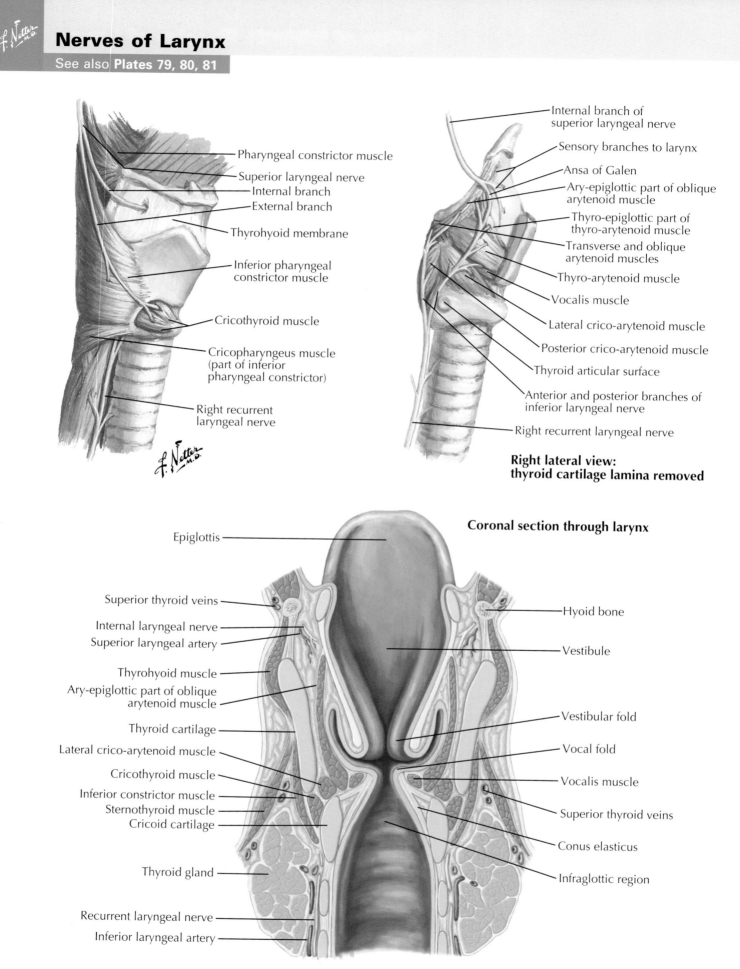

Pharyngeal constrictor muscle

Superior laryngeal nerve

Internal branch

External branch

Thyrohyoid membrane

Inferior pharyngeal constrictor muscle

Cricothyroid muscle

Cricopharyngeus muscle (part of inferior pharyngeal constrictor)

Right recurrent laryngeal nerve

Internal branch of superior laryngeal nerve

Sensory branches to larynx

Ansa of Galen

Ary-epiglottic part of oblique arytenoid muscle

Thyro-epiglottic part of thyro-arytenoid muscle

Transverse and oblique arytenoid muscles

Thyro-arytenoid muscle

Vocalis muscle

Lateral crico-arytenoid muscle

Posterior crico-arytenoid muscle

Thyroid articular surface

Anterior and posterior branches of inferior laryngeal nerve

Right recurrent laryngeal nerve

**Right lateral view: thyroid cartilage lamina removed**

**Coronal section through larynx**

Epiglottis

Superior thyroid veins

Internal laryngeal nerve

Superior laryngeal artery

Thyrohyoid muscle

Ary-epiglottic part of oblique arytenoid muscle

Thyroid cartilage

Lateral crico-arytenoid muscle

Cricothyroid muscle

Inferior constrictor muscle

Sternothyroid muscle

Cricoid cartilage

Thyroid gland

Recurrent laryngeal nerve

Inferior laryngeal artery

Hyoid bone

Vestibule

Vestibular fold

Vocal fold

Vocalis muscle

Superior thyroid veins

Conus elasticus

Infraglottic region

**Plate 82**

**Thyroid Gland and Larynx**

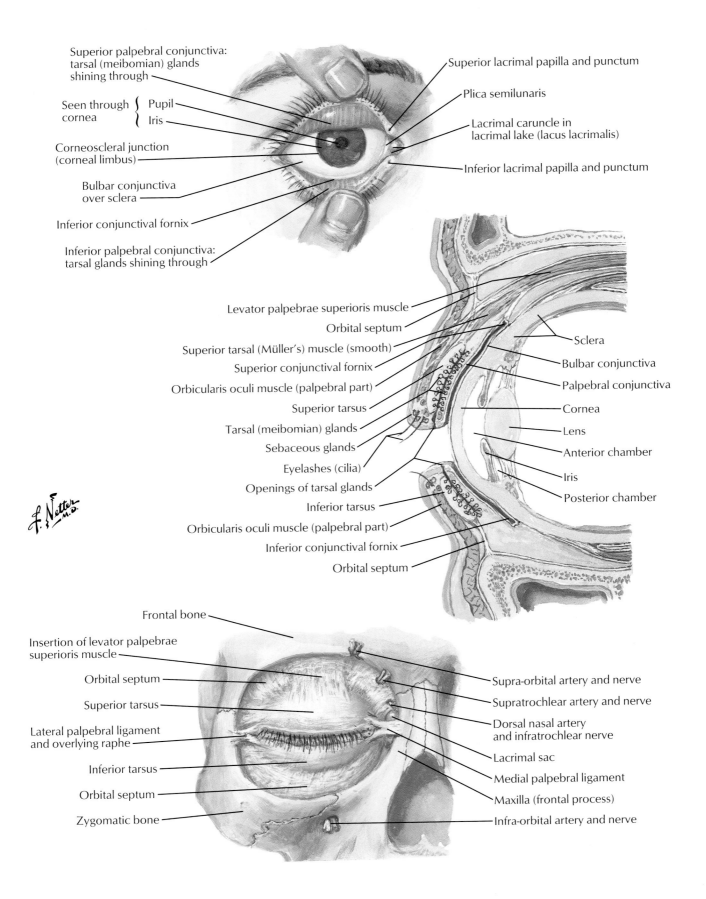

Superior palpebral conjunctiva: tarsal (meibomian) glands shining through

Seen through cornea { Pupil / Iris

Corneoscleral junction (corneal limbus)

Bulbar conjunctiva over sclera

Inferior conjunctival fornix

Inferior palpebral conjunctiva: tarsal glands shining through

Superior lacrimal papilla and punctum

Plica semilunaris

Lacrimal caruncle in lacrimal lake (lacus lacrimalis)

Inferior lacrimal papilla and punctum

Levator palpebrae superioris muscle

Orbital septum

Superior tarsal (Müller's) muscle (smooth)

Superior conjunctival fornix

Orbicularis oculi muscle (palpebral part)

Superior tarsus

Tarsal (meibomian) glands

Sebaceous glands

Eyelashes (cilia)

Openings of tarsal glands

Inferior tarsus

Orbicularis oculi muscle (palpebral part)

Inferior conjunctival fornix

Orbital septum

Sclera

Bulbar conjunctiva

Palpebral conjunctiva

Cornea

Lens

Anterior chamber

Iris

Posterior chamber

Frontal bone

Insertion of levator palpebrae superioris muscle

Orbital septum

Superior tarsus

Lateral palpebral ligament and overlying raphe

Inferior tarsus

Orbital septum

Zygomatic bone

Supra-orbital artery and nerve

Supratrochlear artery and nerve

Dorsal nasal artery and infratrochlear nerve

Lacrimal sac

Medial palpebral ligament

Maxilla (frontal process)

Infra-orbital artery and nerve

**Orbit and Contents**

**Plate 83**

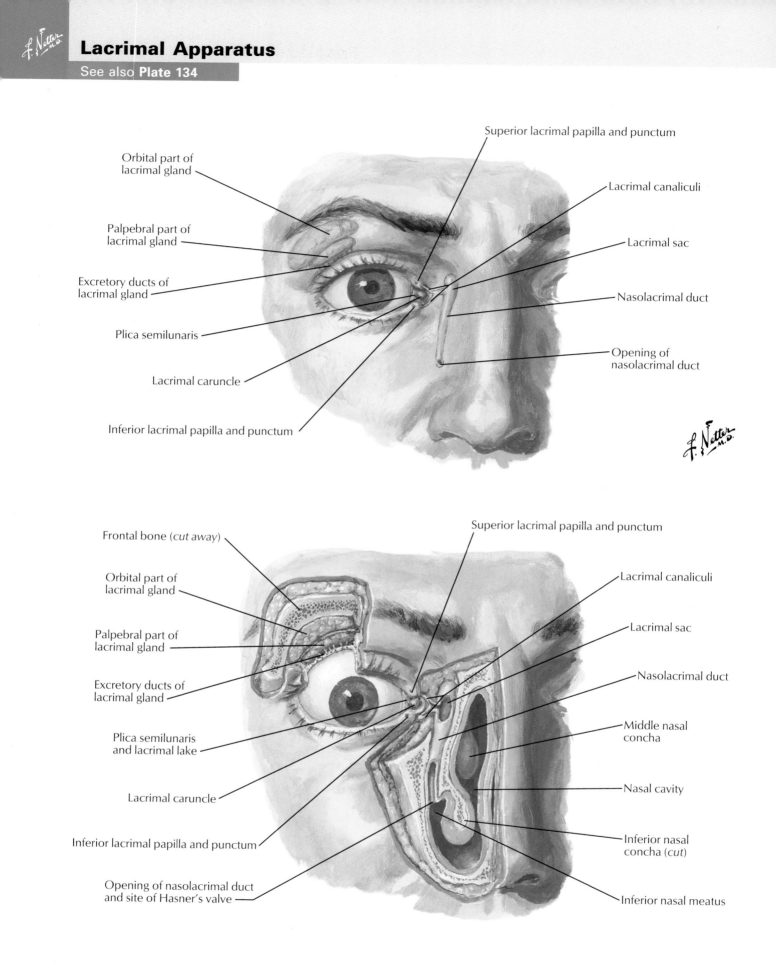

Orbital part of
lacrimal gland

Palpebral part of
lacrimal gland

Excretory ducts of
lacrimal gland

Plica semilunaris

Lacrimal caruncle

Inferior lacrimal papilla and punctum

Superior lacrimal papilla and punctum

Lacrimal canaliculi

Lacrimal sac

Nasolacrimal duct

Opening of
nasolacrimal duct

Frontal bone (*cut away*)

Orbital part of
lacrimal gland

Palpebral part of
lacrimal gland

Excretory ducts of
lacrimal gland

Plica semilunaris
and lacrimal lake

Lacrimal caruncle

Inferior lacrimal papilla and punctum

Opening of nasolacrimal duct
and site of Hasner's valve

Superior lacrimal papilla and punctum

Lacrimal canaliculi

Lacrimal sac

Nasolacrimal duct

Middle nasal
concha

Nasal cavity

Inferior nasal
concha (cut)

Inferior nasal meatus

**Plate 84**

**Orbit and Contents**

**Horizontal section**

Tarsus of eyelid

Palpebral conjunctiva

Bulbar conjunctiva

Lens

Cornea

Medial palpebral ligament

Lateral palpebral ligament

Nasal cavity

Check ligament of lateral rectus muscle

Check ligament of medial rectus muscle

Periorbita

Ethmoidal cells

Sclera

Periorbita

Fascial sheath of eyeball (Tenon's capsule)

Medial rectus muscle and fascial sheath

Episcleral space

Fascial sheath of eyeball (Tenon's capsule)

Lateral rectus muscle and fascial sheath

Sclera

Retrobulbar fat (orbital fat body)

Episcleral space

Optic nerve (II) and meningeal sheath

Common tendinous ring (of Zinn)

Sphenoidal sinus

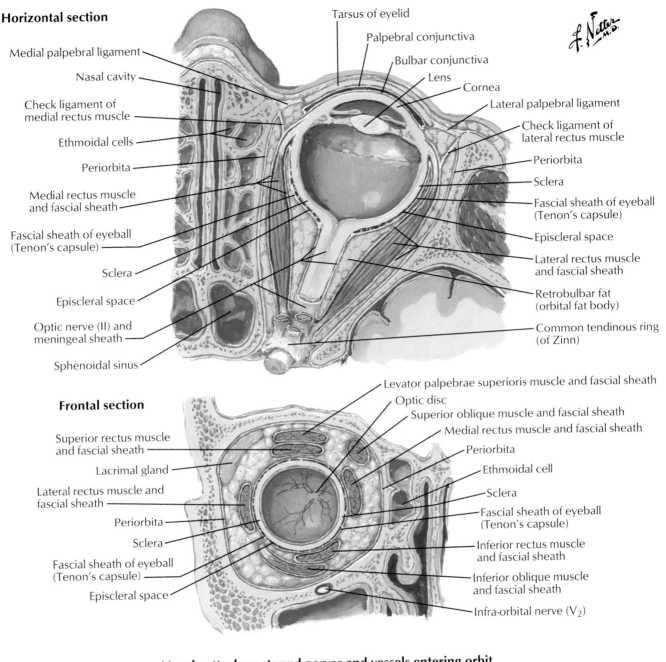

Levator palpebrae superioris muscle and fascial sheath

Optic disc

**Frontal section**

Superior oblique muscle and fascial sheath

Medial rectus muscle and fascial sheath

Superior rectus muscle and fascial sheath

Periorbita

Lacrimal gland

Ethmoidal cell

Lateral rectus muscle and fascial sheath

Sclera

Periorbita

Fascial sheath of eyeball (Tenon's capsule)

Sclera

Inferior rectus muscle and fascial sheath

Fascial sheath of eyeball (Tenon's capsule)

Inferior oblique muscle and fascial sheath

Episcleral space

Infra-orbital nerve (V₂)

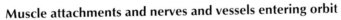

**Muscle attachments and nerves and vessels entering orbit**

Superior orbital fissure

Levator palpebrae superioris muscle

Lacrimal nerve (V₁)

Superior oblique muscle

Frontal nerve (V₁)

Superior rectus muscle

Trochlear nerve (IV)

Medial rectus muscle

Superior ophthalmic vein

Optic nerve (II)

Ophthalmic artery

in optic canal

Lateral rectus muscle

Superior branch of oculomotor nerve (III)

Inferior rectus muscle

Inferior orbital fissure

Inferior branch of oculomotor nerve (III)

Abducent nerve (VI)

Nasociliary nerve (V₁)

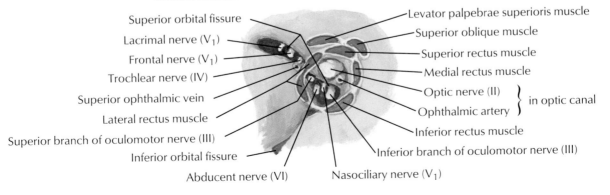

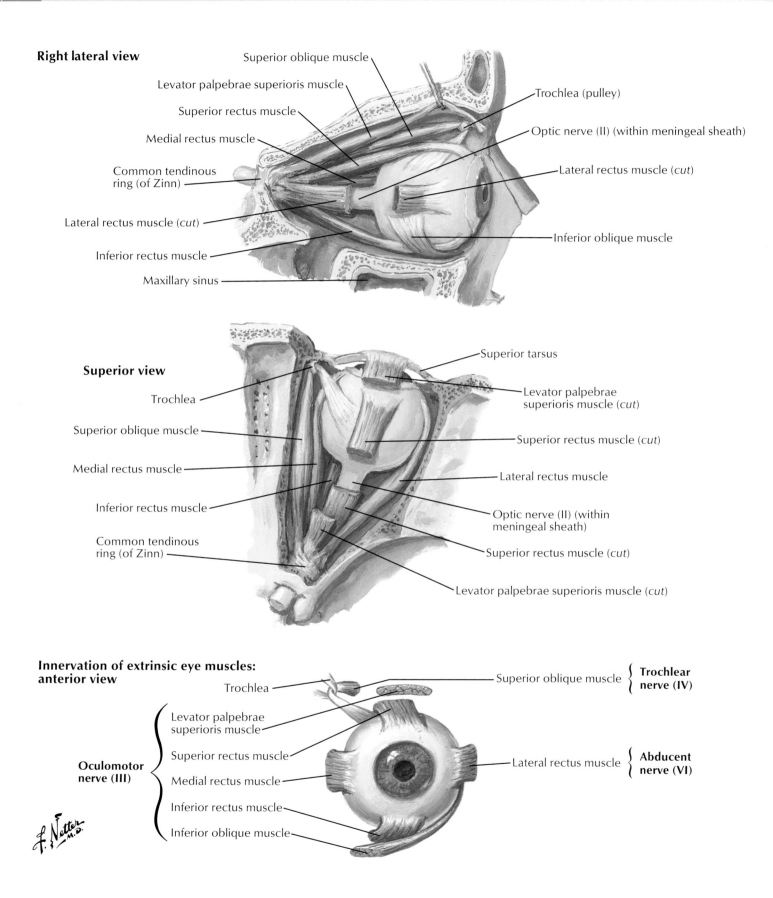

**Right lateral view**

Superior oblique muscle

Levator palpebrae superioris muscle

Superior rectus muscle

Medial rectus muscle

Common tendinous ring (of Zinn)

Lateral rectus muscle (*cut*)

Inferior rectus muscle

Maxillary sinus

Trochlea (pulley)

Optic nerve (II) (within meningeal sheath)

Lateral rectus muscle (*cut*)

Inferior oblique muscle

**Superior view**

Trochlea

Superior oblique muscle

Medial rectus muscle

Inferior rectus muscle

Common tendinous ring (of Zinn)

Superior tarsus

Levator palpebrae superioris muscle (*cut*)

Superior rectus muscle (*cut*)

Lateral rectus muscle

Optic nerve (II) (within meningeal sheath)

Superior rectus muscle (*cut*)

Levator palpebrae superioris muscle (*cut*)

**Innervation of extrinsic eye muscles: anterior view**

Trochlea

Levator palpebrae superioris muscle

Superior rectus muscle

Medial rectus muscle

Inferior rectus muscle

Inferior oblique muscle

Oculomotor nerve (III)

Superior oblique muscle { **Trochlear nerve (IV)**

Lateral rectus muscle { **Abducent nerve (VI)**

**Plate 86**

**Orbit and Contents**

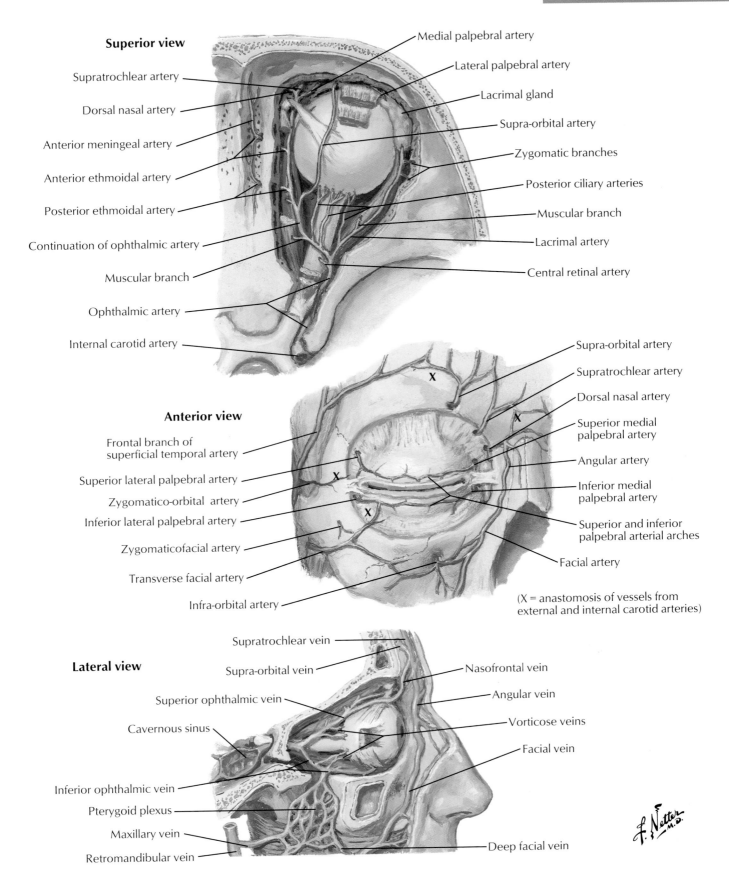

**Superior view**

Supratrochlear artery

Dorsal nasal artery

Anterior meningeal artery

Anterior ethmoidal artery

Posterior ethmoidal artery

Continuation of ophthalmic artery

Muscular branch

Ophthalmic artery

Internal carotid artery

Medial palpebral artery

Lateral palpebral artery

Lacrimal gland

Supra-orbital artery

Zygomatic branches

Posterior ciliary arteries

Muscular branch

Lacrimal artery

Central retinal artery

**Anterior view**

Frontal branch of
superficial temporal artery

Superior lateral palpebral artery

Zygomatico-orbital artery

Inferior lateral palpebral artery

Zygomaticofacial artery

Transverse facial artery

Infra-orbital artery

Supra-orbital artery

Supratrochlear artery

Dorsal nasal artery

Superior medial
palpebral artery

Angular artery

Inferior medial
palpebral artery

Superior and inferior
palpebral arterial arches

Facial artery

(X = anastomosis of vessels from
external and internal carotid arteries)

**Lateral view**

Supratrochlear vein

Supra-orbital vein

Superior ophthalmic vein

Cavernous sinus

Inferior ophthalmic vein

Pterygoid plexus

Maxillary vein

Retromandibular vein

Nasofrontal vein

Angular vein

Vorticose veins

Facial vein

Deep facial vein

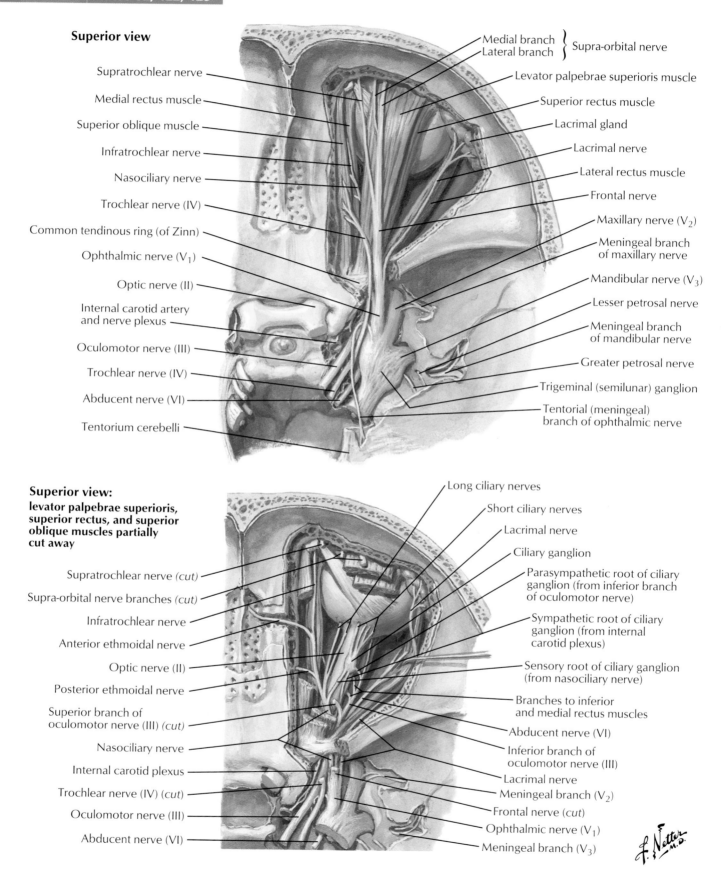

**Superior view**

Supratrochlear nerve

Medial rectus muscle

Superior oblique muscle

Infratrochlear nerve

Nasociliary nerve

Trochlear nerve (IV)

Common tendinous ring (of Zinn)

Ophthalmic nerve (V₁)

Optic nerve (II)

Internal carotid artery and nerve plexus

Oculomotor nerve (III)

Trochlear nerve (IV)

Abducent nerve (VI)

Tentorium cerebelli

Medial branch } Supra-orbital nerve
Lateral branch

Levator palpebrae superioris muscle

Superior rectus muscle

Lacrimal gland

Lacrimal nerve

Lateral rectus muscle

Frontal nerve

Maxillary nerve (V₂)

Meningeal branch of maxillary nerve

Mandibular nerve (V₃)

Lesser petrosal nerve

Meningeal branch of mandibular nerve

Greater petrosal nerve

Trigeminal (semilunar) ganglion

Tentorial (meningeal) branch of ophthalmic nerve

**Superior view:**
**levator palpebrae superioris, superior rectus, and superior oblique muscles partially cut away**

Supratrochlear nerve (cut)

Supra-orbital nerve branches (cut)

Infratrochlear nerve

Anterior ethmoidal nerve

Optic nerve (II)

Posterior ethmoidal nerve

Superior branch of oculomotor nerve (III) (cut)

Nasociliary nerve

Internal carotid plexus

Trochlear nerve (IV) (cut)

Oculomotor nerve (III)

Abducent nerve (VI)

Long ciliary nerves

Short ciliary nerves

Lacrimal nerve

Ciliary ganglion

Parasympathetic root of ciliary ganglion (from inferior branch of oculomotor nerve)

Sympathetic root of ciliary ganglion (from internal carotid plexus)

Sensory root of ciliary ganglion (from nasociliary nerve)

Branches to inferior and medial rectus muscles

Abducent nerve (VI)

Inferior branch of oculomotor nerve (III)

Lacrimal nerve

Meningeal branch (V₂)

Frontal nerve (cut)

Ophthalmic nerve (V₁)

Meningeal branch (V₃)

**Plate 88**

**Orbit and Contents**

**Horizontal section**

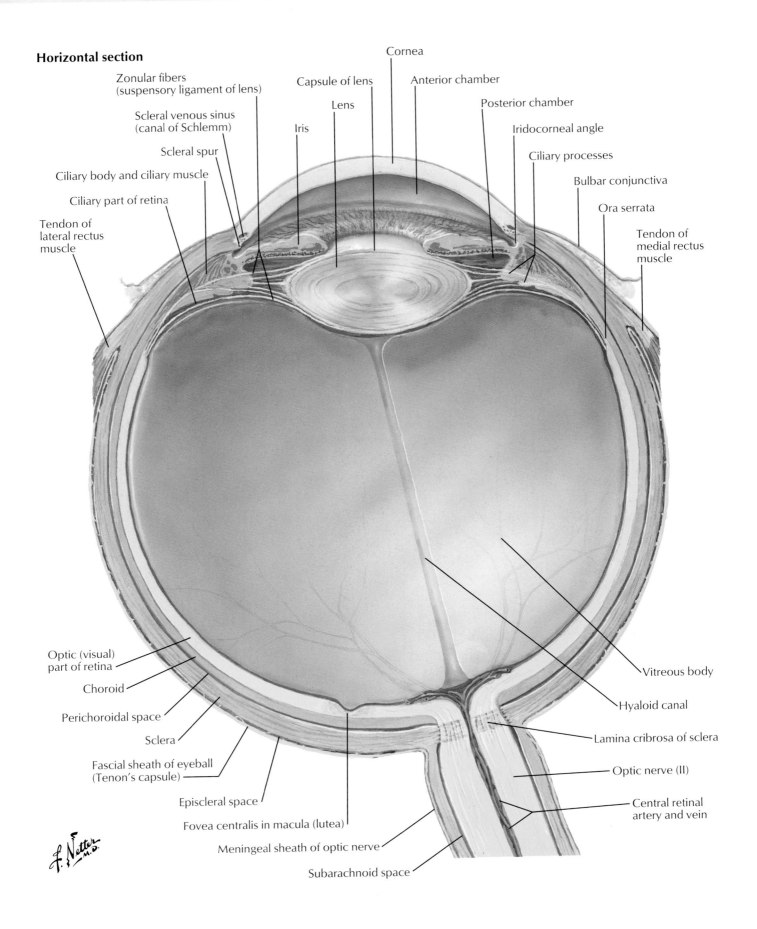

Zonular fibers
(suspensory ligament of lens)

Scleral venous sinus
(canal of Schlemm)

Scleral spur

Ciliary body and ciliary muscle

Ciliary part of retina

Tendon of
lateral rectus
muscle

Capsule of lens

Iris

Lens

Cornea

Anterior chamber

Posterior chamber

Iridocorneal angle

Ciliary processes

Bulbar conjunctiva

Ora serrata

Tendon of
medial rectus
muscle

Optic (visual)
part of retina

Choroid

Perichoroidal space

Sclera

Fascial sheath of eyeball
(Tenon's capsule)

Episcleral space

Fovea centralis in macula (lutea)

Meningeal sheath of optic nerve

Subarachnoid space

Vitreous body

Hyaloid canal

Lamina cribrosa of sclera

Optic nerve (II)

Central retinal
artery and vein

*f. Netter*
*m.d.*

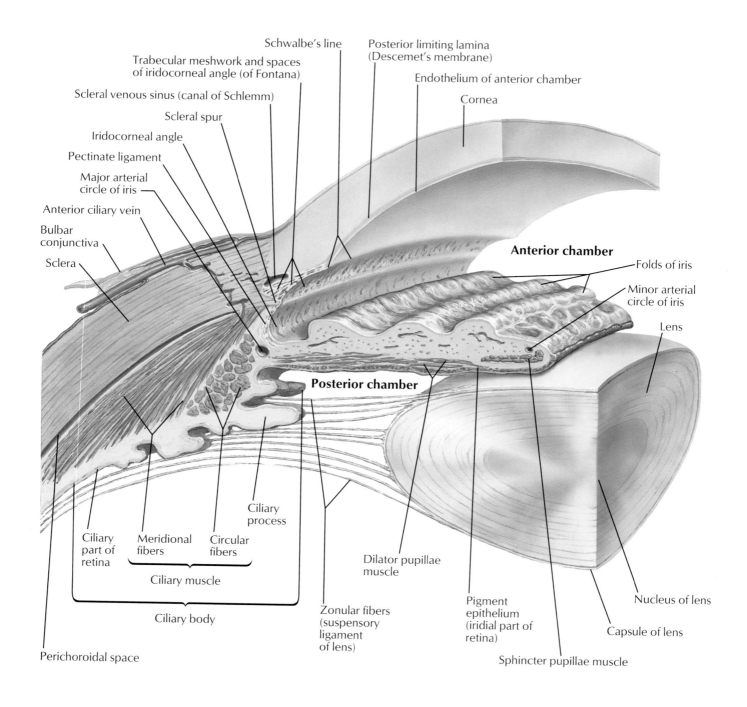

Schwalbe's line

Posterior limiting lamina (Descemet's membrane)

Trabecular meshwork and spaces of iridocorneal angle (of Fontana)

Endothelium of anterior chamber

Scleral venous sinus (canal of Schlemm)

Cornea

Scleral spur

Iridocorneal angle

Pectinate ligament

Major arterial circle of iris

Anterior ciliary vein

Bulbar conjunctiva

Sclera

Anterior chamber

Folds of iris

Minor arterial circle of iris

Lens

Posterior chamber

Ciliary process

Ciliary part of retina

Meridional fibers

Circular fibers

Dilator pupillae muscle

Ciliary muscle

Pigment epithelium (iridial part of retina)

Nucleus of lens

Ciliary body

Zonular fibers (suspensory ligament of lens)

Capsule of lens

Perichoroidal space

Sphincter pupillae muscle

*Note: For clarity, only single plane of zonular fibers shown; actually, fibers surround entire circumference of lens.*

**Plate 90**

**Orbit and Contents**

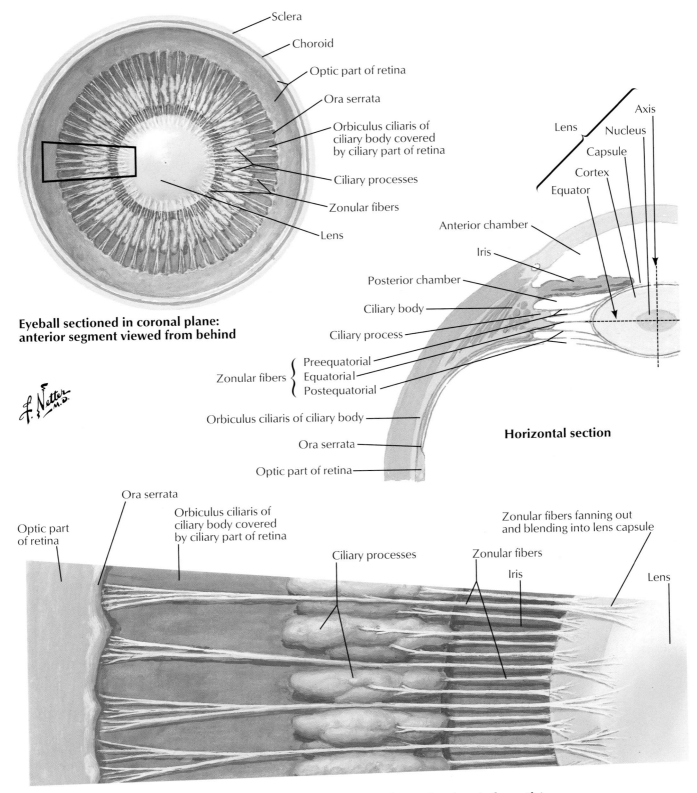

Sclera

Choroid

Optic part of retina

Ora serrata

Orbiculus ciliaris of
ciliary body covered
by ciliary part of retina

Ciliary processes

Zonular fibers

Lens

**Eyeball sectioned in coronal plane:
anterior segment viewed from behind**

Axis

Lens Nucleus

Capsule

Cortex

Equator

Anterior chamber

Iris

Posterior chamber

Ciliary body

Ciliary process

Zonular fibers { Preequatorial
Equatorial
Postequatorial

Orbiculus ciliaris of ciliary body

Ora serrata

Optic part of retina

**Horizontal section**

Ora serrata

Orbiculus ciliaris of
ciliary body covered
by ciliary part of retina

Zonular fibers fanning out
and blending into lens capsule

Optic part
of retina

Ciliary processes

Zonular fibers

Iris

Lens

**Enlargement of segment outlined in top illustration (semischematic)**

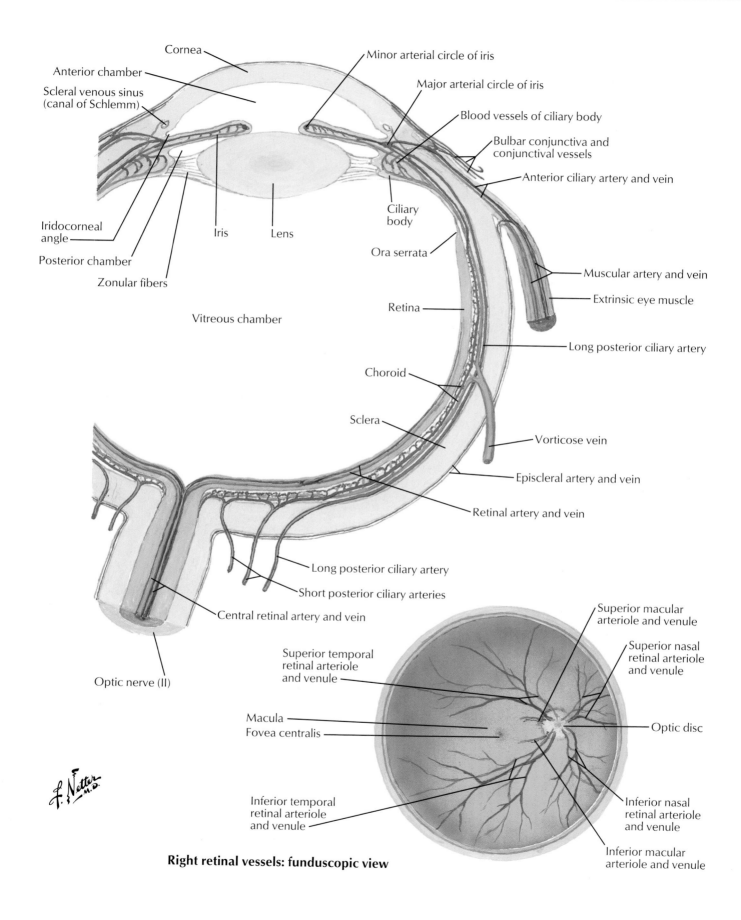

Cornea

Anterior chamber

Scleral venous sinus
(canal of Schlemm)

Minor arterial circle of iris

Major arterial circle of iris

Blood vessels of ciliary body

Bulbar conjunctiva and
conjunctival vessels

Anterior ciliary artery and vein

Iridocorneal
angle

Iris

Lens

Ciliary
body

Ora serrata

Muscular artery and vein

Extrinsic eye muscle

Posterior chamber

Zonular fibers

Retina

Long posterior ciliary artery

Vitreous chamber

Choroid

Sclera

Vorticose vein

Episcleral artery and vein

Retinal artery and vein

Long posterior ciliary artery

Short posterior ciliary arteries

Central retinal artery and vein

Optic nerve (II)

Superior temporal
retinal arteriole
and venule

Macula

Fovea centralis

Inferior temporal
retinal arteriole
and venule

Superior macular
arteriole and venule

Superior nasal
retinal arteriole
and venule

Optic disc

Inferior nasal
retinal arteriole
and venule

Inferior macular
arteriole and venule

**Right retinal vessels: funduscopic view**

**Plate 92**

**Orbit and Contents**

**Vascular arrangements within the choroid (vascular tunic) of the eyeball**

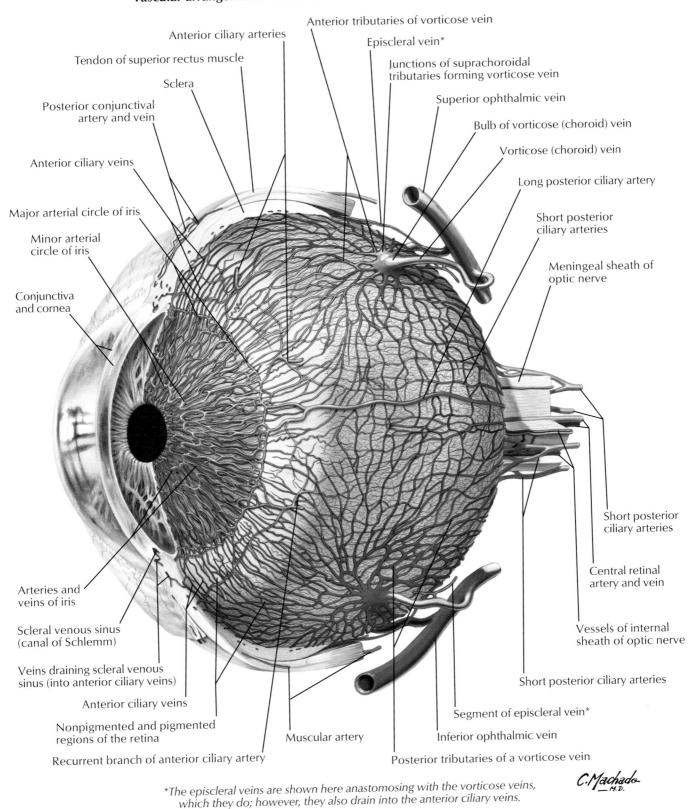

Anterior ciliary arteries

Tendon of superior rectus muscle

Sclera

Posterior conjunctival artery and vein

Anterior ciliary veins

Major arterial circle of iris

Minor arterial circle of iris

Conjunctiva and cornea

Arteries and veins of iris

Scleral venous sinus (canal of Schlemm)

Veins draining scleral venous sinus (into anterior ciliary veins)

Anterior ciliary veins

Nonpigmented and pigmented regions of the retina

Recurrent branch of anterior ciliary artery

Muscular artery

Anterior tributaries of vorticose vein

Episcleral vein*

Junctions of suprachoroidal tributaries forming vorticose vein

Superior ophthalmic vein

Bulb of vorticose (choroid) vein

Vorticose (choroid) vein

Long posterior ciliary artery

Short posterior ciliary arteries

Meningeal sheath of optic nerve

Short posterior ciliary arteries

Central retinal artery and vein

Vessels of internal sheath of optic nerve

Short posterior ciliary arteries

Segment of episcleral vein*

Inferior ophthalmic vein

Posterior tributaries of a vorticose vein

*The episcleral veins are shown here anastomosing with the vorticose veins, which they do; however, they also drain into the anterior ciliary veins.*

C.Machado M.D.

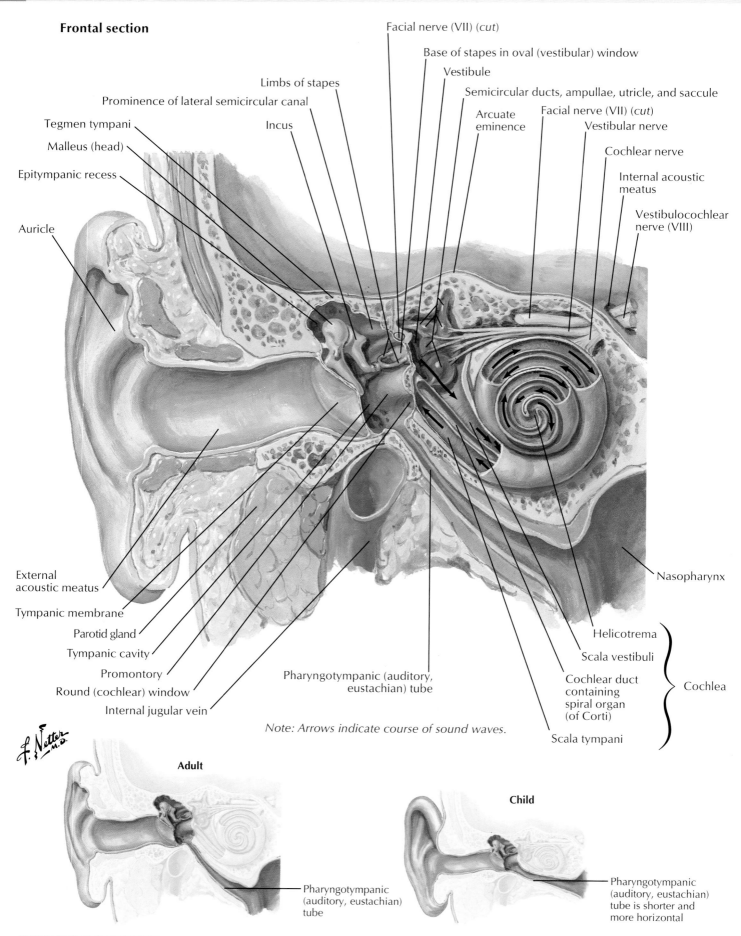

**Frontal section**

Facial nerve (VII) (*cut*)

Base of stapes in oval (vestibular) window

Vestibule

Semicircular ducts, ampullae, utricle, and saccule

Limbs of stapes

Prominence of lateral semicircular canal

Arcuate eminence

Facial nerve (VII) (*cut*)

Tegmen tympani

Incus

Vestibular nerve

Malleus (head)

Cochlear nerve

Epitympanic recess

Internal acoustic meatus

Auricle

Vestibulocochlear nerve (VIII)

External acoustic meatus

Nasopharynx

Tympanic membrane

Parotid gland

Tympanic cavity

Helicotrema

Promontory

Scala vestibuli

Round (cochlear) window

Cochlear duct containing spiral organ (of Corti)

Internal jugular vein

Pharyngotympanic (auditory, eustachian) tube

*Note: Arrows indicate course of sound waves.*

Scala tympani

Cochlea

**Adult**

**Child**

Pharyngotympanic (auditory, eustachian) tube

Pharyngotympanic (auditory, eustachian) tube is shorter and more horizontal

**Plate 94**

**Ear**

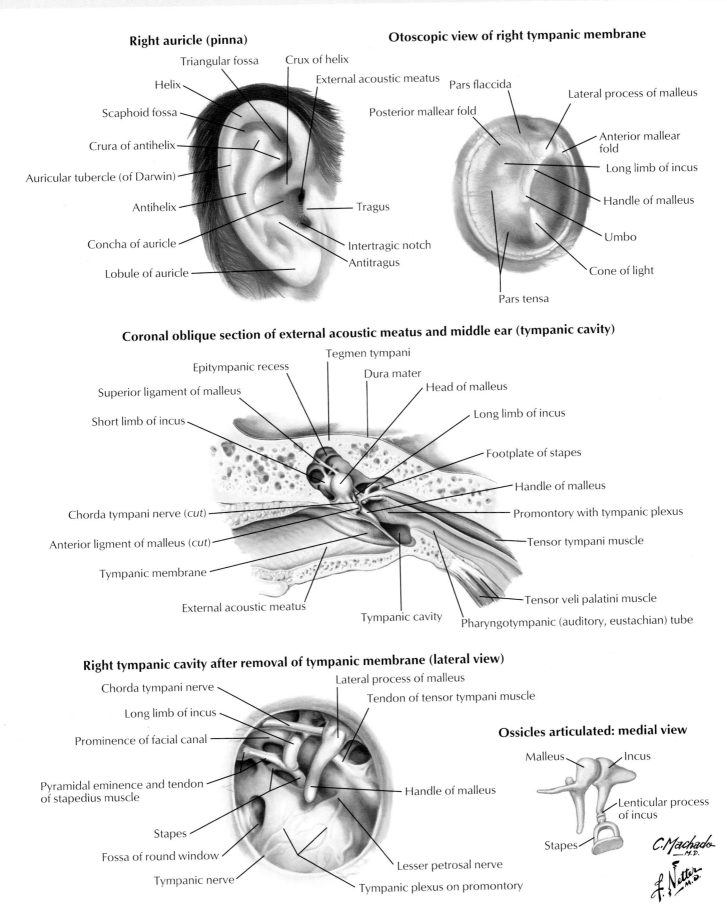

## Right auricle (pinna)

Triangular fossa
Crux of helix
Helix
External acoustic meatus
Scaphoid fossa
Crura of antihelix
Auricular tubercle (of Darwin)
Antihelix
Tragus
Concha of auricle
Intertragic notch
Antitragus
Lobule of auricle

## Otoscopic view of right tympanic membrane

Pars flaccida
Lateral process of malleus
Posterior mallear fold
Anterior mallear fold
Long limb of incus
Handle of malleus
Umbo
Cone of light
Pars tensa

## Coronal oblique section of external acoustic meatus and middle ear (tympanic cavity)

Tegmen tympani
Epitympanic recess
Dura mater
Superior ligament of malleus
Head of malleus
Short limb of incus
Long limb of incus
Footplate of stapes
Handle of malleus
Chorda tympani nerve (cut)
Promontory with tympanic plexus
Anterior ligment of malleus (cut)
Tensor tympani muscle
Tympanic membrane
Tensor veli palatini muscle
External acoustic meatus
Tympanic cavity
Pharyngotympanic (auditory, eustachian) tube

## Right tympanic cavity after removal of tympanic membrane (lateral view)

Lateral process of malleus
Chorda tympani nerve
Tendon of tensor tympani muscle
Long limb of incus
Prominence of facial canal

### Ossicles articulated: medial view

Malleus
Incus
Pyramidal eminence and tendon of stapedius muscle
Lenticular process of incus
Handle of malleus
Stapes
Fossa of round window
Lesser petrosal nerve
Tympanic nerve
Tympanic plexus on promontory
Stapes

C. Machado M.D.
F. Netter M.D.

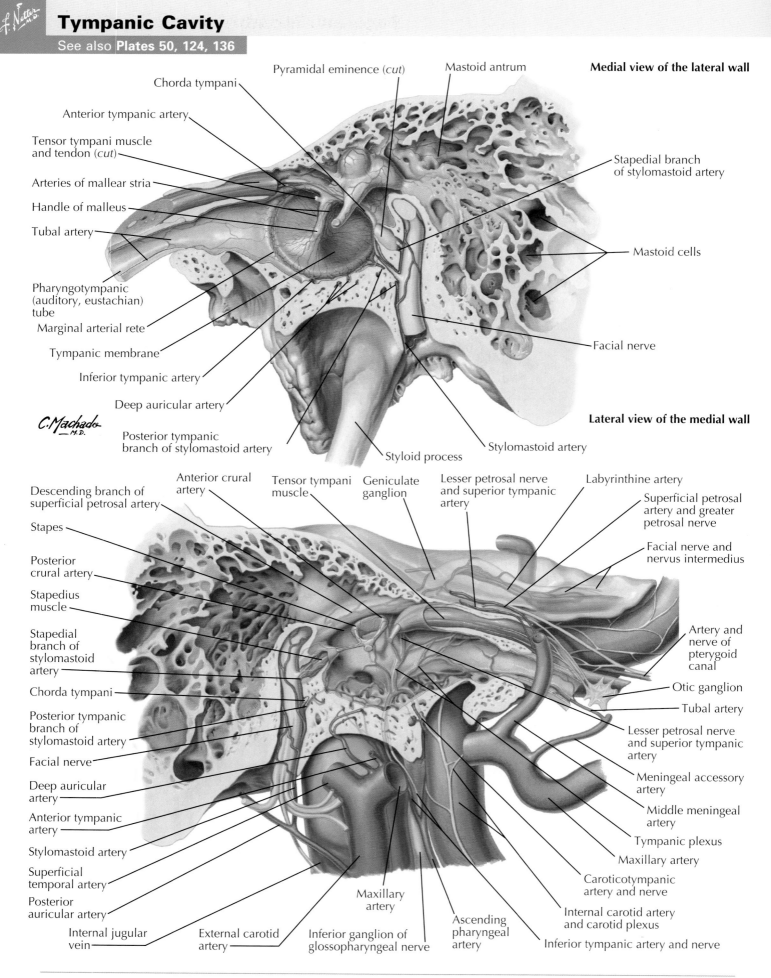

Medial view of the lateral wall

Pyramidal eminence (cut)

Mastoid antrum

Chorda tympani

Anterior tympanic artery

Tensor tympani muscle and tendon (cut)

Arteries of mallear stria

Handle of malleus

Tubal artery

Pharyngotympanic (auditory, eustachian) tube

Marginal arterial rete

Tympanic membrane

Inferior tympanic artery

Deep auricular artery

Posterior tympanic branch of stylomastoid artery

Stapedial branch of stylomastoid artery

Mastoid cells

Facial nerve

Lateral view of the medial wall

Styloid process

Stylomastoid artery

C. Machado — M.D.

Anterior crural artery

Tensor tympani muscle

Geniculate ganglion

Lesser petrosal nerve and superior tympanic artery

Labyrinthine artery

Superficial petrosal artery and greater petrosal nerve

Descending branch of superficial petrosal artery

Stapes

Posterior crural artery

Stapedius muscle

Stapedial branch of stylomastoid artery

Chorda tympani

Posterior tympanic branch of stylomastoid artery

Facial nerve

Deep auricular artery

Anterior tympanic artery

Stylomastoid artery

Superficial temporal artery

Posterior auricular artery

Internal jugular vein

External carotid artery

Inferior ganglion of glossopharyngeal nerve

Maxillary artery

Ascending pharyngeal artery

Facial nerve and nervus intermedius

Artery and nerve of pterygoid canal

Otic ganglion

Tubal artery

Lesser petrosal nerve and superior tympanic artery

Meningeal accessory artery

Middle meningeal artery

Tympanic plexus

Maxillary artery

Caroticotympanic artery and nerve

Internal carotid artery and carotid plexus

Inferior tympanic artery and nerve

**Plate 96**

**Ear**

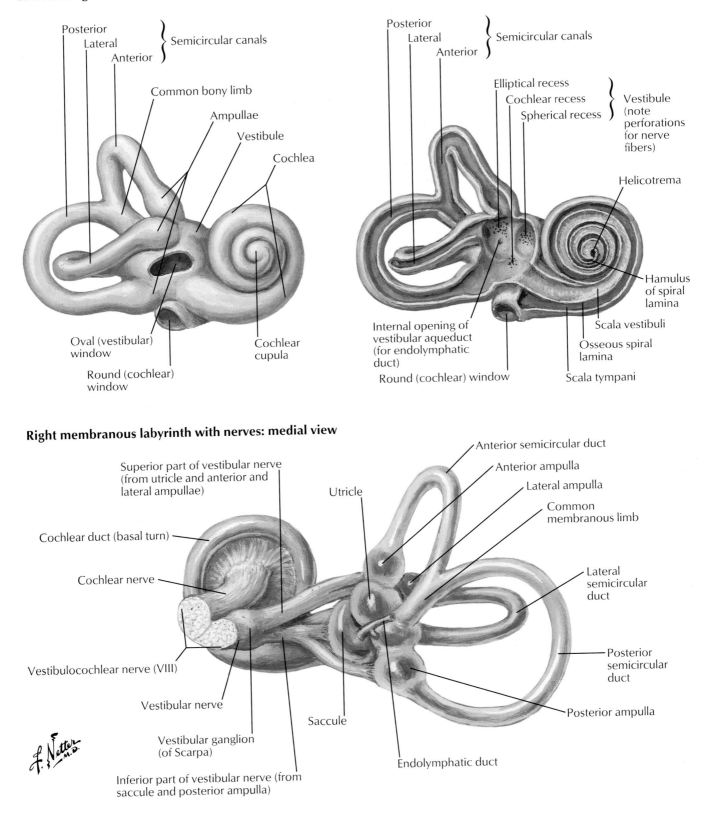

**Right bony labyrinth (otic capsule), anterolateral view: surrounding cancellous bone removed**

Posterior
Lateral } Semicircular canals
Anterior }

Common bony limb

Ampullae

Vestibule

Cochlea

Oval (vestibular) window

Round (cochlear) window

Cochlear cupula

**Dissected right bony labyrinth (otic capsule): membranous labyrinth removed**

Posterior
Lateral } Semicircular canals
Anterior }

Elliptical recess
Cochlear recess } Vestibule (note perforations for nerve fibers)
Spherical recess

Helicotrema

Internal opening of vestibular aqueduct (for endolymphatic duct)

Round (cochlear) window

Hamulus of spiral lamina

Scala vestibuli

Osseous spiral lamina

Scala tympani

**Right membranous labyrinth with nerves: medial view**

Superior part of vestibular nerve (from utricle and anterior and lateral ampullae)

Utricle

Anterior semicircular duct

Anterior ampulla

Lateral ampulla

Common membranous limb

Cochlear duct (basal turn)

Cochlear nerve

Lateral semicircular duct

Vestibulocochlear nerve (VIII)

Posterior semicircular duct

Vestibular nerve

Vestibular ganglion (of Scarpa)

Saccule

Endolymphatic duct

Posterior ampulla

Inferior part of vestibular nerve (from saccule and posterior ampulla)

## Bony and membranous labyrinths: schema

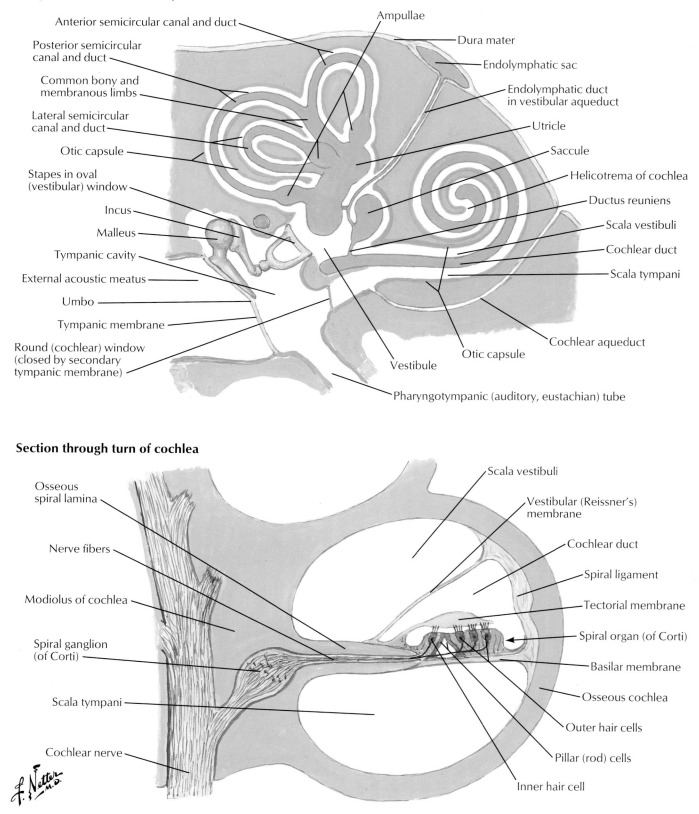

Anterior semicircular canal and duct

Posterior semicircular canal and duct

Common bony and membranous limbs

Lateral semicircular canal and duct

Otic capsule

Stapes in oval (vestibular) window

Incus

Malleus

Tympanic cavity

External acoustic meatus

Umbo

Tympanic membrane

Round (cochlear) window (closed by secondary tympanic membrane)

Ampullae

Dura mater

Endolymphatic sac

Endolymphatic duct in vestibular aqueduct

Utricle

Saccule

Helicotrema of cochlea

Ductus reuniens

Scala vestibuli

Cochlear duct

Scala tympani

Cochlear aqueduct

Otic capsule

Vestibule

Pharyngotympanic (auditory, eustachian) tube

## Section through turn of cochlea

Osseous spiral lamina

Nerve fibers

Modiolus of cochlea

Spiral ganglion (of Corti)

Scala tympani

Cochlear nerve

Scala vestibuli

Vestibular (Reissner's) membrane

Cochlear duct

Spiral ligament

Tectorial membrane

Spiral organ (of Corti)

Basilar membrane

Osseous cochlea

Outer hair cells

Pillar (rod) cells

Inner hair cell

**Plate 98**

**Ear**

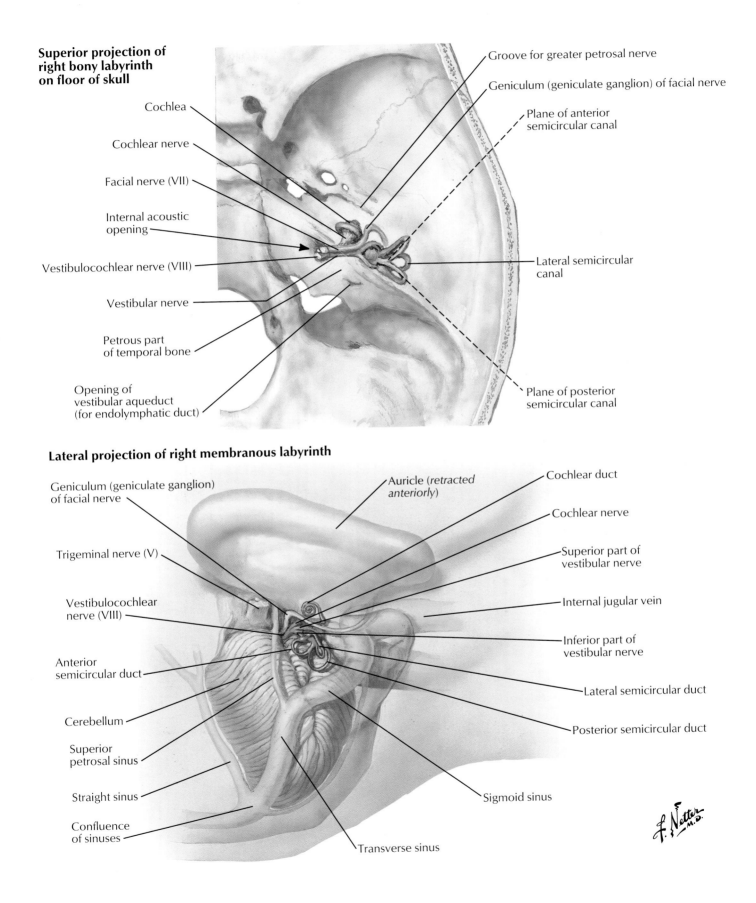

**Superior projection of right bony labyrinth on floor of skull**

Cochlea

Cochlear nerve

Facial nerve (VII)

Internal acoustic opening

Vestibulocochlear nerve (VIII)

Vestibular nerve

Petrous part of temporal bone

Opening of vestibular aqueduct (for endolymphatic duct)

Groove for greater petrosal nerve

Geniculum (geniculate ganglion) of facial nerve

Plane of anterior semicircular canal

Lateral semicircular canal

Plane of posterior semicircular canal

**Lateral projection of right membranous labyrinth**

Geniculum (geniculate ganglion) of facial nerve

Trigeminal nerve (V)

Vestibulocochlear nerve (VIII)

Anterior semicircular duct

Cerebellum

Superior petrosal sinus

Straight sinus

Confluence of sinuses

Auricle (*retracted anteriorly*)

Cochlear duct

Cochlear nerve

Superior part of vestibular nerve

Internal jugular vein

Inferior part of vestibular nerve

Lateral semicircular duct

Posterior semicircular duct

Sigmoid sinus

Transverse sinus

**Cartilaginous part of pharyngotympanic (auditory, eustachian) tube at base of skull: inferior view**

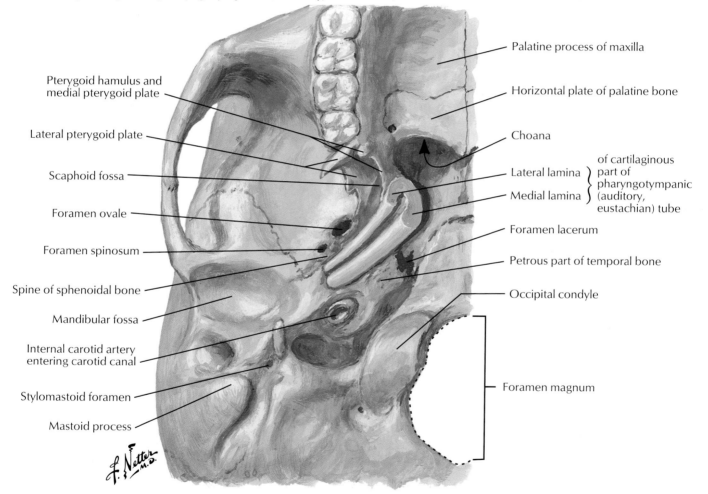

Pterygoid hamulus and medial pterygoid plate

Lateral pterygoid plate

Scaphoid fossa

Foramen ovale

Foramen spinosum

Spine of sphenoidal bone

Mandibular fossa

Internal carotid artery entering carotid canal

Stylomastoid foramen

Mastoid process

Palatine process of maxilla

Horizontal plate of palatine bone

Choana

Lateral lamina
Medial lamina
of cartilaginous part of pharyngotympanic (auditory, eustachian) tube

Foramen lacerum

Petrous part of temporal bone

Occipital condyle

Foramen magnum

**Plate 100**

**Ear**

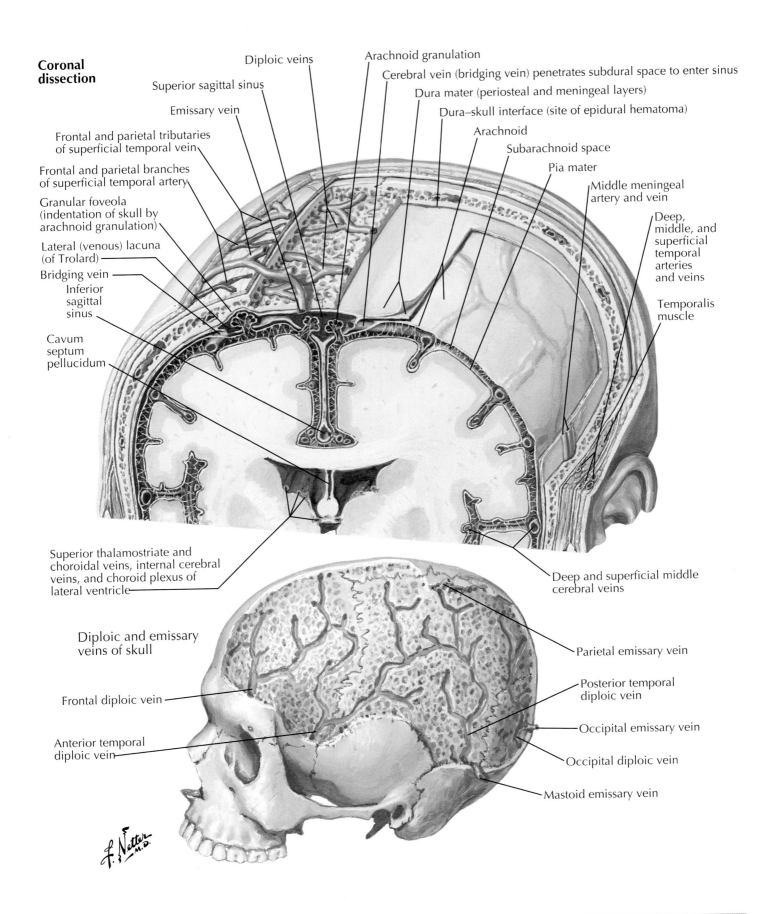

**Coronal dissection**

Diploic veins

Superior sagittal sinus

Emissary vein

Frontal and parietal tributaries of superficial temporal vein

Frontal and parietal branches of superficial temporal artery

Granular foveola (indentation of skull by arachnoid granulation)

Lateral (venous) lacuna (of Trolard)

Bridging vein

Inferior sagittal sinus

Cavum septum pellucidum

Arachnoid granulation

Cerebral vein (bridging vein) penetrates subdural space to enter sinus

Dura mater (periosteal and meningeal layers)

Dura–skull interface (site of epidural hematoma)

Arachnoid

Subarachnoid space

Pia mater

Middle meningeal artery and vein

Deep, middle, and superficial temporal arteries and veins

Temporalis muscle

Superior thalamostriate and choroidal veins, internal cerebral veins, and choroid plexus of lateral ventricle

Deep and superficial middle cerebral veins

Diploic and emissary veins of skull

Frontal diploic vein

Anterior temporal diploic vein

Parietal emissary vein

Posterior temporal diploic vein

Occipital emissary vein

Occipital diploic vein

Mastoid emissary vein

**Meninges and Brain**

**Plate 101**

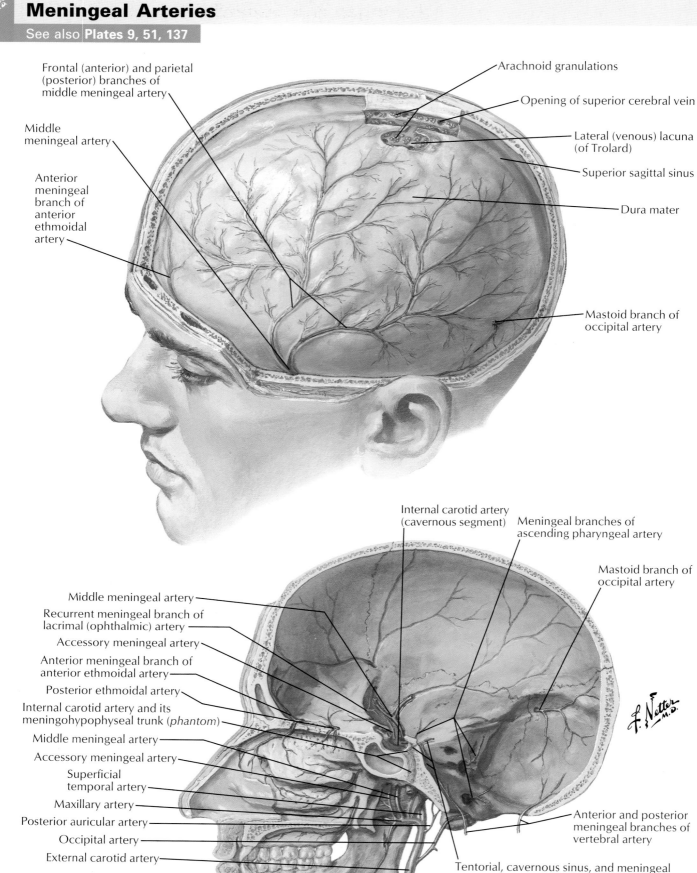

Frontal (anterior) and parietal (posterior) branches of middle meningeal artery

Middle meningeal artery

Anterior meningeal branch of anterior ethmoidal artery

Arachnoid granulations

Opening of superior cerebral vein

Lateral (venous) lacuna (of Trolard)

Superior sagittal sinus

Dura mater

Mastoid branch of occipital artery

Internal carotid artery (cavernous segment)

Meningeal branches of ascending pharyngeal artery

Mastoid branch of occipital artery

Middle meningeal artery

Recurrent meningeal branch of lacrimal (ophthalmic) artery

Accessory meningeal artery

Anterior meningeal branch of anterior ethmoidal artery

Posterior ethmoidal artery

Internal carotid artery and its meningohypophyseal trunk (*phantom*)

Middle meningeal artery

Accessory meningeal artery

Superficial temporal artery

Maxillary artery

Posterior auricular artery

Occipital artery

External carotid artery

Anterior and posterior meningeal branches of vertebral artery

Tentorial, cavernous sinus, and meningeal branches of meningohypophyseal trunk

**Plate 102**

**Meninges and Brain**

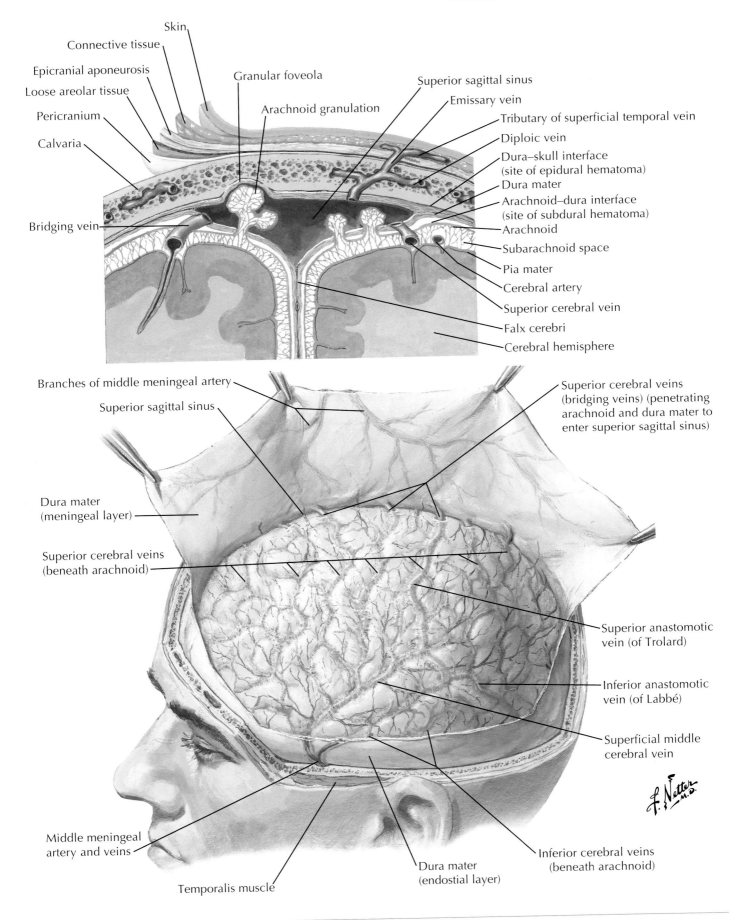

Skin

Connective tissue

Epicranial aponeurosis

Loose areolar tissue

Pericranium

Calvaria

Granular foveola

Arachnoid granulation

Bridging vein

Superior sagittal sinus

Emissary vein

Tributary of superficial temporal vein

Diploic vein

Dura–skull interface (site of epidural hematoma)

Dura mater

Arachnoid–dura interface (site of subdural hematoma)

Arachnoid

Subarachnoid space

Pia mater

Cerebral artery

Superior cerebral vein

Falx cerebri

Cerebral hemisphere

Branches of middle meningeal artery

Superior sagittal sinus

Dura mater (meningeal layer)

Superior cerebral veins (beneath arachnoid)

Superior cerebral veins (bridging veins) (penetrating arachnoid and dura mater to enter superior sagittal sinus)

Superior anastomotic vein (of Trolard)

Inferior anastomotic vein (of Labbé)

Superficial middle cerebral vein

Middle meningeal artery and veins

Temporalis muscle

Dura mater (endostial layer)

Inferior cerebral veins (beneath arachnoid)

**Meninges and Brain**

**Plate 103**

**Sagittal section**

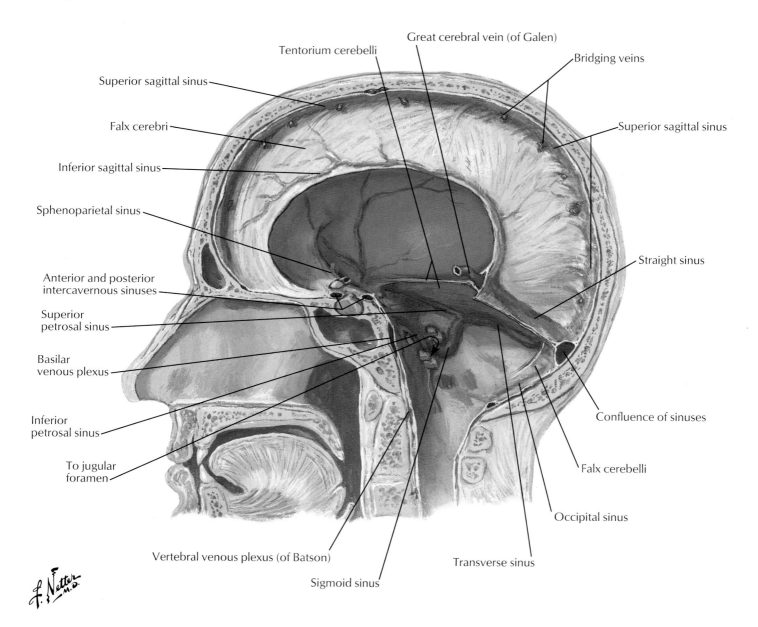

Tentorium cerebelli

Great cerebral vein (of Galen)

Bridging veins

Superior sagittal sinus

Falx cerebri

Superior sagittal sinus

Inferior sagittal sinus

Sphenoparietal sinus

Straight sinus

Anterior and posterior intercavernous sinuses

Superior petrosal sinus

Basilar venous plexus

Confluence of sinuses

Inferior petrosal sinus

Falx cerebelli

To jugular foramen

Occipital sinus

Vertebral venous plexus (of Batson)

Transverse sinus

Sigmoid sinus

**Plate 104**

**Meninges and Brain**

**Skull sectioned horizontally: superior view**

Superior sagittal sinus (*cut*)

Falx cerebri (*cut*)

Superior ophthalmic vein

Anterior and posterior intercavernous sinuses

Superficial middle cerebral vein (*cut*)

Cavernous sinus

Basilar venous plexus

Superior petrosal sinus

Inferior petrosal sinus

Tentorial artery

Tentorium cerebelli

Inferior cerebral vein (*cut*)

Transverse sinus

Inferior sagittal sinus (*cut*)

Straight sinus

Falx cerebri (*cut*)

Confluence of sinuses

Superior sagittal sinus (*cut*)

Hypophysis (pituitary gland)

Optic nerve (II)

Internal carotid artery (cavernous segment)

Oculomotor nerve (III)

Sphenoparietal sinus

Trochlear nerve (IV)

Ophthalmic nerve ($V_1$)

Maxillary nerve ($V_2$)

Trigeminal ganglion (gasserian)

Mandibular nerve ($V_3$)

Middle meningeal artery

Abducent nerve (VI)

Petrosal vein

Facial nerve (VII), intermediate nerve (of Wrisberg), and vestibulocochlear nerve (VIII)

Glossopharyngeal (IX) and vagus (X) nerves

Jugular foramen

Sigmoid sinus (continuation of transverse sinus)

Transverse sinus

Accessory nerve (XI)

Hypoglossal nerve (XII)

Great cerebral vein (of Galen)

Cavernous sinus

Oculomotor nerve (III)

Trochlear nerve (IV)

Abducent nerve (VI)

Ophthalmic nerve ($V_1$)

Maxillary nerve ($V_2$)

Optic chiasm

Posterior communicating artery

Internal carotid artery (cavernous segment)

Hypophysis (pituitary gland)

Sphenoidal sinus

Nasopharynx

**Coronal section through cavernous sinus: posterior view**

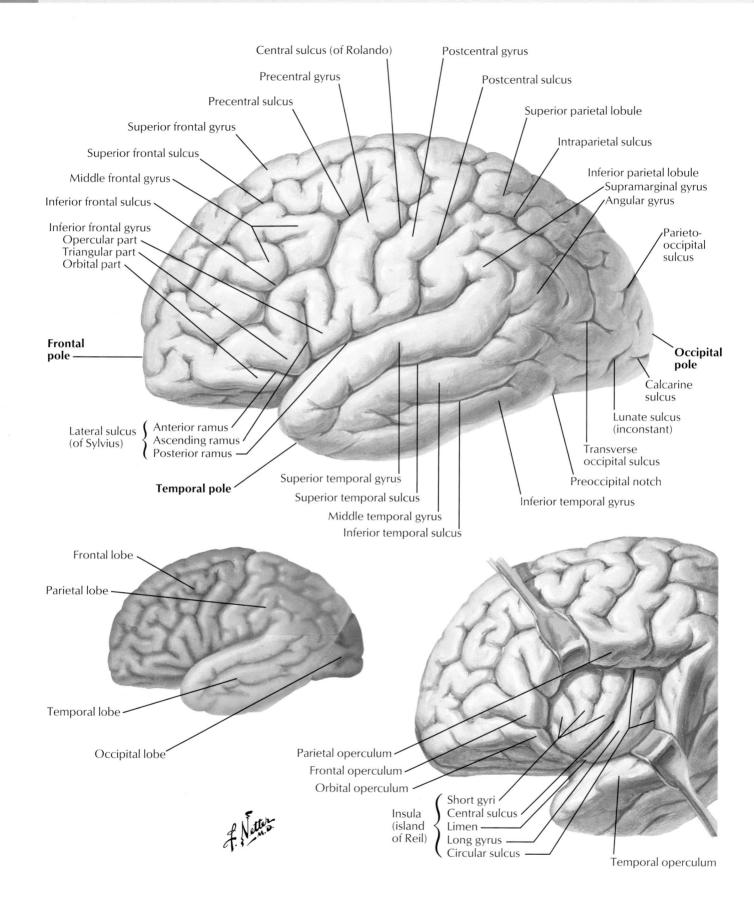

Central sulcus (of Rolando)
Precentral gyrus
Precentral sulcus
Superior frontal gyrus
Superior frontal sulcus
Middle frontal gyrus
Inferior frontal sulcus
Inferior frontal gyrus
Opercular part
Triangular part
Orbital part

Postcentral gyrus
Postcentral sulcus
Superior parietal lobule
Intraparietal sulcus
Inferior parietal lobule
Supramarginal gyrus
Angular gyrus

Frontal pole

Parieto-occipital sulcus

Occipital pole

Calcarine sulcus

Lunate sulcus (inconstant)

Lateral sulcus (of Sylvius) { Anterior ramus / Ascending ramus / Posterior ramus

Temporal pole

Superior temporal gyrus
Superior temporal sulcus
Middle temporal gyrus
Inferior temporal sulcus

Transverse occipital sulcus
Preoccipital notch
Inferior temporal gyrus

Frontal lobe
Parietal lobe

Temporal lobe

Occipital lobe

Parietal operculum
Frontal operculum
Orbital operculum

Insula (island of Reil) { Short gyri / Central sulcus / Limen / Long gyrus / Circular sulcus

Temporal operculum

**Plate 106**

**Meninges and Brain**

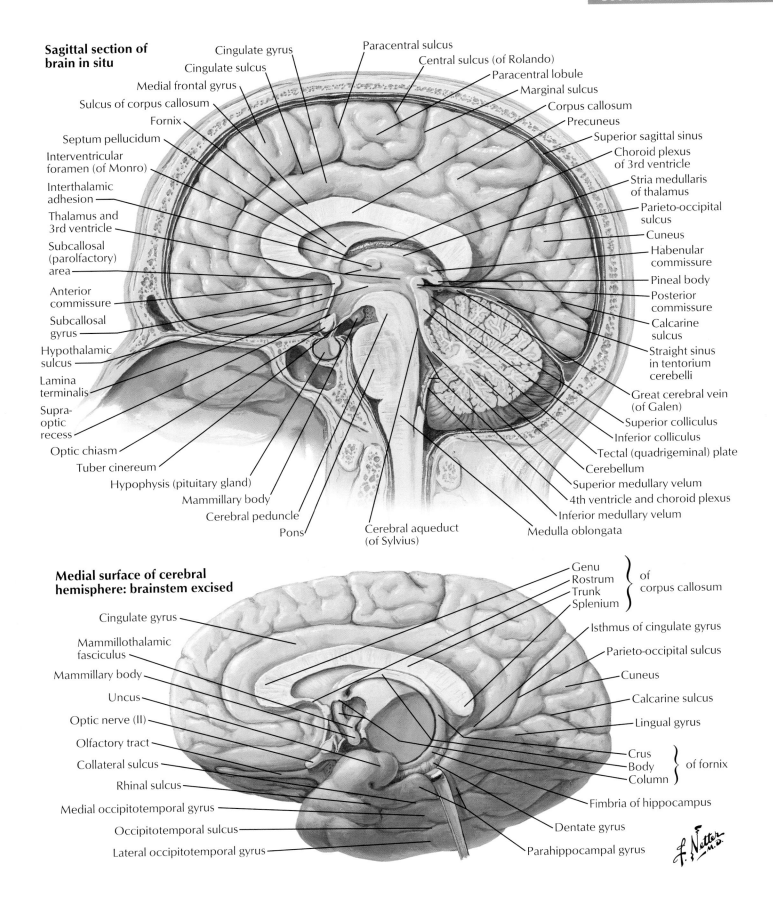

**Sagittal section of brain in situ**

Cingulate gyrus
Cingulate sulcus
Medial frontal gyrus
Sulcus of corpus callosum
Fornix
Septum pellucidum
Interventricular foramen (of Monro)
Interthalamic adhesion
Thalamus and 3rd ventricle
Subcallosal (parolfactory) area
Anterior commissure
Subcallosal gyrus
Hypothalamic sulcus
Lamina terminalis
Supra-optic recess
Optic chiasm
Tuber cinereum
Hypophysis (pituitary gland)
Mammillary body
Cerebral peduncle
Pons

Paracentral sulcus
Central sulcus (of Rolando)
Paracentral lobule
Marginal sulcus
Corpus callosum
Precuneus
Superior sagittal sinus
Choroid plexus of 3rd ventricle
Stria medullaris of thalamus
Parieto-occipital sulcus
Cuneus
Habenular commissure
Pineal body
Posterior commissure
Calcarine sulcus
Straight sinus in tentorium cerebelli
Great cerebral vein (of Galen)
Superior colliculus
Inferior colliculus
Tectal (quadrigeminal) plate
Cerebellum
Superior medullary velum
4th ventricle and choroid plexus
Inferior medullary velum
Medulla oblongata

Cerebral aqueduct (of Sylvius)

**Medial surface of cerebral hemisphere: brainstem excised**

Cingulate gyrus
Mammillothalamic fasciculus
Mammillary body
Uncus
Optic nerve (II)
Olfactory tract
Collateral sulcus
Rhinal sulcus
Medial occipitotemporal gyrus
Occipitotemporal sulcus
Lateral occipitotemporal gyrus

Genu
Rostrum
Trunk
Splenium
} of corpus callosum

Isthmus of cingulate gyrus
Parieto-occipital sulcus
Cuneus
Calcarine sulcus
Lingual gyrus
Crus
Body
Column
} of fornix
Fimbria of hippocampus
Dentate gyrus
Parahippocampal gyrus

*f. Netter. M.D.*

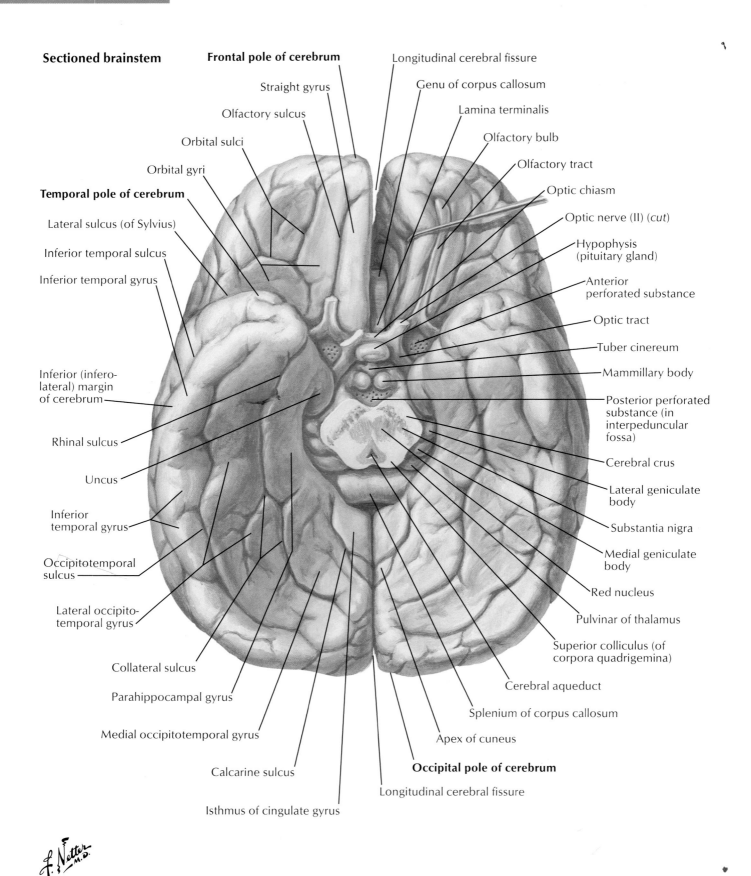

Sectioned brainstem

Frontal pole of cerebrum

Straight gyrus

Olfactory sulcus

Orbital sulci

Orbital gyri

Temporal pole of cerebrum

Lateral sulcus (of Sylvius)

Inferior temporal sulcus

Inferior temporal gyrus

Inferior (infero-lateral) margin of cerebrum

Rhinal sulcus

Uncus

Inferior temporal gyrus

Occipitotemporal sulcus

Lateral occipito-temporal gyrus

Collateral sulcus

Parahippocampal gyrus

Medial occipitotemporal gyrus

Calcarine sulcus

Isthmus of cingulate gyrus

Longitudinal cerebral fissure

Genu of corpus callosum

Lamina terminalis

Olfactory bulb

Olfactory tract

Optic chiasm

Optic nerve (II) (cut)

Hypophysis (pituitary gland)

Anterior perforated substance

Optic tract

Tuber cinereum

Mammillary body

Posterior perforated substance (in interpeduncular fossa)

Cerebral crus

Lateral geniculate body

Substantia nigra

Medial geniculate body

Red nucleus

Pulvinar of thalamus

Superior colliculus (of corpora quadrigemina)

Cerebral aqueduct

Splenium of corpus callosum

Apex of cuneus

Occipital pole of cerebrum

Longitudinal cerebral fissure

Plate 108

Meninges and Brain

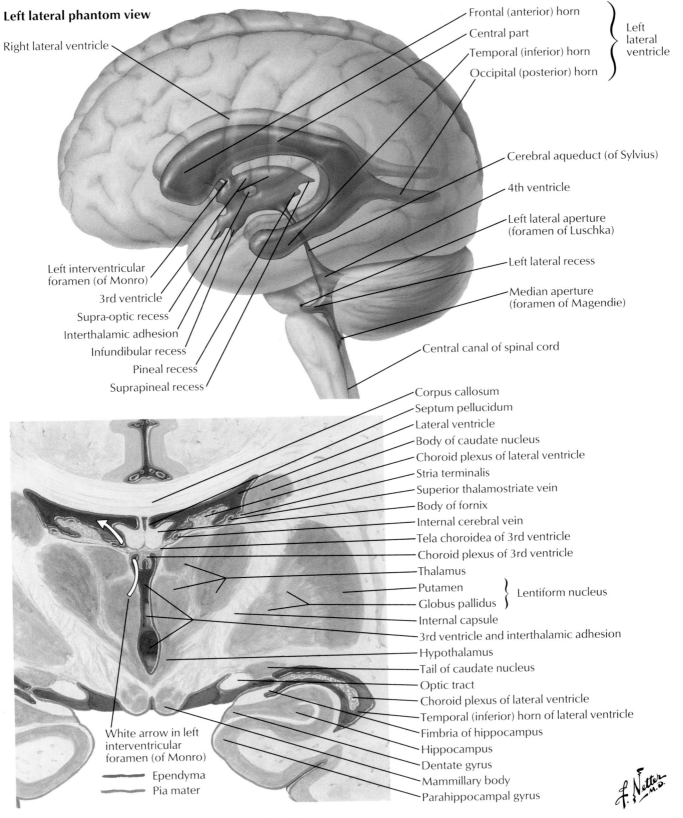

**Left lateral phantom view**

Right lateral ventricle

Frontal (anterior) horn
Central part
Temporal (inferior) horn
Occipital (posterior) horn

Left lateral ventricle

Cerebral aqueduct (of Sylvius)

4th ventricle

Left lateral aperture (foramen of Luschka)

Left lateral recess

Median aperture (foramen of Magendie)

Central canal of spinal cord

Left interventricular foramen (of Monro)
3rd ventricle
Supra-optic recess
Interthalamic adhesion
Infundibular recess
Pineal recess
Suprapineal recess

Corpus callosum
Septum pellucidum
Lateral ventricle
Body of caudate nucleus
Choroid plexus of lateral ventricle
Stria terminalis
Superior thalamostriate vein
Body of fornix
Internal cerebral vein
Tela choroidea of 3rd ventricle
Choroid plexus of 3rd ventricle
Thalamus
Putamen
Globus pallidus
Internal capsule
3rd ventricle and interthalamic adhesion
Hypothalamus
Tail of caudate nucleus
Optic tract
Choroid plexus of lateral ventricle
Temporal (inferior) horn of lateral ventricle
Fimbria of hippocampus
Hippocampus
Dentate gyrus
Mammillary body
Parahippocampal gyrus

Lentiform nucleus

White arrow in left interventricular foramen (of Monro)

Ependyma
Pia mater

**Coronal section of brain: posterior view**

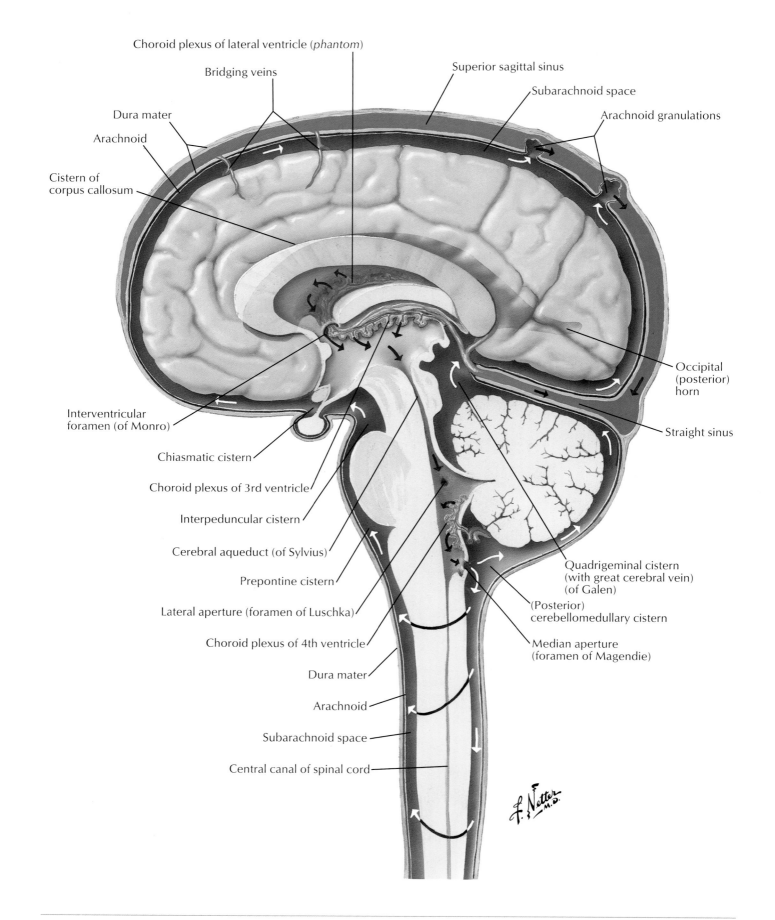

Choroid plexus of lateral ventricle (*phantom*)

Bridging veins

Dura mater

Arachnoid

Cistern of corpus callosum

Superior sagittal sinus

Subarachnoid space

Arachnoid granulations

Interventricular foramen (of Monro)

Chiasmatic cistern

Choroid plexus of 3rd ventricle

Interpeduncular cistern

Cerebral aqueduct (of Sylvius)

Prepontine cistern

Lateral aperture (foramen of Luschka)

Choroid plexus of 4th ventricle

Dura mater

Arachnoid

Subarachnoid space

Central canal of spinal cord

Occipital (posterior) horn

Straight sinus

Quadrigeminal cistern (with great cerebral vein) (of Galen)

(Posterior) cerebellomedullary cistern

Median aperture (foramen of Magendie)

**Plate 110**

**Meninges and Brain**

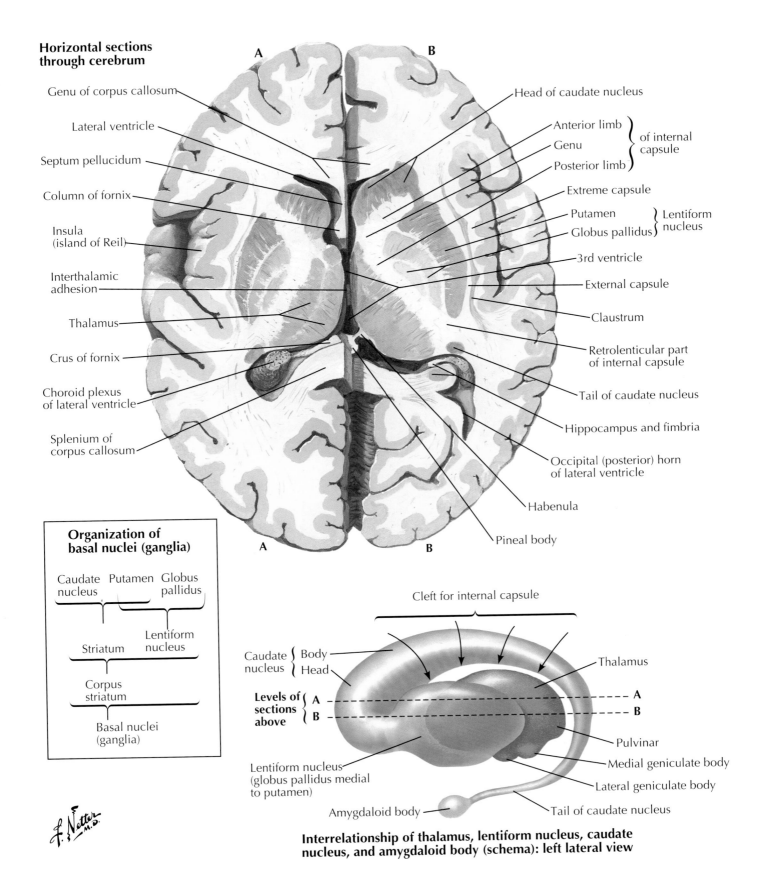

**Horizontal sections through cerebrum**

Genu of corpus callosum

Lateral ventricle

Septum pellucidum

Column of fornix

Insula (island of Reil)

Interthalamic adhesion

Thalamus

Crus of fornix

Choroid plexus of lateral ventricle

Splenium of corpus callosum

Head of caudate nucleus

Anterior limb ⎱
Genu ⎰ of internal capsule
Posterior limb ⎰

Extreme capsule

Putamen ⎱ Lentiform
Globus pallidus ⎰ nucleus

3rd ventricle

External capsule

Claustrum

Retrolenticular part of internal capsule

Tail of caudate nucleus

Hippocampus and fimbria

Occipital (posterior) horn of lateral ventricle

Habenula

Pineal body

**Organization of basal nuclei (ganglia)**

Caudate nucleus — Putamen — Globus pallidus

Striatum — Lentiform nucleus

Corpus striatum

Basal nuclei (ganglia)

Cleft for internal capsule

Caudate ⎰ Body
nucleus ⎱ Head

Thalamus

Levels of ⎰ A
sections ⎱ B
above

A
B

Pulvinar

Medial geniculate body

Lateral geniculate body

Tail of caudate nucleus

Lentiform nucleus (globus pallidus medial to putamen)

Amygdaloid body

**Interrelationship of thalamus, lentiform nucleus, caudate nucleus, and amygdaloid body (schema): left lateral view**

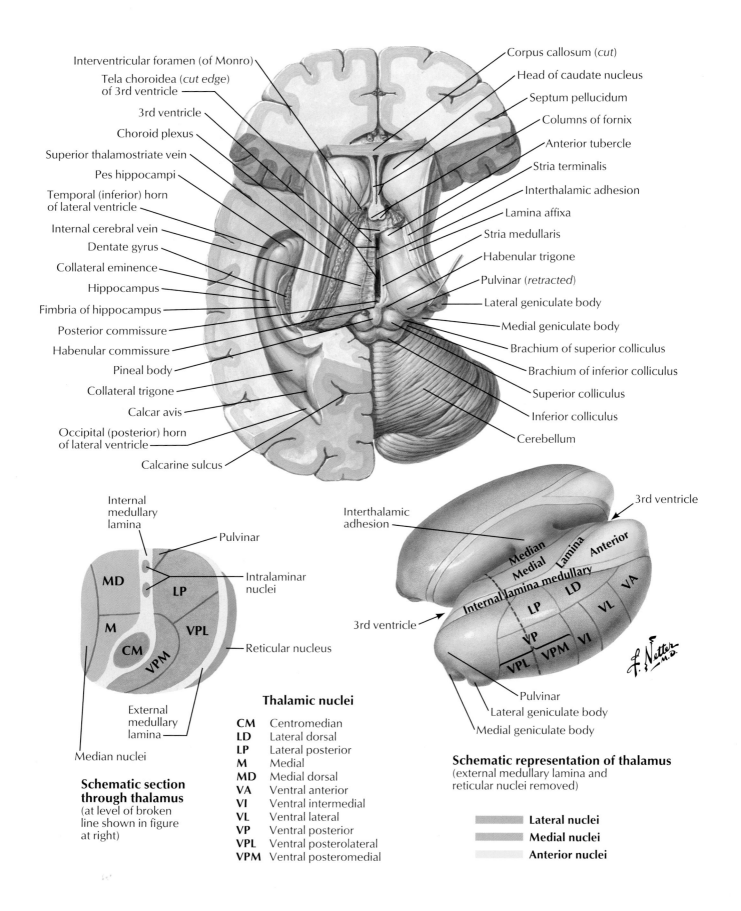

Interventricular foramen (of Monro)

Tela choroidea (*cut edge*) of 3rd ventricle

3rd ventricle

Choroid plexus

Superior thalamostriate vein

Pes hippocampi

Temporal (inferior) horn of lateral ventricle

Internal cerebral vein

Dentate gyrus

Collateral eminence

Hippocampus

Fimbria of hippocampus

Posterior commissure

Habenular commissure

Pineal body

Collateral trigone

Calcar avis

Occipital (posterior) horn of lateral ventricle

Calcarine sulcus

Corpus callosum (*cut*)

Head of caudate nucleus

Septum pellucidum

Columns of fornix

Anterior tubercle

Stria terminalis

Interthalamic adhesion

Lamina affixa

Stria medullaris

Habenular trigone

Pulvinar (*retracted*)

Lateral geniculate body

Medial geniculate body

Brachium of superior colliculus

Brachium of inferior colliculus

Superior colliculus

Inferior colliculus

Cerebellum

Internal medullary lamina

Pulvinar

Intralaminar nuclei

Reticular nucleus

MD

LP

M

VPL

CM

VPM

External medullary lamina

Median nuclei

**Schematic section through thalamus**
(at level of broken line shown in figure at right)

## Thalamic nuclei

| | |
|---|---|
| CM | Centromedian |
| LD | Lateral dorsal |
| LP | Lateral posterior |
| M | Medial |
| MD | Medial dorsal |
| VA | Ventral anterior |
| VI | Ventral intermedial |
| VL | Ventral lateral |
| VP | Ventral posterior |
| VPL | Ventral posterolateral |
| VPM | Ventral posteromedial |

Interthalamic adhesion

3rd ventricle

3rd ventricle

Median
Medial
Lamina
Anterior
Internal lamina medullary
LP
LD
VA
VL
VP
VI
VPL
VPM

Pulvinar

Lateral geniculate body

Medial geniculate body

**Schematic representation of thalamus**
(external medullary lamina and reticular nuclei removed)

Lateral nuclei
Medial nuclei
Anterior nuclei

**Plate 112**

**Meninges and Brain**

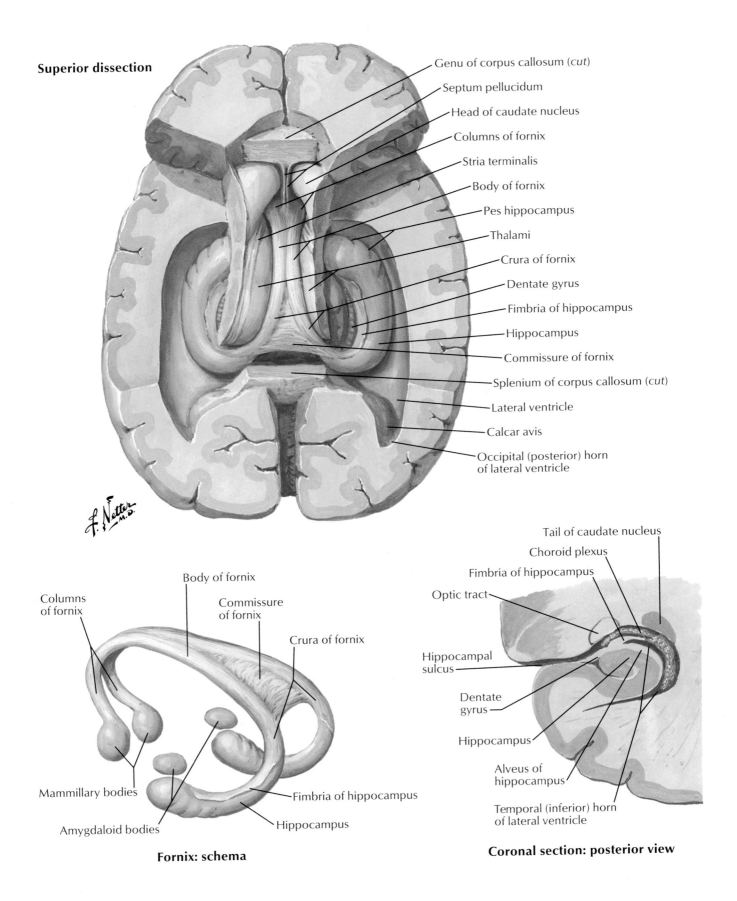

**Superior dissection**

Genu of corpus callosum (*cut*)

Septum pellucidum

Head of caudate nucleus

Columns of fornix

Stria terminalis

Body of fornix

Pes hippocampus

Thalami

Crura of fornix

Dentate gyrus

Fimbria of hippocampus

Hippocampus

Commissure of fornix

Splenium of corpus callosum (*cut*)

Lateral ventricle

Calcar avis

Occipital (posterior) horn of lateral ventricle

Columns of fornix

Body of fornix

Commissure of fornix

Crura of fornix

Mammillary bodies

Amygdaloid bodies

Fimbria of hippocampus

Hippocampus

**Fornix: schema**

Tail of caudate nucleus

Choroid plexus

Fimbria of hippocampus

Optic tract

Hippocampal sulcus

Dentate gyrus

Hippocampus

Alveus of hippocampus

Temporal (inferior) horn of lateral ventricle

**Coronal section: posterior view**

**Meninges and Brain**

**Plate 113**

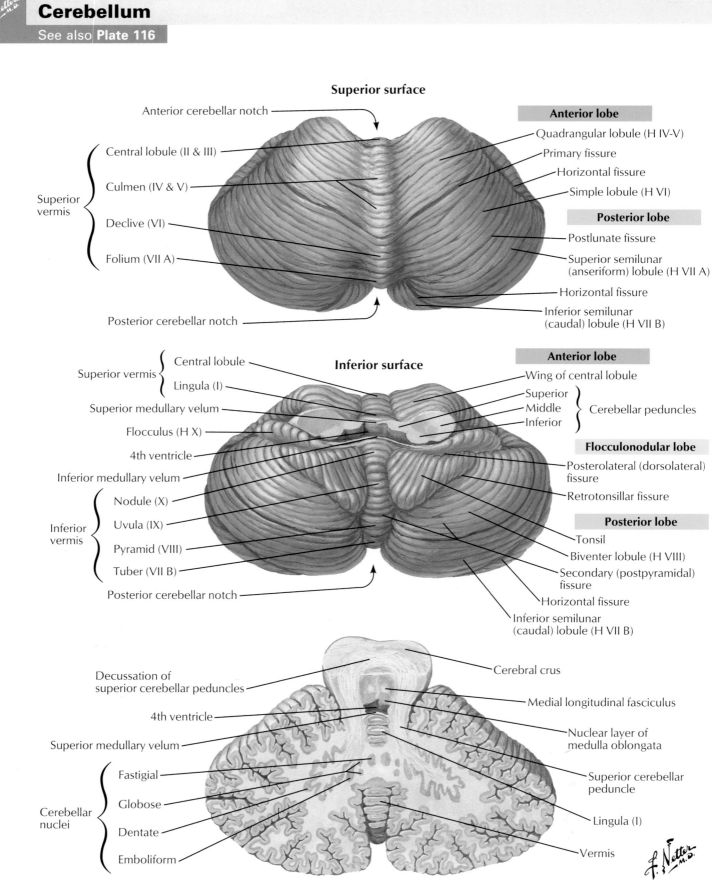

**Superior surface**

Anterior cerebellar notch

**Anterior lobe**

Quadrangular lobule (H IV-V)

Primary fissure

Horizontal fissure

Simple lobule (H VI)

Superior vermis
- Central lobule (II & III)
- Culmen (IV & V)
- Declive (VI)
- Folium (VII A)

**Posterior lobe**

Postlunate fissure

Superior semilunar (anseriform) lobule (H VII A)

Horizontal fissure

Inferior semilunar (caudal) lobule (H VII B)

Posterior cerebellar notch

**Inferior surface**

Superior vermis
- Central lobule
- Lingula (I)

Superior medullary velum

Flocculus (H X)

4th ventricle

Inferior medullary velum

Inferior vermis
- Nodule (X)
- Uvula (IX)
- Pyramid (VIII)
- Tuber (VII B)

Posterior cerebellar notch

**Anterior lobe**

Wing of central lobule

Cerebellar peduncles
- Superior
- Middle
- Inferior

**Flocculonodular lobe**

Posterolateral (dorsolateral) fissure

Retrotonsillar fissure

**Posterior lobe**

Tonsil

Biventer lobule (H VIII)

Secondary (postpyramidal) fissure

Horizontal fissure

Inferior semilunar (caudal) lobule (H VII B)

Decussation of superior cerebellar peduncles

4th ventricle

Superior medullary velum

Cerebellar nuclei
- Fastigial
- Globose
- Dentate
- Emboliform

Cerebral crus

Medial longitudinal fasciculus

Nuclear layer of medulla oblongata

Superior cerebellar peduncle

Lingula (I)

Vermis

**Section in plane of superior cerebellar peduncle**

**Plate 114**

**Meninges and Brain**

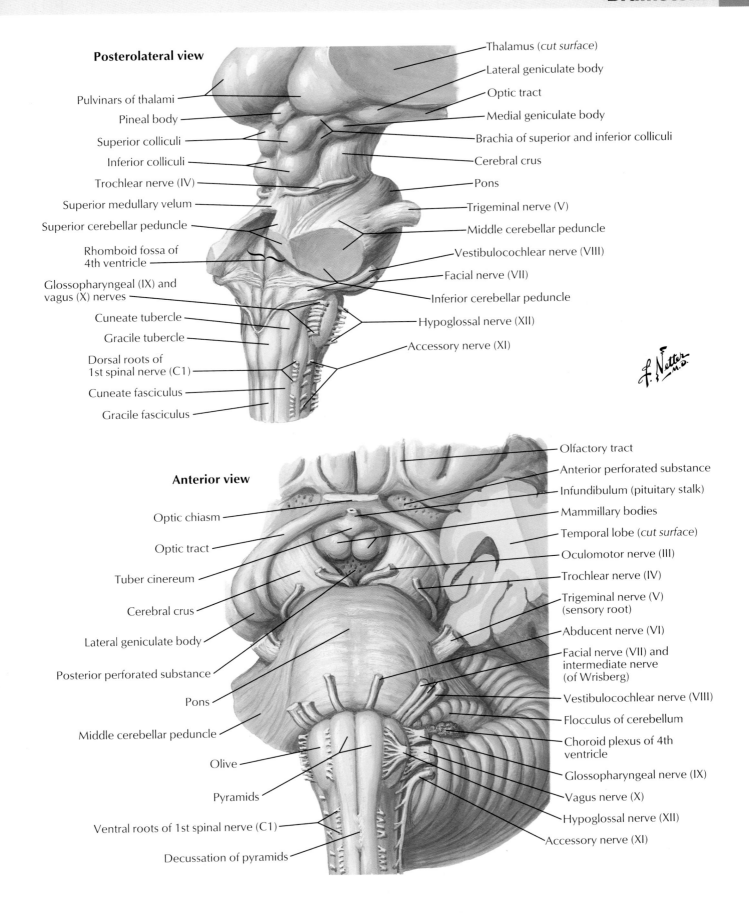

**Posterolateral view**

Pulvinars of thalami
Pineal body
Superior colliculi
Inferior colliculi
Trochlear nerve (IV)
Superior medullary velum
Superior cerebellar peduncle
Rhomboid fossa of 4th ventricle
Glossopharyngeal (IX) and vagus (X) nerves
Cuneate tubercle
Gracile tubercle
Dorsal roots of 1st spinal nerve (C1)
Cuneate fasciculus
Gracile fasciculus

Thalamus (*cut surface*)
Lateral geniculate body
Optic tract
Medial geniculate body
Brachia of superior and inferior colliculi
Cerebral crus
Pons
Trigeminal nerve (V)
Middle cerebellar peduncle
Vestibulocochlear nerve (VIII)
Facial nerve (VII)
Inferior cerebellar peduncle
Hypoglossal nerve (XII)
Accessory nerve (XI)

*f. Netter*
*M.D.*

**Anterior view**

Optic chiasm
Optic tract
Tuber cinereum
Cerebral crus
Lateral geniculate body
Posterior perforated substance
Pons
Middle cerebellar peduncle
Olive
Pyramids
Ventral roots of 1st spinal nerve (C1)
Decussation of pyramids

Olfactory tract
Anterior perforated substance
Infundibulum (pituitary stalk)
Mammillary bodies
Temporal lobe (*cut surface*)
Oculomotor nerve (III)
Trochlear nerve (IV)
Trigeminal nerve (V) (sensory root)
Abducent nerve (VI)
Facial nerve (VII) and intermediate nerve (of Wrisberg)
Vestibulocochlear nerve (VIII)
Flocculus of cerebellum
Choroid plexus of 4th ventricle
Glossopharyngeal nerve (IX)
Vagus nerve (X)
Hypoglossal nerve (XII)
Accessory nerve (XI)

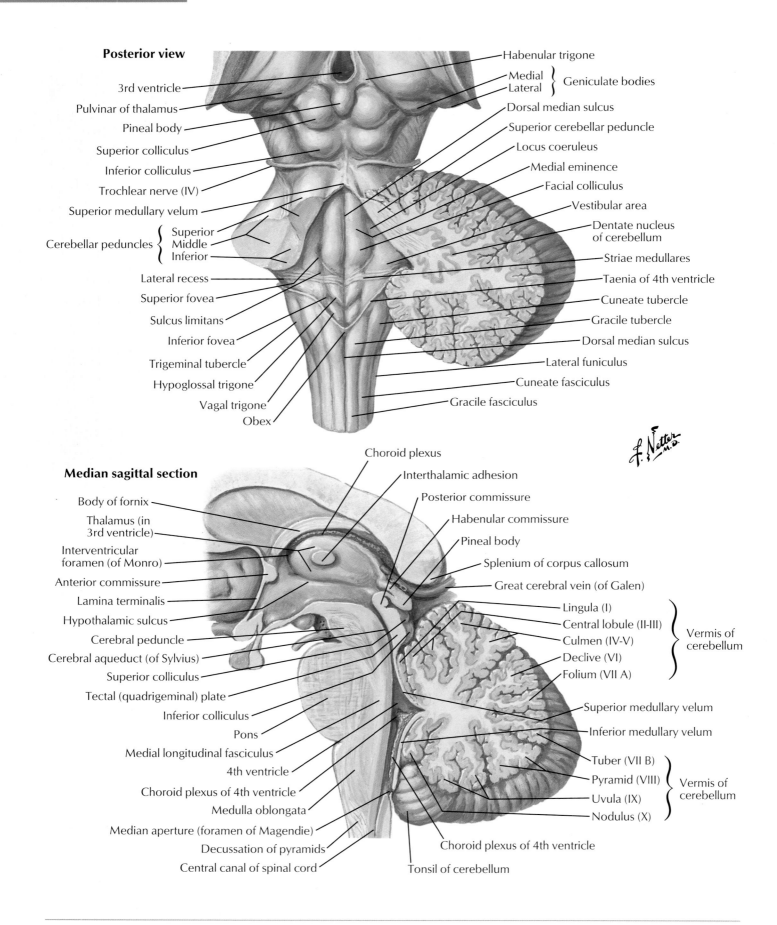

**Posterior view**

3rd ventricle
Pulvinar of thalamus
Pineal body
Superior colliculus
Inferior colliculus
Trochlear nerve (IV)
Superior medullary velum

Cerebellar peduncles { Superior / Middle / Inferior }

Lateral recess
Superior fovea
Sulcus limitans
Inferior fovea
Trigeminal tubercle
Hypoglossal trigone
Vagal trigone
Obex

Habenular trigone
Medial } Geniculate bodies
Lateral }
Dorsal median sulcus
Superior cerebellar peduncle
Locus coeruleus
Medial eminence
Facial colliculus
Vestibular area
Dentate nucleus of cerebellum
Striae medullares
Taenia of 4th ventricle
Cuneate tubercle
Gracile tubercle
Dorsal median sulcus
Lateral funiculus
Cuneate fasciculus
Gracile fasciculus

**Median sagittal section**

Choroid plexus
Interthalamic adhesion
Posterior commissure
Habenular commissure
Pineal body
Splenium of corpus callosum
Great cerebral vein (of Galen)

Body of fornix
Thalamus (in 3rd ventricle)
Interventricular foramen (of Monro)
Anterior commissure
Lamina terminalis
Hypothalamic sulcus
Cerebral peduncle
Cerebral aqueduct (of Sylvius)
Superior colliculus
Tectal (quadrigeminal) plate
Inferior colliculus
Pons
Medial longitudinal fasciculus
4th ventricle
Choroid plexus of 4th ventricle
Medulla oblongata
Median aperture (foramen of Magendie)
Decussation of pyramids
Central canal of spinal cord

Lingula (I)
Central lobule (II-III)
Culmen (IV-V)
Declive (VI)
Folium (VII A)
} Vermis of cerebellum

Superior medullary velum
Inferior medullary velum

Tuber (VII B)
Pyramid (VIII)
Uvula (IX)
Nodulus (X)
} Vermis of cerebellum

Choroid plexus of 4th ventricle
Tonsil of cerebellum

**Plate 116**                    **Meninges and Brain**

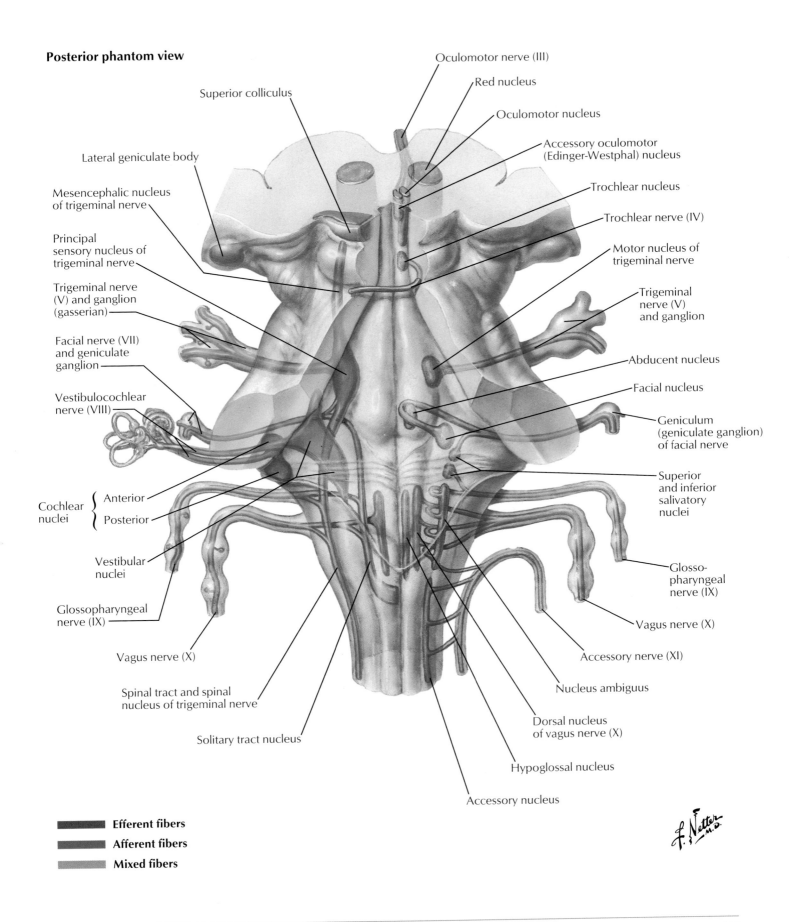

**Posterior phantom view**

Superior colliculus

Lateral geniculate body

Mesencephalic nucleus of trigeminal nerve

Principal sensory nucleus of trigeminal nerve

Trigeminal nerve (V) and ganglion (gasserian)

Facial nerve (VII) and geniculate ganglion

Vestibulocochlear nerve (VIII)

Cochlear nuclei { Anterior / Posterior }

Vestibular nuclei

Glossopharyngeal nerve (IX)

Vagus nerve (X)

Spinal tract and spinal nucleus of trigeminal nerve

Solitary tract nucleus

Oculomotor nerve (III)

Red nucleus

Oculomotor nucleus

Accessory oculomotor (Edinger-Westphal) nucleus

Trochlear nucleus

Trochlear nerve (IV)

Motor nucleus of trigeminal nerve

Trigeminal nerve (V) and ganglion

Abducent nucleus

Facial nucleus

Geniculum (geniculate ganglion) of facial nerve

Superior and inferior salivatory nuclei

Glosso-pharyngeal nerve (IX)

Vagus nerve (X)

Accessory nerve (XI)

Nucleus ambiguus

Dorsal nucleus of vagus nerve (X)

Hypoglossal nucleus

Accessory nucleus

■ Efferent fibers
■ Afferent fibers
■ Mixed fibers

**Medial dissection**

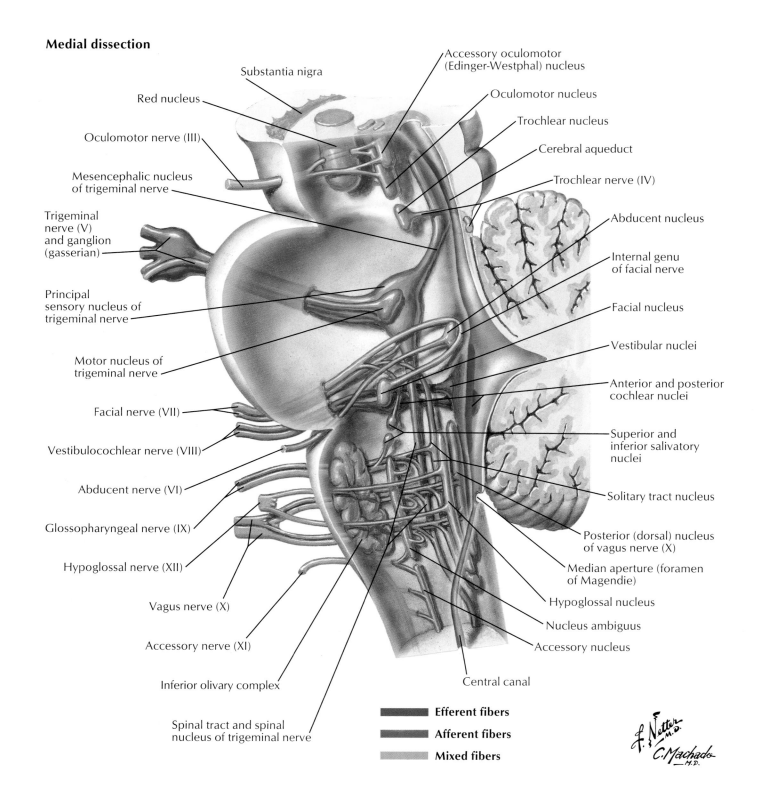

Substantia nigra

Red nucleus

Oculomotor nerve (III)

Mesencephalic nucleus
of trigeminal nerve

Trigeminal
nerve (V)
and ganglion
(gasserian)

Principal
sensory nucleus of
trigeminal nerve

Motor nucleus of
trigeminal nerve

Facial nerve (VII)

Vestibulocochlear nerve (VIII)

Abducent nerve (VI)

Glossopharyngeal nerve (IX)

Hypoglossal nerve (XII)

Vagus nerve (X)

Accessory nerve (XI)

Inferior olivary complex

Spinal tract and spinal
nucleus of trigeminal nerve

Accessory oculomotor
(Edinger-Westphal) nucleus

Oculomotor nucleus

Trochlear nucleus

Cerebral aqueduct

Trochlear nerve (IV)

Abducent nucleus

Internal genu
of facial nerve

Facial nucleus

Vestibular nuclei

Anterior and posterior
cochlear nuclei

Superior and
inferior salivatory
nuclei

Solitary tract nucleus

Posterior (dorsal) nucleus
of vagus nerve (X)

Median aperture (foramen
of Magendie)

Hypoglossal nucleus

Nucleus ambiguus

Accessory nucleus

Central canal

Efferent fibers

Afferent fibers

Mixed fibers

**Plate 118**

**Cranial and Cervical Nerves**

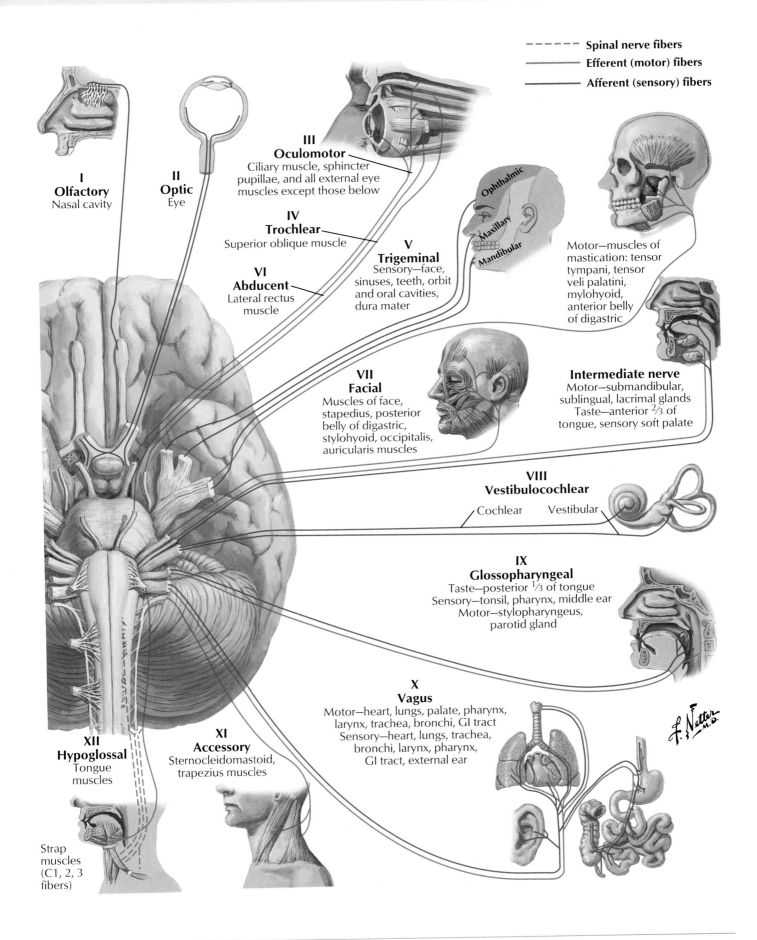

- - - - - Spinal nerve fibers
───── Efferent (motor) fibers
───── Afferent (sensory) fibers

**I**
**Olfactory**
Nasal cavity

**II**
**Optic**
Eye

**III**
**Oculomotor**
Ciliary muscle, sphincter pupillae, and all external eye muscles except those below

**IV**
**Trochlear**
Superior oblique muscle

**VI**
**Abducent**
Lateral rectus muscle

Ophthalmic
Maxillary
Mandibular

**V**
**Trigeminal**
Sensory—face, sinuses, teeth, orbit and oral cavities, dura mater

Motor—muscles of mastication: tensor tympani, tensor veli palatini, mylohyoid, anterior belly of digastric

**VII**
**Facial**
Muscles of face, stapedius, posterior belly of digastric, stylohyoid, occipitalis, auricularis muscles

**Intermediate nerve**
Motor—submandibular, sublingual, lacrimal glands
Taste—anterior ⅔ of tongue, sensory soft palate

**VIII**
**Vestibulocochlear**
Cochlear     Vestibular

**IX**
**Glossopharyngeal**
Taste—posterior ⅓ of tongue
Sensory—tonsil, pharynx, middle ear
Motor—stylopharyngeus, parotid gland

**X**
**Vagus**
Motor—heart, lungs, palate, pharynx, larynx, trachea, bronchi, GI tract
Sensory—heart, lungs, trachea, bronchi, larynx, pharynx, GI tract, external ear

**XII**
**Hypoglossal**
Tongue muscles

Strap muscles (C1, 2, 3 fibers)

**XI**
**Accessory**
Sternocleidomastoid, trapezius muscles

F. Netter M.D.

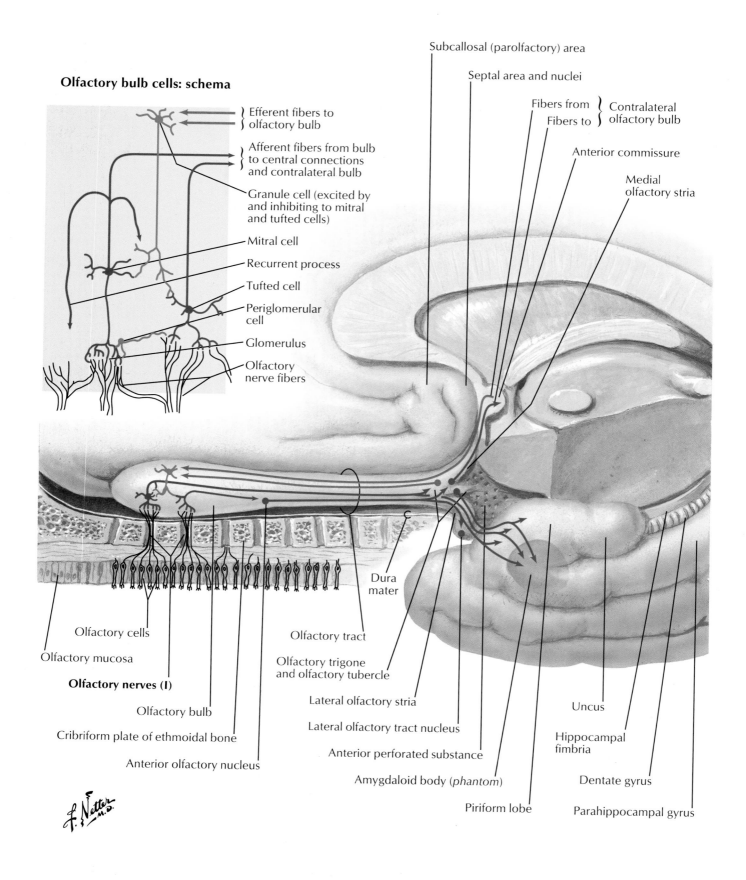

## Olfactory bulb cells: schema

} Efferent fibers to olfactory bulb

} Afferent fibers from bulb to central connections and contralateral bulb

Granule cell (excited by and inhibiting to mitral and tufted cells)

Mitral cell

Recurrent process

Tufted cell

Periglomerular cell

Glomerulus

Olfactory nerve fibers

Subcallosal (parolfactory) area

Septal area and nuclei

Fibers from } Contralateral
Fibers to } olfactory bulb

Anterior commissure

Medial olfactory stria

Dura mater

Olfactory cells

Olfactory mucosa

**Olfactory nerves (I)**

Olfactory bulb

Cribriform plate of ethmoidal bone

Anterior olfactory nucleus

Olfactory tract

Olfactory trigone and olfactory tubercle

Lateral olfactory stria

Lateral olfactory tract nucleus

Anterior perforated substance

Amygdaloid body (*phantom*)

Piriform lobe

Uncus

Hippocampal fimbria

Dentate gyrus

Parahippocampal gyrus

**Plate 120**

**Cranial and Cervical Nerves**

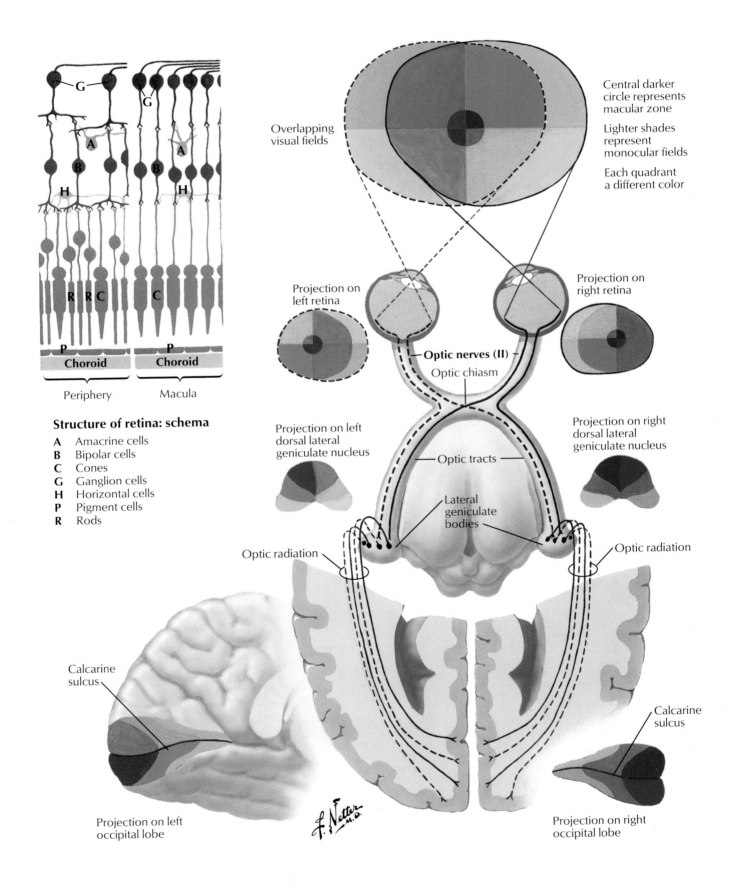

**Overlapping visual fields**

Central darker circle represents macular zone

Lighter shades represent monocular fields

Each quadrant a different color

Projection on left retina

Projection on right retina

**Optic nerves (II)**

Optic chiasm

Projection on left dorsal lateral geniculate nucleus

Projection on right dorsal lateral geniculate nucleus

Optic tracts

Lateral geniculate bodies

Optic radiation

Optic radiation

Calcarine sulcus

Calcarine sulcus

Projection on left occipital lobe

Projection on right occipital lobe

G

G

A

A

B

B

H

H

R R C

C

P

P

**Choroid**

**Choroid**

Periphery

Macula

## Structure of retina: schema

**A**  Amacrine cells
**B**  Bipolar cells
**C**  Cones
**G**  Ganglion cells
**H**  Horizontal cells
**P**  Pigment cells
**R**  Rods

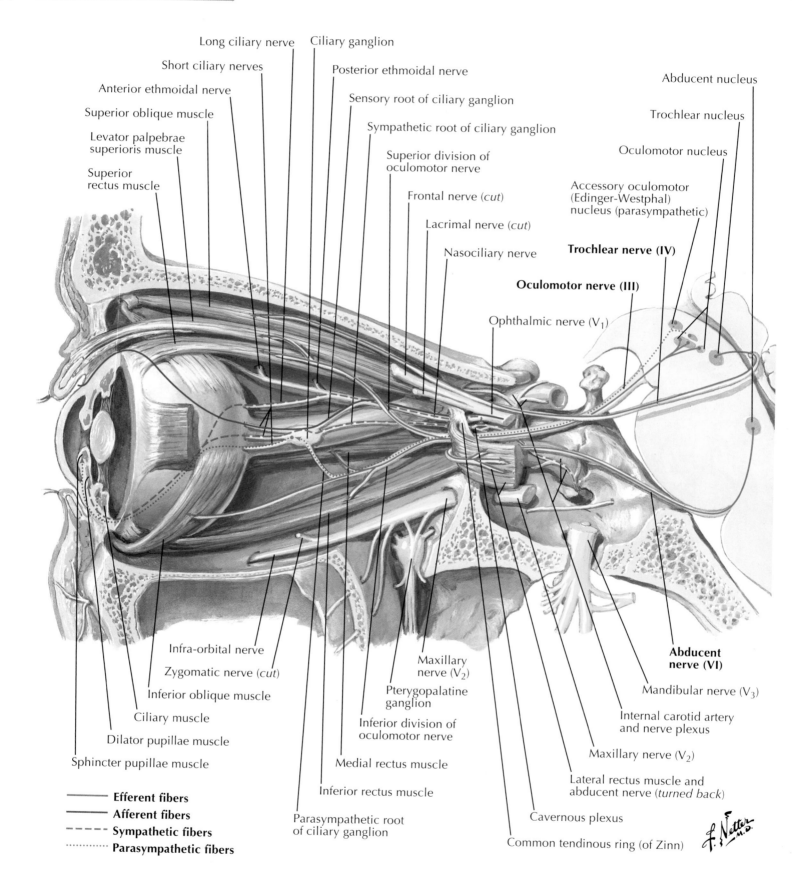

Long ciliary nerve

Short ciliary nerves

Anterior ethmoidal nerve

Superior oblique muscle

Levator palpebrae superioris muscle

Superior rectus muscle

Ciliary ganglion

Posterior ethmoidal nerve

Sensory root of ciliary ganglion

Sympathetic root of ciliary ganglion

Superior division of oculomotor nerve

Frontal nerve (cut)

Lacrimal nerve (cut)

Nasociliary nerve

Abducent nucleus

Trochlear nucleus

Oculomotor nucleus

Accessory oculomotor (Edinger-Westphal) nucleus (parasympathetic)

**Trochlear nerve (IV)**

**Oculomotor nerve (III)**

Ophthalmic nerve (V₁)

Infra-orbital nerve

Zygomatic nerve (cut)

Inferior oblique muscle

Ciliary muscle

Dilator pupillae muscle

Sphincter pupillae muscle

Maxillary nerve (V₂)

Pterygopalatine ganglion

Inferior division of oculomotor nerve

Medial rectus muscle

Inferior rectus muscle

Parasympathetic root of ciliary ganglion

**Abducent nerve (VI)**

Mandibular nerve (V₃)

Internal carotid artery and nerve plexus

Maxillary nerve (V₂)

Lateral rectus muscle and abducent nerve (turned back)

Cavernous plexus

Common tendinous ring (of Zinn)

———— **Efferent fibers**
———— **Afferent fibers**
– – – – **Sympathetic fibers**
·········· **Parasympathetic fibers**

**Plate 122**

**Cranial and Cervical Nerves**

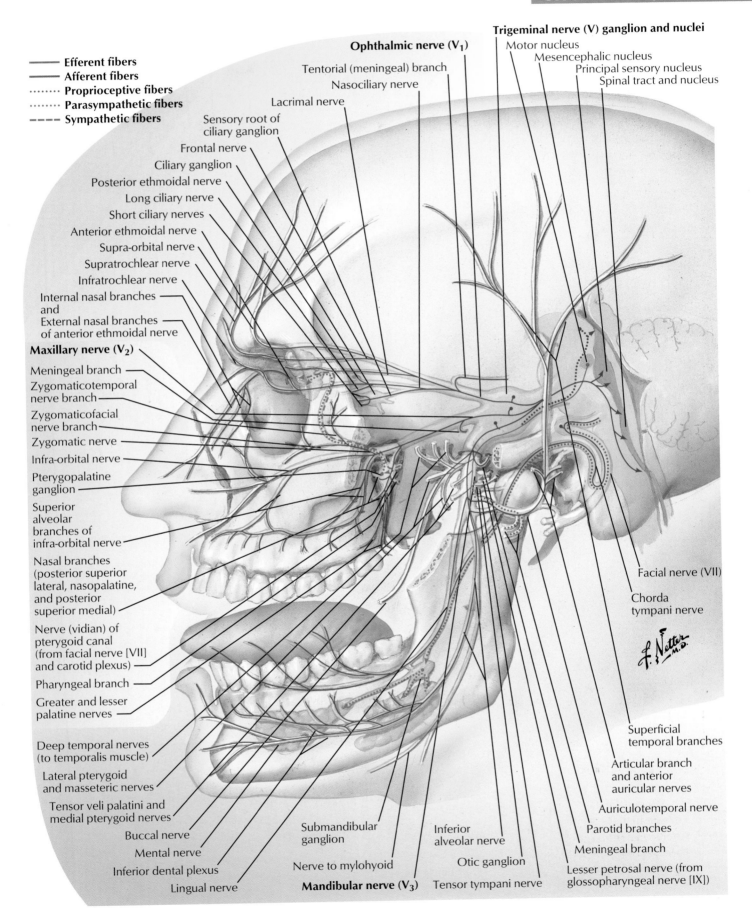

Efferent fibers
Afferent fibers
Proprioceptive fibers
Parasympathetic fibers
Sympathetic fibers

**Ophthalmic nerve (V₁)**

Tentorial (meningeal) branch

Nasociliary nerve

Lacrimal nerve

Sensory root of ciliary ganglion

Frontal nerve

Ciliary ganglion

Posterior ethmoidal nerve

Long ciliary nerve

Short ciliary nerves

Anterior ethmoidal nerve

Supra-orbital nerve

Supratrochlear nerve

Infratrochlear nerve

Internal nasal branches and

External nasal branches of anterior ethmoidal nerve

**Maxillary nerve (V₂)**

Meningeal branch

Zygomaticotemporal nerve branch

Zygomaticofacial nerve branch

Zygomatic nerve

Infra-orbital nerve

Pterygopalatine ganglion

Superior alveolar branches of infra-orbital nerve

Nasal branches (posterior superior lateral, nasopalatine, and posterior superior medial)

Nerve (vidian) of pterygoid canal (from facial nerve [VII] and carotid plexus)

Pharyngeal branch

Greater and lesser palatine nerves

Deep temporal nerves (to temporalis muscle)

Lateral pterygoid and masseteric nerves

Tensor veli palatini and medial pterygoid nerves

Buccal nerve

Mental nerve

Inferior dental plexus

Lingual nerve

Submandibular ganglion

Inferior alveolar nerve

Nerve to mylohyoid

Otic ganglion

**Mandibular nerve (V₃)**

Tensor tympani nerve

**Trigeminal nerve (V) ganglion and nuclei**

Motor nucleus

Mesencephalic nucleus

Principal sensory nucleus

Spinal tract and nucleus

Facial nerve (VII)

Chorda tympani nerve

Superficial temporal branches

Articular branch and anterior auricular nerves

Auriculotemporal nerve

Parotid branches

Meningeal branch

Lesser petrosal nerve (from glossopharyngeal nerve [IX])

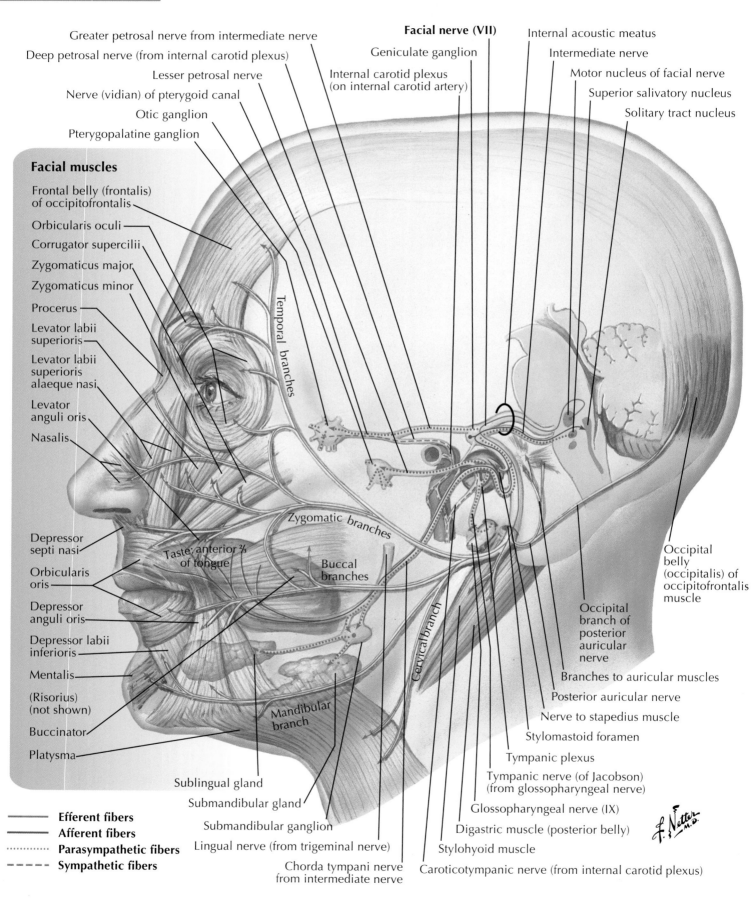

Greater petrosal nerve from intermediate nerve

Deep petrosal nerve (from internal carotid plexus)

Lesser petrosal nerve

Nerve (vidian) of pterygoid canal

Otic ganglion

Pterygopalatine ganglion

**Facial nerve (VII)**

Geniculate ganglion

Internal carotid plexus (on internal carotid artery)

Internal acoustic meatus

Intermediate nerve

Motor nucleus of facial nerve

Superior salivatory nucleus

Solitary tract nucleus

**Facial muscles**

Frontal belly (frontalis) of occipitofrontalis

Orbicularis oculi

Corrugator supercilii

Zygomaticus major

Zygomaticus minor

Procerus

Levator labii superioris

Levator labii superioris alaeque nasi

Levator anguli oris

Nasalis

Depressor septi nasi

Orbicularis oris

Depressor anguli oris

Depressor labii inferioris

Mentalis

(Risorius) (not shown)

Buccinator

Platysma

Temporal branches

Zygomatic branches

Taste: anterior ⅔ of tongue

Buccal branches

Cervical branch

Mandibular branch

Sublingual gland

Submandibular gland

Submandibular ganglion

Lingual nerve (from trigeminal nerve)

Chorda tympani nerve from intermediate nerve

Occipital belly (occipitalis) of occipitofrontalis muscle

Occipital branch of posterior auricular nerve

Branches to auricular muscles

Posterior auricular nerve

Nerve to stapedius muscle

Stylomastoid foramen

Tympanic plexus

Tympanic nerve (of Jacobson) (from glossopharyngeal nerve)

Glossopharyngeal nerve (IX)

Digastric muscle (posterior belly)

Stylohyoid muscle

Caroticotympanic nerve (from internal carotid plexus)

—— Efferent fibers
—— Afferent fibers
·········· Parasympathetic fibers
- - - - Sympathetic fibers

**Plate 124**

**Cranial and Cervical Nerves**

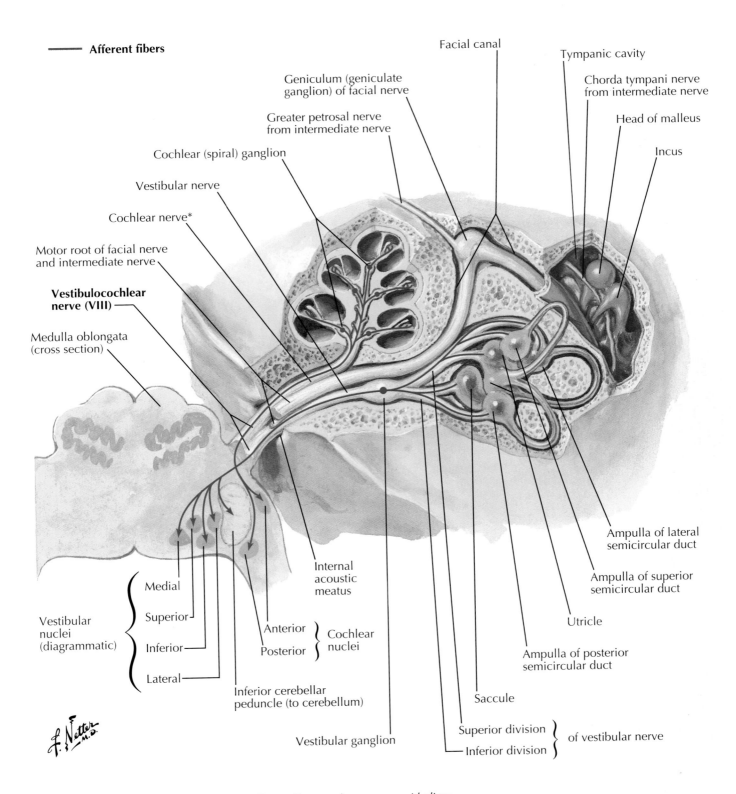

—— **Afferent fibers**

Facial canal

Tympanic cavity

Geniculum (geniculate ganglion) of facial nerve

Chorda tympani nerve from intermediate nerve

Greater petrosal nerve from intermediate nerve

Head of malleus

Cochlear (spiral) ganglion

Incus

Vestibular nerve

Cochlear nerve*

Motor root of facial nerve and intermediate nerve

**Vestibulocochlear nerve (VIII)**

Medulla oblongata (cross section)

Ampulla of lateral semicircular duct

Ampulla of superior semicircular duct

Internal acoustic meatus

Utricle

Medial

Superior

Anterior } Cochlear nuclei

Vestibular nuclei (diagrammatic)

Inferior

Posterior

Ampulla of posterior semicircular duct

Lateral

Inferior cerebellar peduncle (to cerebellum)

Saccule

Superior division } of vestibular nerve

Vestibular ganglion

Inferior division }

*Note: The cochlear nerve also contains efferent fibers to the sensory epithelium. These fibers are derived from the vestibular nerve while in the internal auditory meatus.*

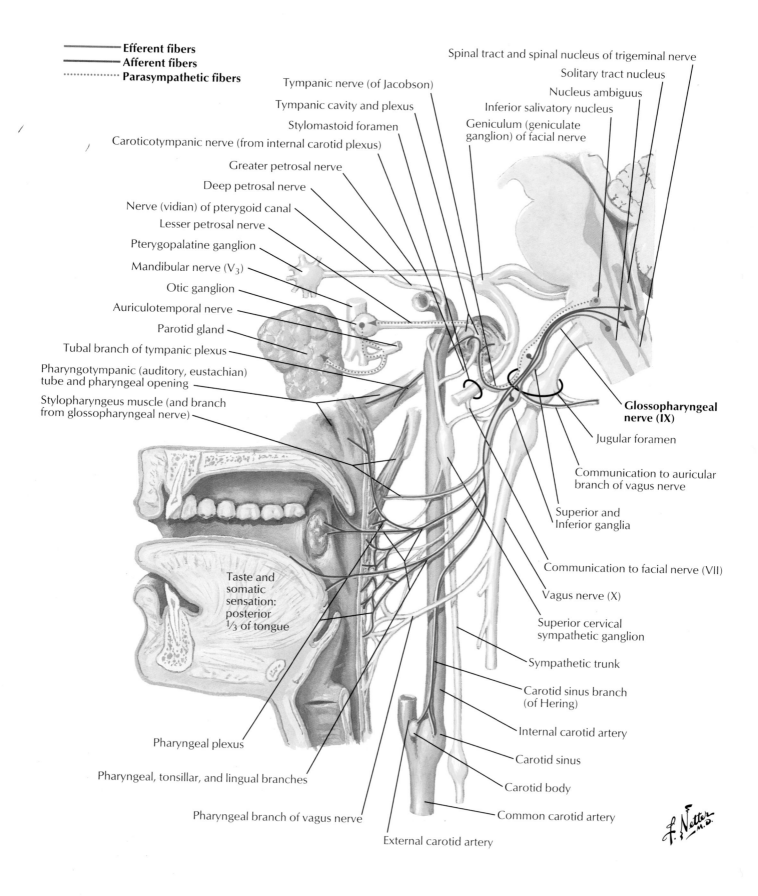

**Efferent fibers**
**Afferent fibers**
**Parasympathetic fibers**

Spinal tract and spinal nucleus of trigeminal nerve

Solitary tract nucleus

Nucleus ambiguus

Inferior salivatory nucleus

Tympanic nerve (of Jacobson)

Tympanic cavity and plexus

Stylomastoid foramen

Geniculum (geniculate ganglion) of facial nerve

Caroticotympanic nerve (from internal carotid plexus)

Greater petrosal nerve

Deep petrosal nerve

Nerve (vidian) of pterygoid canal

Lesser petrosal nerve

Pterygopalatine ganglion

Mandibular nerve (V₃)

Otic ganglion

Auriculotemporal nerve

Parotid gland

Tubal branch of tympanic plexus

Pharyngotympanic (auditory, eustachian) tube and pharyngeal opening

Stylopharyngeus muscle (and branch from glossopharyngeal nerve)

Glossopharyngeal nerve (IX)

Jugular foramen

Communication to auricular branch of vagus nerve

Superior and Inferior ganglia

Communication to facial nerve (VII)

Vagus nerve (X)

Superior cervical sympathetic ganglion

Sympathetic trunk

Carotid sinus branch (of Hering)

Internal carotid artery

Carotid sinus

Carotid body

Common carotid artery

Taste and somatic sensation: posterior ⅓ of tongue

Pharyngeal plexus

Pharyngeal, tonsillar, and lingual branches

Pharyngeal branch of vagus nerve

External carotid artery

**Plate 126**

**Cranial and Cervical Nerves**

Glossopharyngeal nerve (IX)

Meningeal branch of vagus nerve

Auricular branch of vagus nerve

Pharyngotympanic (auditory, eustachian) tube

Levator veli palatini muscle

Salpingopharyngeus muscle

Palatoglossus muscle

Palatopharyngeus muscle

Superior pharyngeal constrictor muscle

Stylopharyngeus muscle

Middle pharyngeal constrictor muscle

Inferior pharyngeal constrictor muscle

Cricothyroid muscle

Trachea

Esophagus

Right subclavian artery

Right recurrent laryngeal nerve

Heart

Hepatic branch of anterior vagal trunk (in lesser omentum)

Celiac branches from anterior and posterior vagal trunks to celiac plexus

Celiac and superior mesenteric ganglia and celiac plexus

Hepatic plexus

Gallbladder and bile ducts

Liver

Pyloric branch from hepatic plexus

Pancreas

Duodenum

Ascending colon

Cecum

Appendix

Dorsal nucleus of vagus nerve (parasympathetic and visceral afferent)

Solitary tract nucleus (visceral afferents including taste)

Spinal tract and spinal nucleus of trigeminal nerve (somatic afferent)

Nucleus ambiguus (motor to pharyngeal and laryngeal muscles)

Cranial root

**Vagus nerve (X)**

Jugular foramen

Superior ganglion of vagus nerve

Inferior ganglion of vagus nerve

Pharyngeal branch of vagus nerve (motor to muscles of palate and pharynx; sensory to lower pharynx)

Communicating branch of vagus nerve to carotid branch of glossopharyngeal nerve

Pharyngeal plexus

Superior laryngeal nerve:
Internal branch (sensory and parasympathetic)
External branch (motor to cricothyroid muscle)

Superior cervical cardiac branch of vagus nerve

Inferior cervical cardiac branch of vagus nerve

Thoracic cardiac branch of vagus nerve

Left recurrent laryngeal nerve (motor to muscles of larynx except cricothyroid; sensory and parasympathetic to larynx below vocal folds; parasympathetic, efferent, and afferent to upper esophagus and trachea)

Pulmonary plexus

Cardiac plexus

Esophageal plexus

Anterior vagal trunk

Gastric branches of anterior vagal trunk (branches from posterior trunk behind stomach)

Vagal fibers (parasympathetic motor, secretomotor, and afferent fibers) accompany superior mesenteric artery and its branches usually as far as left colic (splenic) flexure

Small intestine

Efferent fibers

Afferent fibers

Parasympathetic fibers

*F. Netter M.D.*

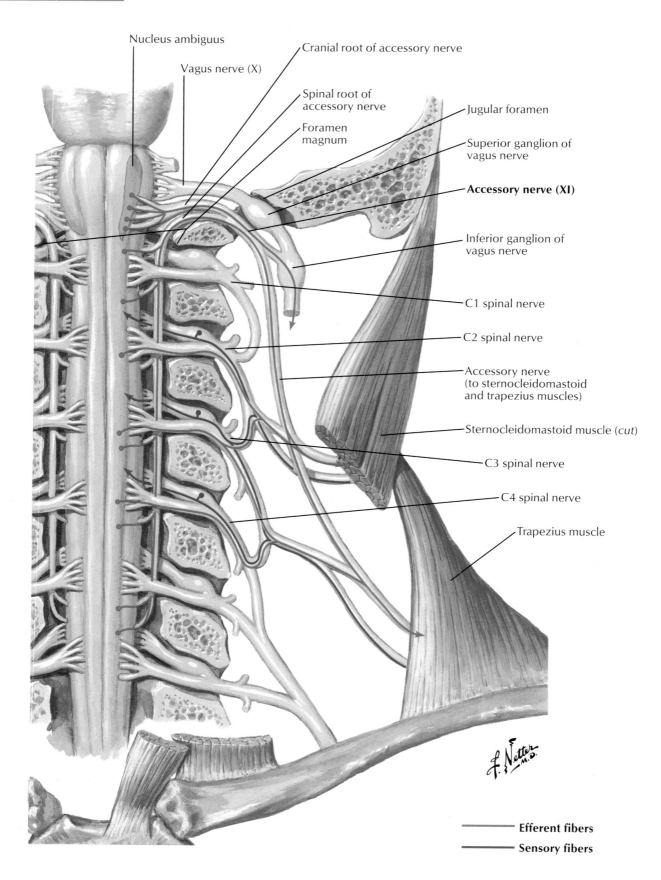

Nucleus ambiguus

Vagus nerve (X)

Cranial root of accessory nerve

Spinal root of accessory nerve

Foramen magnum

Jugular foramen

Superior ganglion of vagus nerve

**Accessory nerve (XI)**

Inferior ganglion of vagus nerve

C1 spinal nerve

C2 spinal nerve

Accessory nerve (to sternocleidomastoid and trapezius muscles)

Sternocleidomastoid muscle (*cut*)

C3 spinal nerve

C4 spinal nerve

Trapezius muscle

——— **Efferent fibers**

——— **Sensory fibers**

**Plate 128**

**Cranial and Cervical Nerves**

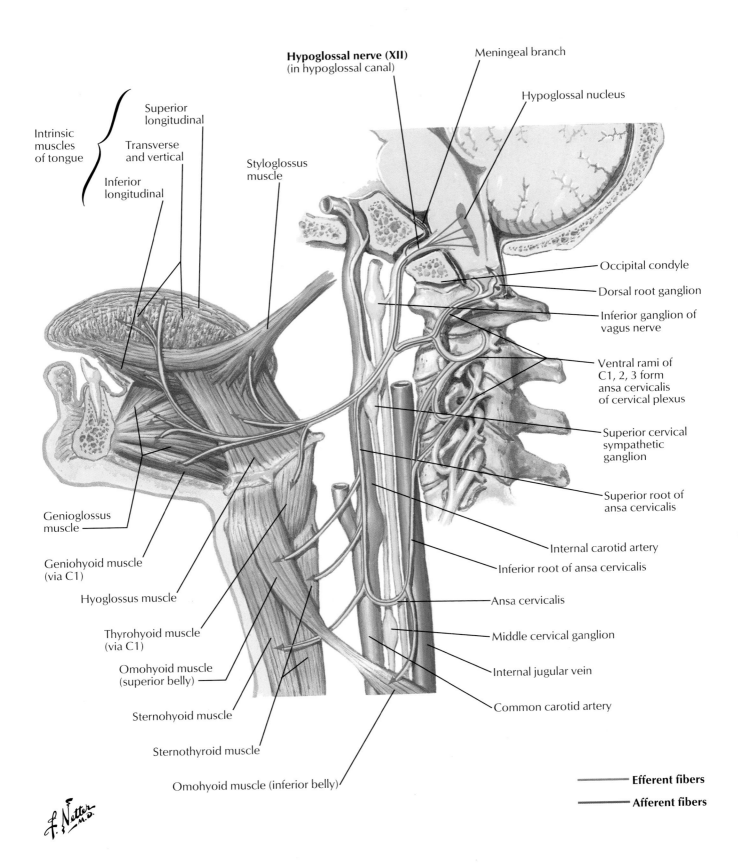

Intrinsic muscles of tongue
- Superior longitudinal
- Transverse and vertical
- Inferior longitudinal

Styloglossus muscle

Hypoglossal nerve (XII) (in hypoglossal canal)

Meningeal branch

Hypoglossal nucleus

Occipital condyle

Dorsal root ganglion

Inferior ganglion of vagus nerve

Ventral rami of C1, 2, 3 form ansa cervicalis of cervical plexus

Superior cervical sympathetic ganglion

Superior root of ansa cervicalis

Internal carotid artery

Inferior root of ansa cervicalis

Ansa cervicalis

Middle cervical ganglion

Internal jugular vein

Common carotid artery

Genioglossus muscle

Geniohyoid muscle (via C1)

Hyoglossus muscle

Thyrohyoid muscle (via C1)

Omohyoid muscle (superior belly)

Sternohyoid muscle

Sternothyroid muscle

Omohyoid muscle (inferior belly)

———— Efferent fibers

———— Afferent fibers

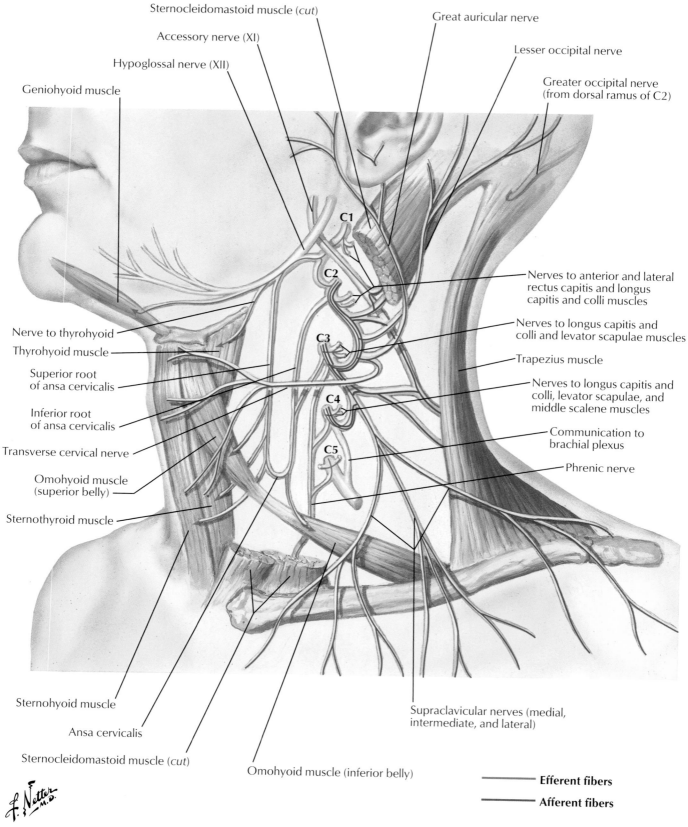

Sternocleidomastoid muscle (cut)

Accessory nerve (XI)

Hypoglossal nerve (XII)

Geniohyoid muscle

Great auricular nerve

Lesser occipital nerve

Greater occipital nerve
(from dorsal ramus of C2)

C1

C2

Nerves to anterior and lateral
rectus capitis and longus
capitis and colli muscles

Nerve to thyrohyoid

Thyrohyoid muscle

Nerves to longus capitis and
colli and levator scapulae muscles

C3

Superior root
of ansa cervicalis

Trapezius muscle

Inferior root
of ansa cervicalis

Nerves to longus capitis and
colli, levator scapulae, and
middle scalene muscles

C4

Transverse cervical nerve

Communication to
brachial plexus

Omohyoid muscle
(superior belly)

C5

Phrenic nerve

Sternothyroid muscle

Sternohyoid muscle

Ansa cervicalis

Supraclavicular nerves (medial,
intermediate, and lateral)

Sternocleidomastoid muscle (cut)

Omohyoid muscle (inferior belly)

——— **Efferent fibers**

——— **Afferent fibers**

**Plate 130**

**Cranial and Cervical Nerves**

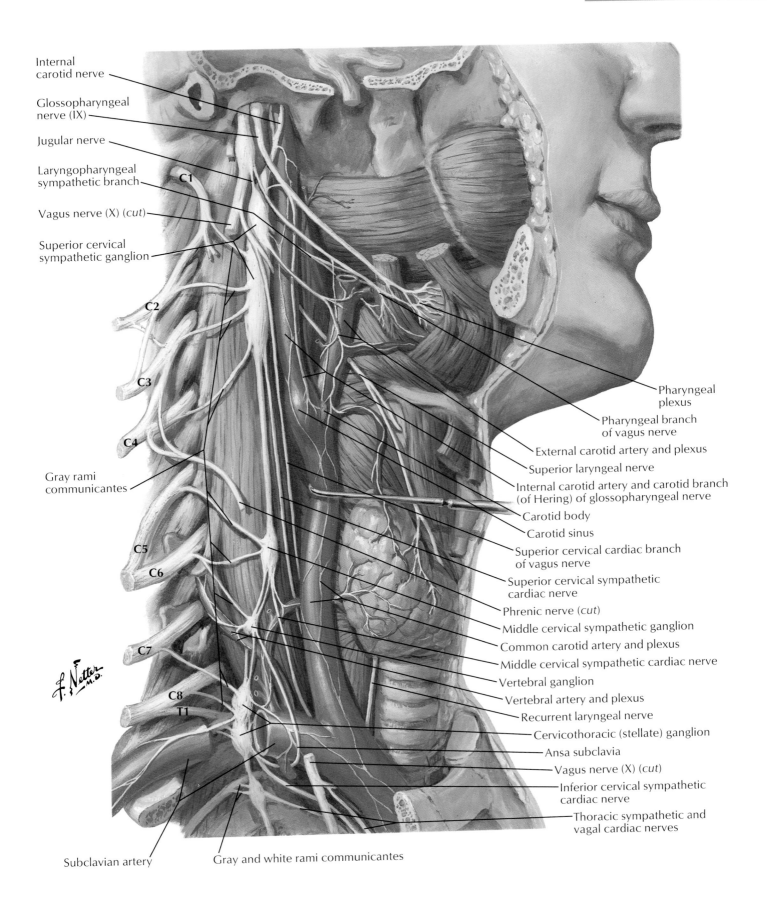

Internal carotid nerve

Glossopharyngeal nerve (IX)

Jugular nerve

Laryngopharyngeal sympathetic branch

Vagus nerve (X) (cut)

Superior cervical sympathetic ganglion

C1

C2

C3

C4

Gray rami communicantes

C5

C6

C7

C8
T1

Subclavian artery

Gray and white rami communicantes

Pharyngeal plexus

Pharyngeal branch of vagus nerve

External carotid artery and plexus

Superior laryngeal nerve

Internal carotid artery and carotid branch (of Hering) of glossopharyngeal nerve

Carotid body

Carotid sinus

Superior cervical cardiac branch of vagus nerve

Superior cervical sympathetic cardiac nerve

Phrenic nerve (cut)

Middle cervical sympathetic ganglion

Common carotid artery and plexus

Middle cervical sympathetic cardiac nerve

Vertebral ganglion

Vertebral artery and plexus

Recurrent laryngeal nerve

Cervicothoracic (stellate) ganglion

Ansa subclavia

Vagus nerve (X) (cut)

Inferior cervical sympathetic cardiac nerve

Thoracic sympathetic and vagal cardiac nerves

**Cranial and Cervical Nerves**

**Plate 131**

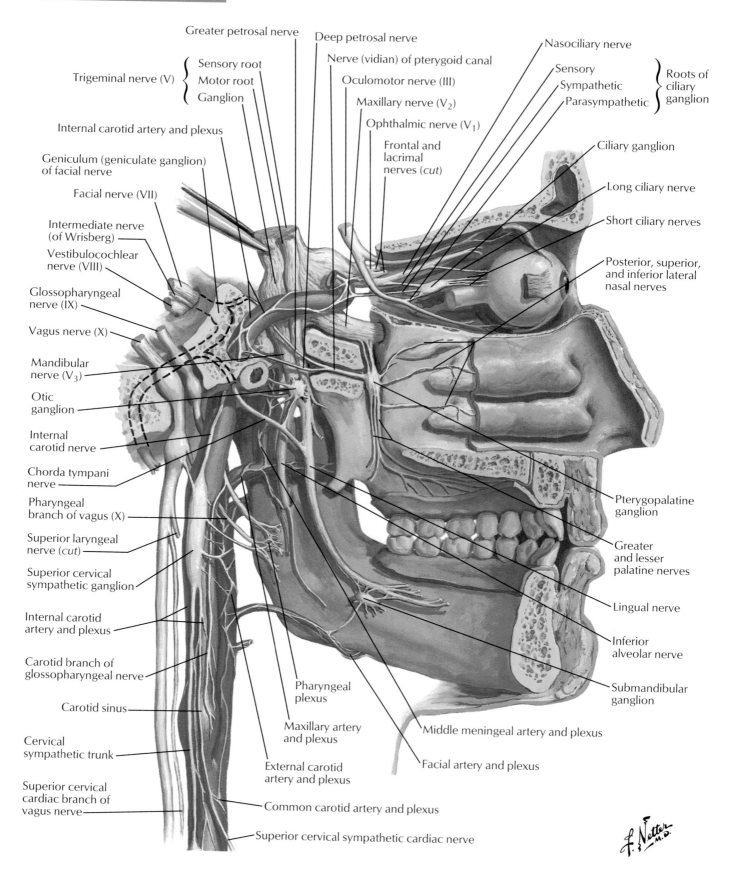

Greater petrosal nerve

Deep petrosal nerve

Nerve (vidian) of pterygoid canal

Nasociliary nerve

Trigeminal nerve (V) { Sensory root / Motor root / Ganglion }

Oculomotor nerve (III)

Sensory
Sympathetic
Parasympathetic } Roots of ciliary ganglion

Internal carotid artery and plexus

Maxillary nerve (V₂)

Ophthalmic nerve (V₁)

Ciliary ganglion

Geniculum (geniculate ganglion) of facial nerve

Frontal and lacrimal nerves (cut)

Long ciliary nerve

Facial nerve (VII)

Short ciliary nerves

Intermediate nerve (of Wrisberg)

Vestibulocochlear nerve (VIII)

Posterior, superior, and inferior lateral nasal nerves

Glossopharyngeal nerve (IX)

Vagus nerve (X)

Mandibular nerve (V₃)

Otic ganglion

Internal carotid nerve

Chorda tympani nerve

Pterygopalatine ganglion

Pharyngeal branch of vagus (X)

Superior laryngeal nerve (cut)

Superior cervical sympathetic ganglion

Greater and lesser palatine nerves

Internal carotid artery and plexus

Lingual nerve

Carotid branch of glossopharyngeal nerve

Inferior alveolar nerve

Carotid sinus

Pharyngeal plexus

Submandibular ganglion

Cervical sympathetic trunk

Maxillary artery and plexus

Middle meningeal artery and plexus

Superior cervical cardiac branch of vagus nerve

External carotid artery and plexus

Facial artery and plexus

Common carotid artery and plexus

Superior cervical sympathetic cardiac nerve

**Plate 132**

**Cranial and Cervical Nerves**

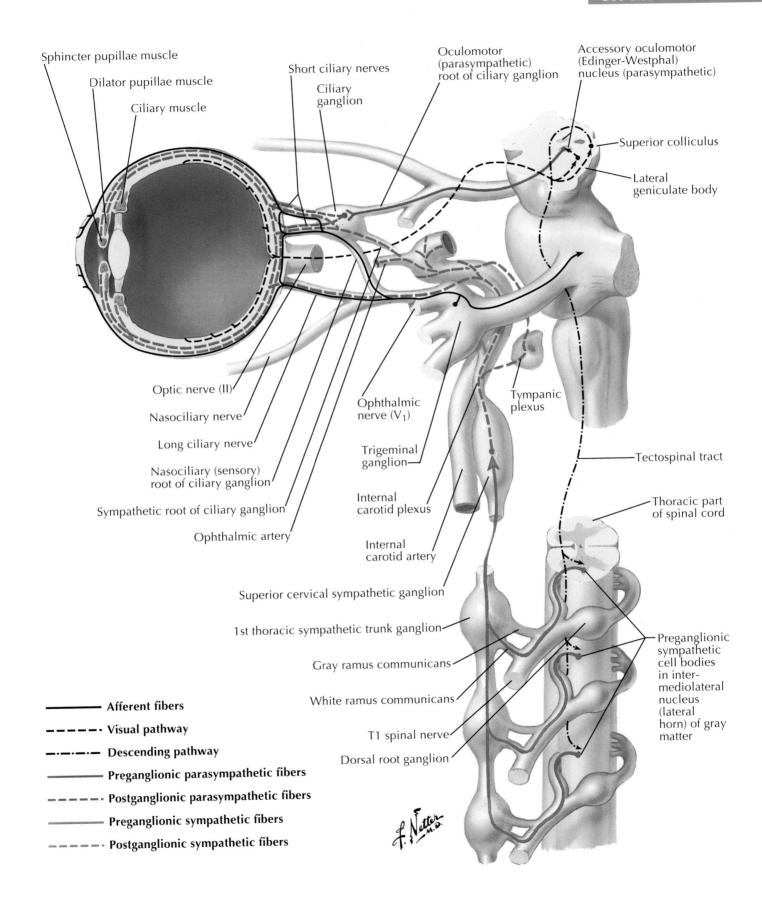

Sphincter pupillae muscle

Dilator pupillae muscle

Ciliary muscle

Short ciliary nerves

Ciliary ganglion

Oculomotor (parasympathetic) root of ciliary ganglion

Accessory oculomotor (Edinger-Westphal) nucleus (parasympathetic)

Superior colliculus

Lateral geniculate body

Optic nerve (II)

Nasociliary nerve

Long ciliary nerve

Nasociliary (sensory) root of ciliary ganglion

Sympathetic root of ciliary ganglion

Ophthalmic artery

Ophthalmic nerve (V$_1$)

Trigeminal ganglion

Internal carotid plexus

Internal carotid artery

Tympanic plexus

Tectospinal tract

Thoracic part of spinal cord

Superior cervical sympathetic ganglion

1st thoracic sympathetic trunk ganglion

Gray ramus communicans

White ramus communicans

T1 spinal nerve

Dorsal root ganglion

Preganglionic sympathetic cell bodies in intermediolateral nucleus (lateral horn) of gray matter

—— Afferent fibers

- - - - Visual pathway

—·—·— Descending pathway

—— Preganglionic parasympathetic fibers

- - - - Postganglionic parasympathetic fibers

—— Preganglionic sympathetic fibers

- - - - Postganglionic sympathetic fibers

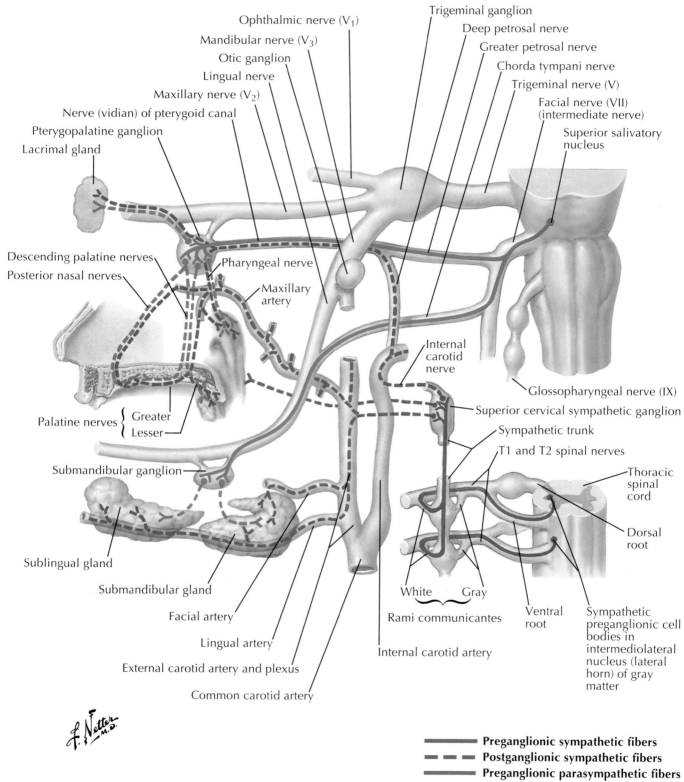

Ophthalmic nerve (V₁)
Mandibular nerve (V₃)
Otic ganglion
Lingual nerve
Maxillary nerve (V₂)
Nerve (vidian) of pterygoid canal
Pterygopalatine ganglion
Lacrimal gland

Trigeminal ganglion
Deep petrosal nerve
Greater petrosal nerve
Chorda tympani nerve
Trigeminal nerve (V)
Facial nerve (VII) (intermediate nerve)
Superior salivatory nucleus

Descending palatine nerves
Posterior nasal nerves
Pharyngeal nerve
Maxillary artery

Palatine nerves { Greater Lesser

Internal carotid nerve

Glossopharyngeal nerve (IX)
Superior cervical sympathetic ganglion
Sympathetic trunk
T1 and T2 spinal nerves
Thoracic spinal cord
Dorsal root

Submandibular ganglion

Sublingual gland
Submandibular gland
Facial artery
Lingual artery
External carotid artery and plexus
Common carotid artery

White    Gray
Rami communicantes
Internal carotid artery

Ventral root
Sympathetic preganglionic cell bodies in intermediolateral nucleus (lateral horn) of gray matter

——— Preganglionic sympathetic fibers
– – – Postganglionic sympathetic fibers
——— Preganglionic parasympathetic fibers
– – – Postganglionic parasympathetic fibers

**Plate 134**

**Cranial and Cervical Nerves**

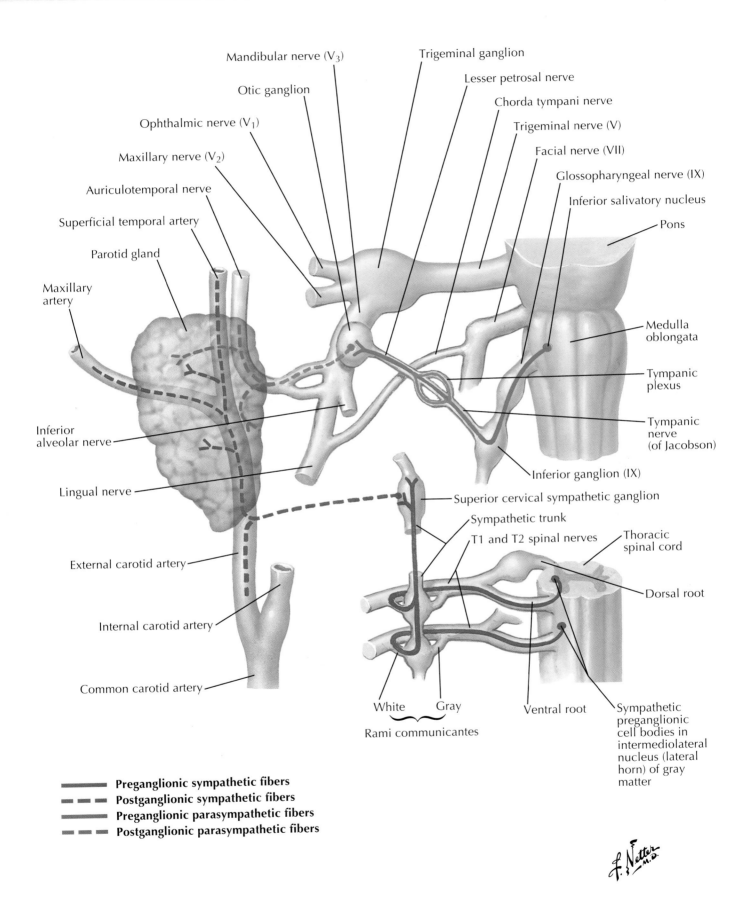

Mandibular nerve (V₃)

Otic ganglion

Ophthalmic nerve (V₁)

Maxillary nerve (V₂)

Auriculotemporal nerve

Superficial temporal artery

Parotid gland

Maxillary artery

Inferior alveolar nerve

Lingual nerve

External carotid artery

Internal carotid artery

Common carotid artery

Trigeminal ganglion

Lesser petrosal nerve

Chorda tympani nerve

Trigeminal nerve (V)

Facial nerve (VII)

Glossopharyngeal nerve (IX)

Inferior salivatory nucleus

Pons

Medulla oblongata

Tympanic plexus

Tympanic nerve (of Jacobson)

Inferior ganglion (IX)

Superior cervical sympathetic ganglion

Sympathetic trunk

T1 and T2 spinal nerves

Thoracic spinal cord

Dorsal root

Ventral root

Sympathetic preganglionic cell bodies in intermediolateral nucleus (lateral horn) of gray matter

White    Gray

Rami communicantes

Preganglionic sympathetic fibers
Postganglionic sympathetic fibers
Preganglionic parasympathetic fibers
Postganglionic parasympathetic fibers

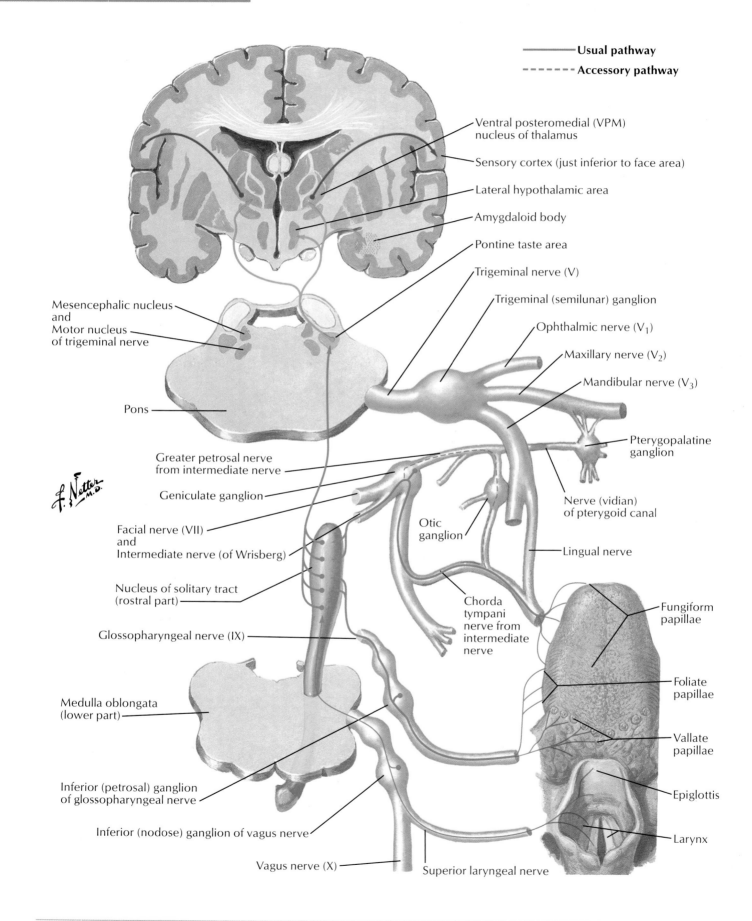

Usual pathway

Accessory pathway

Ventral posteromedial (VPM) nucleus of thalamus

Sensory cortex (just inferior to face area)

Lateral hypothalamic area

Amygdaloid body

Pontine taste area

Trigeminal nerve (V)

Trigeminal (semilunar) ganglion

Ophthalmic nerve (V₁)

Maxillary nerve (V₂)

Mandibular nerve (V₃)

Pterygopalatine ganglion

Nerve (vidian) of pterygoid canal

Lingual nerve

Fungiform papillae

Foliate papillae

Vallate papillae

Epiglottis

Larynx

Mesencephalic nucleus and Motor nucleus of trigeminal nerve

Pons

Greater petrosal nerve from intermediate nerve

Geniculate ganglion

Facial nerve (VII) and Intermediate nerve (of Wrisberg)

Nucleus of solitary tract (rostral part)

Glossopharyngeal nerve (IX)

Otic ganglion

Chorda tympani nerve from intermediate nerve

Medulla oblongata (lower part)

Inferior (petrosal) ganglion of glossopharyngeal nerve

Inferior (nodose) ganglion of vagus nerve

Vagus nerve (X)

Superior laryngeal nerve

**Plate 136**

**Cranial and Cervical Nerves**

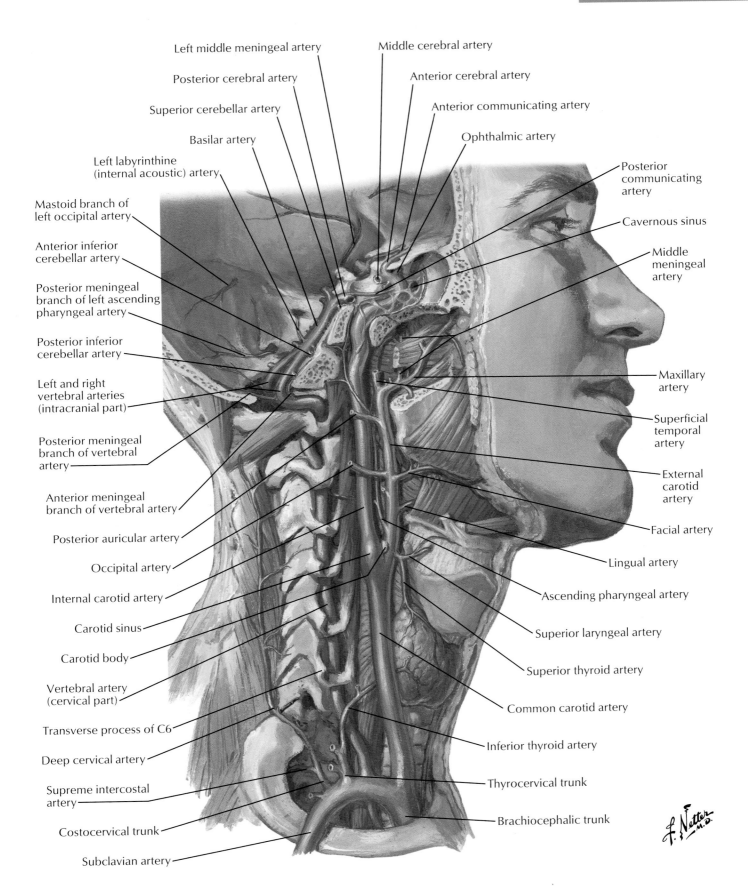

Left middle meningeal artery

Posterior cerebral artery

Superior cerebellar artery

Basilar artery

Left labyrinthine (internal acoustic) artery

Mastoid branch of left occipital artery

Anterior inferior cerebellar artery

Posterior meningeal branch of left ascending pharyngeal artery

Posterior inferior cerebellar artery

Left and right vertebral arteries (intracranial part)

Posterior meningeal branch of vertebral artery

Anterior meningeal branch of vertebral artery

Posterior auricular artery

Occipital artery

Internal carotid artery

Carotid sinus

Carotid body

Vertebral artery (cervical part)

Transverse process of C6

Deep cervical artery

Supreme intercostal artery

Costocervical trunk

Subclavian artery

Middle cerebral artery

Anterior cerebral artery

Anterior communicating artery

Ophthalmic artery

Posterior communicating artery

Cavernous sinus

Middle meningeal artery

Maxillary artery

Superficial temporal artery

External carotid artery

Facial artery

Lingual artery

Ascending pharyngeal artery

Superior laryngeal artery

Superior thyroid artery

Common carotid artery

Inferior thyroid artery

Thyrocervical trunk

Brachiocephalic trunk

*f. Netter*
M.D.

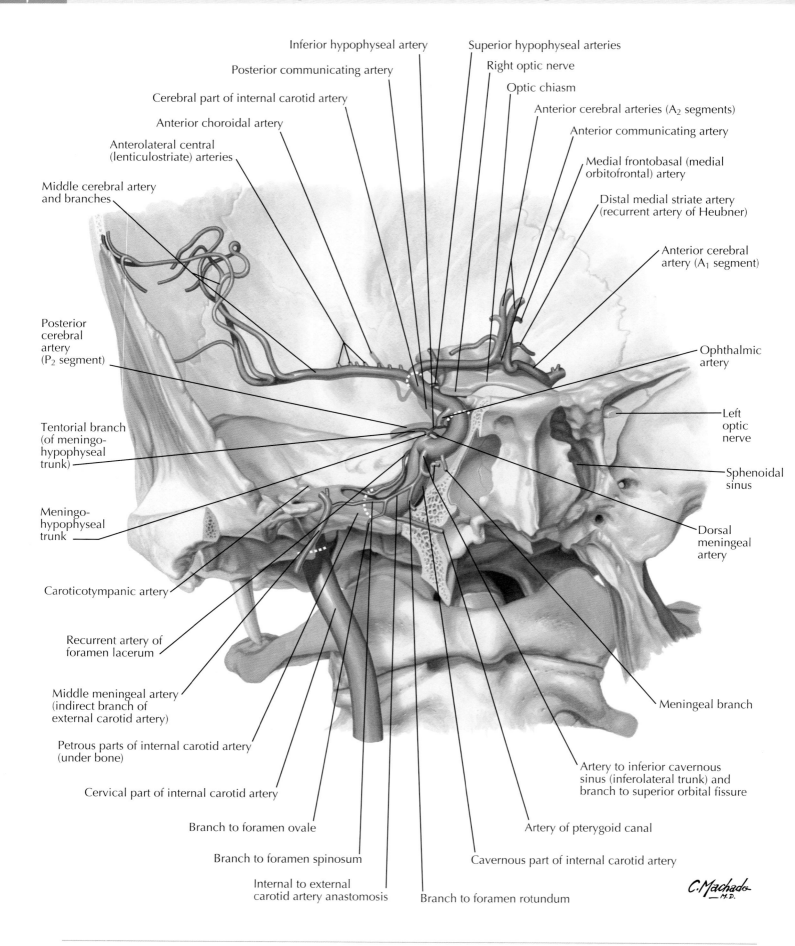

Inferior hypophyseal artery

Superior hypophyseal arteries

Posterior communicating artery

Right optic nerve

Cerebral part of internal carotid artery

Optic chiasm

Anterior choroidal artery

Anterior cerebral arteries (A₂ segments)

Anterolateral central (lenticulostriate) arteries

Anterior communicating artery

Medial frontobasal (medial orbitofrontal) artery

Middle cerebral artery and branches

Distal medial striate artery (recurrent artery of Heubner)

Anterior cerebral artery (A₁ segment)

Posterior cerebral artery (P₂ segment)

Ophthalmic artery

Tentorial branch (of meningo-hypophyseal trunk)

Left optic nerve

Sphenoidal sinus

Meningo-hypophyseal trunk

Dorsal meningeal artery

Caroticotympanic artery

Recurrent artery of foramen lacerum

Middle meningeal artery (indirect branch of external carotid artery)

Meningeal branch

Petrous parts of internal carotid artery (under bone)

Cervical part of internal carotid artery

Artery to inferior cavernous sinus (inferolateral trunk) and branch to superior orbital fissure

Branch to foramen ovale

Artery of pterygoid canal

Branch to foramen spinosum

Cavernous part of internal carotid artery

Internal to external carotid artery anastomosis

Branch to foramen rotundum

**Plate 138**

**Cerebral Vasculature**

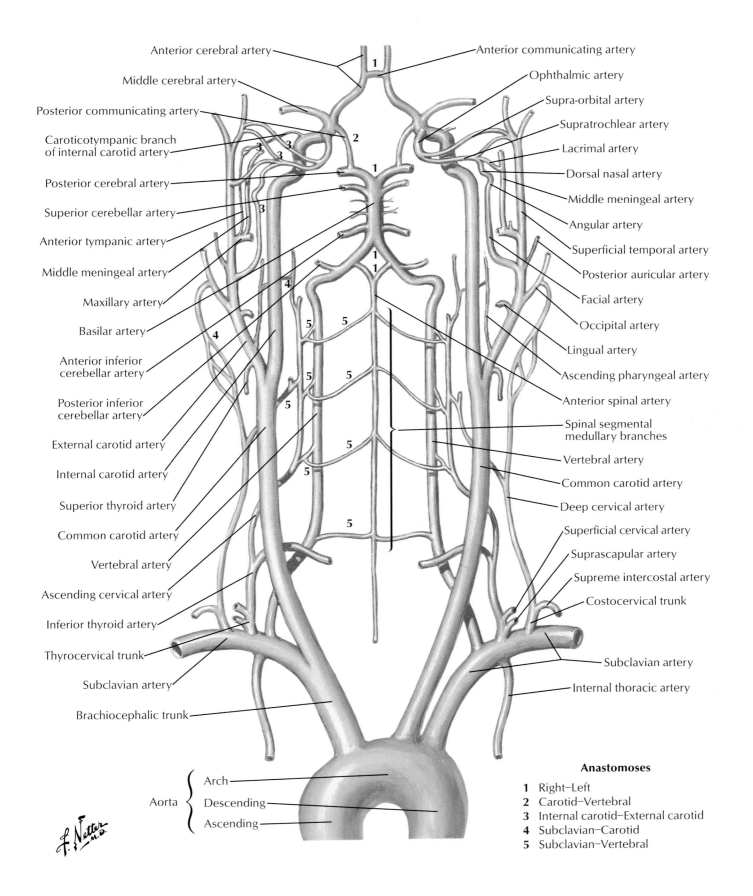

Anterior cerebral artery

Middle cerebral artery

Posterior communicating artery

Caroticotympanic branch of internal carotid artery

Posterior cerebral artery

Superior cerebellar artery

Anterior tympanic artery

Middle meningeal artery

Maxillary artery

Basilar artery

Anterior inferior cerebellar artery

Posterior inferior cerebellar artery

External carotid artery

Internal carotid artery

Superior thyroid artery

Common carotid artery

Vertebral artery

Ascending cervical artery

Inferior thyroid artery

Thyrocervical trunk

Subclavian artery

Brachiocephalic trunk

Anterior communicating artery

Ophthalmic artery

Supra-orbital artery

Supratrochlear artery

Lacrimal artery

Dorsal nasal artery

Middle meningeal artery

Angular artery

Superficial temporal artery

Posterior auricular artery

Facial artery

Occipital artery

Lingual artery

Ascending pharyngeal artery

Anterior spinal artery

Spinal segmental medullary branches

Vertebral artery

Common carotid artery

Deep cervical artery

Superficial cervical artery

Suprascapular artery

Supreme intercostal artery

Costocervical trunk

Subclavian artery

Internal thoracic artery

Aorta { Arch

Descending

Ascending

**Anastomoses**

1  Right–Left
2  Carotid–Vertebral
3  Internal carotid–External carotid
4  Subclavian–Carotid
5  Subclavian–Vertebral

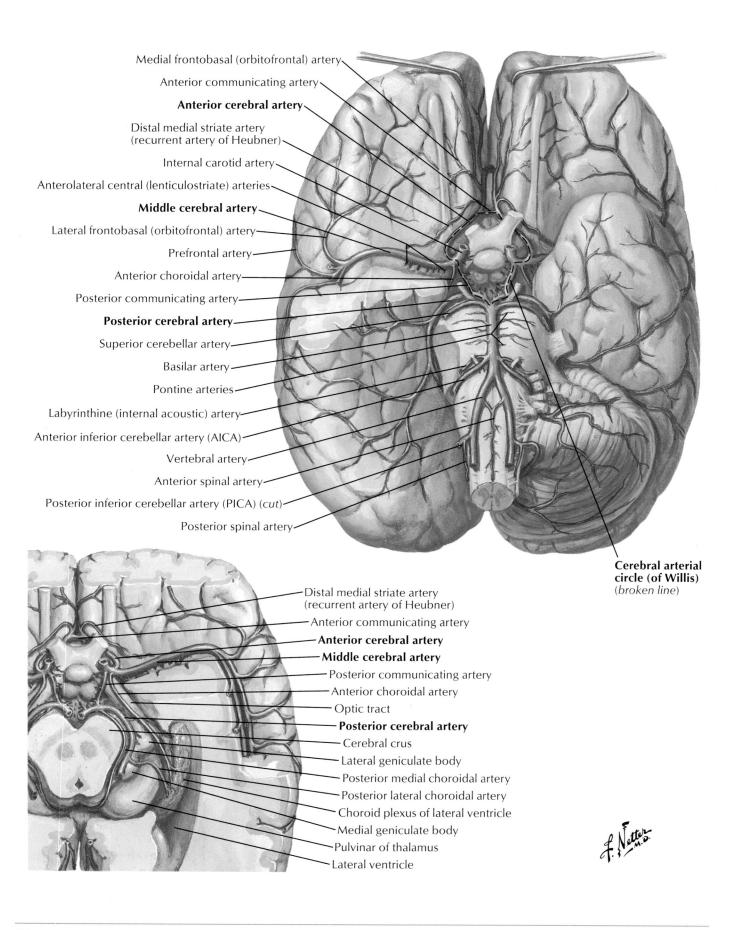

Medial frontobasal (orbitofrontal) artery

Anterior communicating artery

**Anterior cerebral artery**

Distal medial striate artery
(recurrent artery of Heubner)

Internal carotid artery

Anterolateral central (lenticulostriate) arteries

**Middle cerebral artery**

Lateral frontobasal (orbitofrontal) artery

Prefrontal artery

Anterior choroidal artery

Posterior communicating artery

**Posterior cerebral artery**

Superior cerebellar artery

Basilar artery

Pontine arteries

Labyrinthine (internal acoustic) artery

Anterior inferior cerebellar artery (AICA)

Vertebral artery

Anterior spinal artery

Posterior inferior cerebellar artery (PICA) (*cut*)

Posterior spinal artery

**Cerebral arterial
circle (of Willis)**
(*broken line*)

Distal medial striate artery
(recurrent artery of Heubner)

Anterior communicating artery

**Anterior cerebral artery**

**Middle cerebral artery**

Posterior communicating artery

Anterior choroidal artery

Optic tract

**Posterior cerebral artery**

Cerebral crus

Lateral geniculate body

Posterior medial choroidal artery

Posterior lateral choroidal artery

Choroid plexus of lateral ventricle

Medial geniculate body

Pulvinar of thalamus

Lateral ventricle

**Plate 140**

**Cerebral Vasculature**

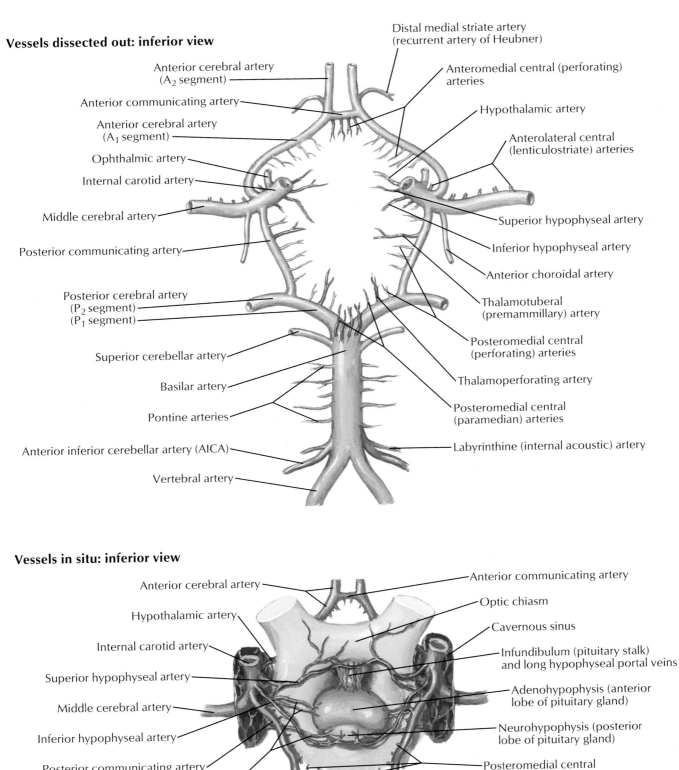

**Vessels dissected out: inferior view**

Anterior cerebral artery (A₂ segment)

Anterior communicating artery

Anterior cerebral artery (A₁ segment)

Ophthalmic artery

Internal carotid artery

Middle cerebral artery

Posterior communicating artery

Posterior cerebral artery (P₂ segment) (P₁ segment)

Superior cerebellar artery

Basilar artery

Pontine arteries

Anterior inferior cerebellar artery (AICA)

Vertebral artery

Distal medial striate artery (recurrent artery of Heubner)

Anteromedial central (perforating) arteries

Hypothalamic artery

Anterolateral central (lenticulostriate) arteries

Superior hypophyseal artery

Inferior hypophyseal artery

Anterior choroidal artery

Thalamotuberal (premammillary) artery

Posteromedial central (perforating) arteries

Thalamoperforating artery

Posteromedial central (paramedian) arteries

Labyrinthine (internal acoustic) artery

**Vessels in situ: inferior view**

Anterior cerebral artery

Hypothalamic artery

Internal carotid artery

Superior hypophyseal artery

Middle cerebral artery

Inferior hypophyseal artery

Posterior communicating artery

Efferent hypophyseal veins

Posterior cerebral artery

Anterior communicating artery

Optic chiasm

Cavernous sinus

Infundibulum (pituitary stalk) and long hypophyseal portal veins

Adenohypophysis (anterior lobe of pituitary gland)

Neurohypophysis (posterior lobe of pituitary gland)

Posteromedial central (perforating) arteries

Superior cerebellar artery

Basilar artery

*F. Netter M.D.*

**Cerebral Vasculature**

**Plate 141**

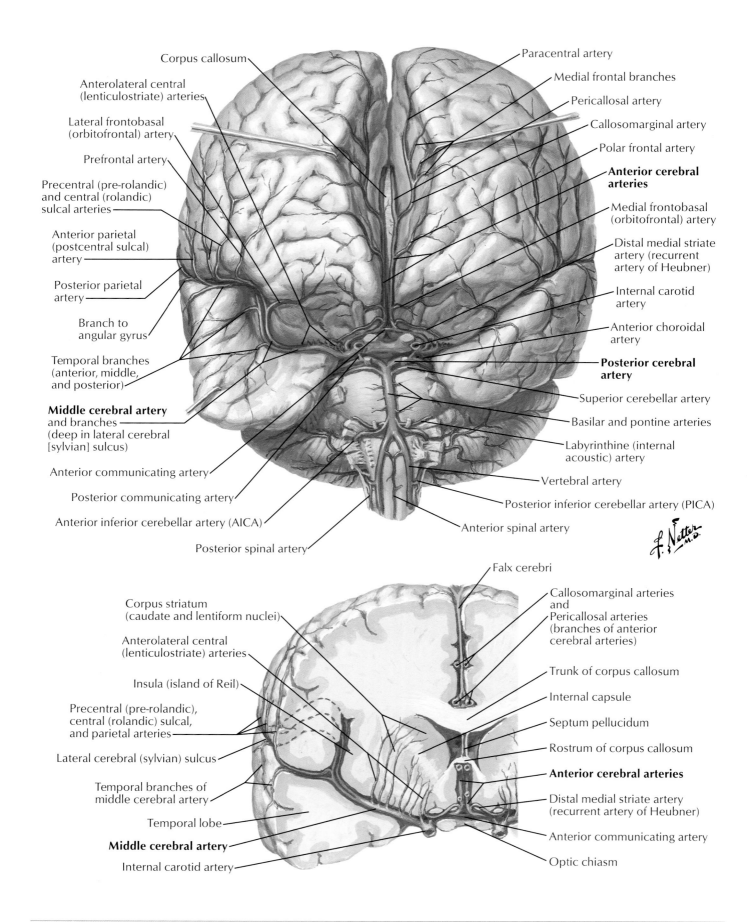

Corpus callosum

Anterolateral central (lenticulostriate) arteries

Lateral frontobasal (orbitofrontal) artery

Prefrontal artery

Precentral (pre-rolandic) and central (rolandic) sulcal arteries

Anterior parietal (postcentral sulcal) artery

Posterior parietal artery

Branch to angular gyrus

Temporal branches (anterior, middle, and posterior)

**Middle cerebral artery** and branches (deep in lateral cerebral [sylvian] sulcus)

Anterior communicating artery

Posterior communicating artery

Anterior inferior cerebellar artery (AICA)

Posterior spinal artery

Paracentral artery

Medial frontal branches

Pericallosal artery

Callosomarginal artery

Polar frontal artery

**Anterior cerebral arteries**

Medial frontobasal (orbitofrontal) artery

Distal medial striate artery (recurrent artery of Heubner)

Internal carotid artery

Anterior choroidal artery

**Posterior cerebral artery**

Superior cerebellar artery

Basilar and pontine arteries

Labyrinthine (internal acoustic) artery

Vertebral artery

Posterior inferior cerebellar artery (PICA)

Anterior spinal artery

Falx cerebri

Corpus striatum (caudate and lentiform nuclei)

Anterolateral central (lenticulostriate) arteries

Insula (island of Reil)

Precentral (pre-rolandic), central (rolandic) sulcal, and parietal arteries

Lateral cerebral (sylvian) sulcus

Temporal branches of middle cerebral artery

Temporal lobe

**Middle cerebral artery**

Internal carotid artery

Callosomarginal arteries and Pericallosal arteries (branches of anterior cerebral arteries)

Trunk of corpus callosum

Internal capsule

Septum pellucidum

Rostrum of corpus callosum

**Anterior cerebral arteries**

Distal medial striate artery (recurrent artery of Heubner)

Anterior communicating artery

Optic chiasm

**Plate 142**     **Cerebral Vasculature**

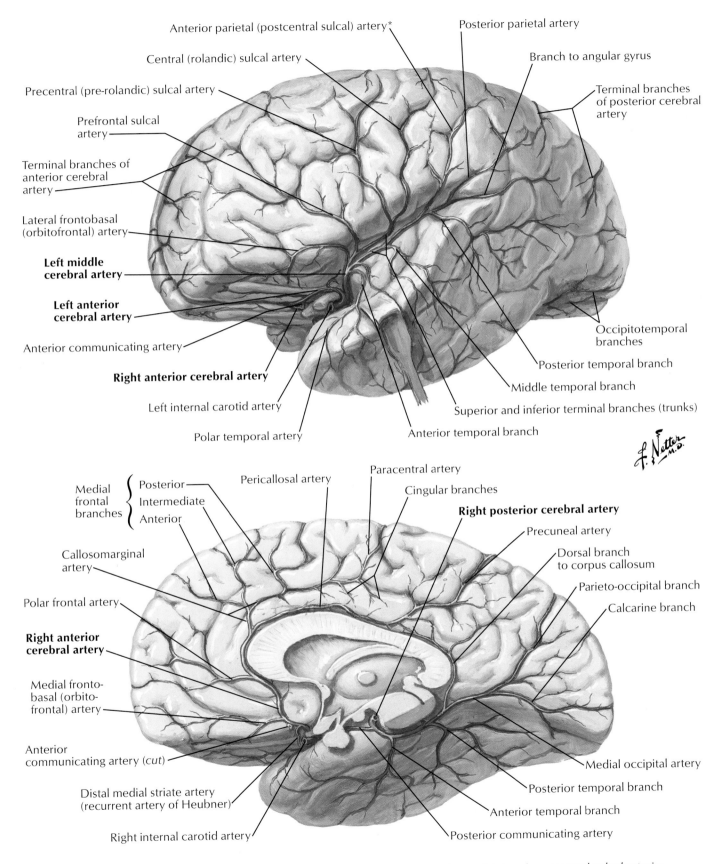

Anterior parietal (postcentral sulcal) artery*

Posterior parietal artery

Central (rolandic) sulcal artery

Branch to angular gyrus

Precentral (pre-rolandic) sulcal artery

Terminal branches of posterior cerebral artery

Prefrontal sulcal artery

Terminal branches of anterior cerebral artery

Lateral frontobasal (orbitofrontal) artery

**Left middle cerebral artery**

**Left anterior cerebral artery**

Occipitotemporal branches

Anterior communicating artery

Posterior temporal branch

**Right anterior cerebral artery**

Middle temporal branch

Left internal carotid artery

Superior and inferior terminal branches (trunks)

Polar temporal artery

Anterior temporal branch

Paracentral artery

Medial frontal branches { Posterior — Intermediate — Anterior

Pericallosal artery

Cingular branches

**Right posterior cerebral artery**

Precuneal artery

Callosomarginal artery

Dorsal branch to corpus callosum

Polar frontal artery

Parieto-occipital branch

**Right anterior cerebral artery**

Calcarine branch

Medial fronto-basal (orbito-frontal) artery

Anterior communicating artery (*cut*)

Distal medial striate artery (recurrent artery of Heubner)

Medial occipital artery

Posterior temporal branch

Anterior temporal branch

Right internal carotid artery

Posterior communicating artery

*Note: Anterior parietal (postcentral sulcal) artery also occurs as separate anterior parietal and postcentral sulcal arteries.*

**Cerebral Vasculature**

**Plate 143**

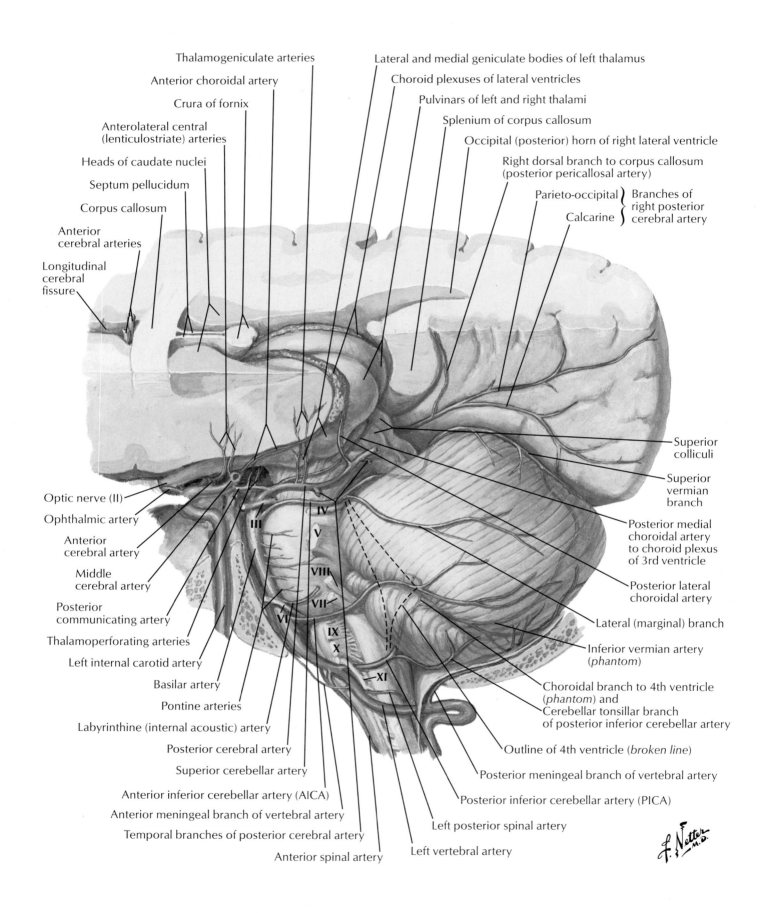

Thalamogeniculate arteries

Anterior choroidal artery

Crura of fornix

Anterolateral central (lenticulostriate) arteries

Heads of caudate nuclei

Septum pellucidum

Corpus callosum

Anterior cerebral arteries

Longitudinal cerebral fissure

Lateral and medial geniculate bodies of left thalamus

Choroid plexuses of lateral ventricles

Pulvinars of left and right thalami

Splenium of corpus callosum

Occipital (posterior) horn of right lateral ventricle

Right dorsal branch to corpus callosum (posterior pericallosal artery)

Parieto-occipital

Calcarine

Branches of right posterior cerebral artery

Superior colliculi

Superior vermian branch

Posterior medial choroidal artery to choroid plexus of 3rd ventricle

Posterior lateral choroidal artery

Lateral (marginal) branch

Inferior vermian artery (*phantom*)

Choroidal branch to 4th ventricle (*phantom*) and Cerebellar tonsillar branch of posterior inferior cerebellar artery

Outline of 4th ventricle (*broken line*)

Posterior meningeal branch of vertebral artery

Posterior inferior cerebellar artery (PICA)

Left posterior spinal artery

Left vertebral artery

Optic nerve (II)

Ophthalmic artery

Anterior cerebral artery

Middle cerebral artery

Posterior communicating artery

Thalamoperforating arteries

Left internal carotid artery

Basilar artery

Pontine arteries

Labyrinthine (internal acoustic) artery

Posterior cerebral artery

Superior cerebellar artery

Anterior inferior cerebellar artery (AICA)

Anterior meningeal branch of vertebral artery

Temporal branches of posterior cerebral artery

Anterior spinal artery

III

IV

V

VIII

VII

VI

IX

X

XI

**Plate 144**

**Cerebral Vasculature**

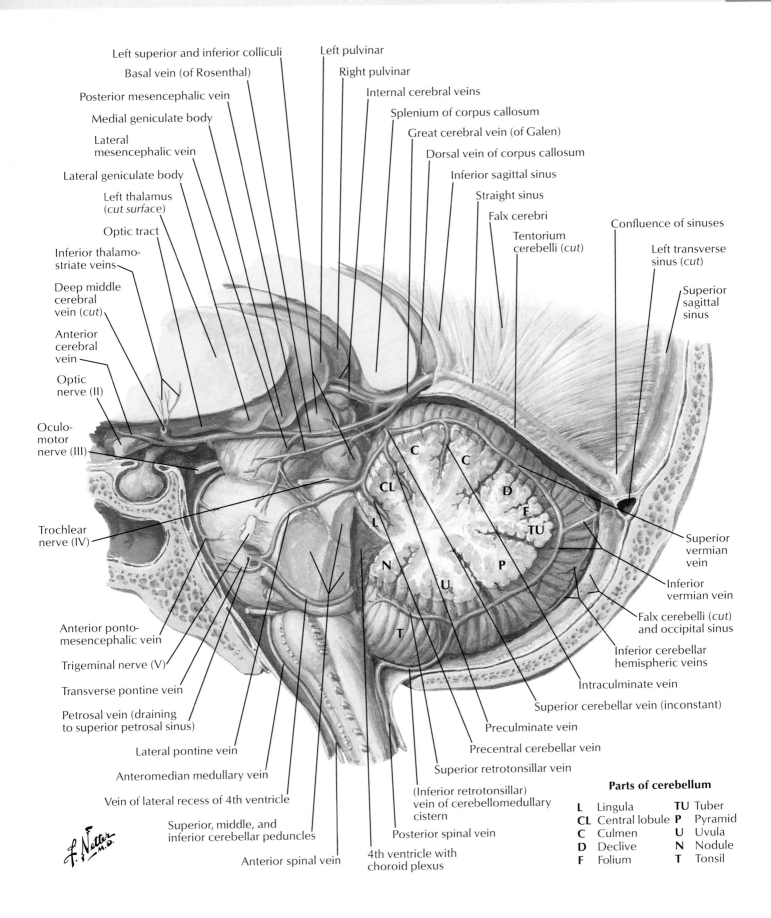

Left superior and inferior colliculi

Basal vein (of Rosenthal)

Posterior mesencephalic vein

Medial geniculate body

Lateral mesencephalic vein

Lateral geniculate body

Left thalamus (*cut surface*)

Optic tract

Inferior thalamo-striate veins

Deep middle cerebral vein (*cut*)

Anterior cerebral vein

Optic nerve (II)

Oculo-motor nerve (III)

Trochlear nerve (IV)

Anterior ponto-mesencephalic vein

Trigeminal nerve (V)

Transverse pontine vein

Petrosal vein (draining to superior petrosal sinus)

Lateral pontine vein

Anteromedian medullary vein

Vein of lateral recess of 4th ventricle

Superior, middle, and inferior cerebellar peduncles

Anterior spinal vein

Left pulvinar

Right pulvinar

Internal cerebral veins

Splenium of corpus callosum

Great cerebral vein (of Galen)

Dorsal vein of corpus callosum

Inferior sagittal sinus

Straight sinus

Falx cerebri

Tentorium cerebelli (*cut*)

Confluence of sinuses

Left transverse sinus (*cut*)

Superior sagittal sinus

Superior vermian vein

Inferior vermian vein

Falx cerebelli (*cut*) and occipital sinus

Inferior cerebellar hemispheric veins

Intraculminate vein

Superior cerebellar vein (inconstant)

Preculminate vein

Precentral cerebellar vein

Superior retrotonsillar vein

(Inferior retrotonsillar) vein of cerebellomedullary cistern

Posterior spinal vein

4th ventricle with choroid plexus

**Parts of cerebellum**

| | | | |
|---|---|---|---|
| **L** | Lingula | **TU** | Tuber |
| **CL** | Central lobule | **P** | Pyramid |
| **C** | Culmen | **U** | Uvula |
| **D** | Declive | **N** | Nodule |
| **F** | Folium | **T** | Tonsil |

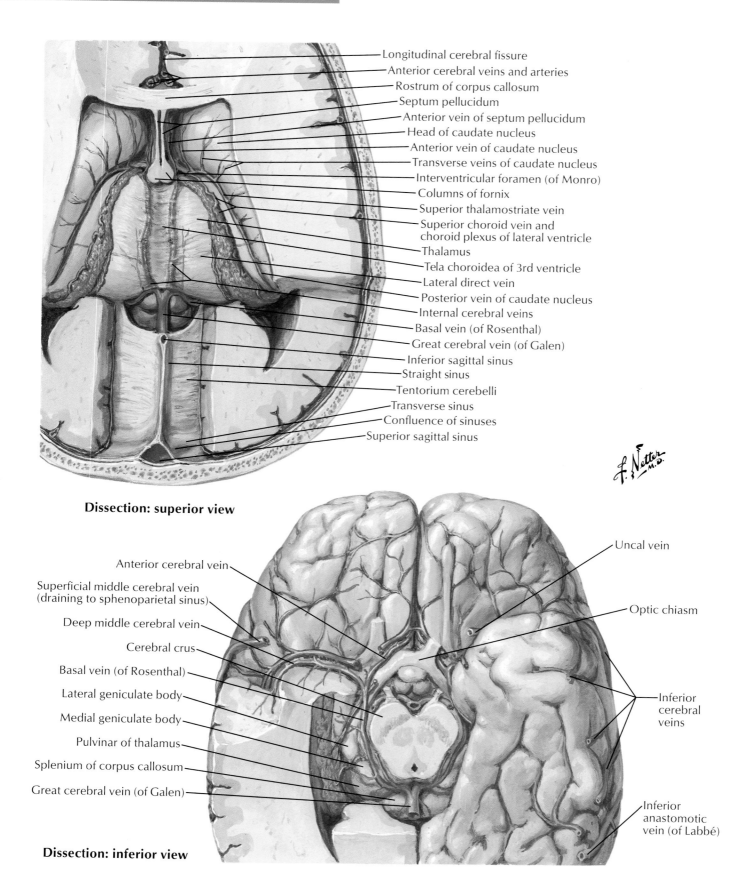

Longitudinal cerebral fissure
Anterior cerebral veins and arteries
Rostrum of corpus callosum
Septum pellucidum
Anterior vein of septum pellucidum
Head of caudate nucleus
Anterior vein of caudate nucleus
Transverse veins of caudate nucleus
Interventricular foramen (of Monro)
Columns of fornix
Superior thalamostriate vein
Superior choroid vein and choroid plexus of lateral ventricle
Thalamus
Tela choroidea of 3rd ventricle
Lateral direct vein
Posterior vein of caudate nucleus
Internal cerebral veins
Basal vein (of Rosenthal)
Great cerebral vein (of Galen)
Inferior sagittal sinus
Straight sinus
Tentorium cerebelli
Transverse sinus
Confluence of sinuses
Superior sagittal sinus

**Dissection: superior view**

Anterior cerebral vein
Superficial middle cerebral vein (draining to sphenoparietal sinus)
Deep middle cerebral vein
Cerebral crus
Basal vein (of Rosenthal)
Lateral geniculate body
Medial geniculate body
Pulvinar of thalamus
Splenium of corpus callosum
Great cerebral vein (of Galen)

Uncal vein
Optic chiasm
Inferior cerebral veins
Inferior anastomotic vein (of Labbé)

**Dissection: inferior view**

**Plate 146**

**Cerebral Vasculature**

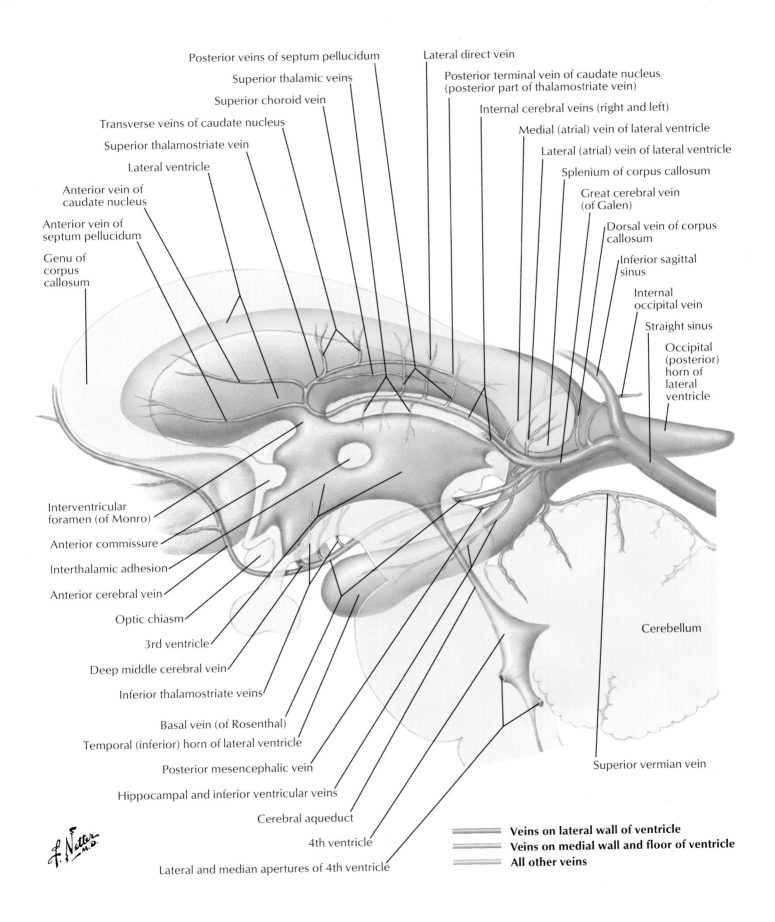

Posterior veins of septum pellucidum

Superior thalamic veins

Superior choroid vein

Transverse veins of caudate nucleus

Superior thalamostriate vein

Lateral ventricle

Anterior vein of caudate nucleus

Anterior vein of septum pellucidum

Genu of corpus callosum

Lateral direct vein

Posterior terminal vein of caudate nucleus (posterior part of thalamostriate vein)

Internal cerebral veins (right and left)

Medial (atrial) vein of lateral ventricle

Lateral (atrial) vein of lateral ventricle

Splenium of corpus callosum

Great cerebral vein (of Galen)

Dorsal vein of corpus callosum

Inferior sagittal sinus

Internal occipital vein

Straight sinus

Occipital (posterior) horn of lateral ventricle

Interventricular foramen (of Monro)

Anterior commissure

Interthalamic adhesion

Anterior cerebral vein

Optic chiasm

3rd ventricle

Deep middle cerebral vein

Inferior thalamostriate veins

Basal vein (of Rosenthal)

Temporal (inferior) horn of lateral ventricle

Posterior mesencephalic vein

Hippocampal and inferior ventricular veins

Cerebral aqueduct

4th ventricle

Lateral and median apertures of 4th ventricle

Cerebellum

Superior vermian vein

Veins on lateral wall of ventricle
Veins on medial wall and floor of ventricle
All other veins

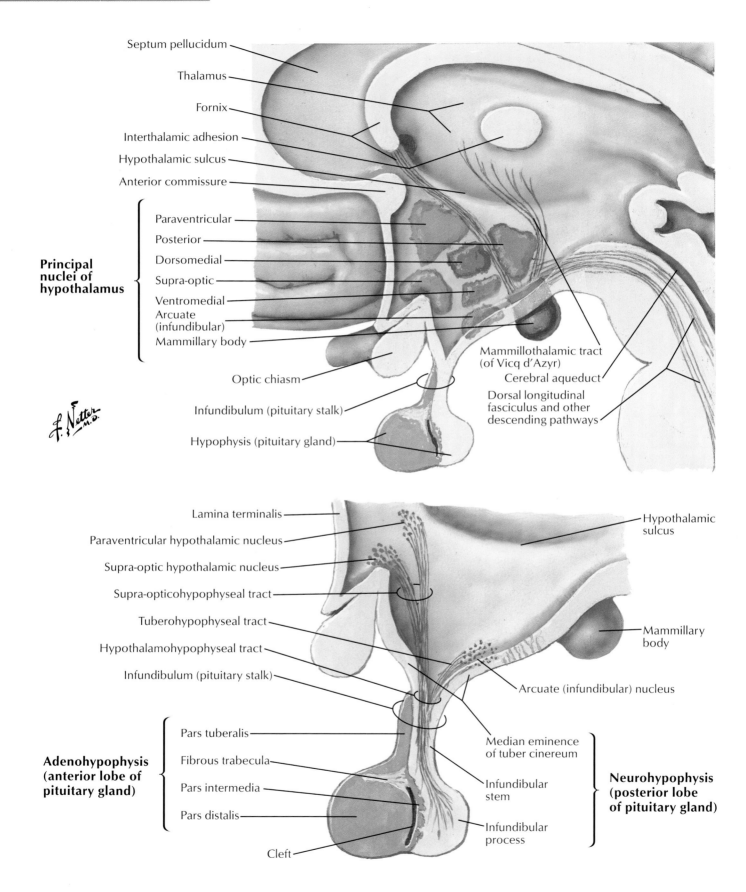

Septum pellucidum

Thalamus

Fornix

Interthalamic adhesion

Hypothalamic sulcus

Anterior commissure

**Principal nuclei of hypothalamus**

Paraventricular

Posterior

Dorsomedial

Supra-optic

Ventromedial

Arcuate (infundibular)

Mammillary body

Optic chiasm

Infundibulum (pituitary stalk)

Hypophysis (pituitary gland)

Mammillothalamic tract (of Vicq d'Azyr)

Cerebral aqueduct

Dorsal longitudinal fasciculus and other descending pathways

Lamina terminalis

Paraventricular hypothalamic nucleus

Supra-optic hypothalamic nucleus

Supra-opticohypophyseal tract

Tuberohypophyseal tract

Hypothalamohypophyseal tract

Infundibulum (pituitary stalk)

Hypothalamic sulcus

Mammillary body

Arcuate (infundibular) nucleus

**Adenohypophysis (anterior lobe of pituitary gland)**

Pars tuberalis

Fibrous trabecula

Pars intermedia

Pars distalis

Cleft

Median eminence of tuber cinereum

Infundibular stem

Infundibular process

**Neurohypophysis (posterior lobe of pituitary gland)**

**Plate 148**                                                                    **Cerebral Vasculature**

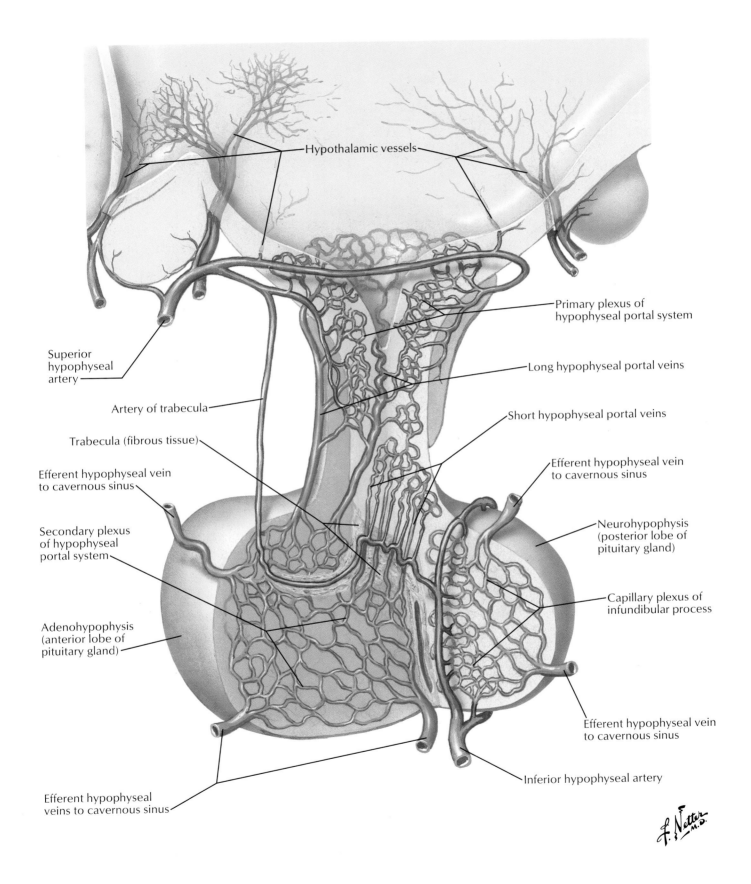

Hypothalamic vessels

Primary plexus of hypophyseal portal system

Superior hypophyseal artery

Long hypophyseal portal veins

Artery of trabecula

Short hypophyseal portal veins

Trabecula (fibrous tissue)

Efferent hypophyseal vein to cavernous sinus

Efferent hypophyseal vein to cavernous sinus

Secondary plexus of hypophyseal portal system

Neurohypophysis (posterior lobe of pituitary gland)

Capillary plexus of infundibular process

Adenohypophysis (anterior lobe of pituitary gland)

Efferent hypophyseal vein to cavernous sinus

Inferior hypophyseal artery

Efferent hypophyseal veins to cavernous sinus

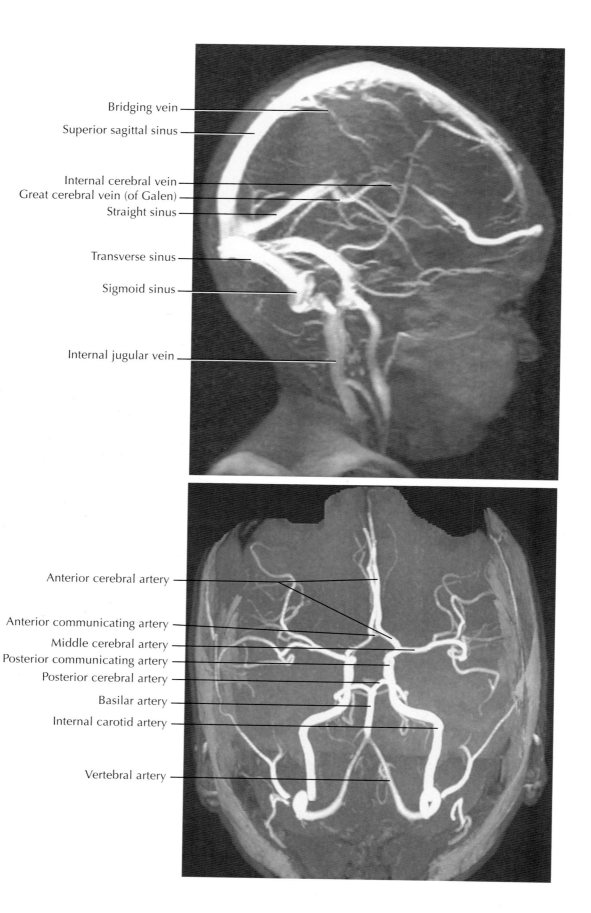

Bridging vein

Superior sagittal sinus

Internal cerebral vein
Great cerebral vein (of Galen)
Straight sinus

Transverse sinus

Sigmoid sinus

Internal jugular vein

Anterior cerebral artery

Anterior communicating artery
Middle cerebral artery
Posterior communicating artery
Posterior cerebral artery
Basilar artery
Internal carotid artery

Vertebral artery

**Plate 150**

**Regional Scans**

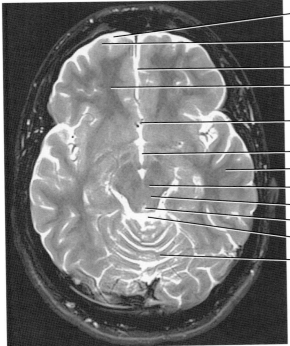

- Subarachnoid space
- Gray matter
- Longitudinal fissure
- White matter
- Anterior cerebral artery
- Third ventricle
- Temporal lobe
- Red nucleus
- Midbrain
- Cerebral aqueduct
- Quadrigeminal cistern
- Cerebellum

Superior sagittal sinus
Corpus callosum

Head of caudate
Lateral ventricle
Third ventricle

Pons
Basilar artery
Vertebral artery

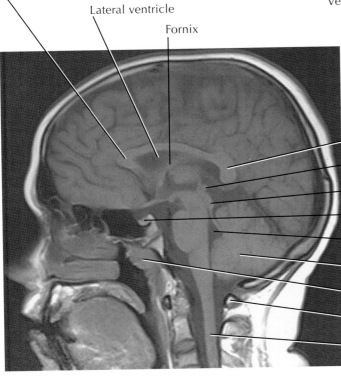

Genu of corpus callosum
Lateral ventricle
Fornix

- Splenium of corpus callosum
- Pineal gland
- Tectum
- Pituitary gland
- Fourth ventricle
- Cerebellum
- Pharyngeal tonsil
- Posterior arch of atlas
- Spinal cord

| MUSCLE | PROXIMAL ATTACHMENT (ORIGIN) | DISTAL ATTACHMENT (INSERTION) | INNERVATION | MAIN ACTIONS | BLOOD SUPPLY | MUSCLE GROUP |
|---|---|---|---|---|---|---|
| Auricularis anterior | Temporal fascia, epicranial aponeurosis | Anterior part of medial surface of helix of ear | Posterior auricular and temporal branches of facial nerve | Elevates and draws ear forward | Auricular branch of posterior auricular artery, parietal branch of superficial temporal artery | External ear |
| Auricularis posterior | Base of mastoid process | Lower part of cranial surface of auricle | Posterior auricular and temporal branches of facial nerve | Retracts and elevates ear | Auricular branch of posterior auricular artery, parietal branch of superficial temporal artery | External ear |
| Auricularis superior | Temporal fascia, epicranial aponeurosis | Upper part of medial surface of auricle | Posterior auricular and temporal branches of facial nerve | Retracts and elevates ear | Auricular branch of posterior auricular artery, parietal branch of superficial temporal artery | External ear |
| Buccinator | Posterior portion of alveolar process of maxilla and mandible opposite sockets of molar teeth, anterior border of pterygomandibular raphe | Angle of mouth | Buccal branches of facial nerve | Compresses cheeks, expels air between lips, aids in mastication | Muscular branches of facial artery, buccal branch of maxillary artery | Facial expression |
| Ciliary | Corneoscleral junction | Ciliary body | Parasympathetic fibers via short ciliary nerves (CN III) | Constricts ciliary body and lens rounds up (accommodation) | Ophthalmic artery | Intrinsic eye |
| Corrugator supercilii | Medial part of supra-orbital margin | Skin of medial half of eyebrow | Zygomatic and temporal branches of facial nerve | Draws eyebrows downward and medially, produces wrinkles in frowning | Zygomatic and anterior branches of superficial temporal artery | Facial expression |
| Cricothyroid | Anterior cricoid cartilage | Inferior border of thyroid cartilage and its inferior horn | External branch of superior laryngeal nerve | Lengthens and tenses vocal ligaments | Superior and inferior thyroid arteries | Laryngeal |
| Depressor anguli oris | Continuous with platysma on oblique line of mandible | Angle of mouth into orbicularis and skin | Mandibular and buccal branches of facial nerve | Depresses angle of mouth | Inferior labial branch of facial artery | Facial expression |
| Depressor labii inferioris | Lateral surface of mandible between symphysis and mental foramen deep to depressor anguli oris | Skin to lower lip, mingling with orbicularis oris, medial fibers joining those of opposite side | Mandibular and buccal branches of facial nerve | Depresses lower lip and draws it lateralward | Inferior labial branch of facial artery | Facial expression |
| Depressor septi nasi | Incisive fossa of maxilla | Septum and posterior part of ala of nose | Zygomatic and buccal branches of facial nerve | Narrows nostril, draws septum downward | Superior labial branch of facial artery | Facial expression |
| Digastric | *Anterior belly:* digastric fossa of mandible  *Posterior belly:* mastoid notch of temporal bone | Intermediate tendon attached to body of hyoid | *Anterior belly:* nerve to mylohyoid  *Posterior belly:* facial nerve | Raises hyoid bone and base of tongue, steadies hyoid bone, opens mouth by lowering mandible | *Anterior belly:* branches of submental artery  *Posterior belly:* muscular branches of posterior auricular artery, muscular branches of occipital artery | Suprahyoid |
| Dilator pupillae | Radial fibers in iris | Blends with sphincter pupillae fibers | Sympathetic fibers from SCG | Dilates pupil | Ophthalmic artery | Intrinsic eye |
| Frontal belly of occipitofrontalis | Epicranial aponeurosis at level of coronal suture | Skin of frontal region, epicranial aponeurosis | Temporal branches of facial nerve | Wrinkles forehead skin, raises eyebrows | Frontal branch of superficial temporal artery | Facial expression |

Variations in spinal nerve contributions to the innervation of muscles, their arterial supply, their attachments, and their actions are common themes in human anatomy. Therefore, expect differences between texts and realize that anatomical variation is normal.

**Table 1-1**

**Muscle Tables**

| MUSCLE | PROXIMAL ATTACHMENT (ORIGIN) | DISTAL ATTACHMENT (INSERTION) | INNERVATION | MAIN ACTIONS | BLOOD SUPPLY | MUSCLE GROUP |
|---|---|---|---|---|---|---|
| Genioglossus | Mental spine of mandible | Dorsum of tongue, hyoid bone | Hypoglossal nerve (CN XII) | Depresses and protrudes tongue | Sublingual and submental arteries | Extrinsic tongue |
| Geniohyoid | Inferior genial tubercle on back of symphysis of mandible | Anterior surface of body of hyoid bone | Branch of C1 through hypoglossal nerve (CN XII) | Elevates hyoid bone and depresses mandible | Sublingual branch of lingual artery | Suprahyoid |
| Hyoglossus | Body and greater horn of hyoid bone | Lateral and inferior aspect of tongue | Hypoglossal nerve (CN XII) | Depresses and retracts tongue | Sublingual and submental arteries | Extrinsic tongue |
| Inferior longitudinal muscle of tongue | Under surface of tongue between genioglossus and hyoglossus | Tip of tongue blending with styloglossus | Hypoglossal nerve (CN XII) | Shortens tongue, turns tip and sides downward | Deep lingual branch of lingual artery, branches from facial artery | Intrinsic tongue |
| Inferior oblique | Anterior floor of orbit lateral to nasolacrimal canal | Lateral sclera deep to lateral rectus | Oculomotor nerve (CN III), inferior division | Abducts, elevates, and laterally rotates eyeball | Ophthalmic artery | Extra-ocular |
| Inferior pharyngeal constrictor | Oblique line of thyroid cartilage and cricoid cartilage | Median raphe of pharynx | Vagus nerve via pharyngeal plexus | Constricts wall of pharynx during swallowing | Ascending pharyngeal artery, branches of superior thyroid artery | Circular pharyngeal |
| Inferior rectus | Common tendinous ring | Inferior aspect of eyeball, posterior to corneoscleral junction | Oculomotor nerve (CN III), inferior division | Depresses, adducts, and laterally rotates eyeball | Ophthalmic artery | Extra-ocular |
| Lateral crico-arytenoid | Arch of cricoid cartilage | Muscular process of arytenoid cartilage | Recurrent laryngeal nerve | Adducts vocal folds | Superior and inferior thyroid arteries | Laryngeal |
| Lateral pterygoid | *Superior head:* infratemporal surface of greater wing of sphenoid<br><br>*Inferior head:* lateral pterygoid plate | Pterygoid fovea, capsule of temporomandibular joint, articular disc | Mandibular nerve (CN V₃), muscular branches from anterior division | *Bilaterally:* protrude mandible<br><br>*Unilaterally and alternately:* produces side-to-side grinding | Muscular branches of maxillary artery | Mastication |
| Lateral rectus | Common tendinous ring | Lateral aspect of eyeball, posterior to corneoscleral junction | Abducent nerve (CN VI) | Abducts eyeball | Ophthalmic artery | Extra-ocular |
| Levator anguli oris | Canine fossa of maxilla immediately below infra-orbital foramen and under cover of zygomatic head of levator labii superioris | Angle of mouth; fibers intermingle with orbicularis oris, depressor anguli oris, zygomaticus | Zygomatic and buccal branches of facial nerve | Elevates angle of mouth | Superior labial branch of facial artery | Facial expression |
| Levator labii superioris alaeque nasi | *Angular head:* upper part of frontal process of maxilla<br><br>*Infra-orbital head:* orbit above infra-orbital foramen<br><br>*Zygomatic head:* malar surface of zygomatic bone | *Angular head:* into greater alar cartilage, skin of nose, lateral upper lip<br><br>*Infra-orbital head:* into muscular substance of upper lip between angular head and caninus<br><br>*Zygomatic head:* into skin of nasolabial groove and upper lip | Zygomatic and buccal branches of facial nerve | *Angular head:* elevates upper lip and dilates nostril<br><br>*Infra-orbital head:* raises angle of mouth<br><br>*Zygomatic head:* elevates upper lip laterally | Superior labial branch and angular branches of facial artery | Facial expression |

| MUSCLE | PROXIMAL ATTACHMENT (ORIGIN) | DISTAL ATTACHMENT (INSERTION) | INNERVATION | MAIN ACTIONS | BLOOD SUPPLY | MUSCLE GROUP |
|---|---|---|---|---|---|---|
| Levator labii superioris | Maxilla above infra-orbital foramen | Skin of upper lip | Zygomatic and buccal branches of facial nerve | Elevates upper lip, dilates nares | Superior labial artery and angular branches of facial artery | Facial expression |
| Levator palpebrae superioris | Lesser wing of sphenoid, anterior to optic canal | Superior tarsal plate | Oculomotor nerve (CN III), superior division | Raises upper eyelid | Ophthalmic artery | Extra-ocular; eyelid |
| Levator veli palatini | Temporal bone (petrous portion) | Palatine aponeurosis | Vagus nerve via pharyngeal plexus | Elevates soft palate during swallowing | Ascending palatine artery branch of facial artery, descending palatine artery branch of maxillary artery | Palatal |
| Longus capitis | Anterior tubercles of transverse processes of C3–C6 | Inferior surface of basilar part of occipital bone | Ventral rami of cervical nerves (C1–C4) | Flexes and assists in rotating cervical vertebrae and head | Ascending cervical branch of inferior thyroid artery, ascending pharyngeal artery, muscular branches of vertebral artery | Prevertebral |
| Longus colli | *Vertical portion:* C5–T3 vertebrae<br><br>*Inferior oblique portion:* T1–T3 vertebrae<br><br>*Superior oblique portion:* anterior tubercles of transverse processes of C3–C5 vertebrae | *Vertical portion:* into C2–C4 vertebrae<br><br>*Inferior oblique portion* on anterior tubercles of transverse processes of C5–C6 vertebrae<br><br>*Superior oblique portion:* tubercle of anterior arch of atlas | Ventral primary rami of cervical nerves (C2–C8) | *Bilaterally:* flex and assist in rotating cervical vertebrae and head<br><br>*Unilaterally:* flexes vertebral column laterally | Prevertebral branches of ascending pharyngeal artery, muscular branches of ascending cervical and vertebral arteries | Prevertebral |
| Masseter | Zygomatic arch | Ramus of mandible, coronoid process | Mandibular nerve (CN V$_3$), via masseteric nerve | Elevates and protrudes mandible; deep fibers retrude it | Transverse facial artery; masseteric branch of maxillary and facial arteries | Mastication |
| Medial pterygoid | Medial surface of lateral plate of pterygoid, pyramidal process of palatine bone, maxillary tuberosity | Medial surface of ramus and angle of mandible inferior to mandibular foramen | Mandibular nerve (V$_3$), nerve to medial pterygoid | *Bilaterally:* protrude and elevate mandible<br><br>*Unilaterally and alternately:* produces side-to-side movements | Facial and maxillary arteries | Mastication |
| Medial rectus | Common tendinous ring | Medial aspect of eyeball, posterior to corneoscleral junction | Oculomotor nerve (CN III), inferior division | Adducts eyeball | Ophthalmic artery | Extra-ocular |
| Mentalis | Incisive fossa of mandible | Skin of chin | Mandibular branch of facial nerve | Raises and protrudes lower lip | Inferior labial branch of facial artery | Facial expression |
| Middle pharyngeal constrictor | Stylohyoid ligament and horns of hyoid bone | Median raphe of pharynx | Vagus nerve via pharyngeal plexus | Constricts wall of pharynx during swallowing | Ascending pharyngeal artery, ascending palatine and tonsillar branches of facial artery, dorsal lingual branches of lingual artery | Circular pharyngeal |
| Mylohyoid | Mylohyoid line of mandible | Median raphe and body of hyoid bone | Nerve to mylohyoid nerve (branch of trigeminal nerve) | Elevates hyoid bone, base of tongue, floor of mouth; depresses mandible | Sublingual branch of lingual artery, submental branch of facial artery | Suprahyoid |

**Table 1-3**

**Muscle Tables**

| MUSCLE | PROXIMAL ATTACHMENT (ORIGIN) | DISTAL ATTACHMENT (INSERTION) | INNERVATION | MAIN ACTIONS | BLOOD SUPPLY | MUSCLE GROUP |
|---|---|---|---|---|---|---|
| Nasalis | Canine eminence above and lateral to incisive fossa of maxilla | Aponeurosis on nasal cartilages | Zygomatic and buccal branches of facial nerve | Draws ala of nose toward septum, compresses nostrils; alar part opens nostrils | Superior labial, septal, and lateral nasal branches of facial artery | Facial expression |
| Occipital belly (occipitalis) of epicranius | Lateral 2/3 of superior nuchal line and mastoid process | Skin of occipital region, epicranial aponeurosis | Posterior auricular branches of facial nerve | Moves scalp backward | Occipital branch of posterior auricular artery, descending branch of occipital artery | Facial expression |
| Omohyoid | *Inferior belly:* from upper border of scapula and suprascapular ligament, ending in tendon under sternocleidomastoid muscle<br><br>*Superior belly:* from this tendon | *Inferior belly:* to intermediate tendon<br><br>*Superior belly:* to body of hyoid bone | Ansa cervicalis | Steadies hyoid bone and depresses hyoid | Hyoid branch of lingual artery, sternocleidomastoid branch of superior thyroid artery | Infrahyoid |
| Orbicularis oculi | Medial orbital margin, palpebral ligament, lacrimal bone | Skin around orbit, palpebral ligament, upper and lower eyelids | Facial nerve (CN VII) | Closes eyelids | Facial and superficial temporal arteries | Facial expression |
| Orbicularis oris | Maxilla above incisor teeth | Skin around lips | Zygomatic, buccal, and mandibular branches of facial nerve | Compression, contraction, and protrusion of lips | Inferior and superior labial branches of facial artery | Facial expression |
| Palatoglossus | Palatine aponeurosis of soft palate | Lateral aspect of tongue | Vagus nerve via pharyngeal plexus | Elevates posterior tongue, depresses palate | Ascending pharyngeal arteries, palatine branches of facial and maxillary arteries | Palatal |
| Palatopharyngeus | Hard palate, superior palatine aponeurosis | Lateral pharyngeal wall | Vagus nerve via pharyngeal plexus | Tenses soft palate; pulls walls of pharynx superiorly, anteriorly, and medially during swallowing | Ascending palatine artery branch of facial artery, descending palatine artery branch of maxillary artery | Longitudinal pharyngeal |
| Platysma | Skin below clavicle, upper thorax | Mandible, oral muscles | Facial nerve | Tenses skin of neck | Submental and suprascapular arteries | Facial expression |
| Posterior crico-arytenoid | Posterior surface of lamina of cricoid cartilage | Muscular process of arytenoid cartilage | Recurrent laryngeal nerve | Abducts vocal folds | Superior and inferior thyroid arteries | Laryngeal |
| Procerus | Fascia covering lower parts of nasal bone and upper part of lateral nasal cartilage | Skin between and above eyebrow | Temporal and zygomatic branches of facial nerve | Draws down medial angle of eyebrows, produces transverse wrinkles over bridge of nose | Angular and lateral nasal branches of facial artery | Facial expression |
| Rectus capitis anterior | Lateral mass of atlas | Base of occipital bone in front of foramen magnum | Ventral rami of cervical nerves (C1–C2) | Flexes head | Muscular branches of vertebral artery, ascending pharyngeal artery | Prevertebral |
| Rectus capitis lateralis | Upper surface of transverse process of atlas | Inferior surface of jugular process of occipital bone | Ventral rami of cervical nerves (C1–C2) | Flexes head laterally to same side | Muscular branches of vertebral artery, occipital artery, ascending pharyngeal artery | Prevertebral |
| Risorius | Fascia over masseter superficial to platysma | Skin at angle of mouth | Zygomatic and buccal branches of facial nerve | Retracts angle of mouth | Superior labial branch of facial artery | Facial expression |
| Salpingopharyngeus | Pharyngotympanic (auditory, eustachian) tube | Side of pharyngeal wall | Vagus nerve via pharyngeal plexus | Elevates pharynx and larynx during swallowing and speaking | Pharyngeal branch of ascending pharyngeal artery | Longitudinal pharyngeal |

| MUSCLE | PROXIMAL ATTACHMENT (ORIGIN) | DISTAL ATTACHMENT (INSERTION) | INNERVATION | MAIN ACTIONS | BLOOD SUPPLY | MUSCLE GROUP |
|---|---|---|---|---|---|---|
| Scalene (anterior) | Anterior tubercles of transverse processes of C3–C6 | Scalene tubercle on 1st rib | Anterior rami of cervical nerves (C5–C8) | Elevates 1st rib, bends neck | Ascending cervical branch of inferior thyroid artery | Prevertebral |
| Scalene (medius) | Posterior tubercles of transverse processes of C2–C7 | Upper surface of 1st rib (behind subclavian groove) | Anterior rami of cervical nerves (C3–C7) | Elevates 1st rib, bends neck | Muscular branches of ascending cervical artery | Prevertebral |
| Scalene (posterior) | Posterior tubercles of transverse processes of C4–C6 | Outer surface of 2nd rib (behind attachment of serratus anterior) | Anterior rami of lower four cervical nerves | Elevates 2nd rib, bends neck | Muscular branches of ascending cervical division of inferior thyroid artery, superficial branch of transverse cervical artery | Prevertebral |
| Sphincter pupillae | Circular smooth muscle of iris that passes around pupil | Blends with dilator pupillae fibers | Parasympathetic fibers via oculomotor nerve (CN III) | Constricts pupil | Ophthalmic artery | Intrinsic eye |
| Stapedius | Pyramidal eminence of temporal bone | Stapes | Facial nerve | Pulls stapes posteriorly to lessen oscillation of tympanic membrane | Posterior auricular, anterior tympanic, and middle meningeal arteries | Middle ear |
| Sternocleidomastoid | *Sternal head:* anterior surface of manubrium  *Clavicular head:* upper surface of medial 1/3 of clavicle | Lateral surface of mastoid process; lateral half of superior nuchal line of occipital bone | Accessory nerve (CN XI) | *Bilaterally:* flex head, raise thorax  *Unilaterally:* turns face toward opposite side | Sternocleidomastoid branch of superior thyroid and occipital arteries, muscular branch of suprascapular artery, occipital branch of posterior auricular artery | Neck |
| Sternohyoid | Posterior surface of manubrium sterni, posterior sternoclavicular ligament, medial end of clavicle | Medial part of lower border of body of hyoid bone | Ansa cervicalis | Depresses larynx and hyoid bone, steadies hyoid bone | Sternocleidomastoid and hyoid branches of superior thyroid artery, hyoid branch of lingual artery | Infrahyoid |
| Sternothyroid | Posterior surface of manubrium sterni below and deep to origin of sternohyoid, edge of first costal cartilage | Oblique line on lamina of thyroid cartilage | Ansa cervicalis | Depresses larynx and thyroid cartilage | Cricothyroid branch of superior thyroid artery | Infrahyoid |
| Styloglossus | Styloid process and stylohyoid ligament | Lateral and inferior aspect of tongue | Hypoglossal nerve (CN XII) | Retracts tongue and draws it up for swallowing | Sublingual artery | Extrinsic tongue |
| Stylohyoid | Posterior border of styloid process | Body of hyoid bone at junction with greater horn | Facial nerve | Elevates hyoid bone and base of tongue | Muscular branches of facial artery, muscular branches of occipital artery | Suprahyoid |
| Stylopharyngeus | Medial aspect of styloid process | Pharyngeal wall | Glossopharyngeal nerve (CN IX) | Elevates pharynx and larynx during swallowing and speaking | Ascending pharyngeal artery, ascending palatine and tonsillar branches of facial artery, dorsal branches of lingual artery | Longitudinal pharyngeal |
| Subclavius | Upper border of 1st rib and its cartilage | Inferior surface of middle third of clavicle | Nerve to subclavius | Anchors and depresses clavicle | Clavicular branch of thoraco-acromial artery | Neck |
| Superior longitudinal muscle of tongue | Submucous fibers at back of tongue | Tip of tongue; unites with muscle of opposite side | Hypoglossal nerve (CN XII) | Shortens tongue, turns tip and sides upward | Deep lingual branch of lingual artery, branches from facial artery | Intrinsic tongue |
| Superior oblique | Body of sphenoid (above optic foramen), medial to origin of superior rectus | Passes through trochlea, attaches to superior sclera between superior and lateral recti | Trochlear nerve (CN IV) | Abducts, depresses, and medially rotates eyeball | Ophthalmic artery | Extra-ocular |

**Table 1-5**

**Muscle Tables**

| MUSCLE | PROXIMAL ATTACHMENT (ORIGIN) | DISTAL ATTACHMENT (INSERTION) | INNERVATION | MAIN ACTIONS | BLOOD SUPPLY | MUSCLE GROUP |
|---|---|---|---|---|---|---|
| Superior pharyngeal constrictor | Hamulus, pterygomandibular raphe, mylohyoid line of mandible | Median raphe of pharynx | Vagus nerve via pharyngeal plexus | Constricts wall of pharynx during swallowing | Ascending pharyngeal artery, ascending palatine and tonsillar branches of facial artery, dorsal branches of lingual artery | Circular pharyngeal |
| Superior rectus | Common tendinous ring | Superior aspect of eyeball, posterior to the corneoscleral junction | Oculomotor nerve (CN III), superior division | Elevates, adducts, and medially rotates eyeball | Ophthalmic artery | Extra-ocular |
| Temporalis | Floor of temporal fossa, deep temporal fascia | Coronoid process and ramus of mandible | Mandibular nerve (CN V₃), deep temporal nerves | Elevates mandible; posterior fibers retrude mandible | Superficial temporal and maxillary arteries, middle, anterior, and posterior deep temporal arteries | Mastication |
| Tensor tympani | Cartilage of pharyngotympanic (auditory, eustachian) tube | Handle of malleus | Mandibular branch of trigeminal nerve (CN V₃) | Tenses tympanic membrane by drawing it medially | Superior tympanic branch of middle meningeal division of maxillary artery | Middle ear |
| Tensor veli palatini | Scaphoid fossa of medial pterygoid plate, spine of sphenoid, pharyngotympanic (auditory, eustachian) tube | Palatine aponeurosis | Mandibular nerve | Tenses soft palate, opens pharyngotympanic (auditory, eustachian) tube during swallowing and yawning | Ascending palatine artery branch of facial artery, descending palatine artery branch of maxillary artery | Palatal |
| Thyro-arytenoid | Posterior aspect of thyroid cartilage | Muscular process of arytenoid cartilage | Recurrent laryngeal nerve | Shortens and relaxes vocal cords, sphincter of vestibule | Superior and inferior thyroid arteries | Laryngeal |
| Thyrohyoid | Oblique line on lamina of thyroid cartilage | Lower border of body and greater horn of hyoid bone | Thyrohyoid branch of C1 nerve via hypoglossal nerve (CN XII) | Depresses larynx and hyoid bone, elevates thyroid cartilage | Hyoid branch of superior thyroid artery | Infrahyoid |
| Transverse and oblique arytenoid | Arytenoid cartilage | Opposite arytenoid cartilage | Recurrent laryngeal nerve | Closes intercartilaginous portion of rima glottides | Superior and inferior thyroid arteries | Laryngeal |
| Transverse (tongue) | Median fibrous septum of tongue | Dorsum and sides of tongue | Hypoglossal nerve (CN XII) | Narrows and elongates tongue | Deep lingual branch of lingual artery, branches from facial artery | Intrinsic tongue |
| Uvular muscle | Nasal spine, palatine aponeurosis | Mucosa of uvula | Vagus nerve via pharyngeal plexus | Shortens, elevates, and retracts uvula | Ascending palatine artery branch of facial artery, descending palatine artery branch of maxillary artery | Palatal |
| Vertical (tongue) | Mucous membrane on dorsum of forepart of tongue | Fibers extend from dorsum to undersurface of tongue | Hypoglossal nerve (CN XII) | Flattens and broadens tongue | Deep lingual branch of lingual artery, branches from facial artery | Intrinsic tongue |
| Vocalis | Vocal process of arytenoid cartilage | Vocal ligament | Recurrent laryngeal nerve | Tenses anterior vocal ligament, relaxes posterior vocal ligament | Superior and inferior thyroid arteries | Laryngeal |
| Zygomaticus major | Zygomatic arch | Angle of mouth | Zygomatic and buccal branches of facial nerve | Draws angle of mouth backward and upward | Superior labial branch of facial artery | Facial expression |
| Zygomaticus minor | Zygomatic arch | Angle of mouth, upper lip | Zygomatic and buccal branches of facial nerve | Elevates upper lip | Superior labial branch of facial artery | Facial expression |

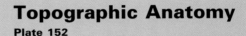

# 2 BACK AND SPINAL CORD

# BACK AND SPINAL CORD

## Muscles and Nerves
**Plates 171–175**

## Cross-Sectional Anatomy
**Plates 176–177**

## Muscle Tables

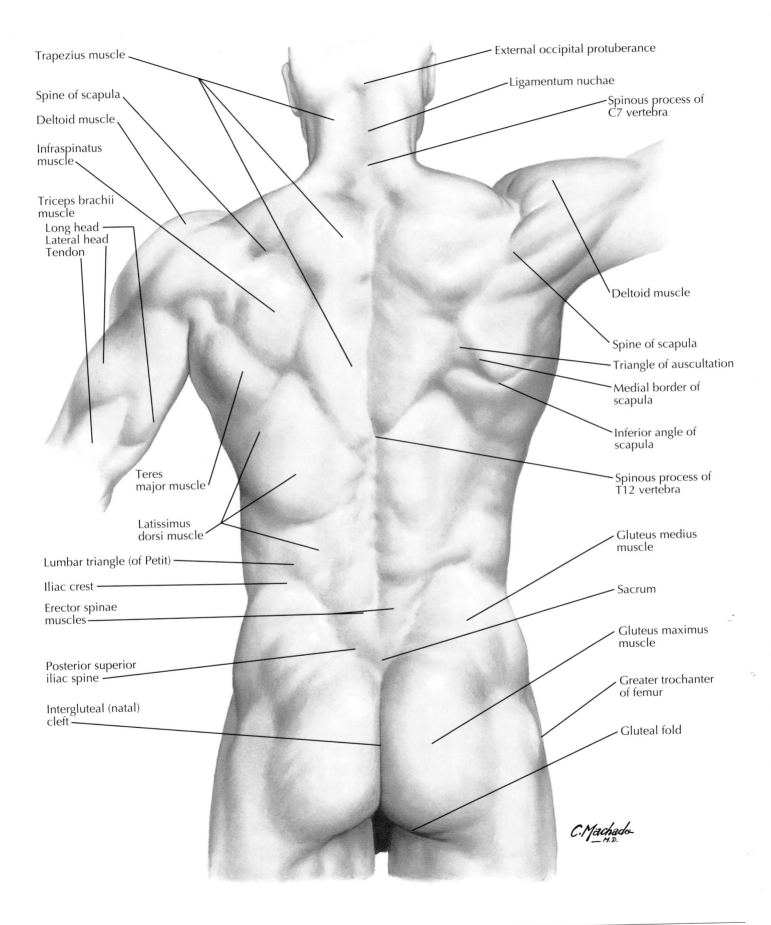

Trapezius muscle

Spine of scapula

Deltoid muscle

Infraspinatus muscle

Triceps brachii muscle
Long head
Lateral head
Tendon

Teres major muscle

Latissimus dorsi muscle

Lumbar triangle (of Petit)

Iliac crest

Erector spinae muscles

Posterior superior iliac spine

Intergluteal (natal) cleft

External occipital protuberance

Ligamentum nuchae

Spinous process of C7 vertebra

Deltoid muscle

Spine of scapula

Triangle of auscultation

Medial border of scapula

Inferior angle of scapula

Spinous process of T12 vertebra

Gluteus medius muscle

Sacrum

Gluteus maximus muscle

Greater trochanter of femur

Gluteal fold

C.Machado
M.D.

**Topographic Anatomy**

**Plate 152**

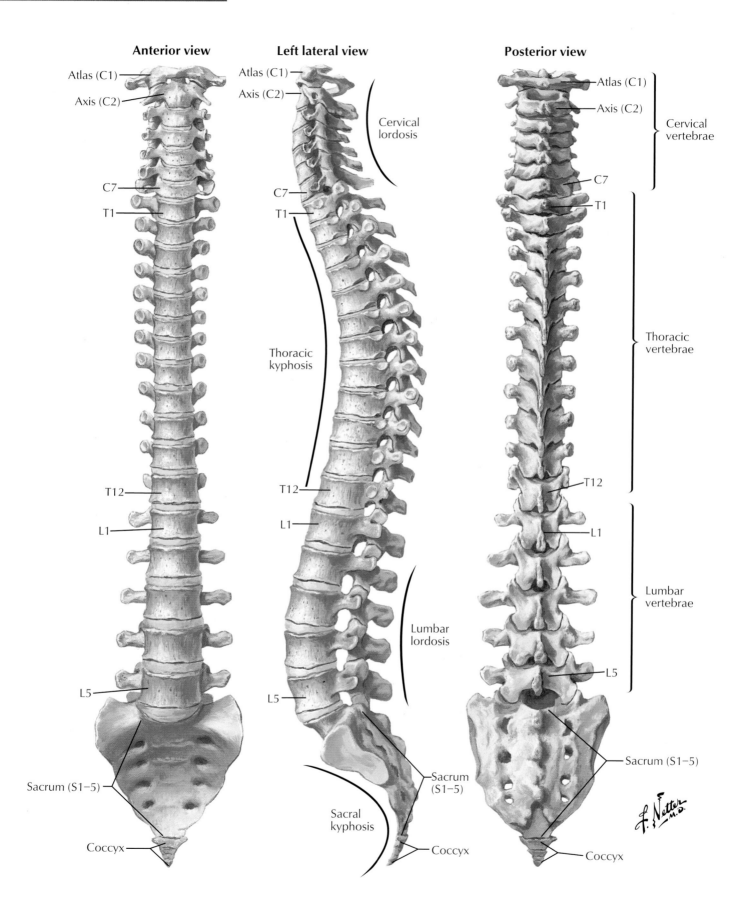

**Anterior view**

Atlas (C1)
Axis (C2)
C7
T1
T12
L1
L5
Sacrum (S1–5)
Coccyx

**Left lateral view**

Atlas (C1)
Axis (C2)
Cervical lordosis
C7
T1
Thoracic kyphosis
T12
L1
Lumbar lordosis
L5
Sacrum (S1–5)
Sacral kyphosis
Coccyx

**Posterior view**

Atlas (C1)
Axis (C2)
Cervical vertebrae
C7
T1
Thoracic vertebrae
T12
L1
Lumbar vertebrae
L5
Sacrum (S1–5)
Coccyx

**Plate 153**

**Bones and Ligaments**

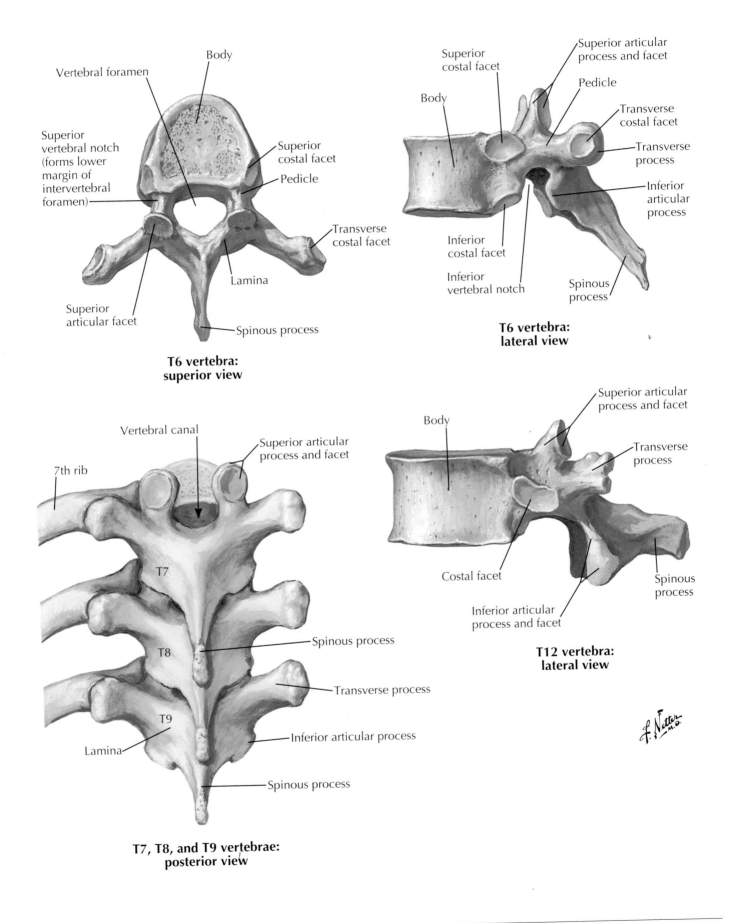

Vertebral foramen

Body

Superior
vertebral notch
(forms lower
margin of
intervertebral
foramen)

Superior
costal facet

Pedicle

Transverse
costal facet

Lamina

Superior
articular facet

Spinous process

**T6 vertebra:
superior view**

Superior
costal facet

Body

Superior articular
process and facet

Pedicle

Transverse
costal facet

Transverse
process

Inferior
costal facet

Inferior
vertebral notch

Inferior
articular
process

Spinous
process

**T6 vertebra:
lateral view**

Vertebral canal

Superior articular
process and facet

7th rib

T7

T8

T9

Lamina

Spinous process

Transverse process

Inferior articular process

Spinous process

**T7, T8, and T9 vertebrae:
posterior view**

Body

Superior articular
process and facet

Transverse
process

Costal facet

Inferior articular
process and facet

Spinous
process

**T12 vertebra:
lateral view**

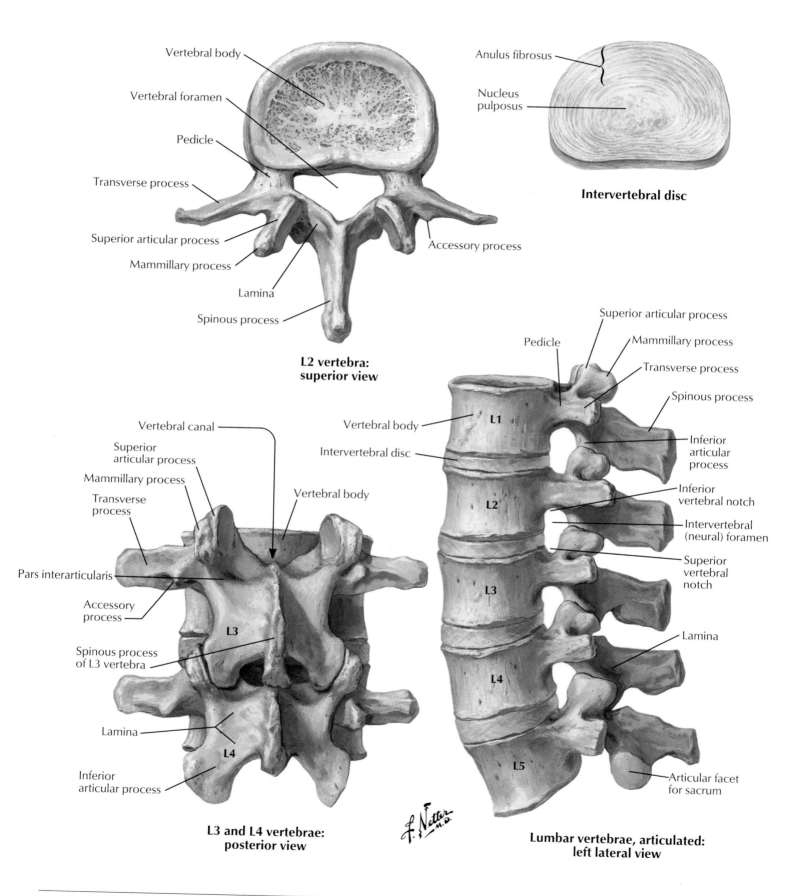

Vertebral body

Vertebral foramen

Pedicle

Transverse process

Superior articular process

Mammillary process

Lamina

Spinous process

**L2 vertebra: superior view**

Anulus fibrosus

Nucleus pulposus

**Intervertebral disc**

Vertebral canal

Superior articular process

Mammillary process

Transverse process

Pars interarticularis

Accessory process

Spinous process of L3 vertebra

Vertebral body

L3

Lamina

L4

Inferior articular process

**L3 and L4 vertebrae: posterior view**

Pedicle

Superior articular process

Mammillary process

Transverse process

Spinous process

Inferior articular process

Inferior vertebral notch

Intervertebral (neural) foramen

Superior vertebral notch

Lamina

Articular facet for sacrum

Vertebral body

Intervertebral disc

L1

L2

L3

L4

L5

**Lumbar vertebrae, articulated: left lateral view**

**Plate 155**

**Bones and Ligaments**

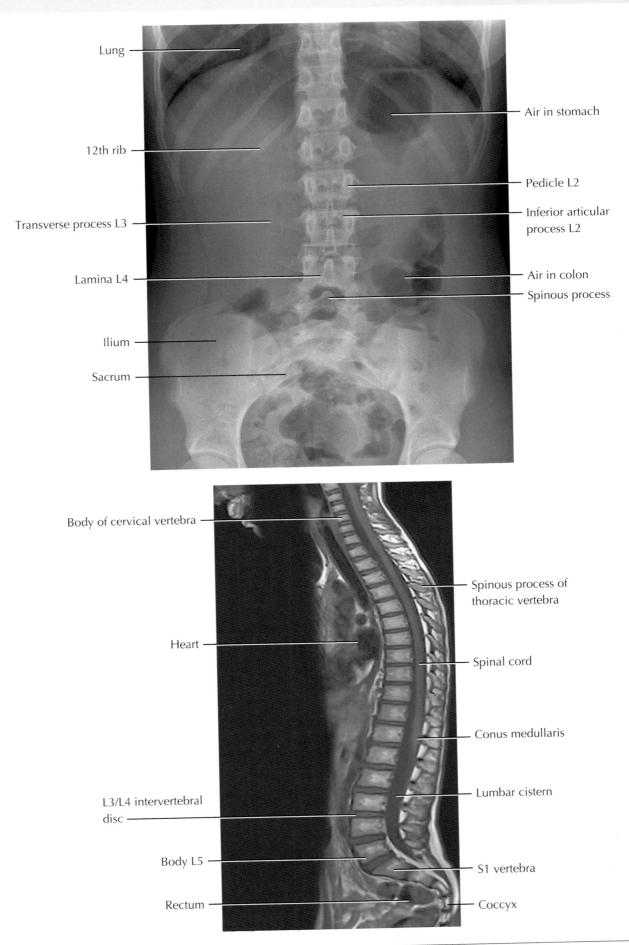

Lung

Air in stomach

12th rib

Pedicle L2

Transverse process L3

Inferior articular process L2

Lamina L4

Air in colon

Spinous process

Ilium

Sacrum

Body of cervical vertebra

Spinous process of thoracic vertebra

Heart

Spinal cord

Conus medullaris

L3/L4 intervertebral disc

Lumbar cistern

Body L5

S1 vertebra

Rectum

Coccyx

**Bones and Ligaments**

**Plate 156**

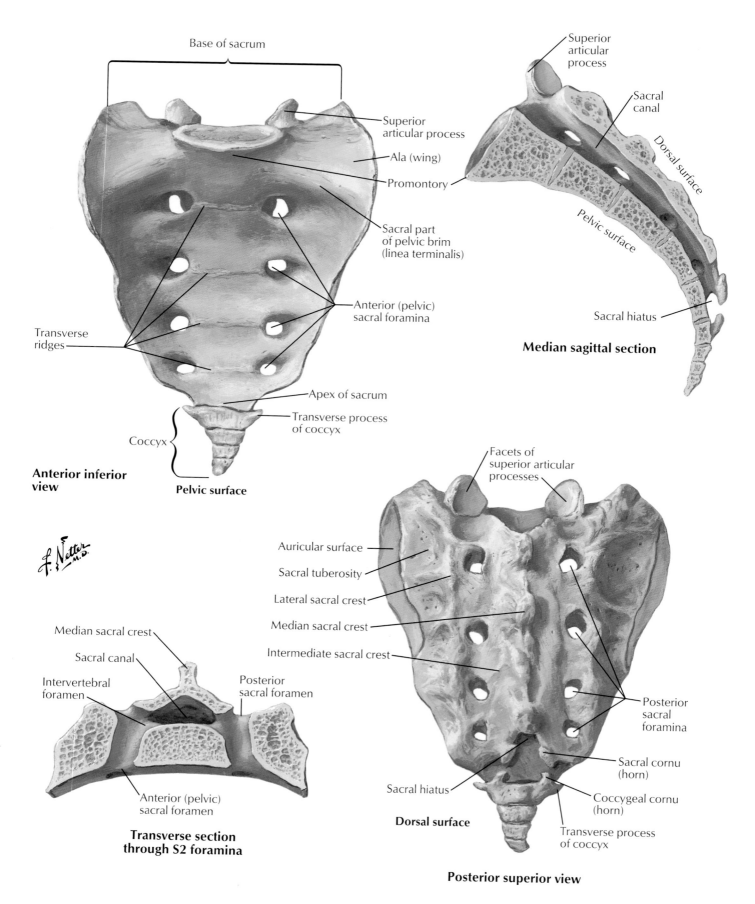

Base of sacrum

Superior articular process

Ala (wing)

Promontory

Sacral part of pelvic brim (linea terminalis)

Anterior (pelvic) sacral foramina

Transverse ridges

Apex of sacrum

Transverse process of coccyx

Coccyx

**Anterior inferior view**

**Pelvic surface**

Superior articular process

Sacral canal

Dorsal surface

Pelvic surface

Sacral hiatus

**Median sagittal section**

Median sacral crest

Sacral canal

Intervertebral foramen

Posterior sacral foramen

Anterior (pelvic) sacral foramen

**Transverse section through S2 foramina**

Facets of superior articular processes

Auricular surface

Sacral tuberosity

Lateral sacral crest

Median sacral crest

Intermediate sacral crest

Posterior sacral foramina

Sacral cornu (horn)

Coccygeal cornu (horn)

Sacral hiatus

Transverse process of coccyx

**Dorsal surface**

**Posterior superior view**

**Plate 157**

**Bones and Ligaments**

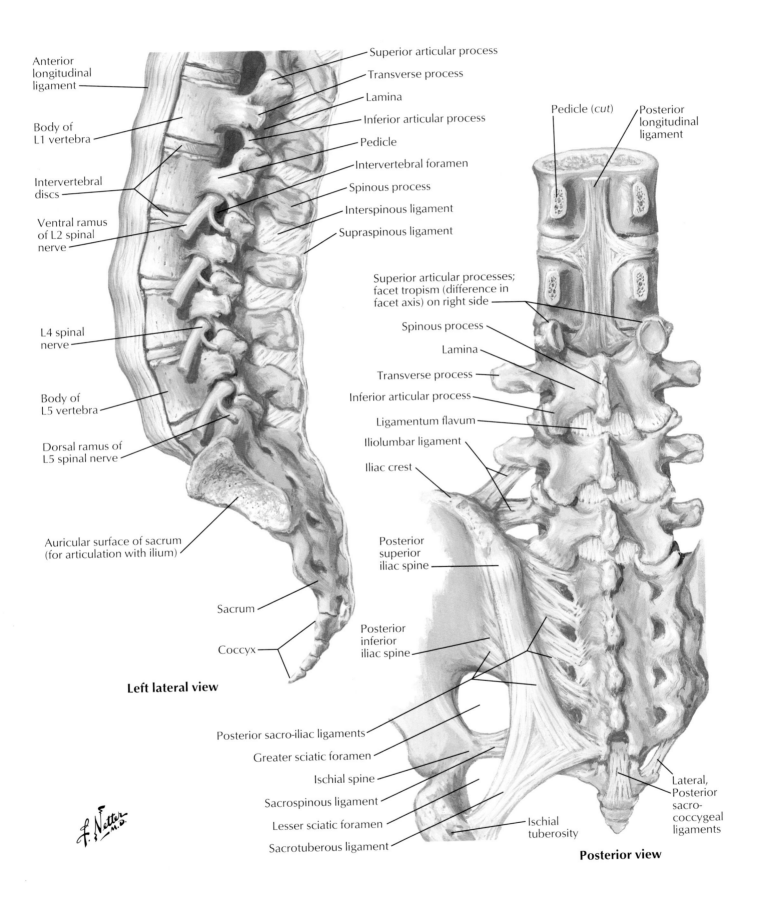

Anterior longitudinal ligament

Body of L1 vertebra

Intervertebral discs

Ventral ramus of L2 spinal nerve

L4 spinal nerve

Body of L5 vertebra

Dorsal ramus of L5 spinal nerve

Superior articular process

Transverse process

Lamina

Inferior articular process

Pedicle

Intervertebral foramen

Spinous process

Interspinous ligament

Supraspinous ligament

Pedicle (cut)

Posterior longitudinal ligament

Auricular surface of sacrum (for articulation with ilium)

Sacrum

Coccyx

**Left lateral view**

Superior articular processes; facet tropism (difference in facet axis) on right side

Spinous process

Lamina

Transverse process

Inferior articular process

Ligamentum flavum

Iliolumbar ligament

Iliac crest

Posterior superior iliac spine

Posterior inferior iliac spine

Posterior sacro-iliac ligaments

Greater sciatic foramen

Ischial spine

Sacrospinous ligament

Lesser sciatic foramen

Sacrotuberous ligament

Ischial tuberosity

Lateral, Posterior sacro-coccygeal ligaments

**Posterior view**

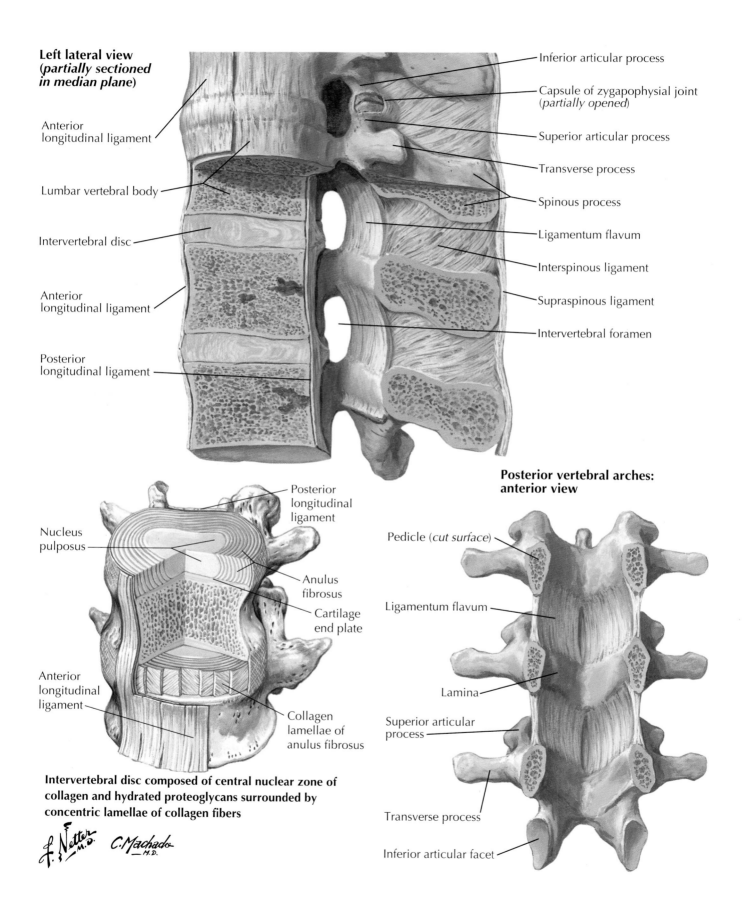

**Left lateral view (*partially sectioned in median plane*)**

Anterior longitudinal ligament

Lumbar vertebral body

Intervertebral disc

Anterior longitudinal ligament

Posterior longitudinal ligament

Inferior articular process

Capsule of zygapophysial joint (*partially opened*)

Superior articular process

Transverse process

Spinous process

Ligamentum flavum

Interspinous ligament

Supraspinous ligament

Intervertebral foramen

Nucleus pulposus

Posterior longitudinal ligament

Anulus fibrosus

Cartilage end plate

Anterior longitudinal ligament

Collagen lamellae of anulus fibrosus

**Intervertebral disc composed of central nuclear zone of collagen and hydrated proteoglycans surrounded by concentric lamellae of collagen fibers**

**Posterior vertebral arches: anterior view**

Pedicle (*cut surface*)

Ligamentum flavum

Lamina

Superior articular process

Transverse process

Inferior articular facet

**Plate 159**

**Bones and Ligaments**

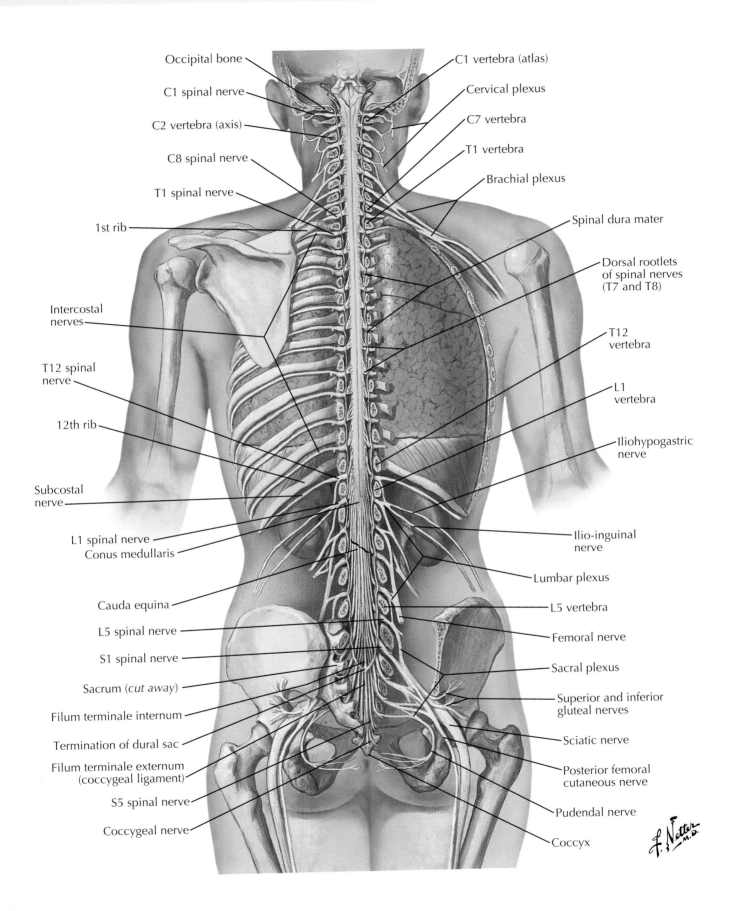

Occipital bone

C1 spinal nerve

C2 vertebra (axis)

C8 spinal nerve

T1 spinal nerve

1st rib

Intercostal nerves

T12 spinal nerve

12th rib

Subcostal nerve

L1 spinal nerve

Conus medullaris

Cauda equina

L5 spinal nerve

S1 spinal nerve

Sacrum (*cut away*)

Filum terminale internum

Termination of dural sac

Filum terminale externum (coccygeal ligament)

S5 spinal nerve

Coccygeal nerve

C1 vertebra (atlas)

Cervical plexus

C7 vertebra

T1 vertebra

Brachial plexus

Spinal dura mater

Dorsal rootlets of spinal nerves (T7 and T8)

T12 vertebra

L1 vertebra

Iliohypogastric nerve

Ilio-inguinal nerve

Lumbar plexus

L5 vertebra

Femoral nerve

Sacral plexus

Superior and inferior gluteal nerves

Sciatic nerve

Posterior femoral cutaneous nerve

Pudendal nerve

Coccyx

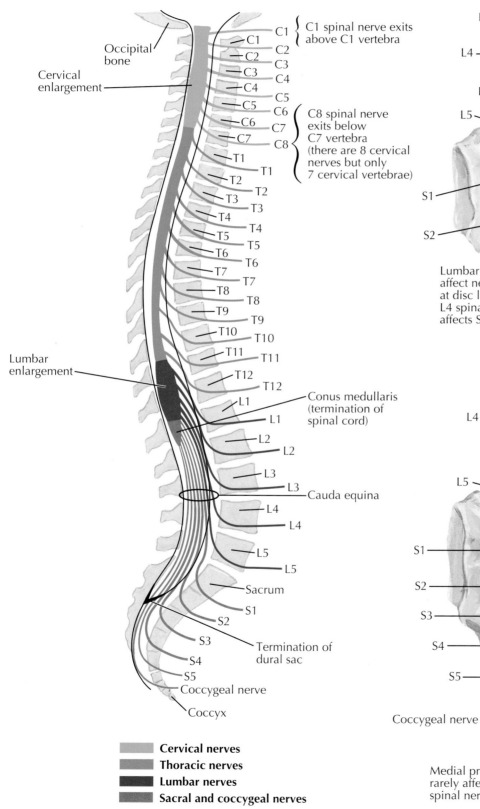

Occipital bone

Cervical enlargement

C1 { C1 spinal nerve exits above C1 vertebra

C1
C2
C2
C3
C3
C4
C4
C5
C5
C6
C6
C7
C7
C8

C8 spinal nerve exits below C7 vertebra (there are 8 cervical nerves but only 7 cervical vertebrae)

T1
T1
T2
T2
T3
T3
T4
T4
T5
T5
T6
T6
T7
T7
T8
T8
T9
T9
T10
T10
T11
T11

Lumbar enlargement

T12
T12
L1

Conus medullaris (termination of spinal cord)

L1
L2
L2
L3
L3

Cauda equina

L4
L4
L5
L5

Sacrum

S1
S2
S3

Termination of dural sac

S4
S5
Coccygeal nerve

Coccyx

Cervical nerves
Thoracic nerves
Lumbar nerves
Sacral and coccygeal nerves

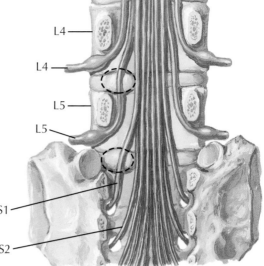

L4

L4

L5

L5

S1

S2

Lumbar disc protrusion (*dashed ovals*) does not usually affect nerve exiting above disc. Lateral protrusion at disc level L4–5 affects L5 spinal nerve, not L4 spinal nerve. Protrusion at disc level L5–S1 affects S1 spinal nerve, not L5 spinal nerve.

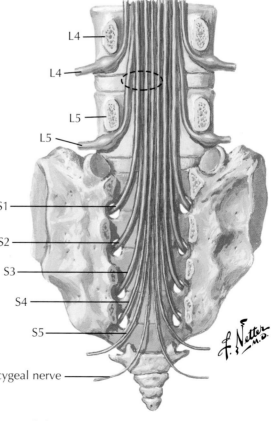

L4

L4

L5

L5

S1

S2

S3

S4

S5

Coccygeal nerve

Medial protrusion at disc level L4–5 (*dashed oval*) rarely affects L4 spinal nerve but may affect L5 spinal nerve and sometimes S1–4 spinal nerves.

**Plate 161**　　　　　　　　　　　　　　　　**Spinal Cord**

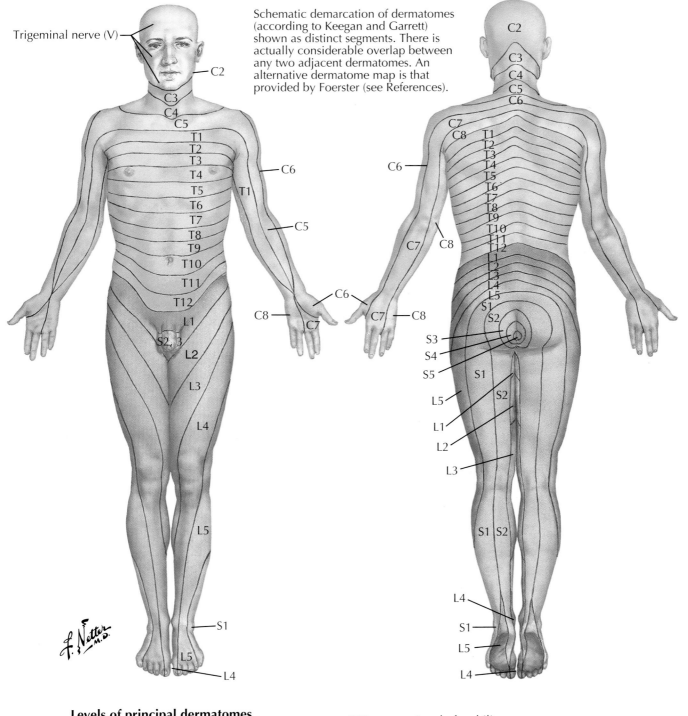

Trigeminal nerve (V)

Schematic demarcation of dermatomes (according to Keegan and Garrett) shown as distinct segments. There is actually considerable overlap between any two adjacent dermatomes. An alternative dermatome map is that provided by Foerster (see References).

## Levels of principal dermatomes

| | |
|---|---|
| **C5** | Clavicles |
| **C5, 6** | Lateral sides of upper limbs |
| **C8, T1** | Medial sides of upper limbs |
| **C6** | Digit I (thumb) |
| **C6, 7, 8** | Hand |
| **C8** | Digits IV and V (ring and little fingers) |
| **T4** | Level of nipples |

| | |
|---|---|
| **T10** | Level of umbilicus |
| **L1** | Inguinal region |
| **L1, 2, 3, 4** | Anterior and inner surfaces of lower limbs |
| **L4, 5, S1** | Foot |
| **L4** | Medial side digit I (great toe) |
| **L5, S1, 2** | Lateral and posterior surfaces of lower limbs |
| **S1** | Lateral margin of foot and digit V (little toe) |
| **S2, 3, 4** | Perineum |

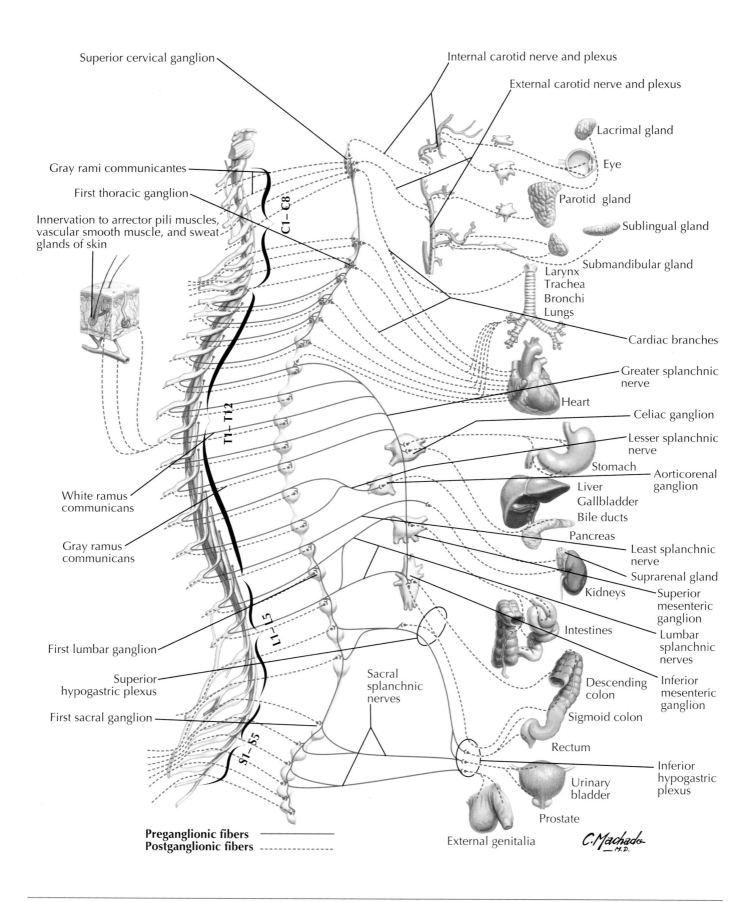

Superior cervical ganglion

Gray rami communicantes

First thoracic ganglion

Innervation to arrector pili muscles, vascular smooth muscle, and sweat glands of skin

White ramus communicans

Gray ramus communicans

First lumbar ganglion

Superior hypogastric plexus

First sacral ganglion

C1–C8

T1–T12

L1–L5

S1–S5

Internal carotid nerve and plexus

External carotid nerve and plexus

Lacrimal gland

Eye

Parotid gland

Sublingual gland

Submandibular gland

Larynx
Trachea
Bronchi
Lungs

Cardiac branches

Greater splanchnic nerve

Heart

Celiac ganglion

Lesser splanchnic nerve

Stomach

Aorticorenal ganglion

Liver
Gallbladder
Bile ducts

Pancreas

Least splanchnic nerve

Suprarenal gland

Kidneys

Superior mesenteric ganglion

Intestines

Lumbar splanchnic nerves

Inferior mesenteric ganglion

Descending colon

Sacral splanchnic nerves

Sigmoid colon

Rectum

Inferior hypogastric plexus

Urinary bladder

Prostate

External genitalia

**Preganglionic fibers** ——————
**Postganglionic fibers** -------------

C. Machado
—M.D.

**Plate 163**

**Spinal Cord**

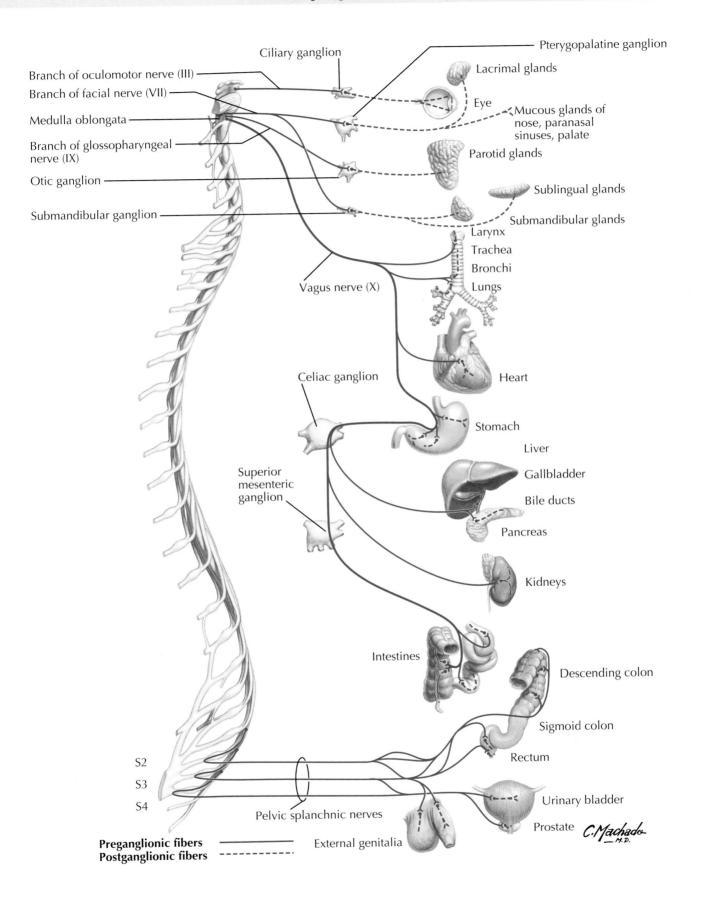

Ciliary ganglion

Pterygopalatine ganglion

Lacrimal glands

Branch of oculomotor nerve (III)

Branch of facial nerve (VII)

Eye

Medulla oblongata

Mucous glands of nose, paranasal sinuses, palate

Branch of glossopharyngeal nerve (IX)

Parotid glands

Otic ganglion

Sublingual glands

Submandibular ganglion

Submandibular glands

Larynx

Trachea

Bronchi

Lungs

Vagus nerve (X)

Heart

Celiac ganglion

Stomach

Liver

Gallbladder

Bile ducts

Superior mesenteric ganglion

Pancreas

Kidneys

Intestines

Descending colon

Sigmoid colon

S2

Rectum

S3

Urinary bladder

S4

Prostate

Pelvic splanchnic nerves

**Preganglionic fibers** ——————

**Postganglionic fibers** - - - - - - -

External genitalia

C. Machado
_M.D._

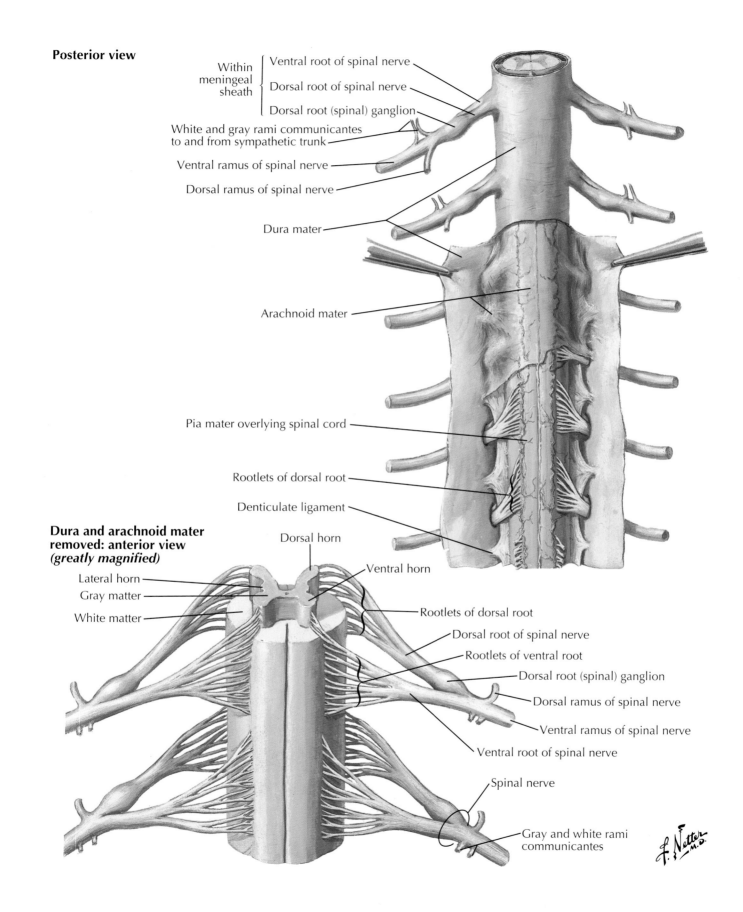

**Posterior view**

Within meningeal sheath
- Ventral root of spinal nerve
- Dorsal root of spinal nerve
- Dorsal root (spinal) ganglion

White and gray rami communicantes to and from sympathetic trunk

Ventral ramus of spinal nerve

Dorsal ramus of spinal nerve

Dura mater

Arachnoid mater

Pia mater overlying spinal cord

Rootlets of dorsal root

Denticulate ligament

**Dura and arachnoid mater removed: anterior view**
*(greatly magnified)*

Dorsal horn

Ventral horn

Lateral horn

Gray matter

White matter

Rootlets of dorsal root

Dorsal root of spinal nerve

Rootlets of ventral root

Dorsal root (spinal) ganglion

Dorsal ramus of spinal nerve

Ventral ramus of spinal nerve

Ventral root of spinal nerve

Spinal nerve

Gray and white rami communicantes

**Plate 165**

**Spinal Cord**

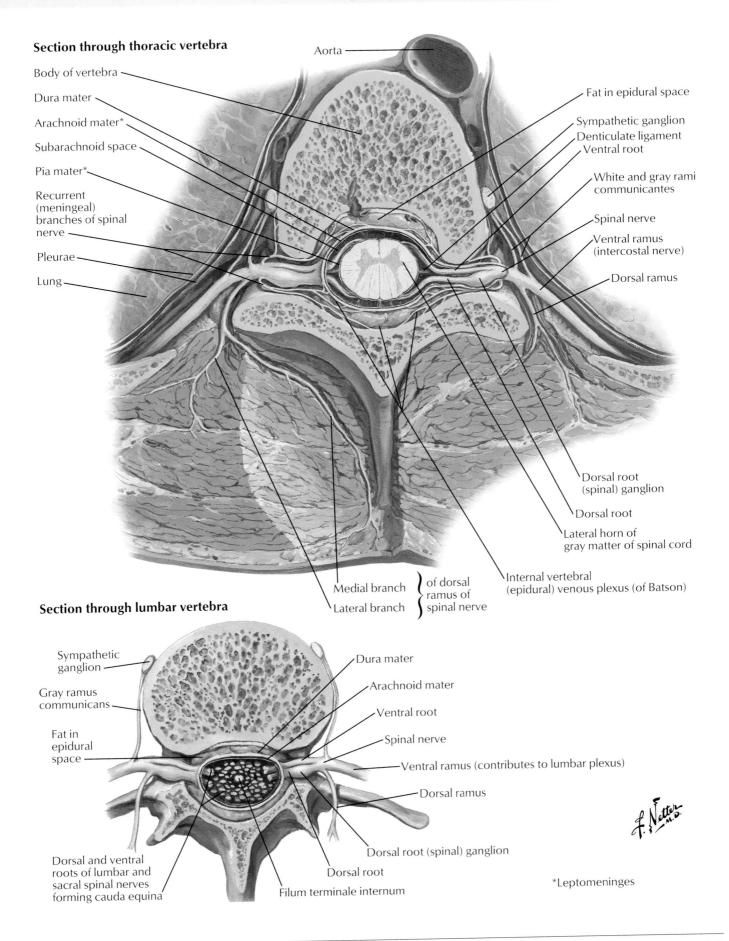

**Section through thoracic vertebra**

Body of vertebra

Dura mater

Arachnoid mater*

Subarachnoid space

Pia mater*

Recurrent (meningeal) branches of spinal nerve

Pleurae

Lung

Aorta

Fat in epidural space

Sympathetic ganglion

Denticulate ligament

Ventral root

White and gray rami communicantes

Spinal nerve

Ventral ramus (intercostal nerve)

Dorsal ramus

Dorsal root (spinal) ganglion

Dorsal root

Lateral horn of gray matter of spinal cord

Internal vertebral (epidural) venous plexus (of Batson)

Medial branch } of dorsal

Lateral branch } ramus of spinal nerve

**Section through lumbar vertebra**

Sympathetic ganglion

Gray ramus communicans

Fat in epidural space

Dura mater

Arachnoid mater

Ventral root

Spinal nerve

Ventral ramus (contributes to lumbar plexus)

Dorsal ramus

Dorsal root (spinal) ganglion

Dorsal root

Dorsal and ventral roots of lumbar and sacral spinal nerves forming cauda equina

Filum terminale internum

*Leptomeninges

**Spinal Cord**

**Plate 166**

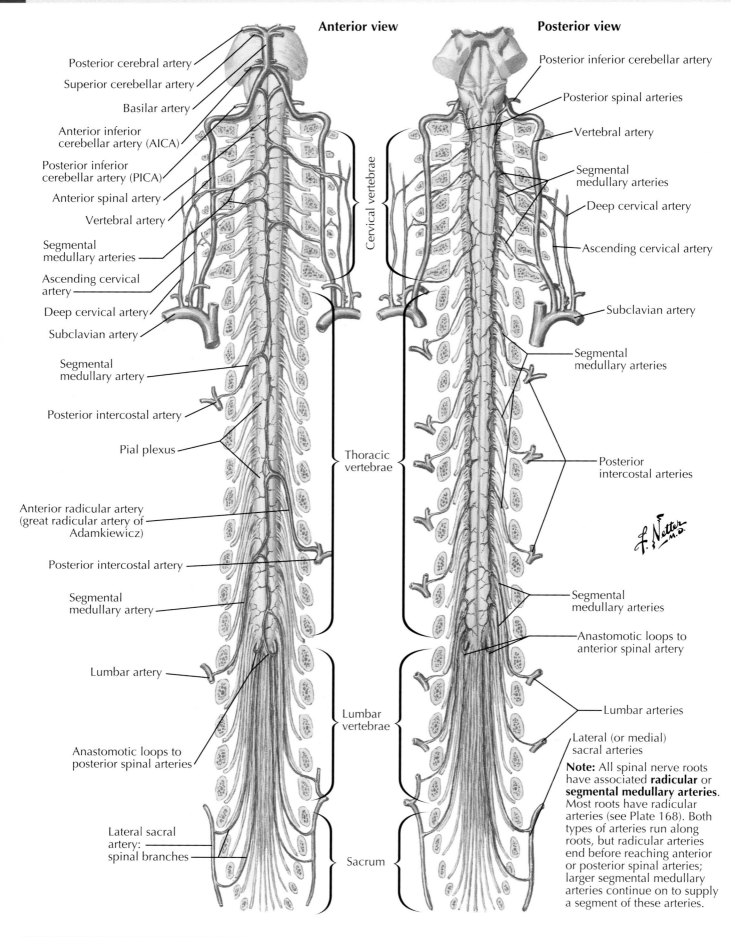

**Anterior view**

Posterior cerebral artery

Superior cerebellar artery

Basilar artery

Anterior inferior cerebellar artery (AICA)

Posterior inferior cerebellar artery (PICA)

Anterior spinal artery

Vertebral artery

Segmental medullary arteries

Ascending cervical artery

Deep cervical artery

Subclavian artery

Segmental medullary artery

Posterior intercostal artery

Pial plexus

Anterior radicular artery (great radicular artery of Adamkiewicz)

Posterior intercostal artery

Segmental medullary artery

Lumbar artery

Anastomotic loops to posterior spinal arteries

Lateral sacral artery: spinal branches

**Posterior view**

Posterior inferior cerebellar artery

Posterior spinal arteries

Vertebral artery

Segmental medullary arteries

Deep cervical artery

Ascending cervical artery

Subclavian artery

Segmental medullary arteries

Posterior intercostal arteries

Segmental medullary arteries

Anastomotic loops to anterior spinal artery

Lumbar arteries

Lateral (or medial) sacral arteries

Cervical vertebrae

Thoracic vertebrae

Lumbar vertebrae

Sacrum

**Note:** All spinal nerve roots have associated **radicular** or **segmental medullary arteries**. Most roots have radicular arteries (see Plate 168). Both types of arteries run along roots, but radicular arteries end before reaching anterior or posterior spinal arteries; larger segmental medullary arteries continue on to supply a segment of these arteries.

**Plate 167**

**Spinal Cord**

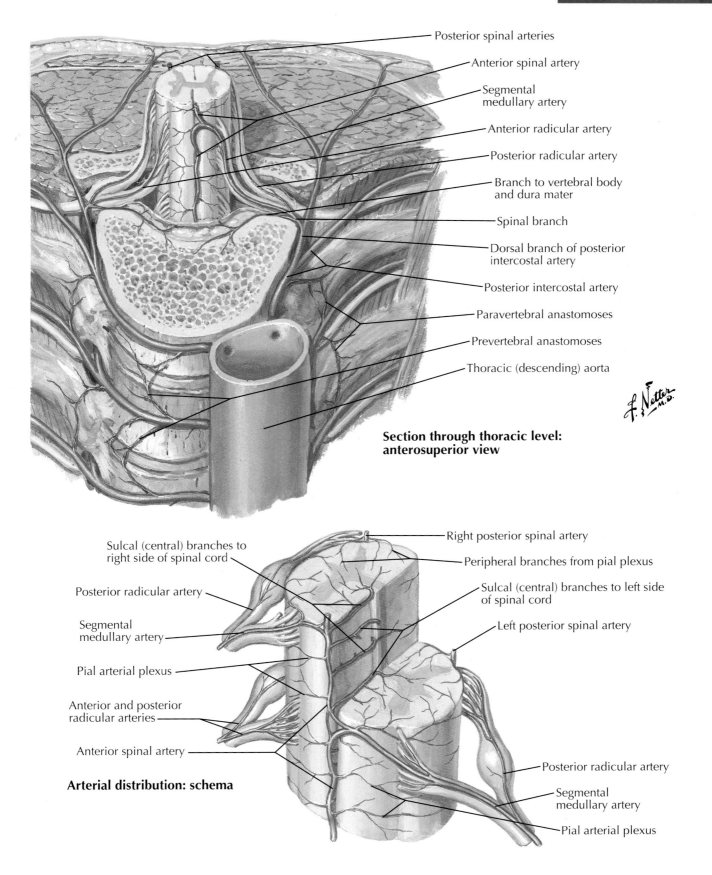

Posterior spinal arteries

Anterior spinal artery

Segmental medullary artery

Anterior radicular artery

Posterior radicular artery

Branch to vertebral body and dura mater

Spinal branch

Dorsal branch of posterior intercostal artery

Posterior intercostal artery

Paravertebral anastomoses

Prevertebral anastomoses

Thoracic (descending) aorta

**Section through thoracic level: anterosuperior view**

Sulcal (central) branches to right side of spinal cord

Posterior radicular artery

Segmental medullary artery

Pial arterial plexus

Anterior and posterior radicular arteries

Anterior spinal artery

**Arterial distribution: schema**

Right posterior spinal artery

Peripheral branches from pial plexus

Sulcal (central) branches to left side of spinal cord

Left posterior spinal artery

Posterior radicular artery

Segmental medullary artery

Pial arterial plexus

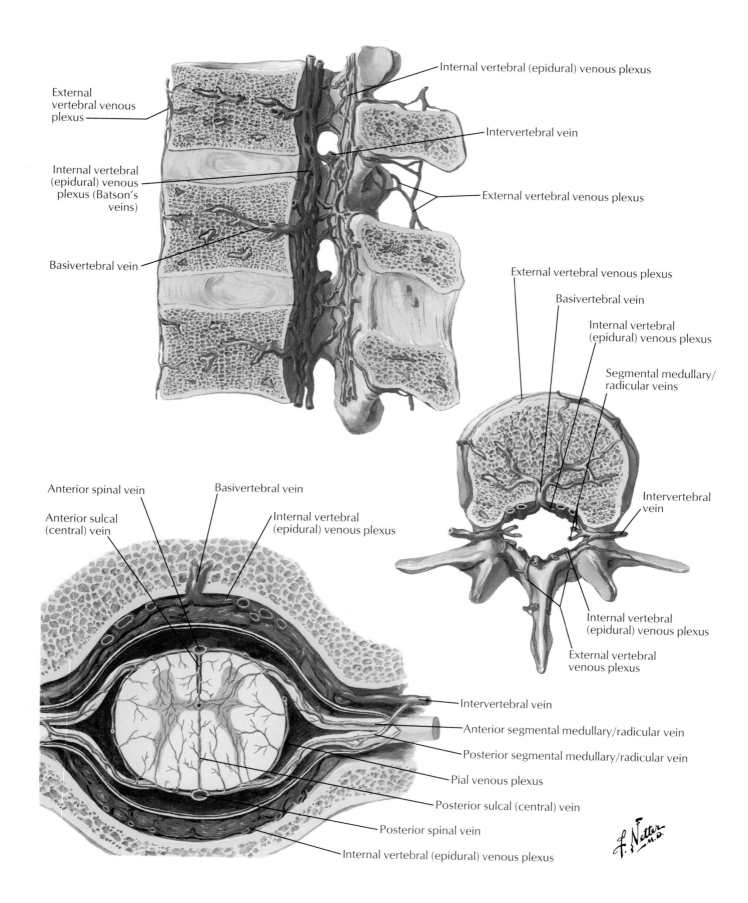

External vertebral venous plexus

Internal vertebral (epidural) venous plexus (Batson's veins)

Basivertebral vein

Internal vertebral (epidural) venous plexus

Intervertebral vein

External vertebral venous plexus

External vertebral venous plexus

Basivertebral vein

Internal vertebral (epidural) venous plexus

Segmental medullary/radicular veins

Intervertebral vein

Internal vertebral (epidural) venous plexus

External vertebral venous plexus

Anterior spinal vein

Anterior sulcal (central) vein

Basivertebral vein

Internal vertebral (epidural) venous plexus

Intervertebral vein

Anterior segmental medullary/radicular vein

Posterior segmental medullary/radicular vein

Pial venous plexus

Posterior sulcal (central) vein

Posterior spinal vein

Internal vertebral (epidural) venous plexus

**Plate 169**

**Spinal Cord**

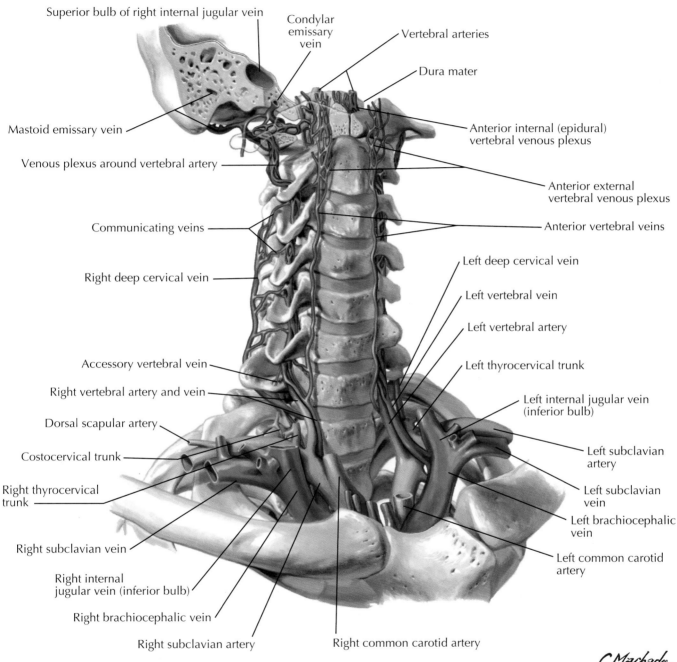

Superior bulb of right internal jugular vein

Condylar emissary vein

Vertebral arteries

Dura mater

Mastoid emissary vein

Anterior internal (epidural) vertebral venous plexus

Venous plexus around vertebral artery

Anterior external vertebral venous plexus

Communicating veins

Anterior vertebral veins

Right deep cervical vein

Left deep cervical vein

Left vertebral vein

Left vertebral artery

Left thyrocervical trunk

Accessory vertebral vein

Right vertebral artery and vein

Left internal jugular vein (inferior bulb)

Dorsal scapular artery

Costocervical trunk

Left subclavian artery

Right thyrocervical trunk

Left subclavian vein

Left brachiocephalic vein

Right subclavian vein

Left common carotid artery

Right internal jugular vein (inferior bulb)

Right brachiocephalic vein

Right subclavian artery

Right common carotid artery

C. Machado
_M.D.

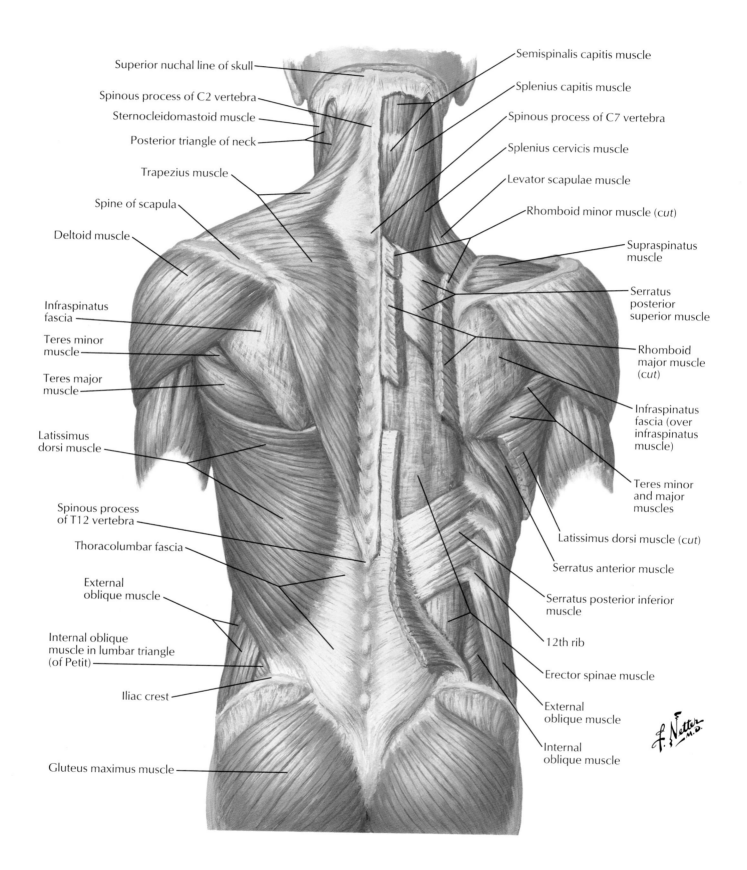

Superior nuchal line of skull

Spinous process of C2 vertebra

Sternocleidomastoid muscle

Posterior triangle of neck

Trapezius muscle

Spine of scapula

Deltoid muscle

Infraspinatus fascia

Teres minor muscle

Teres major muscle

Latissimus dorsi muscle

Spinous process of T12 vertebra

Thoracolumbar fascia

External oblique muscle

Internal oblique muscle in lumbar triangle (of Petit)

Iliac crest

Gluteus maximus muscle

Semispinalis capitis muscle

Splenius capitis muscle

Spinous process of C7 vertebra

Splenius cervicis muscle

Levator scapulae muscle

Rhomboid minor muscle (cut)

Supraspinatus muscle

Serratus posterior superior muscle

Rhomboid major muscle (cut)

Infraspinatus fascia (over infraspinatus muscle)

Teres minor and major muscles

Latissimus dorsi muscle (cut)

Serratus anterior muscle

Serratus posterior inferior muscle

12th rib

Erector spinae muscle

External oblique muscle

Internal oblique muscle

**Plate 171**

**Muscles and Nerves**

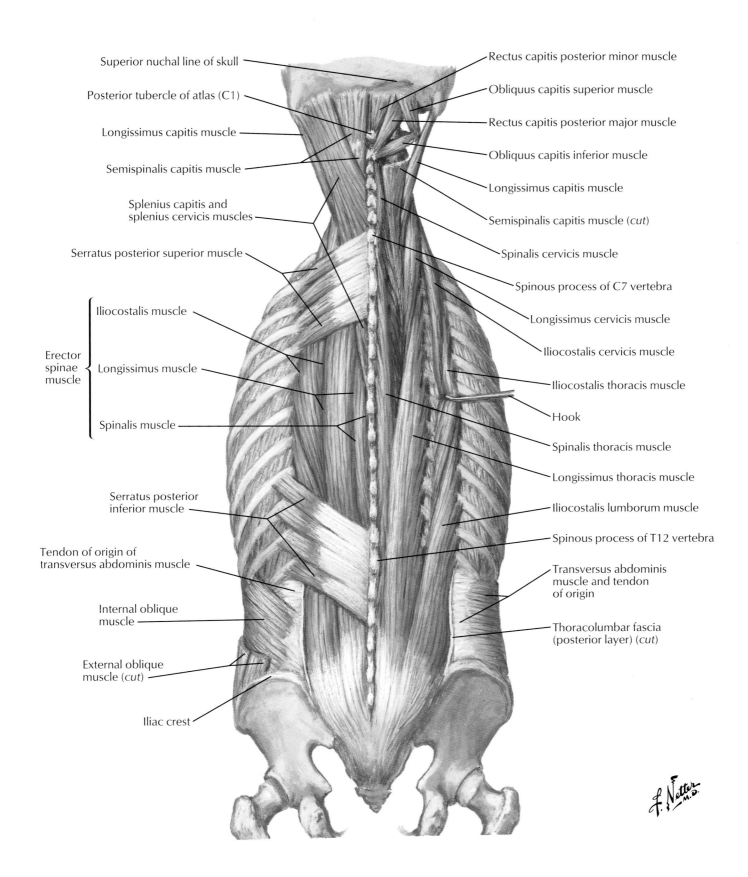

Superior nuchal line of skull

Posterior tubercle of atlas (C1)

Longissimus capitis muscle

Semispinalis capitis muscle

Splenius capitis and splenius cervicis muscles

Serratus posterior superior muscle

Erector spinae muscle {
Iliocostalis muscle

Longissimus muscle

Spinalis muscle
}

Serratus posterior inferior muscle

Tendon of origin of transversus abdominis muscle

Internal oblique muscle

External oblique muscle (cut)

Iliac crest

Rectus capitis posterior minor muscle

Obliquus capitis superior muscle

Rectus capitis posterior major muscle

Obliquus capitis inferior muscle

Longissimus capitis muscle

Semispinalis capitis muscle (cut)

Spinalis cervicis muscle

Spinous process of C7 vertebra

Longissimus cervicis muscle

Iliocostalis cervicis muscle

Iliocostalis thoracis muscle

Hook

Spinalis thoracis muscle

Longissimus thoracis muscle

Iliocostalis lumborum muscle

Spinous process of T12 vertebra

Transversus abdominis muscle and tendon of origin

Thoracolumbar fascia (posterior layer) (cut)

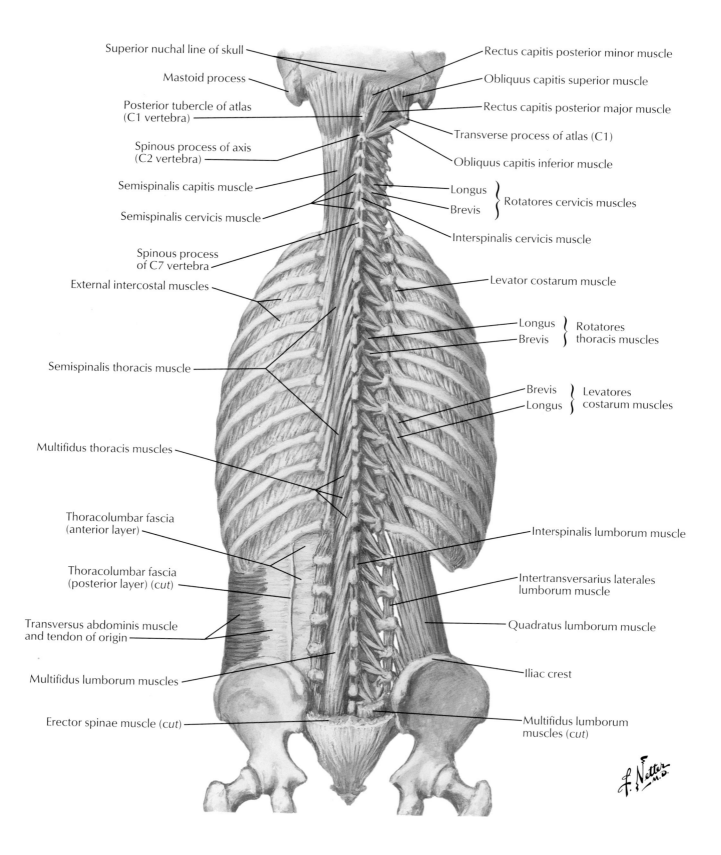

Superior nuchal line of skull

Mastoid process

Posterior tubercle of atlas (C1 vertebra)

Spinous process of axis (C2 vertebra)

Semispinalis capitis muscle

Semispinalis cervicis muscle

Spinous process of C7 vertebra

External intercostal muscles

Semispinalis thoracis muscle

Multifidus thoracis muscles

Thoracolumbar fascia (anterior layer)

Thoracolumbar fascia (posterior layer) (cut)

Transversus abdominis muscle and tendon of origin

Multifidus lumborum muscles

Erector spinae muscle (cut)

Rectus capitis posterior minor muscle

Obliquus capitis superior muscle

Rectus capitis posterior major muscle

Transverse process of atlas (C1)

Obliquus capitis inferior muscle

Longus
Brevis } Rotatores cervicis muscles

Interspinalis cervicis muscle

Levator costarum muscle

Longus
Brevis } Rotatores thoracis muscles

Brevis
Longus } Levatores costarum muscles

Interspinalis lumborum muscle

Intertransversarius laterales lumborum muscle

Quadratus lumborum muscle

Iliac crest

Multifidus lumborum muscles (cut)

**Plate 173**

**Muscles and Nerves**

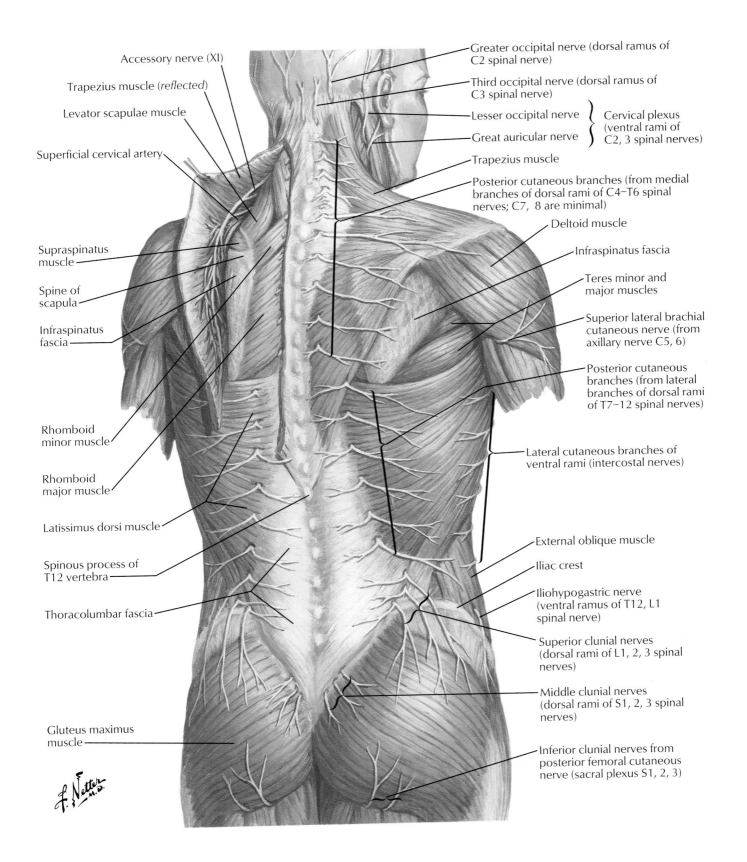

Accessory nerve (XI)

Trapezius muscle (*reflected*)

Levator scapulae muscle

Superficial cervical artery

Supraspinatus muscle

Spine of scapula

Infraspinatus fascia

Rhomboid minor muscle

Rhomboid major muscle

Latissimus dorsi muscle

Spinous process of T12 vertebra

Thoracolumbar fascia

Gluteus maximus muscle

Greater occipital nerve (dorsal ramus of C2 spinal nerve)

Third occipital nerve (dorsal ramus of C3 spinal nerve)

Lesser occipital nerve ⎫ Cervical plexus
Great auricular nerve ⎬ (ventral rami of
⎭ C2, 3 spinal nerves)

Trapezius muscle

Posterior cutaneous branches (from medial branches of dorsal rami of C4–T6 spinal nerves; C7, 8 are minimal)

Deltoid muscle

Infraspinatus fascia

Teres minor and major muscles

Superior lateral brachial cutaneous nerve (from axillary nerve C5, 6)

Posterior cutaneous branches (from lateral branches of dorsal rami of T7–12 spinal nerves)

Lateral cutaneous branches of ventral rami (intercostal nerves)

External oblique muscle

Iliac crest

Iliohypogastric nerve (ventral ramus of T12, L1 spinal nerve)

Superior clunial nerves (dorsal rami of L1, 2, 3 spinal nerves)

Middle clunial nerves (dorsal rami of S1, 2, 3 spinal nerves)

Inferior clunial nerves from posterior femoral cutaneous nerve (sacral plexus S1, 2, 3)

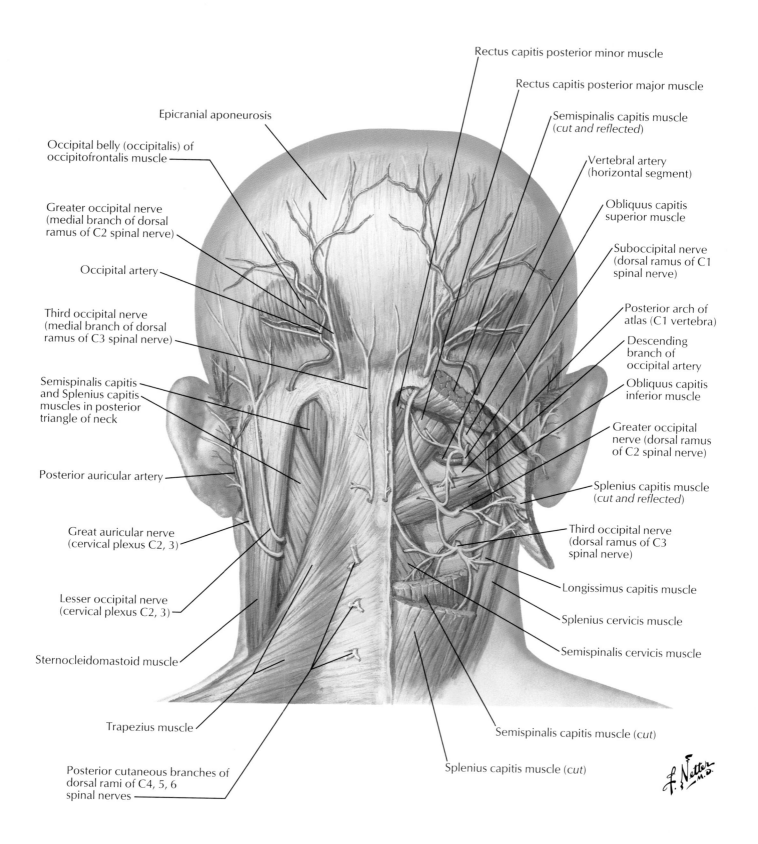

Rectus capitis posterior minor muscle

Rectus capitis posterior major muscle

Semispinalis capitis muscle (*cut and reflected*)

Vertebral artery (horizontal segment)

Obliquus capitis superior muscle

Suboccipital nerve (dorsal ramus of C1 spinal nerve)

Posterior arch of atlas (C1 vertebra)

Descending branch of occipital artery

Obliquus capitis inferior muscle

Greater occipital nerve (dorsal ramus of C2 spinal nerve)

Splenius capitis muscle (*cut and reflected*)

Third occipital nerve (dorsal ramus of C3 spinal nerve)

Longissimus capitis muscle

Splenius cervicis muscle

Semispinalis cervicis muscle

Semispinalis capitis muscle (*cut*)

Splenius capitis muscle (*cut*)

Epicranial aponeurosis

Occipital belly (occipitalis) of occipitofrontalis muscle

Greater occipital nerve (medial branch of dorsal ramus of C2 spinal nerve)

Occipital artery

Third occipital nerve (medial branch of dorsal ramus of C3 spinal nerve)

Semispinalis capitis and Splenius capitis muscles in posterior triangle of neck

Posterior auricular artery

Great auricular nerve (cervical plexus C2, 3)

Lesser occipital nerve (cervical plexus C2, 3)

Sternocleidomastoid muscle

Trapezius muscle

Posterior cutaneous branches of dorsal rami of C4, 5, 6 spinal nerves

**Plate 175**

**Muscles and Nerves**

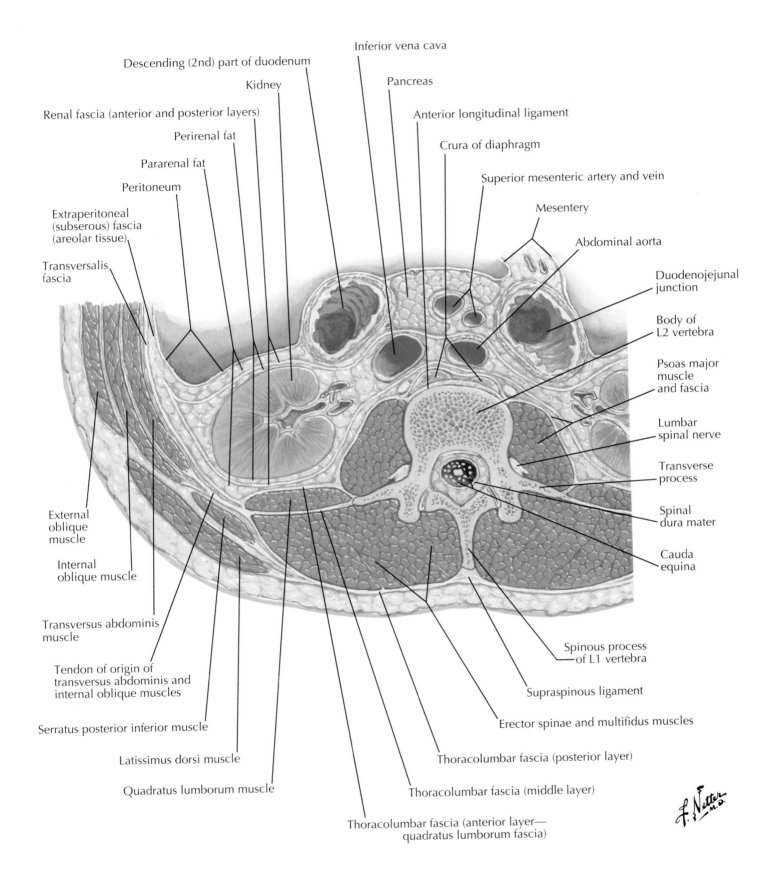

Descending (2nd) part of duodenum

Kidney

Renal fascia (anterior and posterior layers)

Perirenal fat

Pararenal fat

Peritoneum

Extraperitoneal (subserous) fascia (areolar tissue)

Transversalis fascia

External oblique muscle

Internal oblique muscle

Transversus abdominis muscle

Tendon of origin of transversus abdominis and internal oblique muscles

Serratus posterior inferior muscle

Latissimus dorsi muscle

Quadratus lumborum muscle

Inferior vena cava

Pancreas

Anterior longitudinal ligament

Crura of diaphragm

Superior mesenteric artery and vein

Mesentery

Abdominal aorta

Duodenojejunal junction

Body of L2 vertebra

Psoas major muscle and fascia

Lumbar spinal nerve

Transverse process

Spinal dura mater

Cauda equina

Spinous process of L1 vertebra

Supraspinous ligament

Erector spinae and multifidus muscles

Thoracolumbar fascia (posterior layer)

Thoracolumbar fascia (middle layer)

Thoracolumbar fascia (anterior layer— quadratus lumborum fascia)

*f. Netter M.D.*

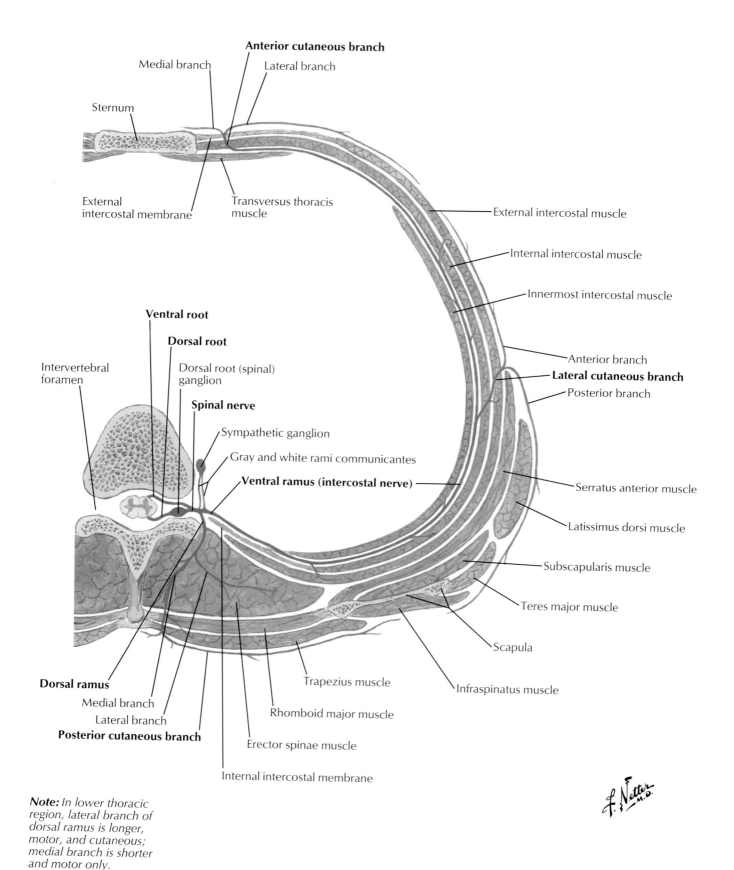

Anterior cutaneous branch

Medial branch

Lateral branch

Sternum

External intercostal membrane

Transversus thoracis muscle

External intercostal muscle

Internal intercostal muscle

Innermost intercostal muscle

Ventral root

Dorsal root

Intervertebral foramen

Dorsal root (spinal) ganglion

Spinal nerve

Sympathetic ganglion

Gray and white rami communicantes

Ventral ramus (intercostal nerve)

Anterior branch

Lateral cutaneous branch

Posterior branch

Serratus anterior muscle

Latissimus dorsi muscle

Subscapularis muscle

Teres major muscle

Scapula

Infraspinatus muscle

Dorsal ramus

Medial branch

Lateral branch

Posterior cutaneous branch

Trapezius muscle

Rhomboid major muscle

Erector spinae muscle

Internal intercostal membrane

**Note:** *In lower thoracic region, lateral branch of dorsal ramus is longer, motor, and cutaneous; medial branch is shorter and motor only.*

**Plate 177**

**Cross-Sectional Anatomy**

| MUSCLE | PROXIMAL ATTACHMENT (ORIGIN) | DISTAL ATTACHMENT (INSERTION) | INNERVATION | MAIN ACTIONS | BLOOD SUPPLY | MUSCLE GROUP |
|---|---|---|---|---|---|---|
| Erector spinae | Posterior sacrum, iliac crest, sacrospinous ligament, supraspinous ligament, spinous processes of lower lumbar and sacral vertebrae | *Iliocostalis:* angles of lower ribs, cervical transverse processes<br><br>*Longissimus:* between tubercles and angles of ribs, transverse processes of thoracic and cervical vertebrae, mastoid process<br><br>*Spinalis:* spinous processes of upper thoracic and midcervical vertebrae | Dorsal rami of each region | Extends and laterally bends vertebral column and head | *Cervical portions:* occipital, deep cervical, and vertebral arteries<br><br>*Thoracic portions:* dorsal branches of posterior intercostal, subcostal, and lumbar arteries<br><br>*Sacral portions:* dorsal branches of lateral sacral arteries | Sacrospinalis |
| Interspinales (cervical, thoracic, lumbar) | Spinous process | Adjacent spinous process | Dorsal rami of spinal nerves | Aid in extension of vertebral column | *Cervical portions:* occipital, deep cervical, and vertebral arteries<br><br>*Thoracic portions:* dorsal branches of posterior intercostal arteries<br><br>*Lumbar portions:* dorsal branches of lumbar arteries | Segmental |
| Intertransversarii (cervical, thoracic, lumbar) | Extend between adjacent transverse processes of vertebrae | Extend between adjacent transverse processes of vertebrae | Dorsal rami of spinal nerves | Assist in lateral flexion of vertebral column | *Cervical portions:* occipital, deep cervical, and vertebral arteries<br><br>*Thoracic portions:* dorsal branches of posterior intercostal, subcostal, and lumbar arteries<br><br>*Lumbar portions:* dorsal branches of lateral lumbar arteries | Segmental |
| Latissimus dorsi | Spinous processes of T7–L5, thoracolumbar fascia, iliac crest, and last three ribs | Humerus (intertubercular sulcus) | Thoracodorsal nerve | Extends, adducts, and medially rotates humerus | Thoracodorsal artery, dorsal perforating branches of 9th, 10th, and 11th posterior intercostal, subcostal, and first three lumbar arteries | Superficial back |
| Levator scapulae | Posterior tubercles of transverse processes of C1–C4 | Medial border of scapula from superior angle to spine | Ventral rami of C3–C4 and dorsal scapular nerve | Elevates scapula medially, inferiorly rotates glenoid cavity | Dorsal scapular artery, transverse cervical artery, ascending cervical artery | Superficial back |
| Multifidus | Sacrum, ilium, transverse processes of T1–T12, and articular processes of C4–C7 | Spinous processes of vertebrae above, spanning two to four segments | Dorsal rami of each region | Stabilizes spine | *Cervical portions:* occipital, deep cervical, and vertebral arteries<br><br>*Thoracic portions:* dorsal branches of posterior intercostal, subcostal, and lumbar arteries<br><br>*Sacral portions:* dorsal branches of lateral sacral arteries | Transversospinalis |
| Obliquus capitis inferior | Spine of axis | Transverse process of atlas | Suboccipital nerve | Rotates atlas to turn face to same side | Vertebral artery, descending branch of occipital artery | Suboccipital |
| Obliquus capitis superior | Transverse process of atlas | Occipital bone | Suboccipital nerve | Extends and bends head laterally | Vertebral artery, descending branch of occipital artery | Suboccipital |
| Rectus capitis posterior major | Spine of axis | Inferior nuchal line | Suboccipital nerve | Extends and rotates head to same side | Vertebral artery, descending branch of occipital artery | Suboccipital |

Variations in spinal nerve contributions to the innervation of muscles, their arterial supply, their attachments, and their actions are common themes in human anatomy. Therefore, expect differences between texts and realize that anatomical variation is normal.

| MUSCLE | PROXIMAL ATTACHMENT (ORIGIN) | DISTAL ATTACHMENT (INSERTION) | INNERVATION | MAIN ACTIONS | BLOOD SUPPLY | MUSCLE GROUP |
|---|---|---|---|---|---|---|
| Rectus capitis posterior minor | Tubercle of posterior arch of atlas | Median inferior nuchal line | Suboccipital nerve | Extends head | Vertebral artery, descending branch of occipital artery | Suboccipital |
| Rhomboid major | Spinous processes of T2–T5 vertebrae | Medial border of scapula below base of spine of scapula | Dorsal scapular nerve | Fixes scapula to thoracic wall and retracts and rotates it to depress glenoid cavity | Dorsal scapular artery *OR* deep branch of transverse cervical artery, dorsal perforating branches of the upper five or six posterior intercostal arteries | Superficial back |
| Rhomboid minor | Ligamentum nuchae, spines of C7 and T1 vertebrae | Medial border of scapula at spine of scapula | Dorsal scapular nerve | Fixes scapula to thoracic wall and retracts and rotates it to depress glenoid cavity | Dorsal scapular artery *OR* deep branch of transverse cervical artery, dorsal perforating branches of the upper five or six posterior intercostal arteries | Superficial back |
| Rotatores | Transverse processes of cervical, thoracic, and lumbar regions | Lamina and transverse process of spine above, spanning one or two segments | Dorsal rami of spinal nerves | Stabilizes, extends, and rotates spine | Dorsal branches of segmental arteries | Transversospinalis |
| Semispinalis | Transverse processes of C4–T12 | Spinous processes of cervical and thoracic regions | Dorsal rami of spinal nerves | Extends head, neck, and thorax and rotates them to opposite side | *Cervical portions:* occipital, deep cervical, and vertebral arteries<br><br>*Thoracic portions:* dorsal branches of posterior intercostal arteries | Transversospinalis |
| Serratus posterior inferior | Spinous processes of T11–L2 | Inferior aspect of ribs 9–12 | Ventral rami of lower thoracic nerves | Depresses ribs | Posterior intercostal arteries | Intermediate back |
| Serratus posterior superior | Ligamentum nuchae, spinous processes of C7–T3 | Superior aspect of ribs 2–4 | Ventral rami of upper thoracic nerves | Elevates ribs | Posterior intercostal arteries | Intermediate back |
| Splenius capitis | Nuchal ligament, spinous process of C7–T3 | Mastoid process of temporal bone, lateral third of superior nuchal line | Dorsal rami of middle cervical nerves | *Bilaterally:* extend head<br><br>*Unilaterally:* laterally bends (flexes) and rotates face to same side | Descending branch of occipital artery, deep cervical artery | Spinotransverse |
| Splenius cervicis | Spinous process of T3–T6 | Transverse processes (C1–C3) | Dorsal rami of lower cervical nerves | *Bilaterally:* extend neck<br><br>*Unilaterally:* laterally bends (flexes) and rotates neck toward same side | Descending branch of occipital artery, deep cervical artery | Spinotransverse |
| Trapezius | Superior nuchal line, external occipital protuberance, nuchal ligament, spinous processes of C7–T12 | Lateral third of clavicle, acromion, spine of scapula | Accessory nerve (CN XI) | Elevates, retracts, and rotates scapula; lower fibers depress scapula | Transverse cervical artery, dorsal perforating branches of posterior intercostal arteries | Superficial back |

**Table 2-2**

**Muscle Tables**

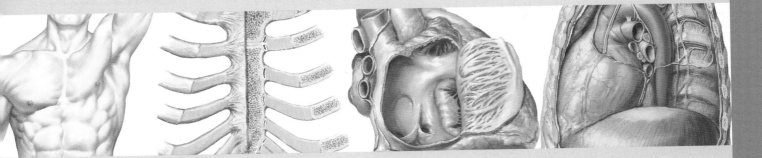

# ³ THORAX

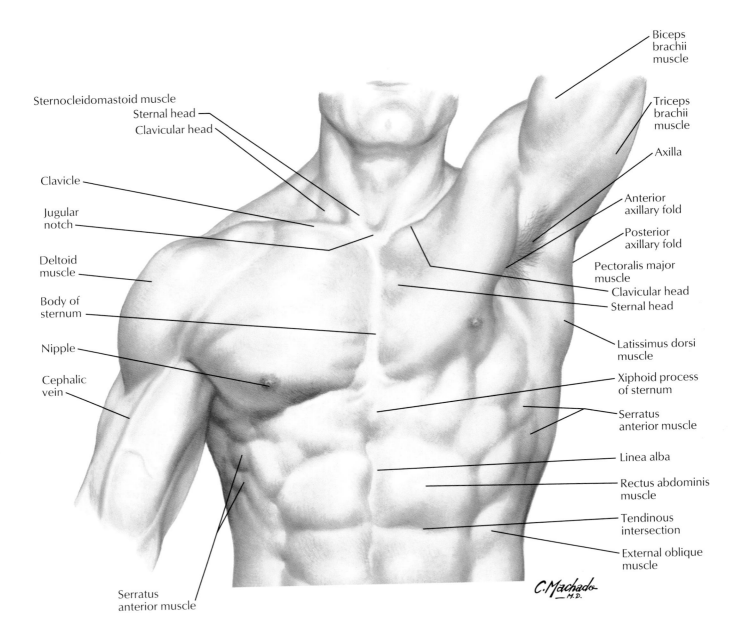

Biceps brachii muscle

Sternocleidomastoid muscle
Sternal head
Clavicular head

Triceps brachii muscle

Axilla

Clavicle

Anterior axillary fold

Jugular notch

Posterior axillary fold

Pectoralis major muscle
Clavicular head
Sternal head

Deltoid muscle

Body of sternum

Latissimus dorsi muscle

Nipple

Xiphoid process of sternum

Cephalic vein

Serratus anterior muscle

Linea alba

Rectus abdominis muscle

Tendinous intersection

External oblique muscle

C. Machado
— M.D.

Serratus anterior muscle

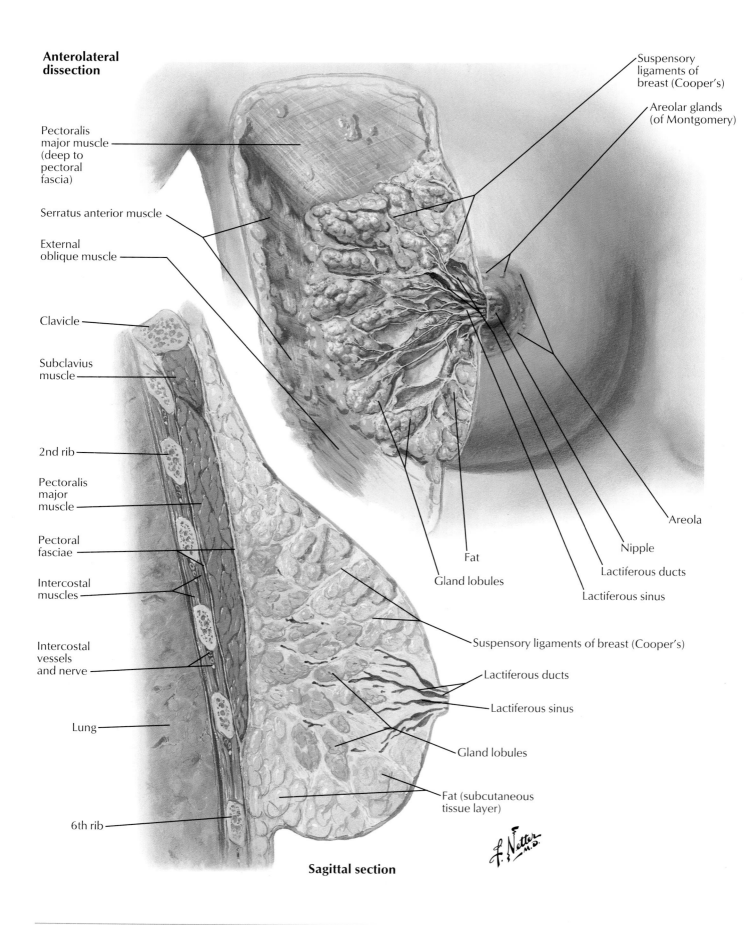

**Anterolateral dissection**

Suspensory ligaments of breast (Cooper's)

Areolar glands (of Montgomery)

Pectoralis major muscle (deep to pectoral fascia)

Serratus anterior muscle

External oblique muscle

Clavicle

Subclavius muscle

2nd rib

Pectoralis major muscle

Pectoral fasciae

Intercostal muscles

Intercostal vessels and nerve

Lung

6th rib

Fat

Gland lobules

Areola

Nipple

Lactiferous ducts

Lactiferous sinus

Suspensory ligaments of breast (Cooper's)

Lactiferous ducts

Lactiferous sinus

Gland lobules

Fat (subcutaneous tissue layer)

**Sagittal section**

**Plate 179**

**Mammary Gland**

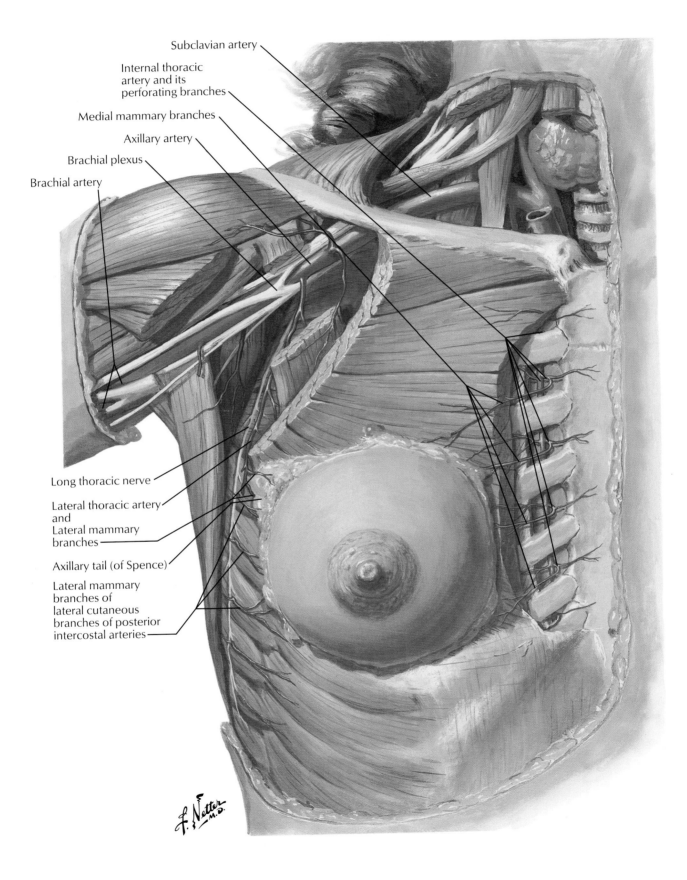

Subclavian artery

Internal thoracic artery and its perforating branches

Medial mammary branches

Axillary artery

Brachial plexus

Brachial artery

Long thoracic nerve

Lateral thoracic artery and Lateral mammary branches

Axillary tail (of Spence)

Lateral mammary branches of lateral cutaneous branches of posterior intercostal arteries

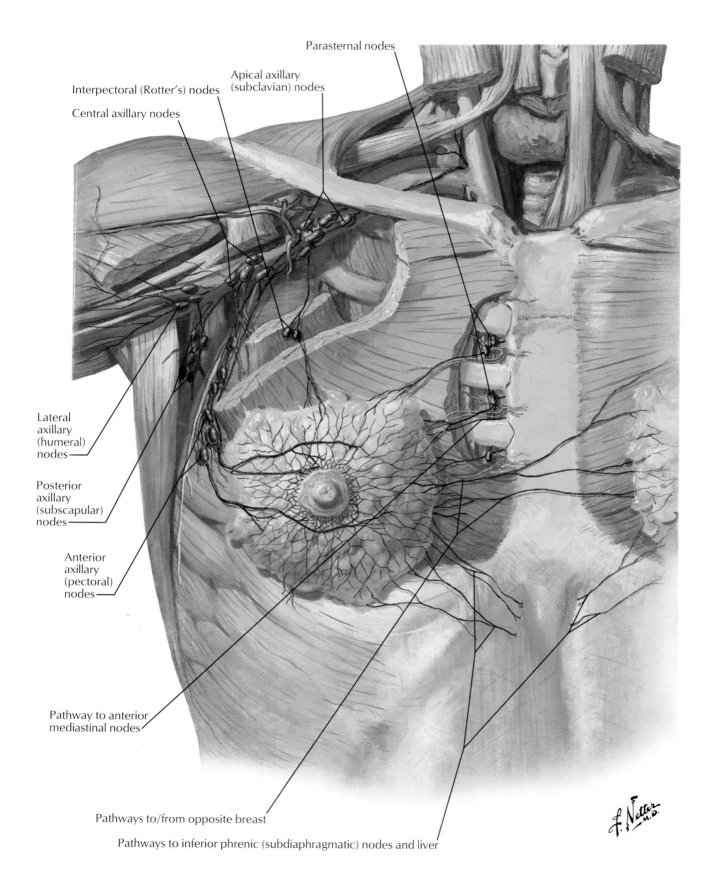

Parasternal nodes

Apical axillary (subclavian) nodes

Interpectoral (Rotter's) nodes

Central axillary nodes

Lateral axillary (humeral) nodes

Posterior axillary (subscapular) nodes

Anterior axillary (pectoral) nodes

Pathway to anterior mediastinal nodes

Pathways to/from opposite breast

Pathways to inferior phrenic (subdiaphragmatic) nodes and liver

**Plate 181**

**Mammary Gland**

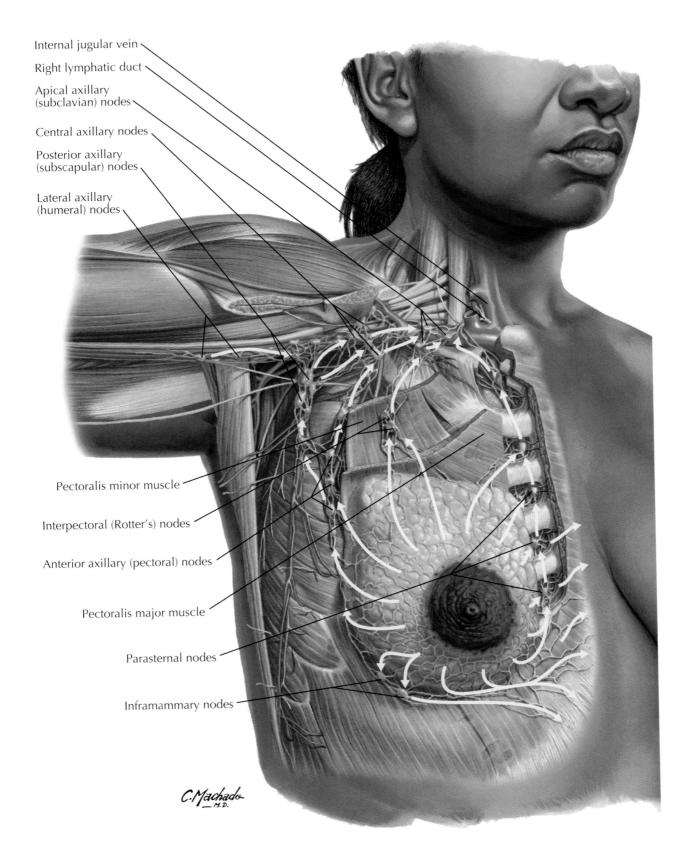

Internal jugular vein

Right lymphatic duct

Apical axillary (subclavian) nodes

Central axillary nodes

Posterior axillary (subscapular) nodes

Lateral axillary (humeral) nodes

Pectoralis minor muscle

Interpectoral (Rotter's) nodes

Anterior axillary (pectoral) nodes

Pectoralis major muscle

Parasternal nodes

Inframammary nodes

C. Machado
M.D.

**Mammary Gland**

**Plate 182**

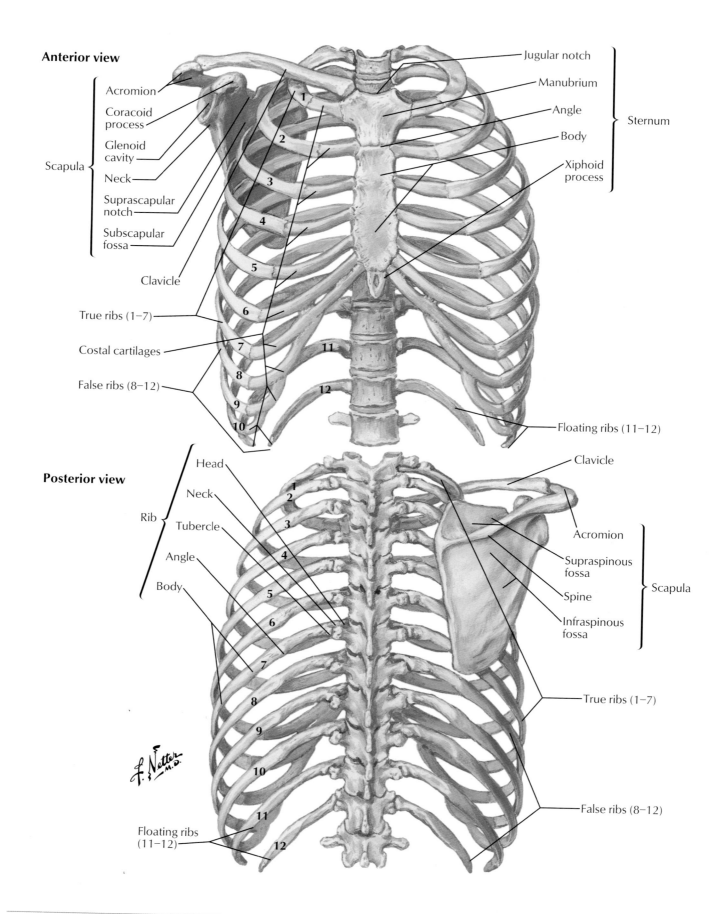

**Anterior view**

Scapula
- Acromion
- Coracoid process
- Glenoid cavity
- Neck
- Suprascapular notch
- Subscapular fossa

Clavicle

True ribs (1–7)

Costal cartilages

False ribs (8–12)

Jugular notch

Sternum
- Manubrium
- Angle
- Body
- Xiphoid process

Floating ribs (11–12)

**Posterior view**

Rib
- Head
- Neck
- Tubercle
- Angle
- Body

Clavicle

Acromion

Scapula
- Supraspinous fossa
- Spine
- Infraspinous fossa

True ribs (1–7)

False ribs (8–12)

Floating ribs (11–12)

**Plate 183**

**Body Wall**

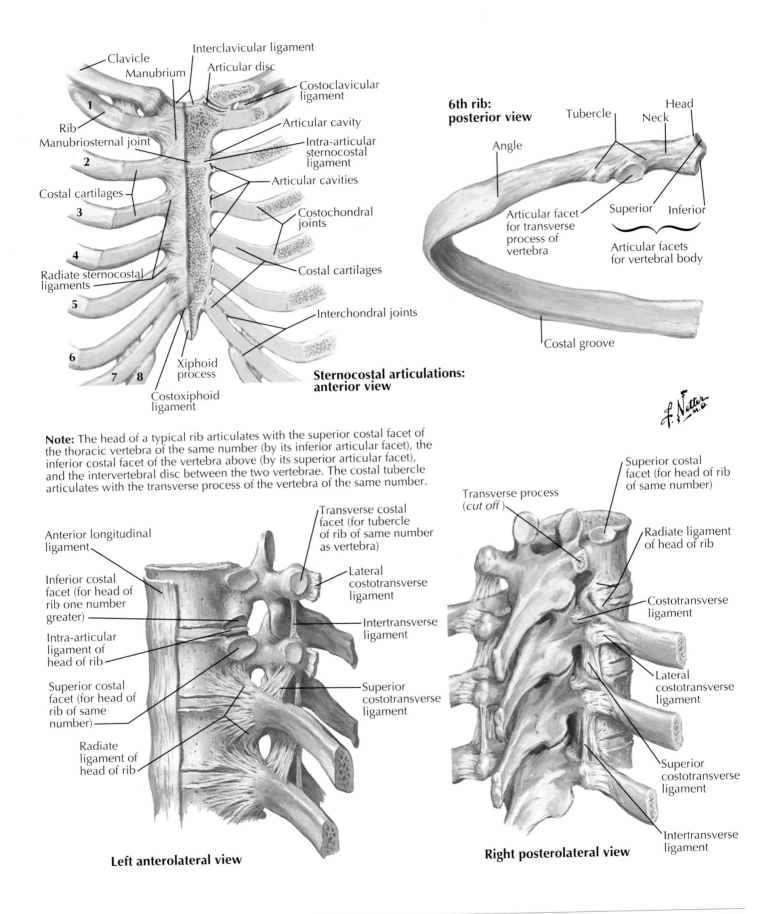

Clavicle
Manubrium
Interclavicular ligament
Articular disc
Costoclavicular ligament
Rib
Manubriosternal joint
Articular cavity
Intra-articular sternocostal ligament
Articular cavities
Costal cartilages
Costochondral joints
Radiate sternocostal ligaments
Costal cartilages
Interchondral joints
Xiphoid process
Costoxiphoid ligament

**Sternocostal articulations: anterior view**

**6th rib: posterior view**
Angle
Tubercle
Neck
Head
Articular facet for transverse process of vertebra
Superior
Inferior
Articular facets for vertebral body
Costal groove

**Note:** The head of a typical rib articulates with the superior costal facet of the thoracic vertebra of the same number (by its inferior articular facet), the inferior costal facet of the vertebra above (by its superior articular facet), and the intervertebral disc between the two vertebrae. The costal tubercle articulates with the transverse process of the vertebra of the same number.

Anterior longitudinal ligament
Inferior costal facet (for head of rib one number greater)
Intra-articular ligament of head of rib
Superior costal facet (for head of rib of same number)
Radiate ligament of head of rib
Transverse costal facet (for tubercle of rib of same number as vertebra)
Lateral costotransverse ligament
Intertransverse ligament
Superior costotransverse ligament

**Left anterolateral view**

Transverse process (cut off)
Superior costal facet (for head of rib of same number)
Radiate ligament of head of rib
Costotransverse ligament
Lateral costotransverse ligament
Superior costotransverse ligament
Intertransverse ligament

**Right posterolateral view**

**Body Wall**

**Plate 184**

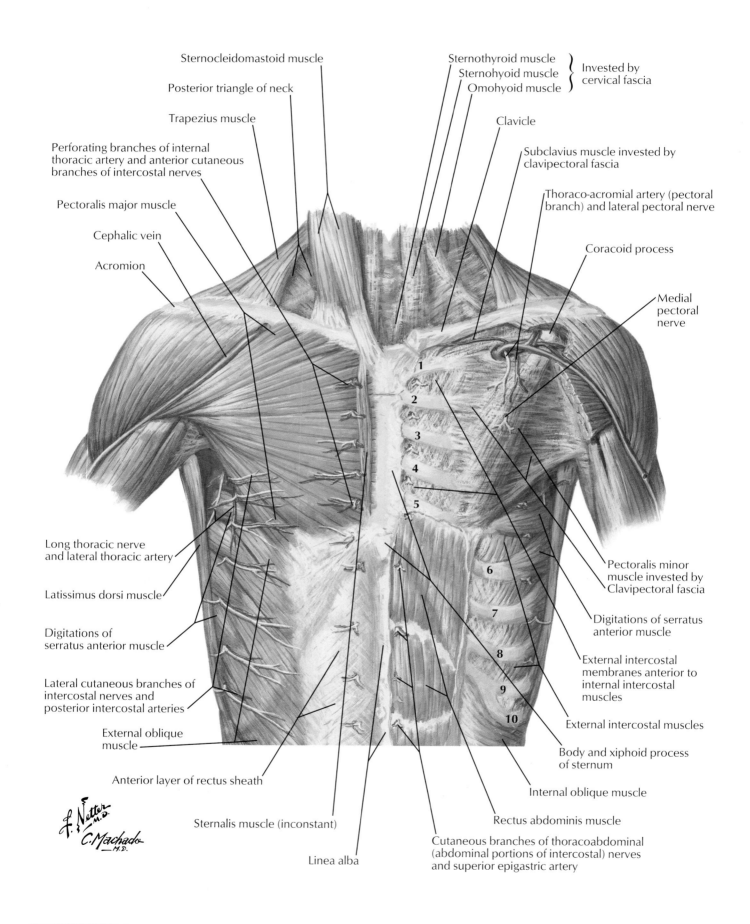

Sternocleidomastoid muscle

Posterior triangle of neck

Trapezius muscle

Perforating branches of internal thoracic artery and anterior cutaneous branches of intercostal nerves

Pectoralis major muscle

Cephalic vein

Acromion

Sternothyroid muscle
Sternohyoid muscle
Omohyoid muscle
} Invested by cervical fascia

Clavicle

Subclavius muscle invested by clavipectoral fascia

Thoraco-acromial artery (pectoral branch) and lateral pectoral nerve

Coracoid process

Medial pectoral nerve

Long thoracic nerve and lateral thoracic artery

Latissimus dorsi muscle

Digitations of serratus anterior muscle

Lateral cutaneous branches of intercostal nerves and posterior intercostal arteries

External oblique muscle

Anterior layer of rectus sheath

Sternalis muscle (inconstant)

Linea alba

Pectoralis minor muscle invested by Clavipectoral fascia

Digitations of serratus anterior muscle

External intercostal membranes anterior to internal intercostal muscles

External intercostal muscles

Body and xiphoid process of sternum

Internal oblique muscle

Rectus abdominis muscle

Cutaneous branches of thoracoabdominal (abdominal portions of intercostal) nerves and superior epigastric artery

**Plate 185**

**Body Wall**

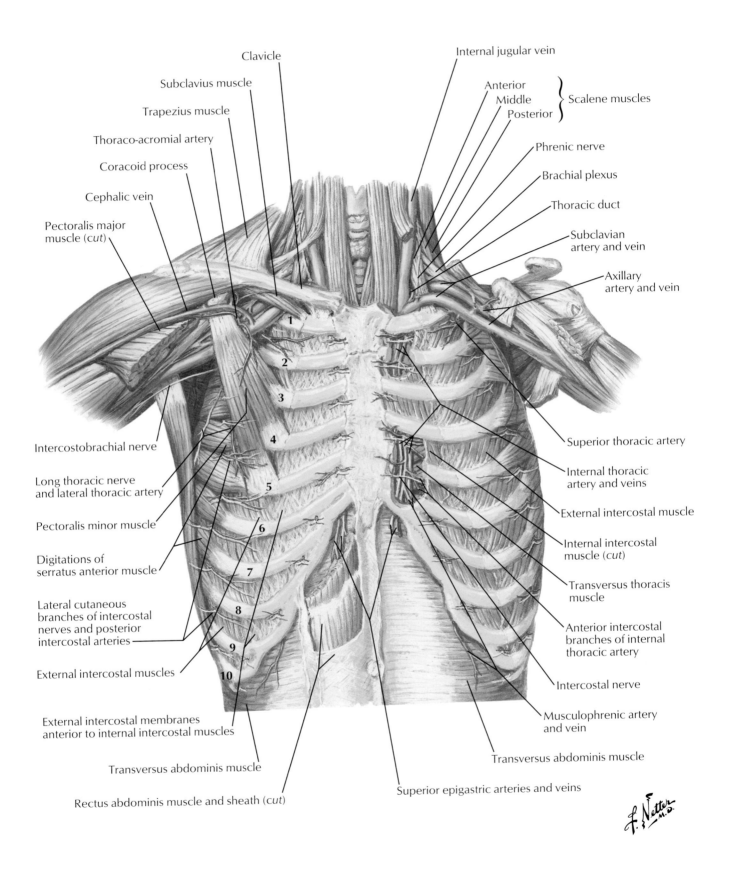

Clavicle

Subclavius muscle

Trapezius muscle

Thoraco-acromial artery

Coracoid process

Cephalic vein

Pectoralis major muscle (cut)

Internal jugular vein

Anterior
Middle } Scalene muscles
Posterior

Phrenic nerve

Brachial plexus

Thoracic duct

Subclavian artery and vein

Axillary artery and vein

Intercostobrachial nerve

Long thoracic nerve and lateral thoracic artery

Pectoralis minor muscle

Digitations of serratus anterior muscle

Lateral cutaneous branches of intercostal nerves and posterior intercostal arteries

External intercostal muscles

External intercostal membranes anterior to internal intercostal muscles

Transversus abdominis muscle

Rectus abdominis muscle and sheath (cut)

Superior thoracic artery

Internal thoracic artery and veins

External intercostal muscle

Internal intercostal muscle (cut)

Transversus thoracis muscle

Anterior intercostal branches of internal thoracic artery

Intercostal nerve

Musculophrenic artery and vein

Transversus abdominis muscle

Superior epigastric arteries and veins

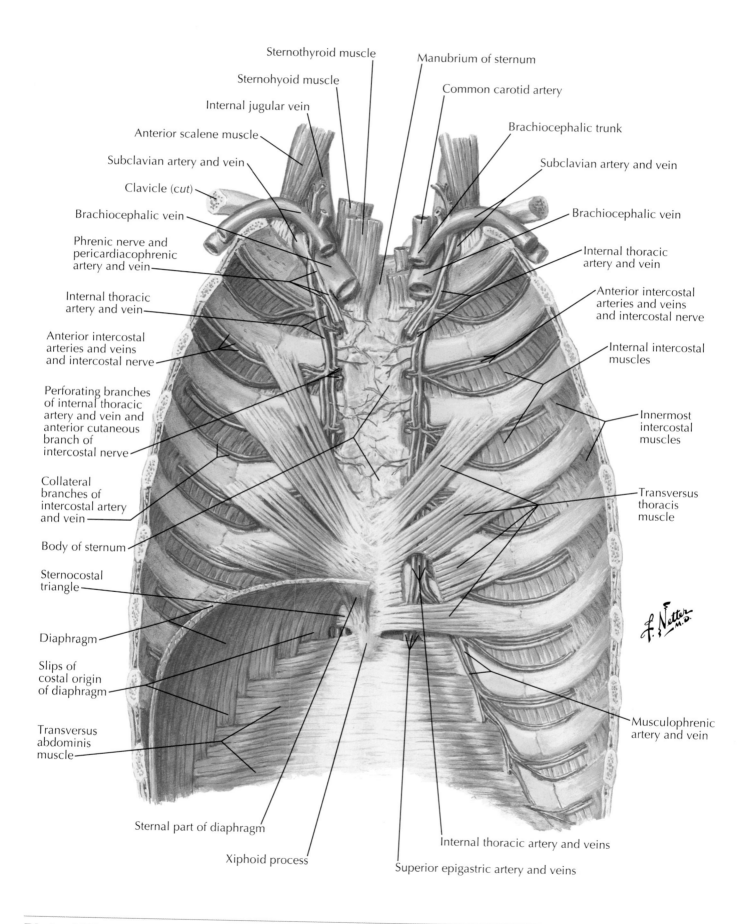

Sternothyroid muscle

Manubrium of sternum

Sternohyoid muscle

Common carotid artery

Internal jugular vein

Anterior scalene muscle

Brachiocephalic trunk

Subclavian artery and vein

Subclavian artery and vein

Clavicle (*cut*)

Brachiocephalic vein

Brachiocephalic vein

Phrenic nerve and pericardiacophrenic artery and vein

Internal thoracic artery and vein

Internal thoracic artery and vein

Anterior intercostal arteries and veins and intercostal nerve

Anterior intercostal arteries and veins and intercostal nerve

Internal intercostal muscles

Perforating branches of internal thoracic artery and vein and anterior cutaneous branch of intercostal nerve

Innermost intercostal muscles

Collateral branches of intercostal artery and vein

Transversus thoracis muscle

Body of sternum

Sternocostal triangle

Diaphragm

Slips of costal origin of diaphragm

Transversus abdominis muscle

Musculophrenic artery and vein

Sternal part of diaphragm

Xiphoid process

Internal thoracic artery and veins

Superior epigastric artery and veins

**Plate 187**

**Body Wall**

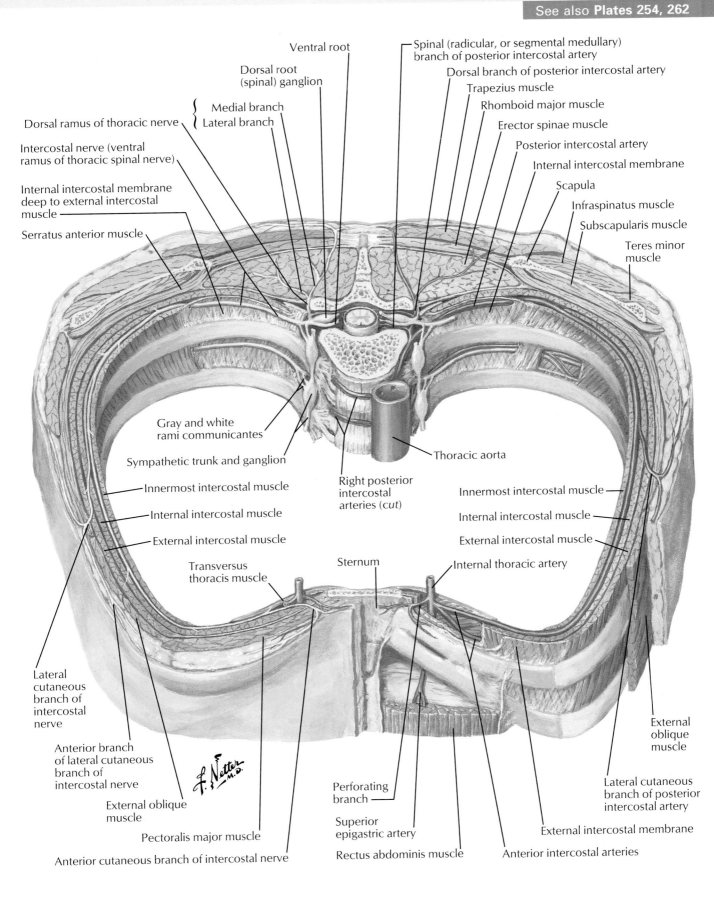

Ventral root

Dorsal root (spinal) ganglion

Medial branch
Lateral branch

Dorsal ramus of thoracic nerve

Intercostal nerve (ventral ramus of thoracic spinal nerve)

Internal intercostal membrane deep to external intercostal muscle

Serratus anterior muscle

Spinal (radicular, or segmental medullary) branch of posterior intercostal artery

Dorsal branch of posterior intercostal artery

Trapezius muscle

Rhomboid major muscle

Erector spinae muscle

Posterior intercostal artery

Internal intercostal membrane

Scapula

Infraspinatus muscle

Subscapularis muscle

Teres minor muscle

Gray and white rami communicantes

Sympathetic trunk and ganglion

Innermost intercostal muscle

Internal intercostal muscle

External intercostal muscle

Thoracic aorta

Right posterior intercostal arteries (cut)

Innermost intercostal muscle

Internal intercostal muscle

External intercostal muscle

Transversus thoracis muscle

Sternum

Internal thoracic artery

Lateral cutaneous branch of intercostal nerve

Anterior branch of lateral cutaneous branch of intercostal nerve

External oblique muscle

Pectoralis major muscle

Anterior cutaneous branch of intercostal nerve

Perforating branch

Superior epigastric artery

Rectus abdominis muscle

External oblique muscle

Lateral cutaneous branch of posterior intercostal artery

External intercostal membrane

Anterior intercostal arteries

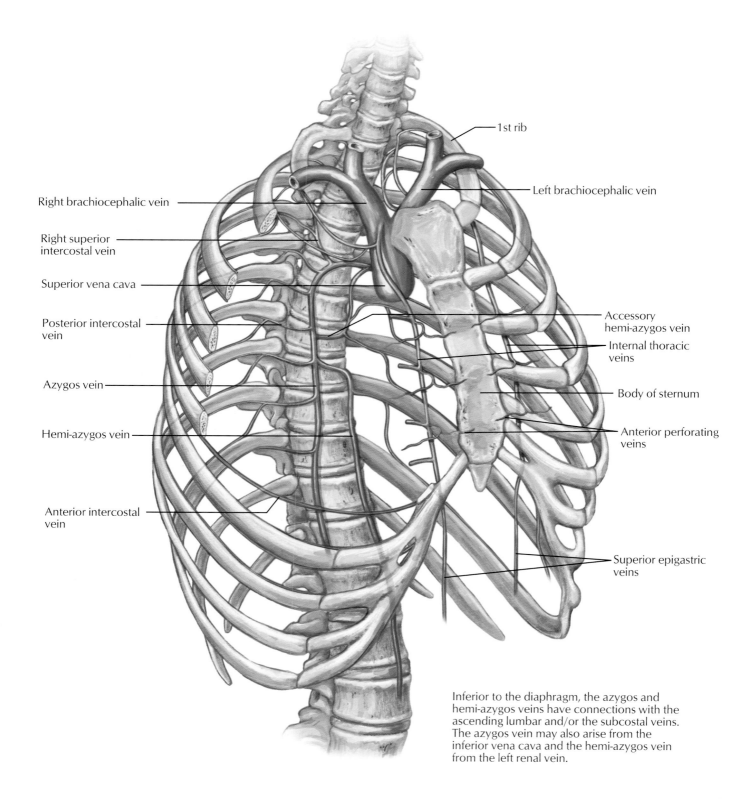

1st rib

Right brachiocephalic vein

Left brachiocephalic vein

Right superior
intercostal vein

Superior vena cava

Accessory
hemi-azygos vein

Posterior intercostal
vein

Internal thoracic
veins

Azygos vein

Body of sternum

Hemi-azygos vein

Anterior perforating
veins

Anterior intercostal
vein

Superior epigastric
veins

Inferior to the diaphragm, the azygos and
hemi-azygos veins have connections with the
ascending lumbar and/or the subcostal veins.
The azygos vein may also arise from the
inferior vena cava and the hemi-azygos vein
from the left renal vein.

**Plate 189**

**Body Wall**

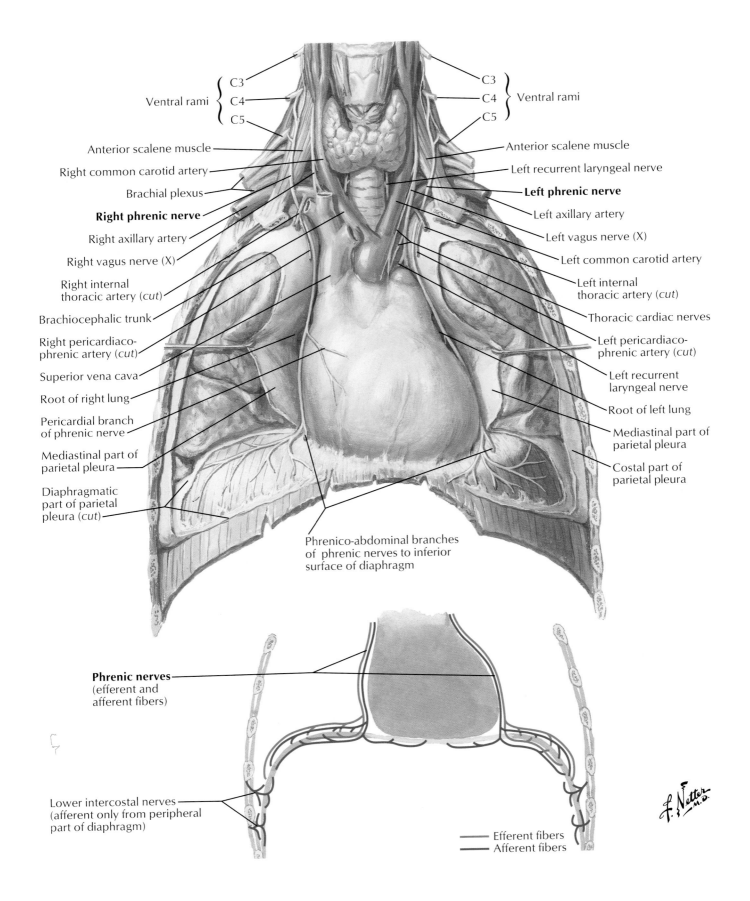

C3
Ventral rami { C4
C5

Anterior scalene muscle

Right common carotid artery

Brachial plexus

**Right phrenic nerve**

Right axillary artery

Right vagus nerve (X)

Right internal thoracic artery (cut)

Brachiocephalic trunk

Right pericardiaco-phrenic artery (cut)

Superior vena cava

Root of right lung

Pericardial branch of phrenic nerve

Mediastinal part of parietal pleura

Diaphragmatic part of parietal pleura (cut)

C3
C4 } Ventral rami
C5

Anterior scalene muscle

Left recurrent laryngeal nerve

**Left phrenic nerve**

Left axillary artery

Left vagus nerve (X)

Left common carotid artery

Left internal thoracic artery (cut)

Thoracic cardiac nerves

Left pericardiaco-phrenic artery (cut)

Left recurrent laryngeal nerve

Root of left lung

Mediastinal part of parietal pleura

Costal part of parietal pleura

Phrenico-abdominal branches of phrenic nerves to inferior surface of diaphragm

**Phrenic nerves** (efferent and afferent fibers)

Lower intercostal nerves (afferent only from peripheral part of diaphragm)

Efferent fibers
Afferent fibers

**Body Wall**

**Plate 190**

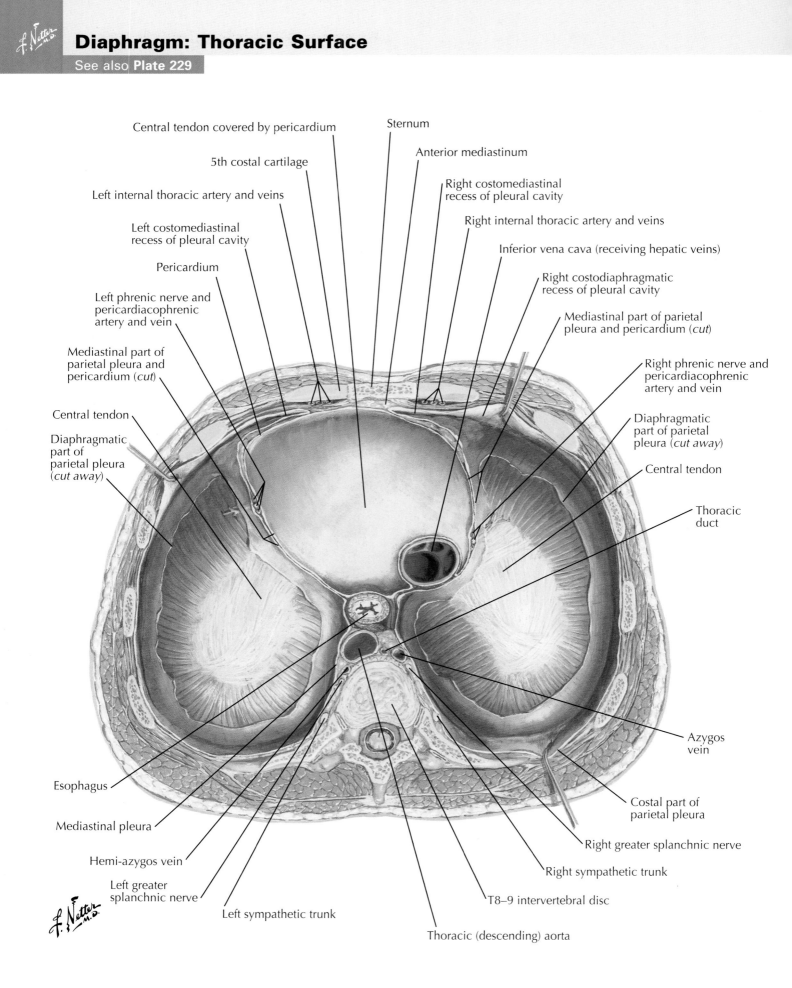

Central tendon covered by pericardium

5th costal cartilage

Left internal thoracic artery and veins

Left costomediastinal recess of pleural cavity

Pericardium

Left phrenic nerve and pericardiacophrenic artery and vein

Mediastinal part of parietal pleura and pericardium (*cut*)

Central tendon

Diaphragmatic part of parietal pleura (*cut away*)

Sternum

Anterior mediastinum

Right costomediastinal recess of pleural cavity

Right internal thoracic artery and veins

Inferior vena cava (receiving hepatic veins)

Right costodiaphragmatic recess of pleural cavity

Mediastinal part of parietal pleura and pericardium (*cut*)

Right phrenic nerve and pericardiacophrenic artery and vein

Diaphragmatic part of parietal pleura (*cut away*)

Central tendon

Thoracic duct

Azygos vein

Costal part of parietal pleura

Right greater splanchnic nerve

Right sympathetic trunk

T8–9 intervertebral disc

Thoracic (descending) aorta

Left sympathetic trunk

Left greater splanchnic nerve

Hemi-azygos vein

Mediastinal pleura

Esophagus

**Plate 191**

**Body Wall**

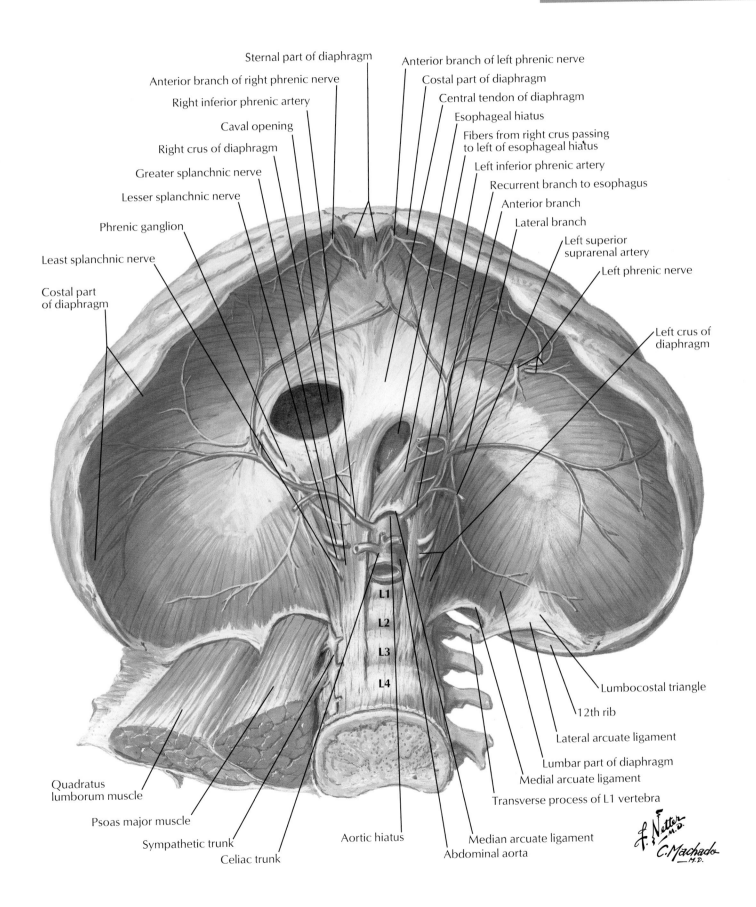

Sternal part of diaphragm

Anterior branch of left phrenic nerve

Anterior branch of right phrenic nerve

Costal part of diaphragm

Right inferior phrenic artery

Central tendon of diaphragm

Caval opening

Esophageal hiatus

Right crus of diaphragm

Fibers from right crus passing to left of esophageal hiatus

Greater splanchnic nerve

Left inferior phrenic artery

Lesser splanchnic nerve

Recurrent branch to esophagus

Phrenic ganglion

Anterior branch

Least splanchnic nerve

Lateral branch

Left superior suprarenal artery

Costal part of diaphragm

Left phrenic nerve

Left crus of diaphragm

L1

L2

L3

L4

Lumbocostal triangle

12th rib

Lateral arcuate ligament

Lumbar part of diaphragm

Medial arcuate ligament

Quadratus lumborum muscle

Transverse process of L1 vertebra

Psoas major muscle

Sympathetic trunk

Median arcuate ligament

Celiac trunk

Aortic hiatus

Abdominal aorta

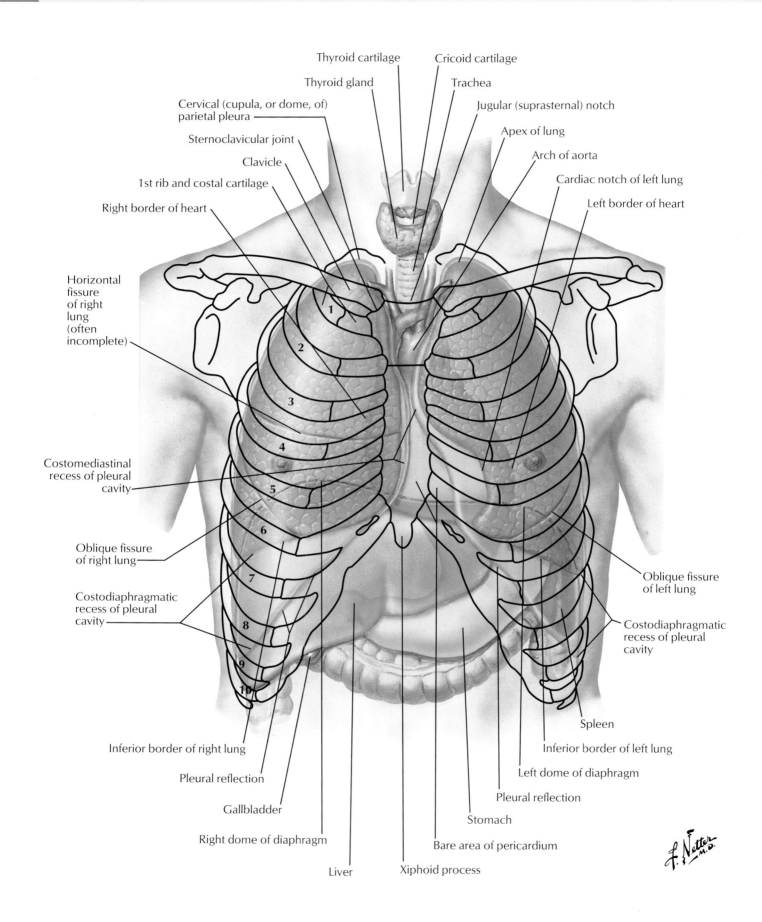

Thyroid cartilage

Cricoid cartilage

Thyroid gland

Trachea

Cervical (cupula, or dome, of) parietal pleura

Jugular (suprasternal) notch

Sternoclavicular joint

Apex of lung

Clavicle

Arch of aorta

1st rib and costal cartilage

Cardiac notch of left lung

Right border of heart

Left border of heart

Horizontal fissure of right lung (often incomplete)

Costomediastinal recess of pleural cavity

Oblique fissure of right lung

Oblique fissure of left lung

Costodiaphragmatic recess of pleural cavity

Costodiaphragmatic recess of pleural cavity

Inferior border of right lung

Spleen

Inferior border of left lung

Pleural reflection

Left dome of diaphragm

Gallbladder

Pleural reflection

Right dome of diaphragm

Stomach

Liver

Bare area of pericardium

Xiphoid process

**Plate 193**

**Lungs**

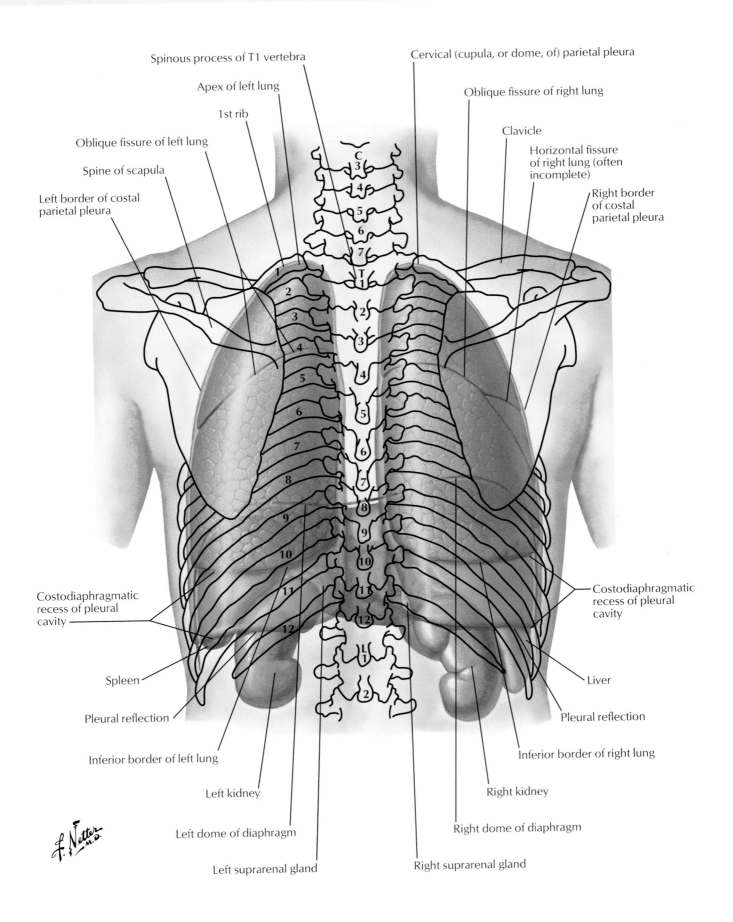

Spinous process of T1 vertebra

Apex of left lung

1st rib

Oblique fissure of left lung

Spine of scapula

Left border of costal parietal pleura

Cervical (cupula, or dome, of) parietal pleura

Oblique fissure of right lung

Clavicle

Horizontal fissure of right lung (often incomplete)

Right border of costal parietal pleura

Costodiaphragmatic recess of pleural cavity

Costodiaphragmatic recess of pleural cavity

Spleen

Liver

Pleural reflection

Pleural reflection

Inferior border of left lung

Inferior border of right lung

Left kidney

Right kidney

Left dome of diaphragm

Right dome of diaphragm

Left suprarenal gland

Right suprarenal gland

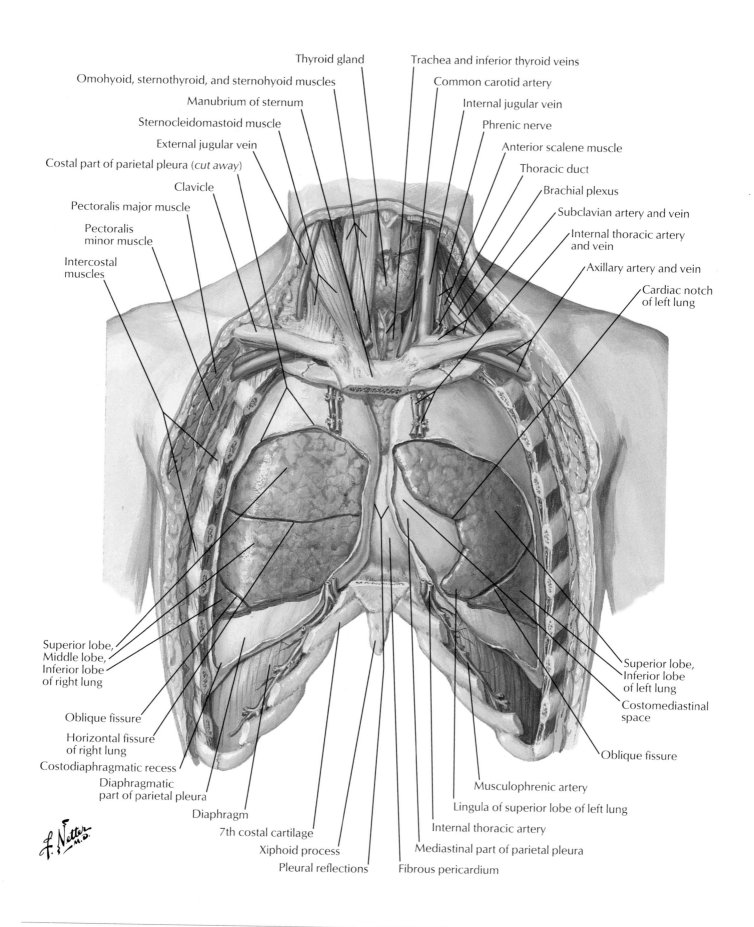

Thyroid gland

Trachea and inferior thyroid veins

Omohyoid, sternothyroid, and sternohyoid muscles

Common carotid artery

Manubrium of sternum

Internal jugular vein

Sternocleidomastoid muscle

Phrenic nerve

External jugular vein

Anterior scalene muscle

Costal part of parietal pleura (*cut away*)

Thoracic duct

Clavicle

Brachial plexus

Pectoralis major muscle

Subclavian artery and vein

Pectoralis minor muscle

Internal thoracic artery and vein

Intercostal muscles

Axillary artery and vein

Cardiac notch of left lung

Superior lobe,
Middle lobe,
Inferior lobe
of right lung

Superior lobe,
Inferior lobe
of left lung

Costomediastinal space

Oblique fissure

Horizontal fissure of right lung

Costodiaphragmatic recess

Oblique fissure

Diaphragmatic part of parietal pleura

Diaphragm

Musculophrenic artery

7th costal cartilage

Lingula of superior lobe of left lung

Xiphoid process

Internal thoracic artery

Pleural reflections

Mediastinal part of parietal pleura

Fibrous pericardium

**Plate 195**

**Lungs**

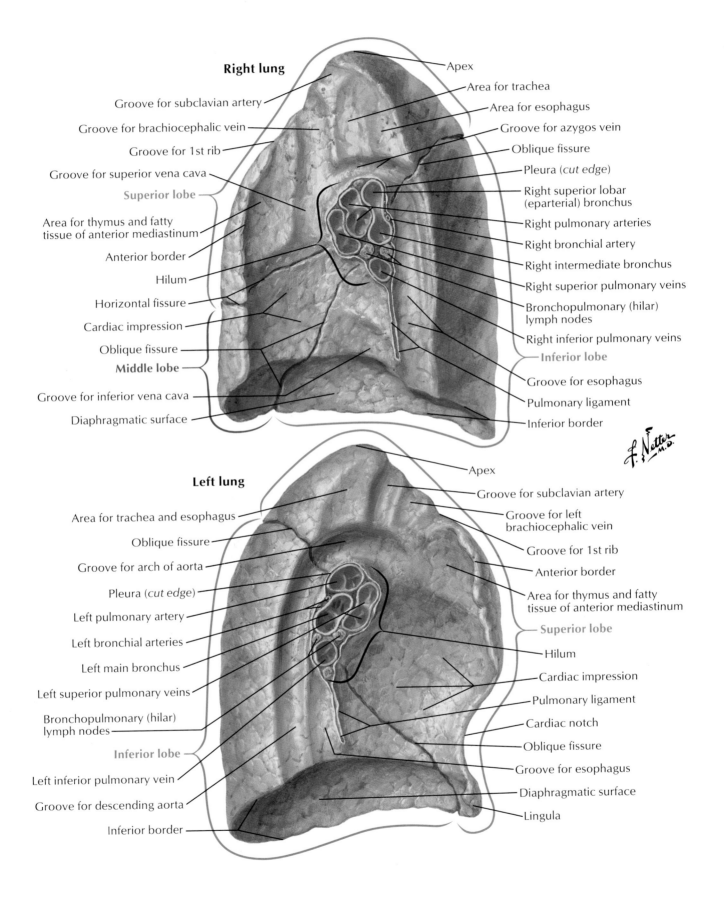

**Right lung**

Groove for subclavian artery

Groove for brachiocephalic vein

Groove for 1st rib

Groove for superior vena cava

Superior lobe

Area for thymus and fatty tissue of anterior mediastinum

Anterior border

Hilum

Horizontal fissure

Cardiac impression

Oblique fissure

**Middle lobe**

Groove for inferior vena cava

Diaphragmatic surface

Apex

Area for trachea

Area for esophagus

Groove for azygos vein

Oblique fissure

Pleura (cut edge)

Right superior lobar (eparterial) bronchus

Right pulmonary arteries

Right bronchial artery

Right intermediate bronchus

Right superior pulmonary veins

Bronchopulmonary (hilar) lymph nodes

Right inferior pulmonary veins

Inferior lobe

Groove for esophagus

Pulmonary ligament

Inferior border

**Left lung**

Area for trachea and esophagus

Oblique fissure

Groove for arch of aorta

Pleura (cut edge)

Left pulmonary artery

Left bronchial arteries

Left main bronchus

Left superior pulmonary veins

Bronchopulmonary (hilar) lymph nodes

Inferior lobe

Left inferior pulmonary vein

Groove for descending aorta

Inferior border

Apex

Groove for subclavian artery

Groove for left brachiocephalic vein

Groove for 1st rib

Anterior border

Area for thymus and fatty tissue of anterior mediastinum

Superior lobe

Hilum

Cardiac impression

Pulmonary ligament

Cardiac notch

Oblique fissure

Groove for esophagus

Diaphragmatic surface

Lingula

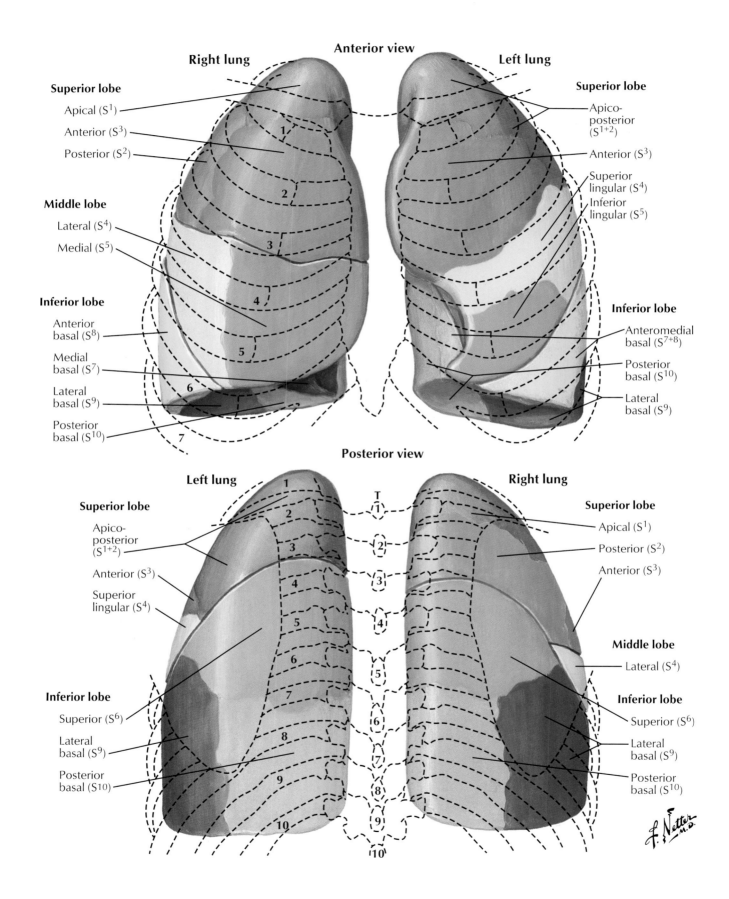

**Anterior view**

**Right lung**

**Superior lobe**
Apical (S$^1$)
Anterior (S$^3$)
Posterior (S$^2$)

**Middle lobe**
Lateral (S$^4$)
Medial (S$^5$)

**Inferior lobe**
Anterior basal (S$^8$)
Medial basal (S$^7$)
Lateral basal (S$^9$)
Posterior basal (S$^{10}$)

**Left lung**

**Superior lobe**
Apico-posterior (S$^{1+2}$)
Anterior (S$^3$)
Superior lingular (S$^4$)
Inferior lingular (S$^5$)

**Inferior lobe**
Anteromedial basal (S$^{7+8}$)
Posterior basal (S$^{10}$)
Lateral basal (S$^9$)

**Posterior view**

**Left lung**

**Superior lobe**
Apico-posterior (S$^{1+2}$)
Anterior (S$^3$)
Superior lingular (S$^4$)

**Inferior lobe**
Superior (S$^6$)
Lateral basal (S$^9$)
Posterior basal (S$^{10}$)

**Right lung**

**Superior lobe**
Apical (S$^1$)
Posterior (S$^2$)
Anterior (S$^3$)

**Middle lobe**
Lateral (S$^4$)

**Inferior lobe**
Superior (S$^6$)
Lateral basal (S$^9$)
Posterior basal (S$^{10}$)

**Plate 197**

**Lungs**

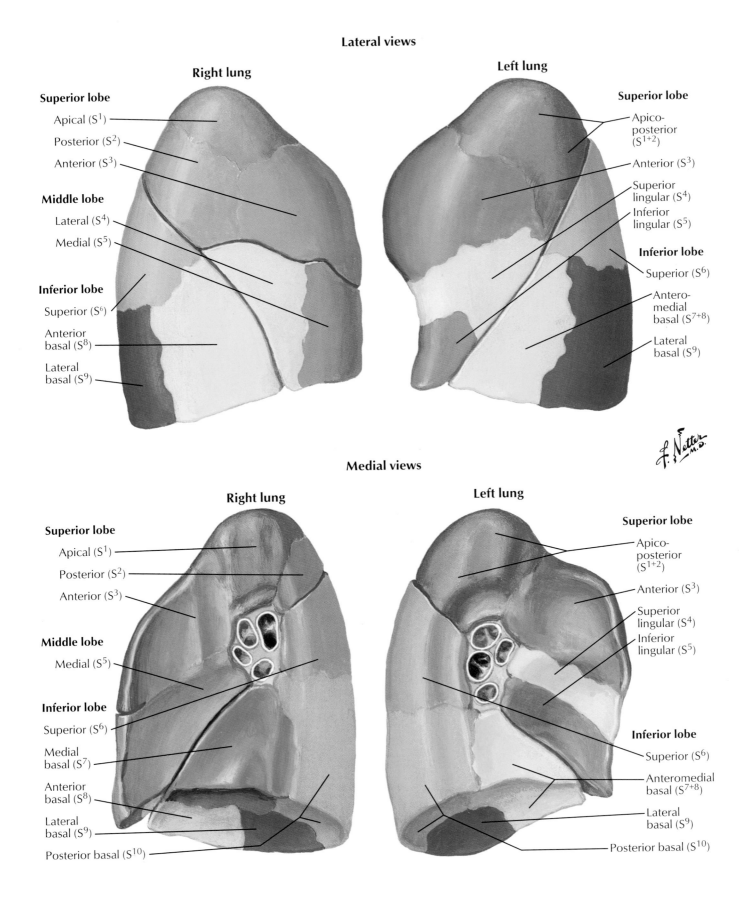

**Lateral views**

**Right lung**

**Left lung**

**Superior lobe**

Apical (S¹)

Posterior (S²)

Anterior (S³)

**Middle lobe**

Lateral (S⁴)

Medial (S⁵)

**Inferior lobe**

Superior (S⁶)

Anterior basal (S⁸)

Lateral basal (S⁹)

**Superior lobe**

Apico-posterior (S¹⁺²)

Anterior (S³)

Superior lingular (S⁴)

Inferior lingular (S⁵)

**Inferior lobe**

Superior (S⁶)

Antero-medial basal (S⁷⁺⁸)

Lateral basal (S⁹)

**Medial views**

**Right lung**

**Left lung**

**Superior lobe**

Apical (S¹)

Posterior (S²)

Anterior (S³)

**Middle lobe**

Medial (S⁵)

**Inferior lobe**

Superior (S⁶)

Medial basal (S⁷)

Anterior basal (S⁸)

Lateral basal (S⁹)

Posterior basal (S¹⁰)

**Superior lobe**

Apico-posterior (S¹⁺²)

Anterior (S³)

Superior lingular (S⁴)

Inferior lingular (S⁵)

**Inferior lobe**

Superior (S⁶)

Anteromedial basal (S⁷⁺⁸)

Lateral basal (S⁹)

Posterior basal (S¹⁰)

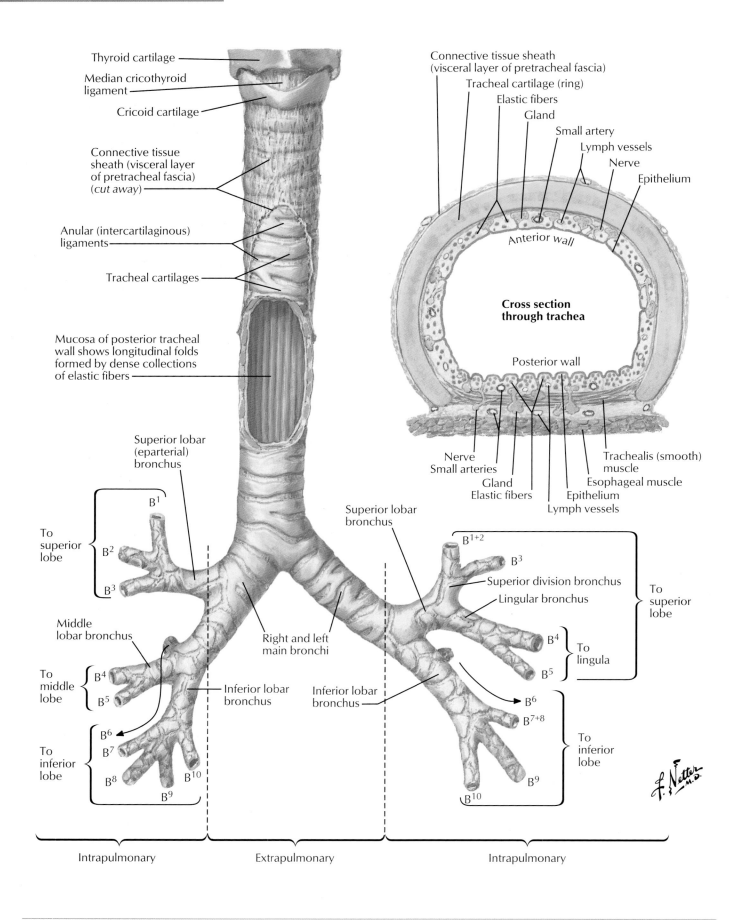

Thyroid cartilage

Median cricothyroid ligament

Cricoid cartilage

Connective tissue sheath (visceral layer of pretracheal fascia) (*cut away*)

Anular (intercartilaginous) ligaments

Tracheal cartilages

Mucosa of posterior tracheal wall shows longitudinal folds formed by dense collections of elastic fibers

Connective tissue sheath (visceral layer of pretracheal fascia)

Tracheal cartilage (ring)

Elastic fibers

Gland

Small artery

Lymph vessels

Nerve

Epithelium

Anterior wall

**Cross section through trachea**

Posterior wall

Nerve
Small arteries

Gland
Elastic fibers

Epithelium
Lymph vessels

Trachealis (smooth) muscle

Esophageal muscle

Superior lobar (eparterial) bronchus

$B^1$

To superior lobe

$B^2$

$B^3$

Middle lobar bronchus

To middle lobe

$B^4$

$B^5$

To inferior lobe

$B^6$

$B^7$

$B^8$

$B^{10}$

$B^9$

Right and left main bronchi

Inferior lobar bronchus

Superior lobar bronchus

$B^{1+2}$

$B^3$

Superior division bronchus

Lingular bronchus

$B^4$

To lingula

$B^5$

To superior lobe

Inferior lobar bronchus

$B^6$

$B^{7+8}$

To inferior lobe

$B^9$

$B^{10}$

Intrapulmonary

Extrapulmonary

Intrapulmonary

**Plate 199**

**Lungs**

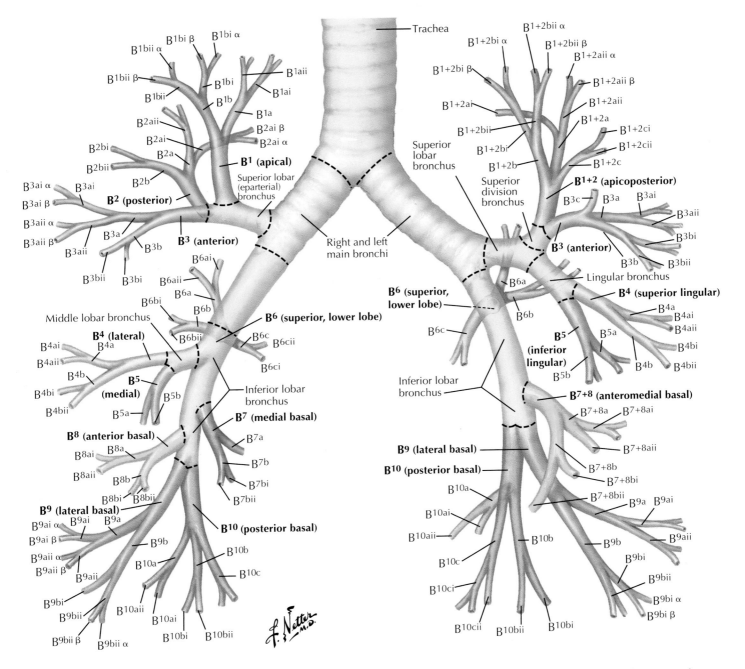

Nomenclature in common usage for bronchopulmonary segments (Plates 197 and 198) is that of Jackson and Huber, and segmental bronchi are named accordingly. Ikeda proposed nomenclature (as demonstrated here) for bronchial subdivisions as far as the 6th generation. For simplification on this illustration, only some bronchial subdivisions are labeled as far as the 5th or 6th generation. Segmental bronchi (B) are numbered from 1 to 10 in each lung, corresponding to pulmonary segments. In the left lung,

$B^1$ and $B^2$ are combined as are $B^7$ and $B^8$. Subsegmental, or 4th order, bronchi are indicated by the addition of lower-case letters a, b, or c when an additional branch is present. Fifth order bronchi are designated by Roman numerals i (anterior) or ii (posterior) and 6th order bronchi by Greek letters α or β. Several texts use alternate numbers (as proposed by Boyden) for segmental bronchi.

Variations of the standard bronchial pattern shown here are common, especially in peripheral airways.

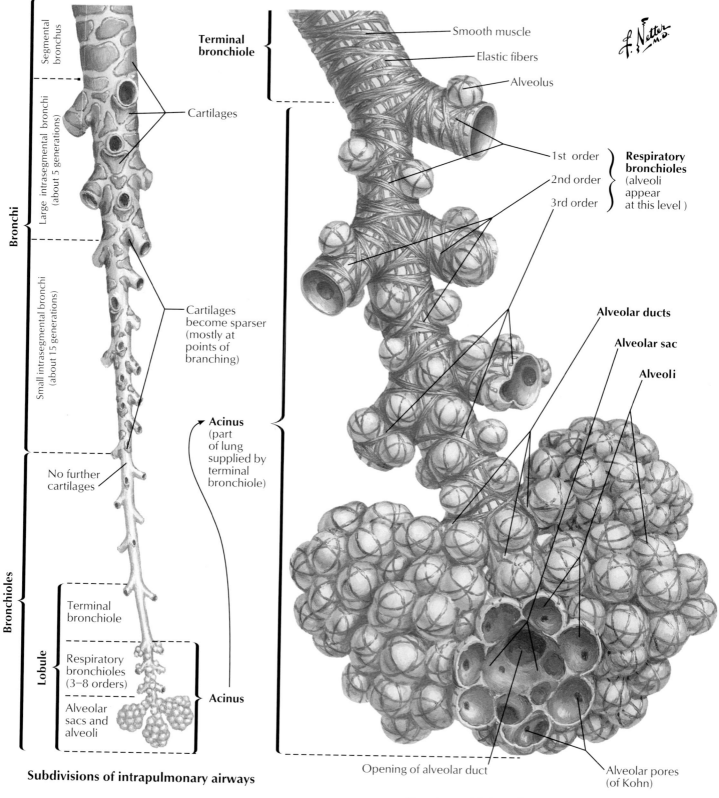

Terminal bronchiole

Cartilages

Smooth muscle

Elastic fibers

Alveolus

1st order
2nd order
3rd order

**Respiratory bronchioles** (alveoli appear at this level )

**Alveolar ducts**

**Alveolar sac**

**Alveoli**

Segmental bronchus

Large intrasegmental bronchi (about 5 generations)

Bronchi

Cartilages

Small intrasegmental bronchi (about 15 generations)

Cartilages become sparser (mostly at points of branching)

No further cartilages

Acinus (part of lung supplied by terminal bronchiole)

Bronchioles

Lobule

Terminal bronchiole

Respiratory bronchioles (3–8 orders)

Alveolar sacs and alveoli

Acinus

**Subdivisions of intrapulmonary airways**

Opening of alveolar duct

Alveolar pores (of Kohn)

**Structure of intrapulmonary airways**

**Plate 201**

**Lungs**

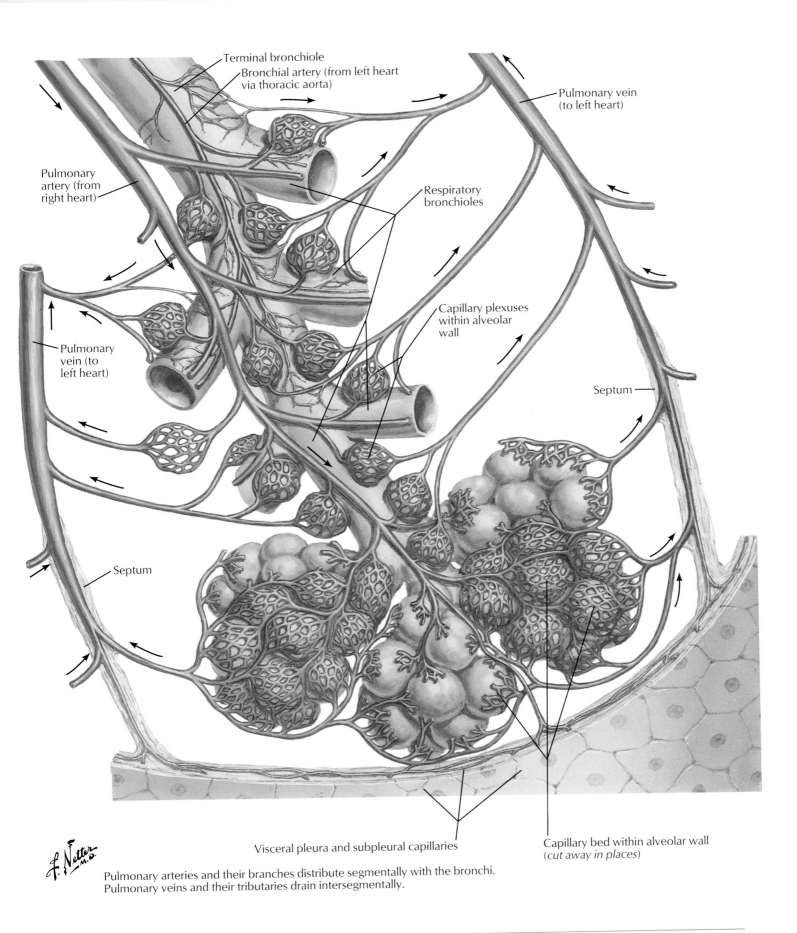

Terminal bronchiole

Bronchial artery (from left heart via thoracic aorta)

Pulmonary vein (to left heart)

Pulmonary artery (from right heart)

Respiratory bronchioles

Pulmonary vein (to left heart)

Capillary plexuses within alveolar wall

Septum

Septum

Visceral pleura and subpleural capillaries

Capillary bed within alveolar wall (*cut away in places*)

Pulmonary arteries and their branches distribute segmentally with the bronchi.
Pulmonary veins and their tributaries drain intersegmentally.

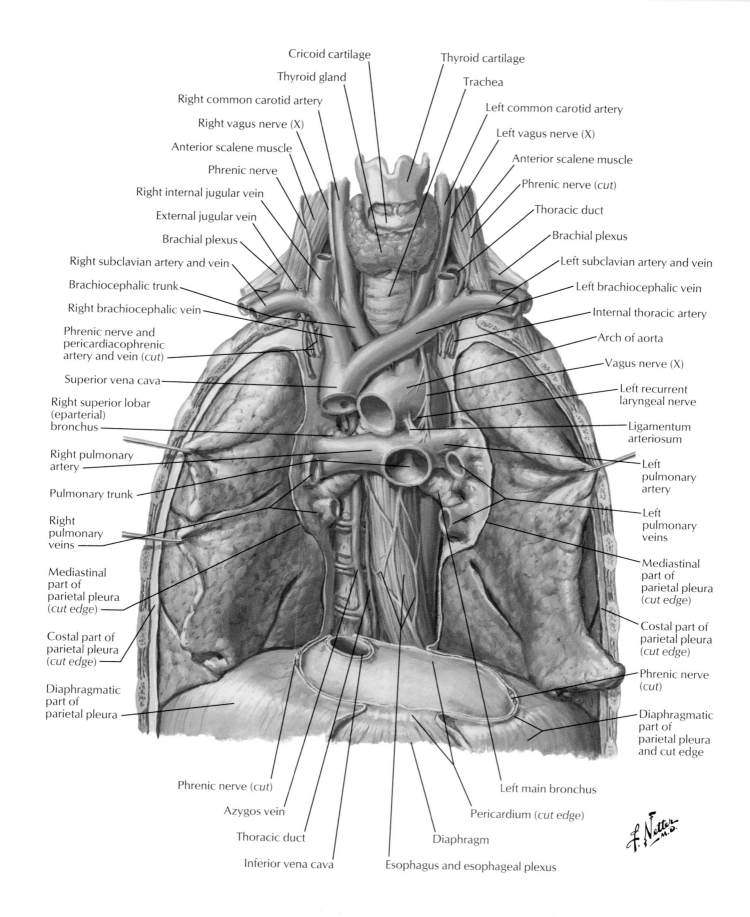

Cricoid cartilage

Thyroid cartilage

Thyroid gland

Trachea

Right common carotid artery

Left common carotid artery

Right vagus nerve (X)

Left vagus nerve (X)

Anterior scalene muscle

Anterior scalene muscle

Phrenic nerve

Phrenic nerve (cut)

Right internal jugular vein

Thoracic duct

External jugular vein

Brachial plexus

Brachial plexus

Right subclavian artery and vein

Left subclavian artery and vein

Brachiocephalic trunk

Left brachiocephalic vein

Right brachiocephalic vein

Internal thoracic artery

Phrenic nerve and pericardiacophrenic artery and vein (cut)

Arch of aorta

Vagus nerve (X)

Superior vena cava

Left recurrent laryngeal nerve

Right superior lobar (eparterial) bronchus

Ligamentum arteriosum

Right pulmonary artery

Left pulmonary artery

Pulmonary trunk

Left pulmonary veins

Right pulmonary veins

Mediastinal part of parietal pleura (cut edge)

Mediastinal part of parietal pleura (cut edge)

Costal part of parietal pleura (cut edge)

Costal part of parietal pleura (cut edge)

Diaphragmatic part of parietal pleura

Phrenic nerve (cut)

Diaphragmatic part of parietal pleura and cut edge

Phrenic nerve (cut)

Left main bronchus

Azygos vein

Pericardium (cut edge)

Thoracic duct

Diaphragm

Inferior vena cava

Esophagus and esophageal plexus

**Plate 203**

**Lungs**

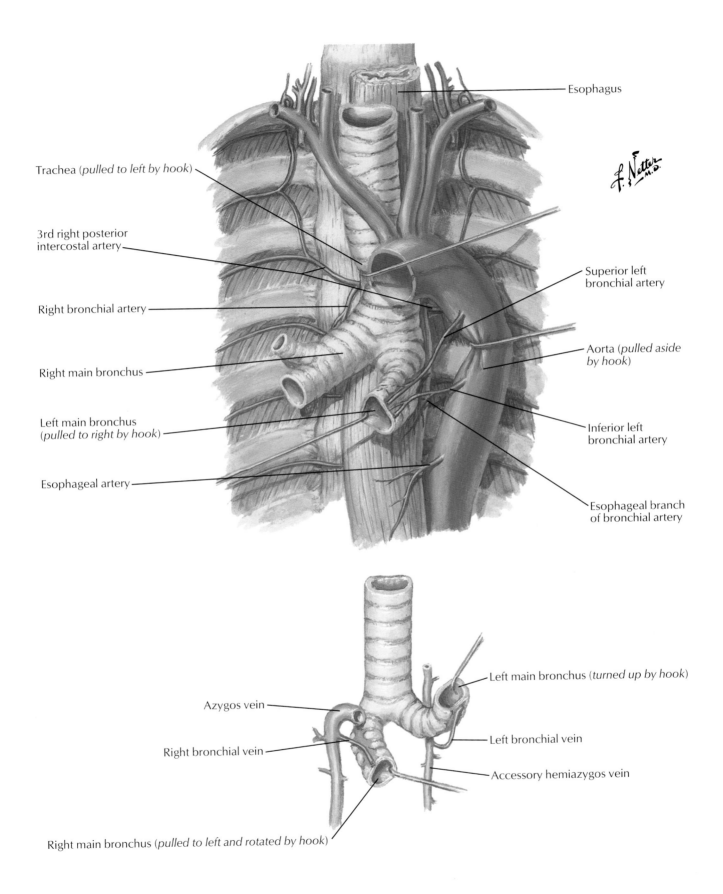

Esophagus

Trachea (*pulled to left by hook*)

3rd right posterior intercostal artery

Right bronchial artery

Right main bronchus

Left main bronchus (*pulled to right by hook*)

Esophageal artery

Superior left bronchial artery

Aorta (*pulled aside by hook*)

Inferior left bronchial artery

Esophageal branch of bronchial artery

Azygos vein

Right bronchial vein

Left main bronchus (*turned up by hook*)

Left bronchial vein

Accessory hemiazygos vein

Right main bronchus (*pulled to left and rotated by hook*)

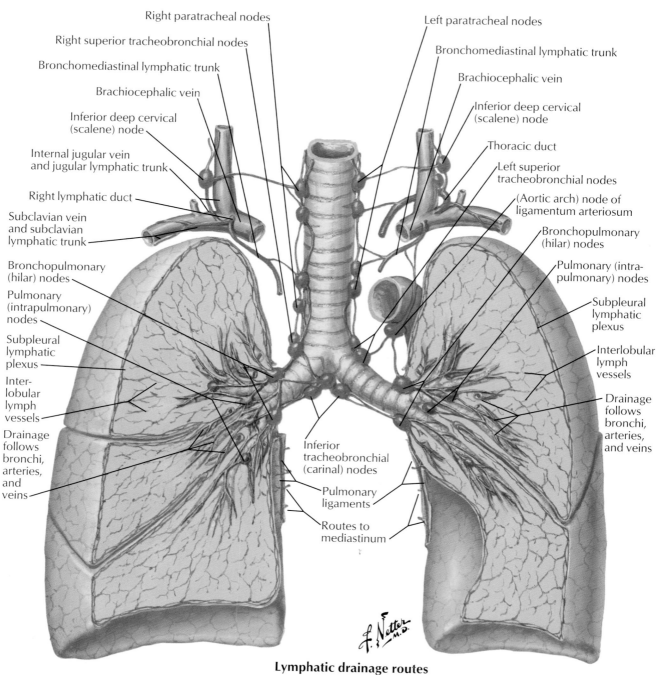

Right paratracheal nodes

Right superior tracheobronchial nodes

Bronchomediastinal lymphatic trunk

Brachiocephalic vein

Inferior deep cervical (scalene) node

Internal jugular vein and jugular lymphatic trunk

Right lymphatic duct

Subclavian vein and subclavian lymphatic trunk

Bronchopulmonary (hilar) nodes

Pulmonary (intrapulmonary) nodes

Subpleural lymphatic plexus

Inter-lobular lymph vessels

Drainage follows bronchi, arteries, and veins

Left paratracheal nodes

Bronchomediastinal lymphatic trunk

Brachiocephalic vein

Inferior deep cervical (scalene) node

Thoracic duct

Left superior tracheobronchial nodes

(Aortic arch) node of ligamentum arteriosum

Bronchopulmonary (hilar) nodes

Pulmonary (intra-pulmonary) nodes

Subpleural lymphatic plexus

Interlobular lymph vessels

Drainage follows bronchi, arteries, and veins

Inferior tracheobronchial (carinal) nodes

Pulmonary ligaments

Routes to mediastinum

**Lymphatic drainage routes**

**Right lung:** All lobes drain to pulmonary and bronchopulmonary (hilar) nodes, then to inferior tracheobronchial (carinal) nodes, right superior tracheobronchial nodes, and right paratracheal nodes on the way to the brachiocephalic vein via the bronchomediastinal lymphatic trunk and/or inferior deep cervical (scalene) node.

**Left lung:** The superior lobe drains to pulmonary and broncho-pulmonary (hilar) nodes, inferior tracheobronchial (carinal) nodes, left superior tracheobronchial nodes, left paratracheal nodes and/or (aortic arch) node of ligamentum arteriosum, then to the brachiocephalic vein via the left bronchomediastinal trunk and thoracic duct. The left inferior lobe also drains to the pulmonary and bronchopulmonary (hilar) nodes and to inferior tracheobronchial (carinal) nodes, but then mostly to right superior tracheobronchial nodes, where it follows the same route as lymph from the right lung.

**Plate 205**

**Lungs**

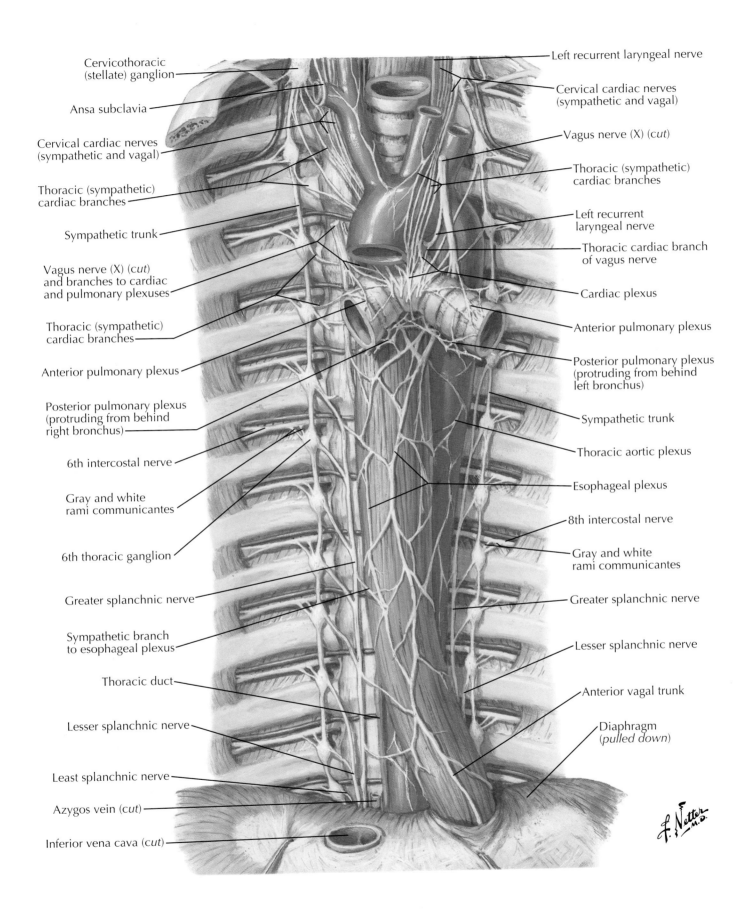

Cervicothoracic (stellate) ganglion

Ansa subclavia

Cervical cardiac nerves (sympathetic and vagal)

Thoracic (sympathetic) cardiac branches

Sympathetic trunk

Vagus nerve (X) (cut) and branches to cardiac and pulmonary plexuses

Thoracic (sympathetic) cardiac branches

Anterior pulmonary plexus

Posterior pulmonary plexus (protruding from behind right bronchus)

6th intercostal nerve

Gray and white rami communicantes

6th thoracic ganglion

Greater splanchnic nerve

Sympathetic branch to esophageal plexus

Thoracic duct

Lesser splanchnic nerve

Least splanchnic nerve

Azygos vein (cut)

Inferior vena cava (cut)

Left recurrent laryngeal nerve

Cervical cardiac nerves (sympathetic and vagal)

Vagus nerve (X) (cut)

Thoracic (sympathetic) cardiac branches

Left recurrent laryngeal nerve

Thoracic cardiac branch of vagus nerve

Cardiac plexus

Anterior pulmonary plexus

Posterior pulmonary plexus (protruding from behind left bronchus)

Sympathetic trunk

Thoracic aortic plexus

Esophageal plexus

8th intercostal nerve

Gray and white rami communicantes

Greater splanchnic nerve

Lesser splanchnic nerve

Anterior vagal trunk

Diaphragm (pulled down)

**Lungs**

**Plate 206**

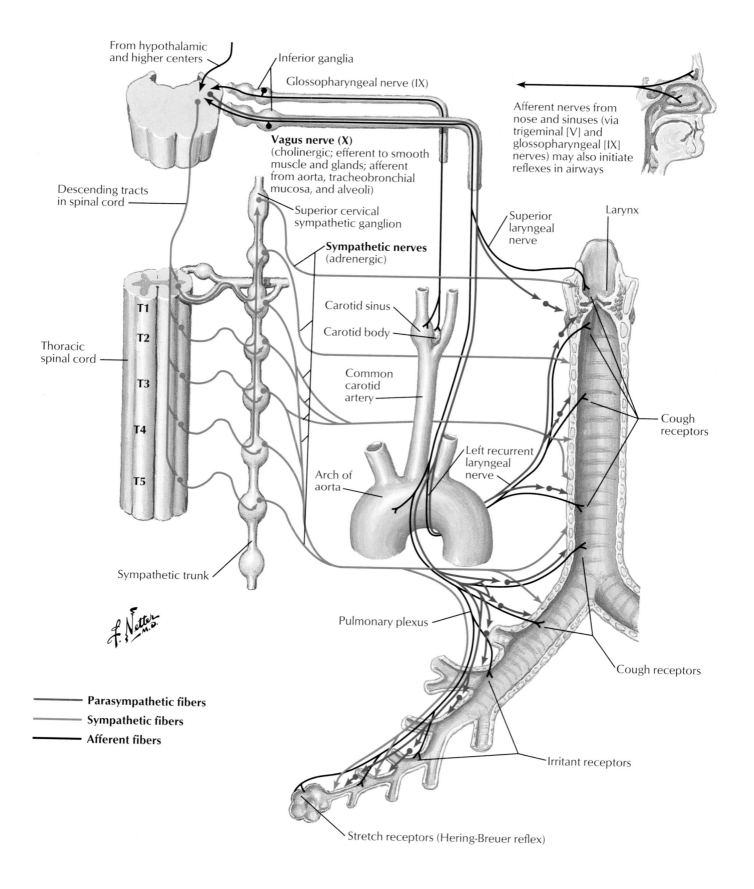

From hypothalamic and higher centers

Inferior ganglia

Glossopharyngeal nerve (IX)

**Vagus nerve (X)**
(cholinergic; efferent to smooth muscle and glands; afferent from aorta, tracheobronchial mucosa, and alveoli)

Afferent nerves from nose and sinuses (via trigeminal [V] and glossopharyngeal [IX] nerves) may also initiate reflexes in airways

Descending tracts in spinal cord

Superior cervical sympathetic ganglion

**Sympathetic nerves**
(adrenergic)

Superior laryngeal nerve

Larynx

T1

T2

Thoracic spinal cord

T3

Carotid sinus

Carotid body

Common carotid artery

Cough receptors

T4

T5

Arch of aorta

Left recurrent laryngeal nerve

Sympathetic trunk

Pulmonary plexus

Cough receptors

Parasympathetic fibers
Sympathetic fibers
Afferent fibers

Irritant receptors

Stretch receptors (Hering-Breuer reflex)

**Plate 207**

**Lungs**

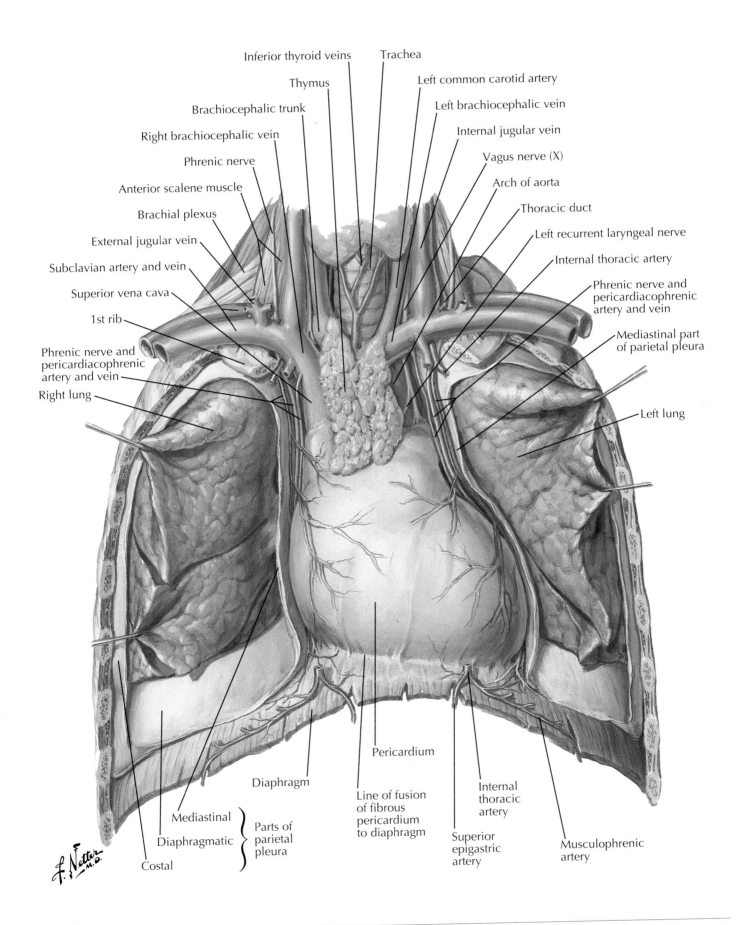

Inferior thyroid veins

Trachea

Thymus

Left common carotid artery

Brachiocephalic trunk

Left brachiocephalic vein

Right brachiocephalic vein

Internal jugular vein

Phrenic nerve

Vagus nerve (X)

Anterior scalene muscle

Arch of aorta

Brachial plexus

Thoracic duct

External jugular vein

Left recurrent laryngeal nerve

Subclavian artery and vein

Internal thoracic artery

Superior vena cava

Phrenic nerve and pericardiacophrenic artery and vein

1st rib

Phrenic nerve and pericardiacophrenic artery and vein

Mediastinal part of parietal pleura

Right lung

Left lung

Diaphragm

Pericardium

Mediastinal

Line of fusion of fibrous pericardium to diaphragm

Internal thoracic artery

Diaphragmatic

Parts of parietal pleura

Costal

Superior epigastric artery

Musculophrenic artery

f. Netter M.D.

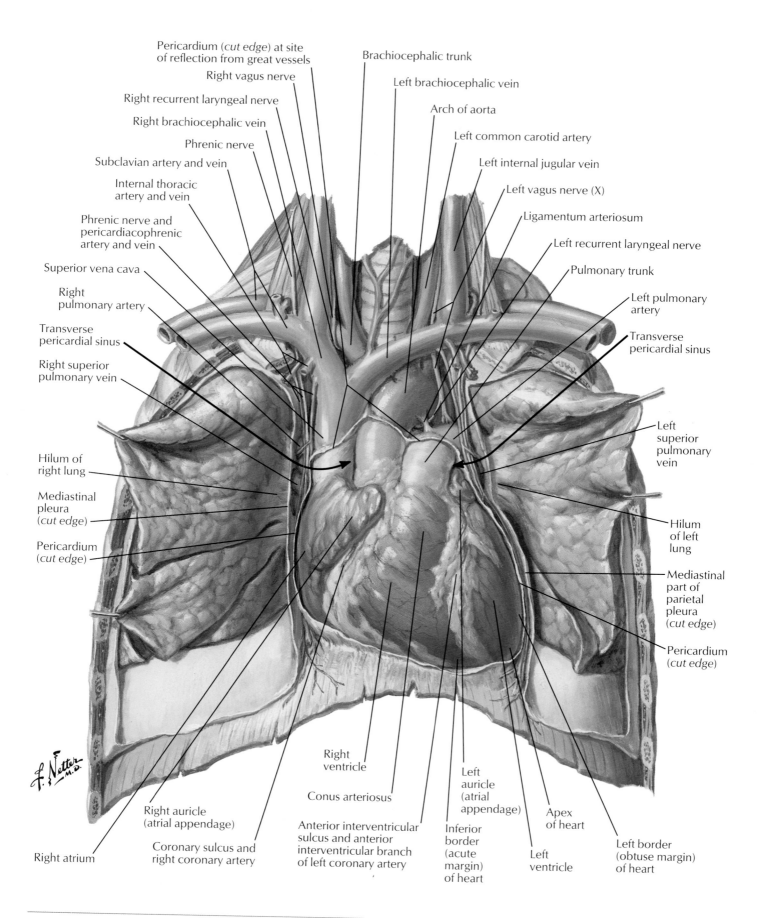

Pericardium (*cut edge*) at site of reflection from great vessels

Right vagus nerve

Right recurrent laryngeal nerve

Right brachiocephalic vein

Phrenic nerve

Subclavian artery and vein

Internal thoracic artery and vein

Phrenic nerve and pericardiacophrenic artery and vein

Superior vena cava

Right pulmonary artery

Transverse pericardial sinus

Right superior pulmonary vein

Hilum of right lung

Mediastinal pleura (*cut edge*)

Pericardium (*cut edge*)

Brachiocephalic trunk

Left brachiocephalic vein

Arch of aorta

Left common carotid artery

Left internal jugular vein

Left vagus nerve (X)

Ligamentum arteriosum

Left recurrent laryngeal nerve

Pulmonary trunk

Left pulmonary artery

Transverse pericardial sinus

Left superior pulmonary vein

Hilum of left lung

Mediastinal part of parietal pleura (*cut edge*)

Pericardium (*cut edge*)

Right ventricle

Conus arteriosus

Anterior interventricular sulcus and anterior interventricular branch of left coronary artery

Inferior border (acute margin) of heart

Left auricle (atrial appendage)

Apex of heart

Left ventricle

Left border (obtuse margin) of heart

Right auricle (atrial appendage)

Coronary sulcus and right coronary artery

Right atrium

**Plate 209**

**Heart**

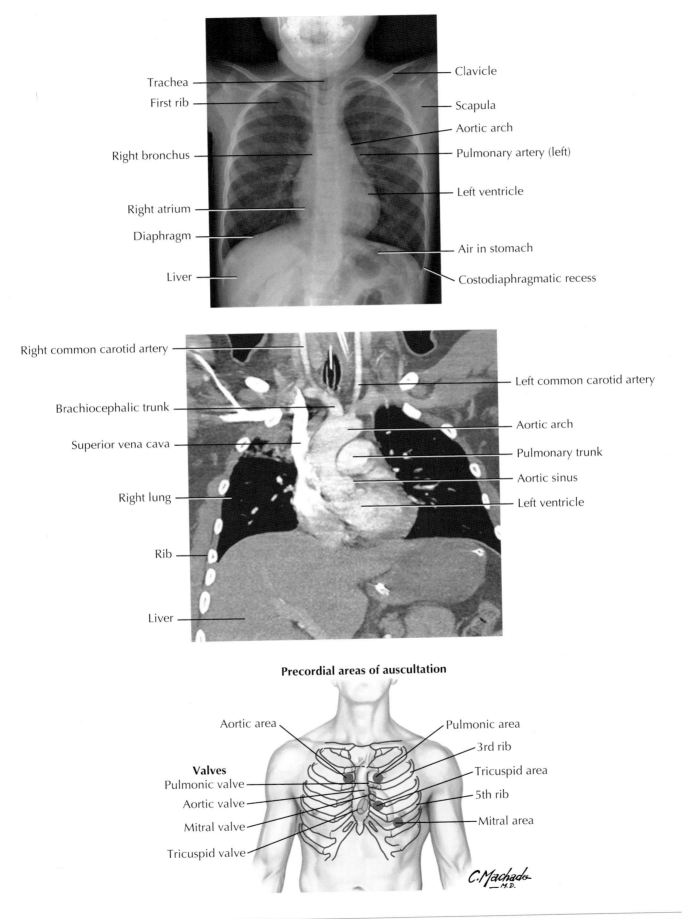

Trachea

First rib

Right bronchus

Right atrium

Diaphragm

Liver

Clavicle

Scapula

Aortic arch

Pulmonary artery (left)

Left ventricle

Air in stomach

Costodiaphragmatic recess

Right common carotid artery

Brachiocephalic trunk

Superior vena cava

Right lung

Rib

Liver

Left common carotid artery

Aortic arch

Pulmonary trunk

Aortic sinus

Left ventricle

**Precordial areas of auscultation**

Aortic area

Pulmonic area

3rd rib

Tricuspid area

5th rib

Mitral area

**Valves**

Pulmonic valve

Aortic valve

Mitral valve

Tricuspid valve

C. Machado
_M.D.

**Heart**

**Plate 210**

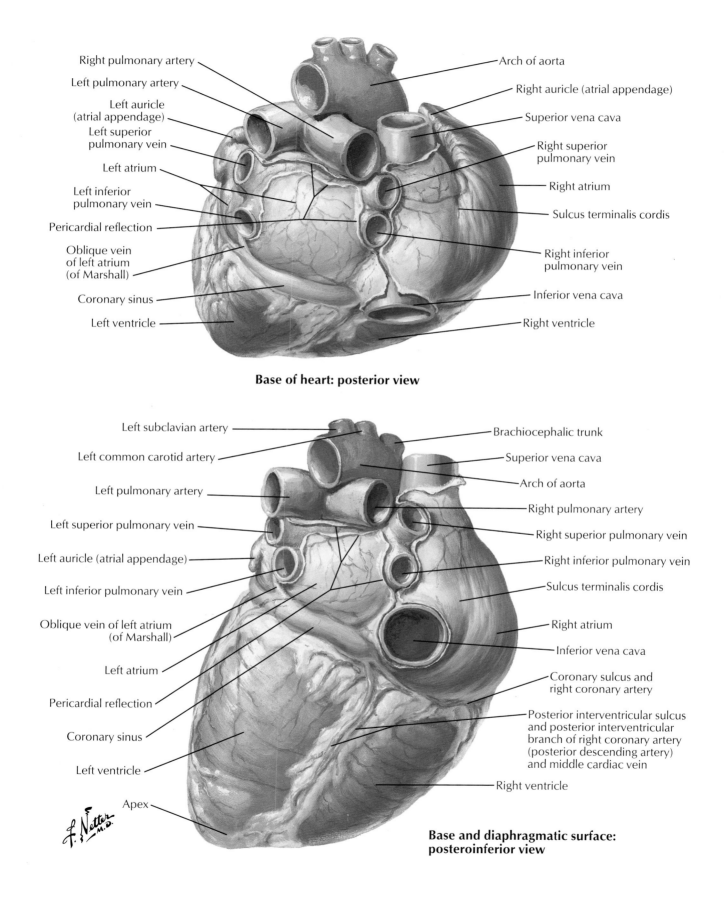

Right pulmonary artery

Left pulmonary artery

Left auricle (atrial appendage)

Left superior pulmonary vein

Left atrium

Left inferior pulmonary vein

Pericardial reflection

Oblique vein of left atrium (of Marshall)

Coronary sinus

Left ventricle

Arch of aorta

Right auricle (atrial appendage)

Superior vena cava

Right superior pulmonary vein

Right atrium

Sulcus terminalis cordis

Right inferior pulmonary vein

Inferior vena cava

Right ventricle

**Base of heart: posterior view**

Left subclavian artery

Left common carotid artery

Left pulmonary artery

Left superior pulmonary vein

Left auricle (atrial appendage)

Left inferior pulmonary vein

Oblique vein of left atrium (of Marshall)

Left atrium

Pericardial reflection

Coronary sinus

Left ventricle

Apex

Brachiocephalic trunk

Superior vena cava

Arch of aorta

Right pulmonary artery

Right superior pulmonary vein

Right inferior pulmonary vein

Sulcus terminalis cordis

Right atrium

Inferior vena cava

Coronary sulcus and right coronary artery

Posterior interventricular sulcus and posterior interventricular branch of right coronary artery (posterior descending artery) and middle cardiac vein

Right ventricle

**Base and diaphragmatic surface: posteroinferior view**

**Plate 211**

**Heart**

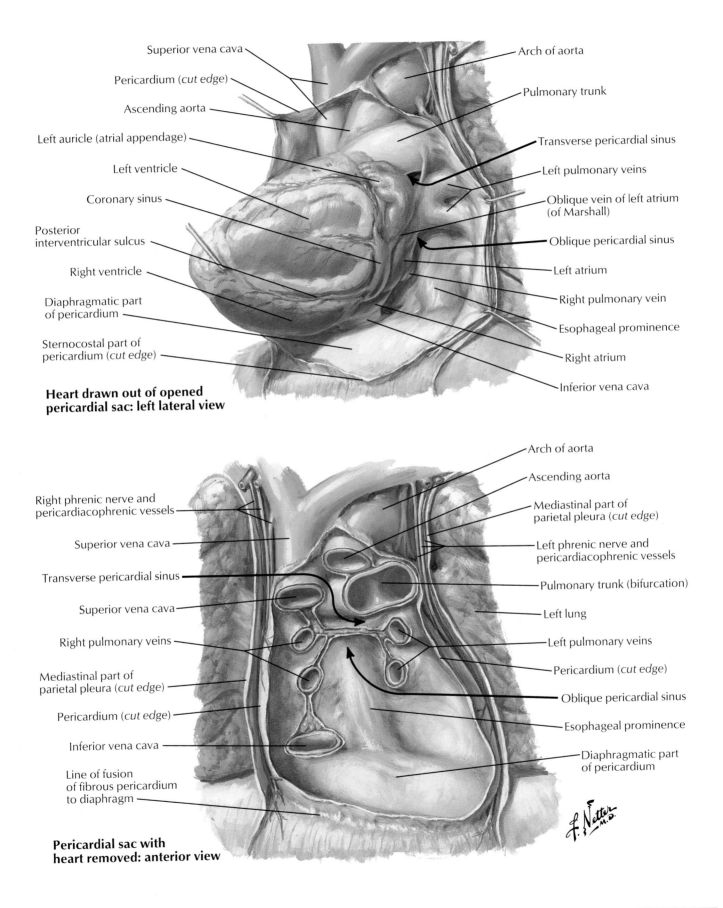

Superior vena cava

Pericardium (*cut edge*)

Ascending aorta

Left auricle (atrial appendage)

Left ventricle

Coronary sinus

Posterior interventricular sulcus

Right ventricle

Diaphragmatic part of pericardium

Sternocostal part of pericardium (*cut edge*)

Arch of aorta

Pulmonary trunk

Transverse pericardial sinus

Left pulmonary veins

Oblique vein of left atrium (of Marshall)

Oblique pericardial sinus

Left atrium

Right pulmonary vein

Esophageal prominence

Right atrium

Inferior vena cava

**Heart drawn out of opened pericardial sac: left lateral view**

Right phrenic nerve and pericardiacophrenic vessels

Superior vena cava

Transverse pericardial sinus

Superior vena cava

Right pulmonary veins

Mediastinal part of parietal pleura (*cut edge*)

Pericardium (*cut edge*)

Inferior vena cava

Line of fusion of fibrous pericardium to diaphragm

Arch of aorta

Ascending aorta

Mediastinal part of parietal pleura (*cut edge*)

Left phrenic nerve and pericardiacophrenic vessels

Pulmonary trunk (bifurcation)

Left lung

Left pulmonary veins

Pericardium (*cut edge*)

Oblique pericardial sinus

Esophageal prominence

Diaphragmatic part of pericardium

**Pericardial sac with heart removed: anterior view**

**Plate 212**

**Heart**

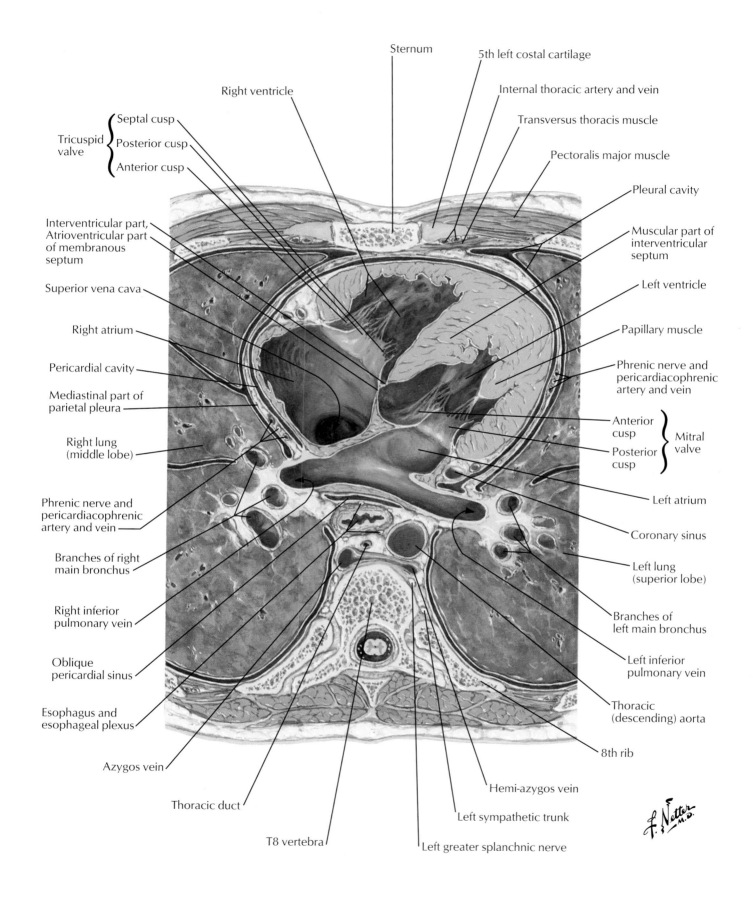

Sternum

5th left costal cartilage

Right ventricle

Internal thoracic artery and vein

Tricuspid valve { Septal cusp / Posterior cusp / Anterior cusp }

Transversus thoracis muscle

Pectoralis major muscle

Pleural cavity

Interventricular part, Atrioventricular part of membranous septum

Muscular part of interventricular septum

Superior vena cava

Left ventricle

Right atrium

Papillary muscle

Pericardial cavity

Phrenic nerve and pericardiacophrenic artery and vein

Mediastinal part of parietal pleura

Anterior cusp

Posterior cusp

Mitral valve

Right lung (middle lobe)

Left atrium

Phrenic nerve and pericardiacophrenic artery and vein

Coronary sinus

Branches of right main bronchus

Left lung (superior lobe)

Right inferior pulmonary vein

Branches of left main bronchus

Oblique pericardial sinus

Left inferior pulmonary vein

Esophagus and esophageal plexus

Thoracic (descending) aorta

Azygos vein

8th rib

Thoracic duct

Hemi-azygos vein

T8 vertebra

Left sympathetic trunk

Left greater splanchnic nerve

**Plate 213**

**Heart**

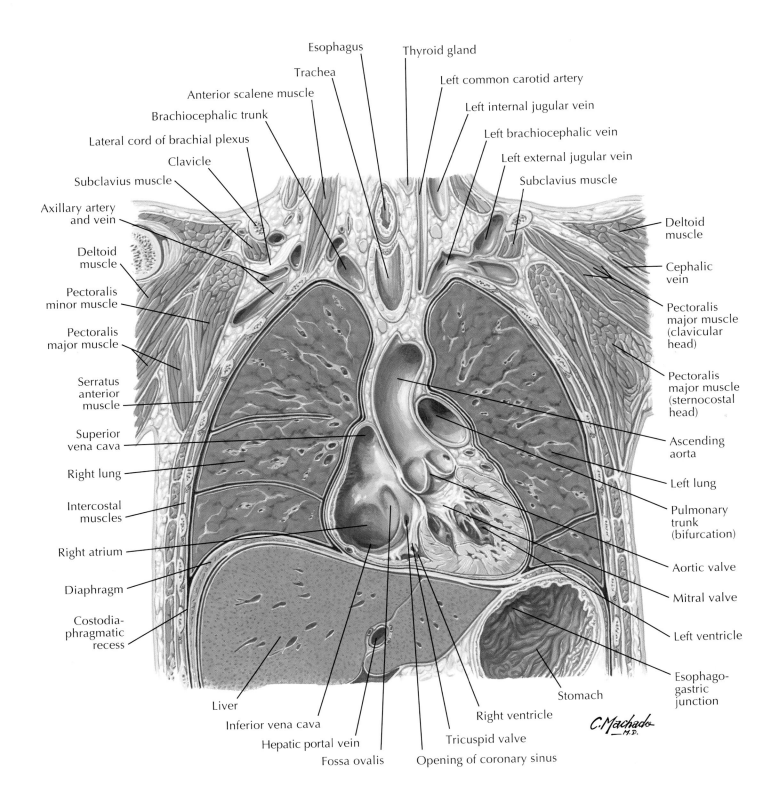

Esophagus

Thyroid gland

Trachea

Left common carotid artery

Anterior scalene muscle

Left internal jugular vein

Brachiocephalic trunk

Left brachiocephalic vein

Lateral cord of brachial plexus

Left external jugular vein

Clavicle

Subclavius muscle

Subclavius muscle

Deltoid muscle

Axillary artery and vein

Cephalic vein

Deltoid muscle

Pectoralis major muscle (clavicular head)

Pectoralis minor muscle

Pectoralis major muscle

Pectoralis major muscle (sternocostal head)

Serratus anterior muscle

Ascending aorta

Superior vena cava

Left lung

Right lung

Pulmonary trunk (bifurcation)

Intercostal muscles

Right atrium

Aortic valve

Diaphragm

Mitral valve

Costodiaphragmatic recess

Left ventricle

Esophagogastric junction

Liver

Stomach

Inferior vena cava

Right ventricle

Hepatic portal vein

Tricuspid valve

Fossa ovalis

Opening of coronary sinus

C.Machado _M.D._

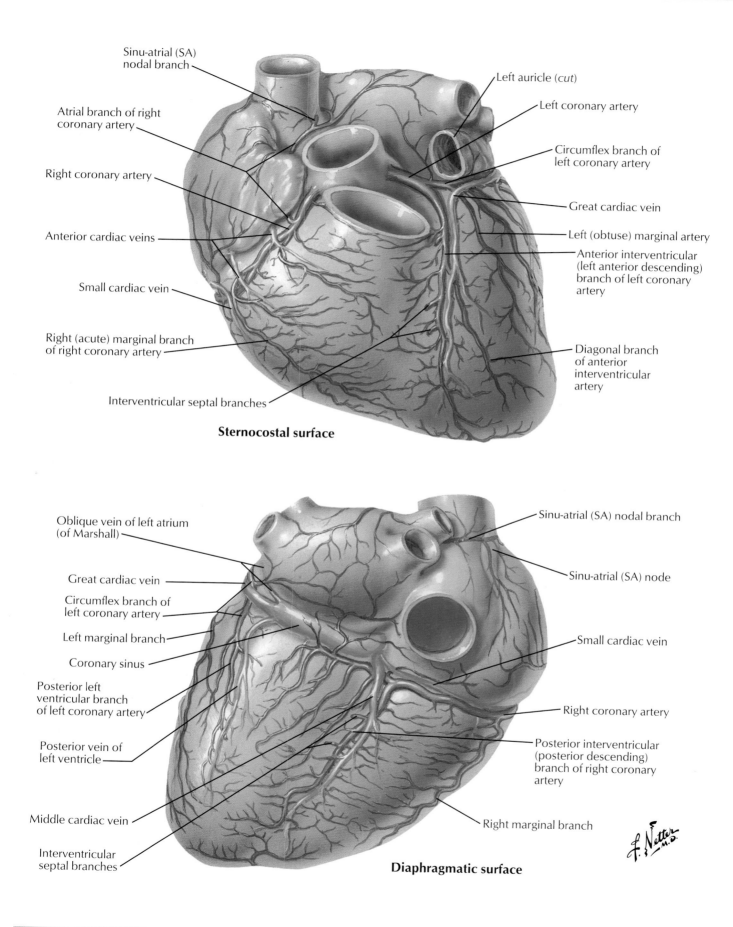

Sinu-atrial (SA) nodal branch

Atrial branch of right coronary artery

Right coronary artery

Anterior cardiac veins

Small cardiac vein

Right (acute) marginal branch of right coronary artery

Interventricular septal branches

Left auricle (*cut*)

Left coronary artery

Circumflex branch of left coronary artery

Great cardiac vein

Left (obtuse) marginal artery

Anterior interventricular (left anterior descending) branch of left coronary artery

Diagonal branch of anterior interventricular artery

**Sternocostal surface**

Oblique vein of left atrium (of Marshall)

Great cardiac vein

Circumflex branch of left coronary artery

Left marginal branch

Coronary sinus

Posterior left ventricular branch of left coronary artery

Posterior vein of left ventricle

Middle cardiac vein

Interventricular septal branches

Sinu-atrial (SA) nodal branch

Sinu-atrial (SA) node

Small cardiac vein

Right coronary artery

Posterior interventricular (posterior descending) branch of right coronary artery

Right marginal branch

**Diaphragmatic surface**

**Plate 215**

**Heart**

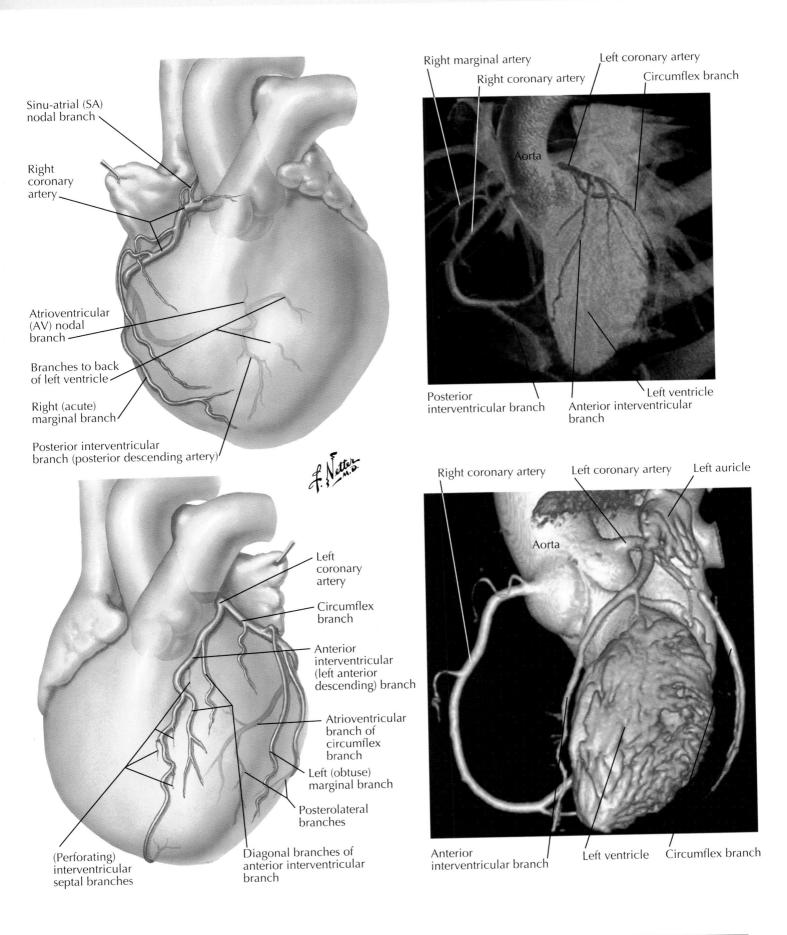

Sinu-atrial (SA) nodal branch

Right coronary artery

Atrioventricular (AV) nodal branch

Branches to back of left ventricle

Right (acute) marginal branch

Posterior interventricular branch (posterior descending artery)

Right marginal artery

Right coronary artery

Left coronary artery

Circumflex branch

Aorta

Posterior interventricular branch

Anterior interventricular branch

Left ventricle

Left coronary artery

Circumflex branch

Anterior interventricular (left anterior descending) branch

Atrioventricular branch of circumflex branch

Left (obtuse) marginal branch

Posterolateral branches

Diagonal branches of anterior interventricular branch

(Perforating) interventricular septal branches

Right coronary artery

Left coronary artery

Left auricle

Aorta

Anterior interventricular branch

Left ventricle

Circumflex branch

**Heart**

**Plate 216**

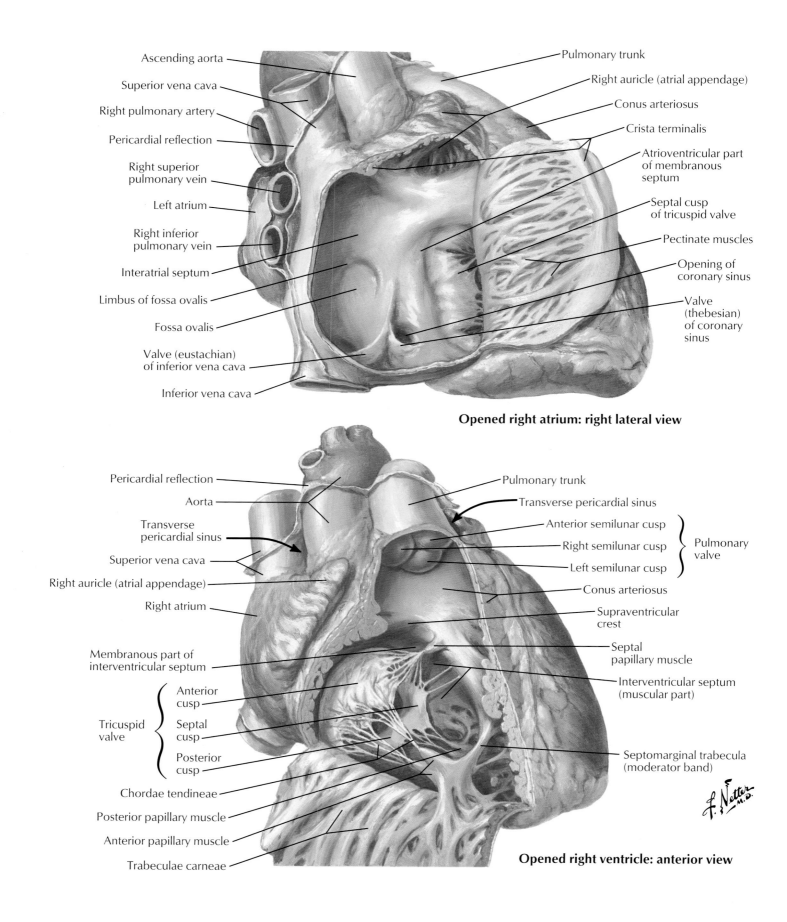

Ascending aorta

Superior vena cava

Right pulmonary artery

Pericardial reflection

Right superior pulmonary vein

Left atrium

Right inferior pulmonary vein

Interatrial septum

Limbus of fossa ovalis

Fossa ovalis

Valve (eustachian) of inferior vena cava

Inferior vena cava

Pulmonary trunk

Right auricle (atrial appendage)

Conus arteriosus

Crista terminalis

Atrioventricular part of membranous septum

Septal cusp of tricuspid valve

Pectinate muscles

Opening of coronary sinus

Valve (thebesian) of coronary sinus

**Opened right atrium: right lateral view**

Pericardial reflection

Aorta

Transverse pericardial sinus

Superior vena cava

Right auricle (atrial appendage)

Right atrium

Membranous part of interventricular septum

Tricuspid valve
- Anterior cusp
- Septal cusp
- Posterior cusp

Chordae tendineae

Posterior papillary muscle

Anterior papillary muscle

Trabeculae carneae

Pulmonary trunk

Transverse pericardial sinus

Anterior semilunar cusp

Right semilunar cusp     Pulmonary valve

Left semilunar cusp

Conus arteriosus

Supraventricular crest

Septal papillary muscle

Interventricular septum (muscular part)

Septomarginal trabecula (moderator band)

**Opened right ventricle: anterior view**

**Plate 217**

**Heart**

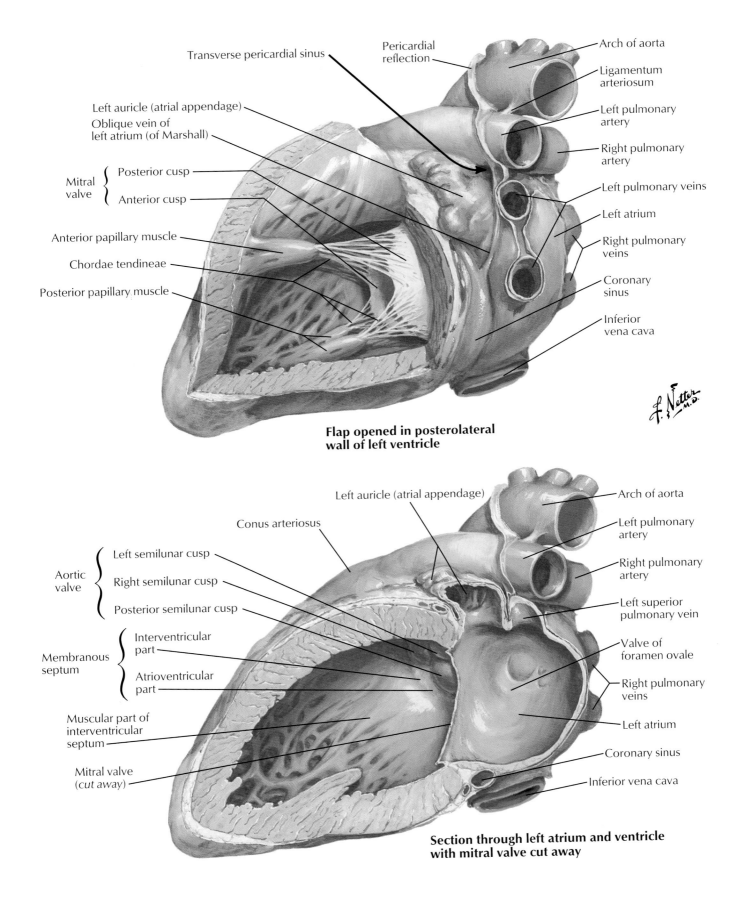

Transverse pericardial sinus

Pericardial reflection

Arch of aorta

Ligamentum arteriosum

Left auricle (atrial appendage)

Left pulmonary artery

Oblique vein of left atrium (of Marshall)

Right pulmonary artery

Mitral valve { Posterior cusp / Anterior cusp }

Left pulmonary veins

Left atrium

Anterior papillary muscle

Right pulmonary veins

Chordae tendineae

Coronary sinus

Posterior papillary muscle

Inferior vena cava

**Flap opened in posterolateral wall of left ventricle**

Left auricle (atrial appendage)

Conus arteriosus

Arch of aorta

Left pulmonary artery

Aortic valve { Left semilunar cusp / Right semilunar cusp / Posterior semilunar cusp }

Right pulmonary artery

Left superior pulmonary vein

Membranous septum { Interventricular part / Atrioventricular part }

Valve of foramen ovale

Right pulmonary veins

Muscular part of interventricular septum

Left atrium

Coronary sinus

Mitral valve (cut away)

Inferior vena cava

**Section through left atrium and ventricle with mitral valve cut away**

**Heart**

**Plate 218**

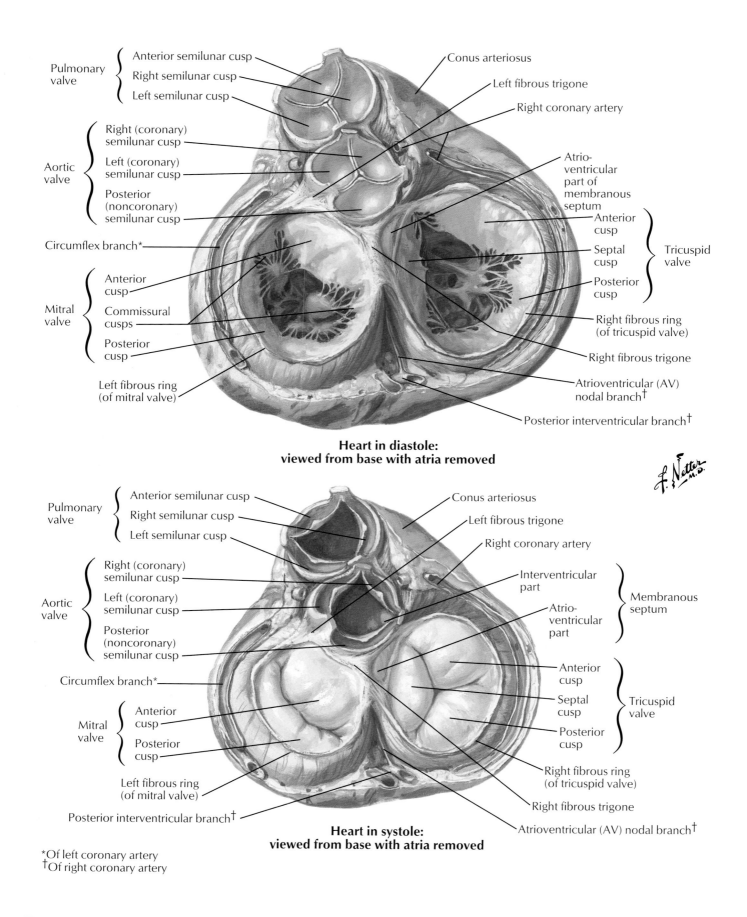

Pulmonary valve
- Anterior semilunar cusp
- Right semilunar cusp
- Left semilunar cusp

Aortic valve
- Right (coronary) semilunar cusp
- Left (coronary) semilunar cusp
- Posterior (noncoronary) semilunar cusp

Circumflex branch*

Mitral valve
- Anterior cusp
- Commissural cusps
- Posterior cusp

Left fibrous ring (of mitral valve)

Conus arteriosus

Left fibrous trigone

Right coronary artery

Atrio-ventricular part of membranous septum

Anterior cusp

Septal cusp

Posterior cusp

Tricuspid valve

Right fibrous ring (of tricuspid valve)

Right fibrous trigone

Atrioventricular (AV) nodal branch†

Posterior interventricular branch†

**Heart in diastole:
viewed from base with atria removed**

Pulmonary valve
- Anterior semilunar cusp
- Right semilunar cusp
- Left semilunar cusp

Aortic valve
- Right (coronary) semilunar cusp
- Left (coronary) semilunar cusp
- Posterior (noncoronary) semilunar cusp

Circumflex branch*

Mitral valve
- Anterior cusp
- Posterior cusp

Left fibrous ring (of mitral valve)

Posterior interventricular branch†

Conus arteriosus

Left fibrous trigone

Right coronary artery

Interventricular part

Atrio-ventricular part

Membranous septum

Anterior cusp

Septal cusp

Posterior cusp

Tricuspid valve

Right fibrous ring (of tricuspid valve)

Right fibrous trigone

Atrioventricular (AV) nodal branch†

**Heart in systole:
viewed from base with atria removed**

*Of left coronary artery
†Of right coronary artery

**Plate 219**

**Heart**

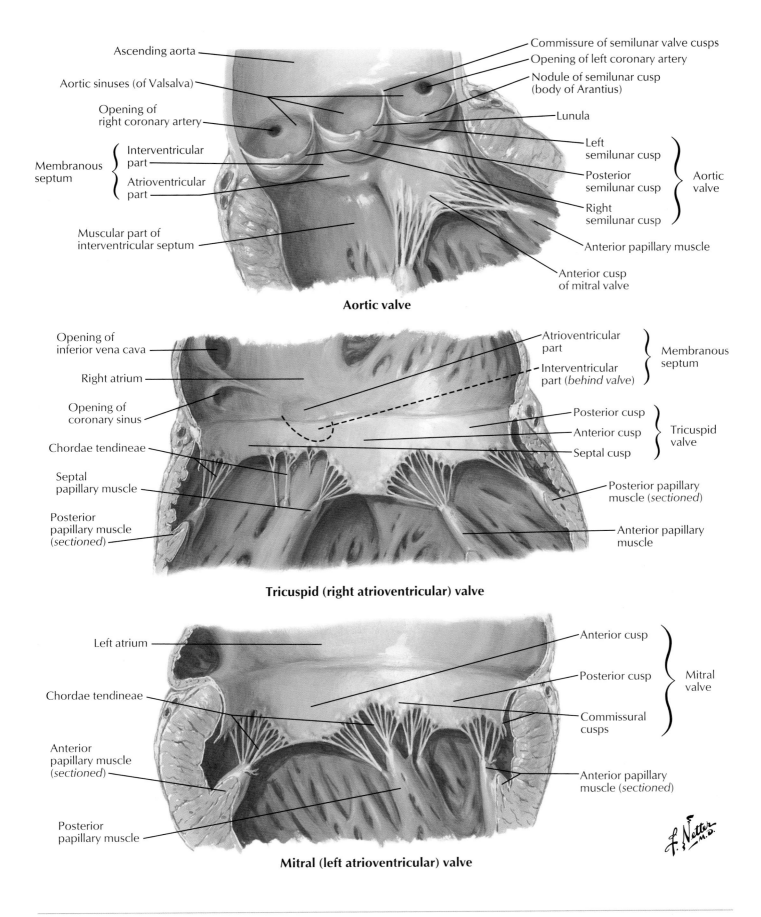

**Aortic valve**

Ascending aorta

Aortic sinuses (of Valsalva)

Opening of right coronary artery

Membranous septum
- Interventricular part
- Atrioventricular part

Muscular part of interventricular septum

Commissure of semilunar valve cusps

Opening of left coronary artery

Nodule of semilunar cusp (body of Arantius)

Lunula

Left semilunar cusp

Posterior semilunar cusp

Right semilunar cusp

Aortic valve

Anterior papillary muscle

Anterior cusp of mitral valve

**Tricuspid (right atrioventricular) valve**

Opening of inferior vena cava

Right atrium

Opening of coronary sinus

Chordae tendineae

Septal papillary muscle

Posterior papillary muscle (sectioned)

Atrioventricular part

Interventricular part (behind valve)

Membranous septum

Posterior cusp

Anterior cusp

Septal cusp

Tricuspid valve

Posterior papillary muscle (sectioned)

Anterior papillary muscle

**Mitral (left atrioventricular) valve**

Left atrium

Chordae tendineae

Anterior papillary muscle (sectioned)

Posterior papillary muscle

Anterior cusp

Posterior cusp

Mitral valve

Commissural cusps

Anterior papillary muscle (sectioned)

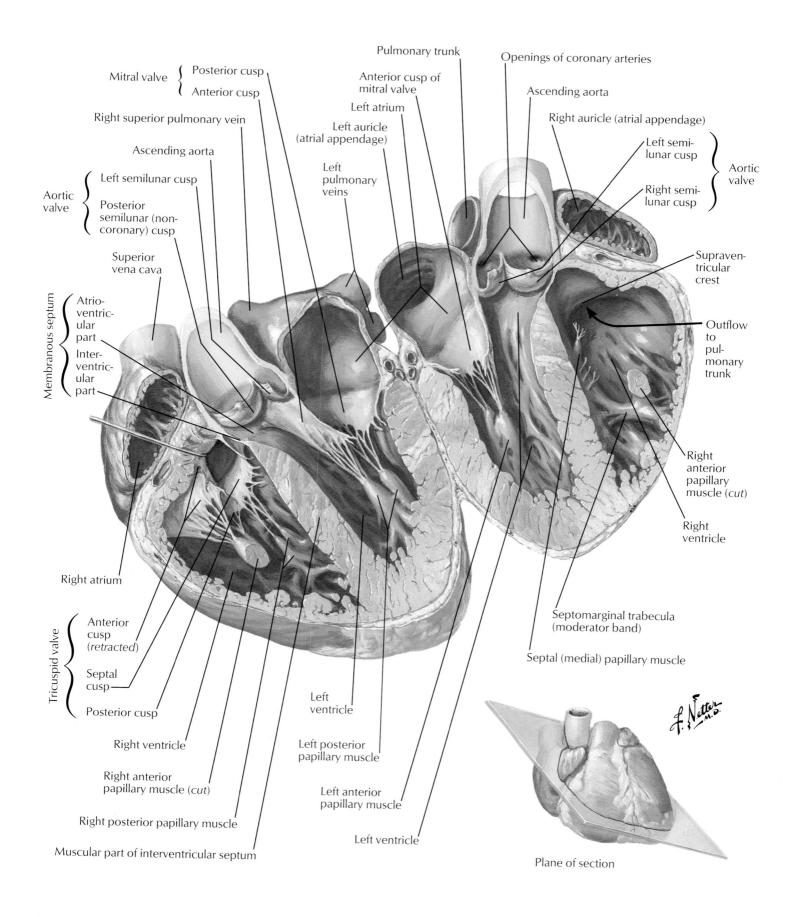

Mitral valve {
Posterior cusp
Anterior cusp

Right superior pulmonary vein

Ascending aorta

Aortic valve {
Left semilunar cusp
Posterior semilunar (non-coronary) cusp

Superior vena cava

Membranous septum {
Atrio-ventricular part
Inter-ventricular part

Right atrium

Tricuspid valve {
Anterior cusp (retracted)
Septal cusp
Posterior cusp

Right ventricle

Right anterior papillary muscle (cut)

Right posterior papillary muscle

Muscular part of interventricular septum

Pulmonary trunk

Anterior cusp of mitral valve

Left atrium

Left auricle (atrial appendage)

Left pulmonary veins

Left ventricle

Left posterior papillary muscle

Left anterior papillary muscle

Left ventricle

Openings of coronary arteries

Ascending aorta

Right auricle (atrial appendage)

Left semilunar cusp
Right semilunar cusp
} Aortic valve

Supraventricular crest

Outflow to pulmonary trunk

Right anterior papillary muscle (cut)

Right ventricle

Septomarginal trabecula (moderator band)

Septal (medial) papillary muscle

Plane of section

**Plate 221**

**Heart**

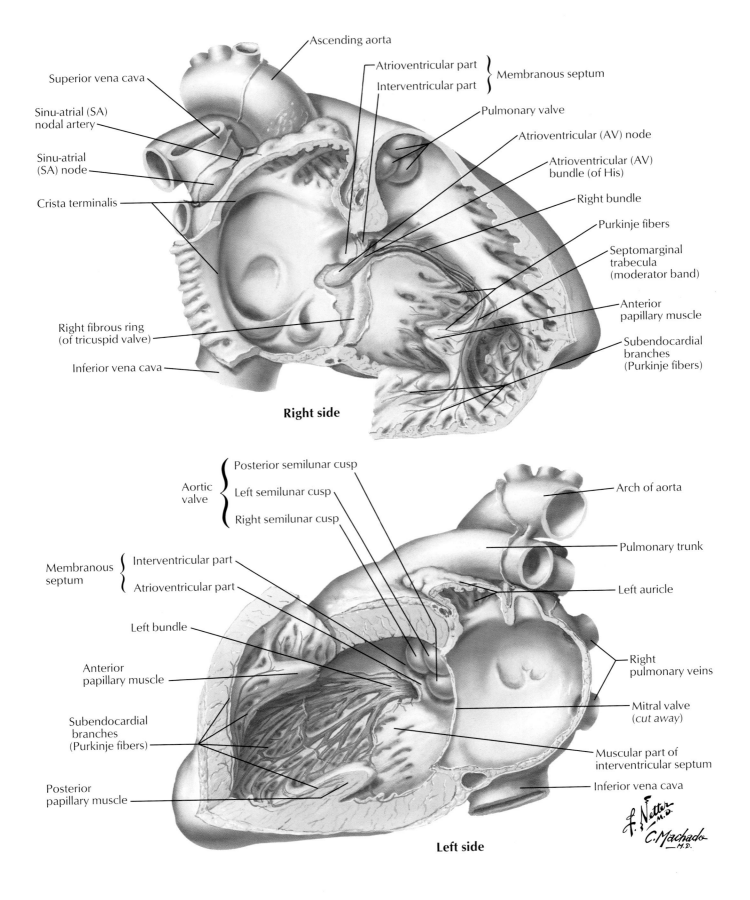

Ascending aorta

Atrioventricular part
Interventricular part
} Membranous septum

Superior vena cava

Pulmonary valve

Sinu-atrial (SA) nodal artery

Atrioventricular (AV) node

Sinu-atrial (SA) node

Atrioventricular (AV) bundle (of His)

Crista terminalis

Right bundle

Purkinje fibers

Septomarginal trabecula (moderator band)

Anterior papillary muscle

Right fibrous ring (of tricuspid valve)

Subendocardial branches (Purkinje fibers)

Inferior vena cava

**Right side**

Posterior semilunar cusp

Aortic valve { Left semilunar cusp

Arch of aorta

Right semilunar cusp

Pulmonary trunk

Membranous septum { Interventricular part

Atrioventricular part

Left auricle

Left bundle

Anterior papillary muscle

Right pulmonary veins

Subendocardial branches (Purkinje fibers)

Mitral valve (cut away)

Muscular part of interventricular septum

Posterior papillary muscle

Inferior vena cava

**Left side**

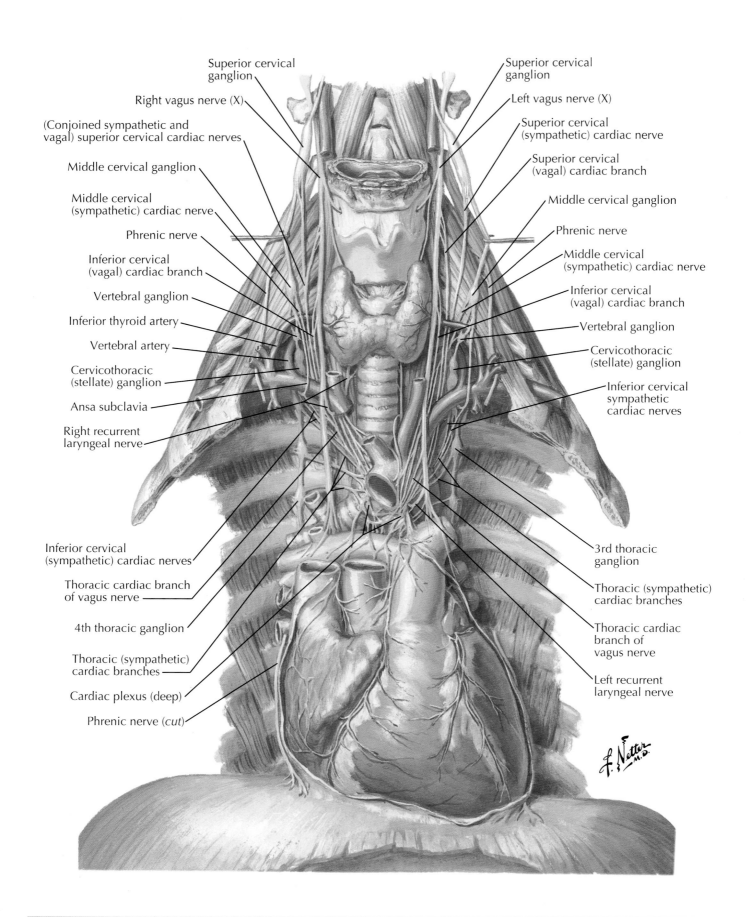

Superior cervical ganglion

Right vagus nerve (X)

(Conjoined sympathetic and vagal) superior cervical cardiac nerves

Middle cervical ganglion

Middle cervical (sympathetic) cardiac nerve

Phrenic nerve

Inferior cervical (vagal) cardiac branch

Vertebral ganglion

Inferior thyroid artery

Vertebral artery

Cervicothoracic (stellate) ganglion

Ansa subclavia

Right recurrent laryngeal nerve

Inferior cervical (sympathetic) cardiac nerves

Thoracic cardiac branch of vagus nerve

4th thoracic ganglion

Thoracic (sympathetic) cardiac branches

Cardiac plexus (deep)

Phrenic nerve (cut)

Superior cervical ganglion

Left vagus nerve (X)

Superior cervical (sympathetic) cardiac nerve

Superior cervical (vagal) cardiac branch

Middle cervical ganglion

Phrenic nerve

Middle cervical (sympathetic) cardiac nerve

Inferior cervical (vagal) cardiac branch

Vertebral ganglion

Cervicothoracic (stellate) ganglion

Inferior cervical sympathetic cardiac nerves

3rd thoracic ganglion

Thoracic (sympathetic) cardiac branches

Thoracic cardiac branch of vagus nerve

Left recurrent laryngeal nerve

**Plate 223**

**Heart**

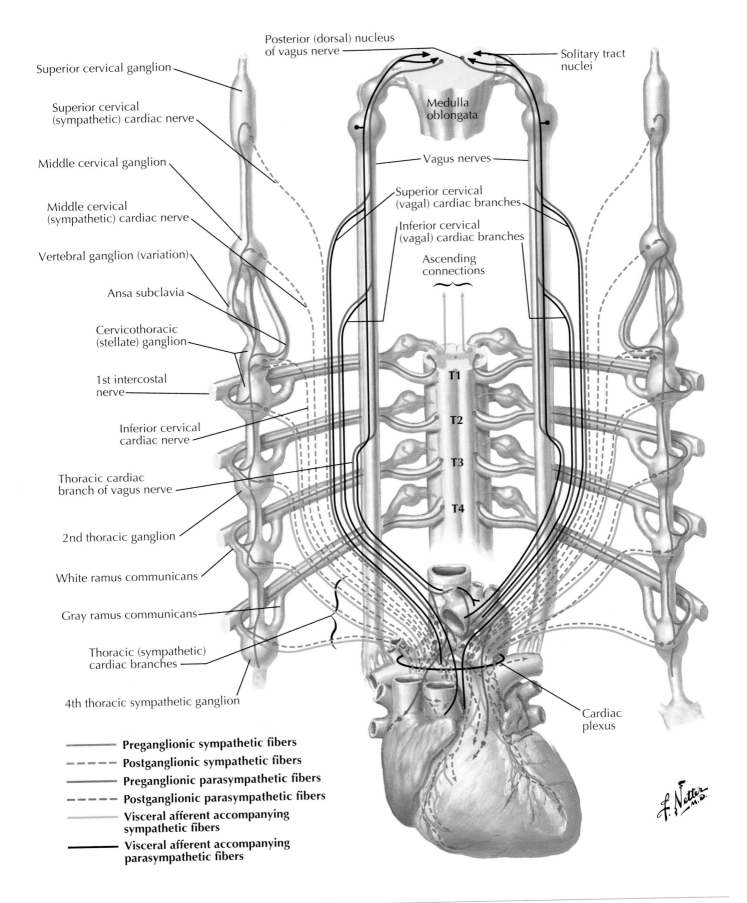

Posterior (dorsal) nucleus of vagus nerve

Solitary tract nuclei

Superior cervical ganglion

Medulla oblongata

Superior cervical (sympathetic) cardiac nerve

Vagus nerves

Middle cervical ganglion

Superior cervical (vagal) cardiac branches

Middle cervical (sympathetic) cardiac nerve

Inferior cervical (vagal) cardiac branches

Vertebral ganglion (variation)

Ascending connections

Ansa subclavia

Cervicothoracic (stellate) ganglion

T1

1st intercostal nerve

T2

Inferior cervical cardiac nerve

T3

Thoracic cardiac branch of vagus nerve

T4

2nd thoracic ganglion

White ramus communicans

Gray ramus communicans

Thoracic (sympathetic) cardiac branches

Cardiac plexus

4th thoracic sympathetic ganglion

—— Preganglionic sympathetic fibers

---- Postganglionic sympathetic fibers

—— Preganglionic parasympathetic fibers

---- Postganglionic parasympathetic fibers

—— Visceral afferent accompanying sympathetic fibers

—— Visceral afferent accompanying parasympathetic fibers

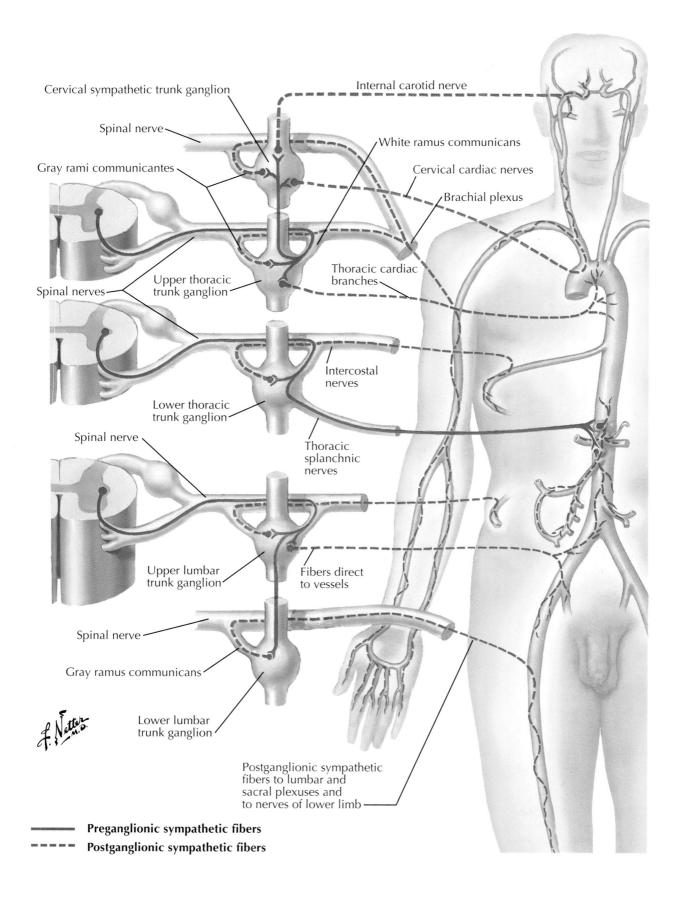

Cervical sympathetic trunk ganglion

Spinal nerve

Gray rami communicantes

Spinal nerves

Upper thoracic trunk ganglion

Lower thoracic trunk ganglion

Spinal nerve

Upper lumbar trunk ganglion

Spinal nerve

Gray ramus communicans

Lower lumbar trunk ganglion

Internal carotid nerve

White ramus communicans

Cervical cardiac nerves

Brachial plexus

Thoracic cardiac branches

Intercostal nerves

Thoracic splanchnic nerves

Fibers direct to vessels

Postganglionic sympathetic fibers to lumbar and sacral plexuses and to nerves of lower limb

——— Preganglionic sympathetic fibers

- - - - - Postganglionic sympathetic fibers

**Plate 225**

**Heart**

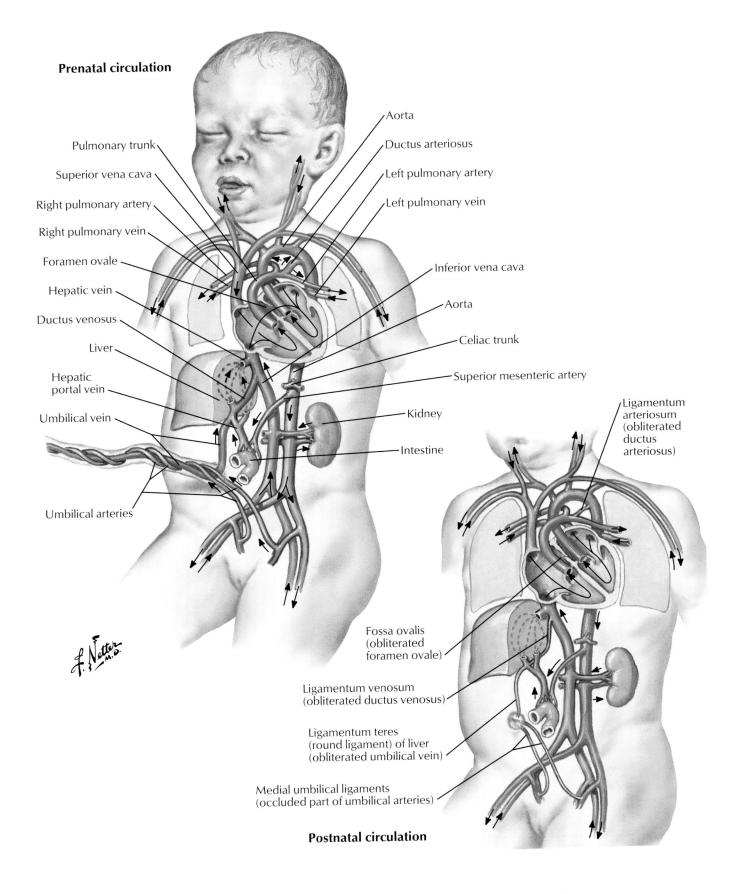

**Prenatal circulation**

Pulmonary trunk

Superior vena cava

Right pulmonary artery

Right pulmonary vein

Foramen ovale

Hepatic vein

Ductus venosus

Liver

Hepatic portal vein

Umbilical vein

Umbilical arteries

Aorta

Ductus arteriosus

Left pulmonary artery

Left pulmonary vein

Inferior vena cava

Aorta

Celiac trunk

Superior mesenteric artery

Kidney

Intestine

Ligamentum arteriosum (obliterated ductus arteriosus)

Fossa ovalis (obliterated foramen ovale)

Ligamentum venosum (obliterated ductus venosus)

Ligamentum teres (round ligament) of liver (obliterated umbilical vein)

Medial umbilical ligaments (occluded part of umbilical arteries)

**Postnatal circulation**

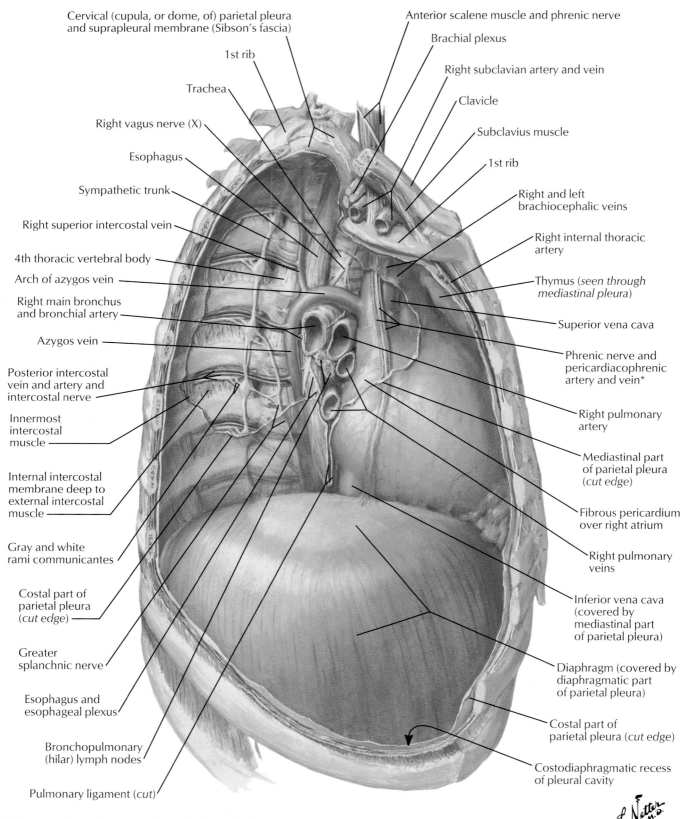

Cervical (cupula, or dome, of) parietal pleura and suprapleural membrane (Sibson's fascia)

1st rib

Trachea

Right vagus nerve (X)

Esophagus

Sympathetic trunk

Right superior intercostal vein

4th thoracic vertebral body

Arch of azygos vein

Right main bronchus and bronchial artery

Azygos vein

Posterior intercostal vein and artery and intercostal nerve

Innermost intercostal muscle

Internal intercostal membrane deep to external intercostal muscle

Gray and white rami communicantes

Costal part of parietal pleura (cut edge)

Greater splanchnic nerve

Esophagus and esophageal plexus

Bronchopulmonary (hilar) lymph nodes

Pulmonary ligament (cut)

Anterior scalene muscle and phrenic nerve

Brachial plexus

Right subclavian artery and vein

Clavicle

Subclavius muscle

1st rib

Right and left brachiocephalic veins

Right internal thoracic artery

Thymus (*seen through mediastinal pleura*)

Superior vena cava

Phrenic nerve and pericardiacophrenic artery and vein*

Right pulmonary artery

Mediastinal part of parietal pleura (*cut edge*)

Fibrous pericardium over right atrium

Right pulmonary veins

Inferior vena cava (covered by mediastinal part of parietal pleura)

Diaphragm (covered by diaphragmatic part of parietal pleura)

Costal part of parietal pleura (*cut edge*)

Costodiaphragmatic recess of pleural cavity

*Nerve and vessels commonly run independently.*

**Plate 227**　　　　　　　　　　　　　　　　　　　　**Mediastinum**

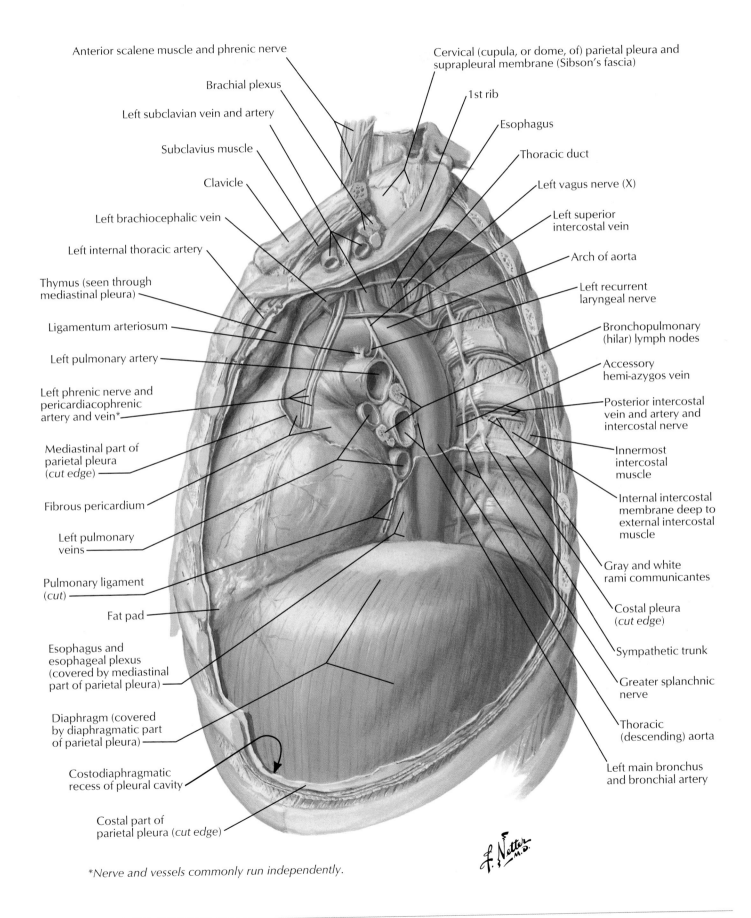

Anterior scalene muscle and phrenic nerve

Brachial plexus

Left subclavian vein and artery

Subclavius muscle

Clavicle

Left brachiocephalic vein

Left internal thoracic artery

Thymus (seen through mediastinal pleura)

Ligamentum arteriosum

Left pulmonary artery

Left phrenic nerve and pericardiacophrenic artery and vein*

Mediastinal part of parietal pleura (*cut edge*)

Fibrous pericardium

Left pulmonary veins

Pulmonary ligament (*cut*)

Fat pad

Esophagus and esophageal plexus (covered by mediastinal part of parietal pleura)

Diaphragm (covered by diaphragmatic part of parietal pleura)

Costodiaphragmatic recess of pleural cavity

Costal part of parietal pleura (*cut edge*)

Cervical (cupula, or dome, of) parietal pleura and suprapleural membrane (Sibson's fascia)

1st rib

Esophagus

Thoracic duct

Left vagus nerve (X)

Left superior intercostal vein

Arch of aorta

Left recurrent laryngeal nerve

Bronchopulmonary (hilar) lymph nodes

Accessory hemi-azygos vein

Posterior intercostal vein and artery and intercostal nerve

Innermost intercostal muscle

Internal intercostal membrane deep to external intercostal muscle

Gray and white rami communicantes

Costal pleura (*cut edge*)

Sympathetic trunk

Greater splanchnic nerve

Thoracic (descending) aorta

Left main bronchus and bronchial artery

*Nerve and vessels commonly run independently.*

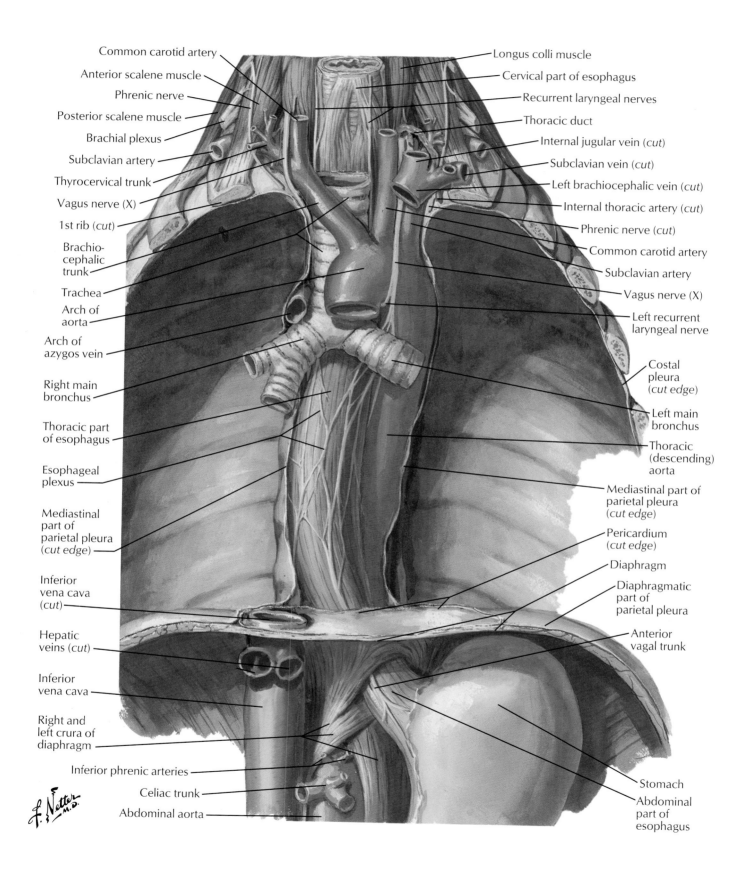

Common carotid artery

Anterior scalene muscle

Phrenic nerve

Posterior scalene muscle

Brachial plexus

Subclavian artery

Thyrocervical trunk

Vagus nerve (X)

1st rib (cut)

Brachio-cephalic trunk

Trachea

Arch of aorta

Arch of azygos vein

Right main bronchus

Thoracic part of esophagus

Esophageal plexus

Mediastinal part of parietal pleura (cut edge)

Inferior vena cava (cut)

Hepatic veins (cut)

Inferior vena cava

Right and left crura of diaphragm

Inferior phrenic arteries

Celiac trunk

Abdominal aorta

Longus colli muscle

Cervical part of esophagus

Recurrent laryngeal nerves

Thoracic duct

Internal jugular vein (cut)

Subclavian vein (cut)

Left brachiocephalic vein (cut)

Internal thoracic artery (cut)

Phrenic nerve (cut)

Common carotid artery

Subclavian artery

Vagus nerve (X)

Left recurrent laryngeal nerve

Costal pleura (cut edge)

Left main bronchus

Thoracic (descending) aorta

Mediastinal part of parietal pleura (cut edge)

Pericardium (cut edge)

Diaphragm

Diaphragmatic part of parietal pleura

Anterior vagal trunk

Stomach

Abdominal part of esophagus

**Plate 229**

**Mediastinum**

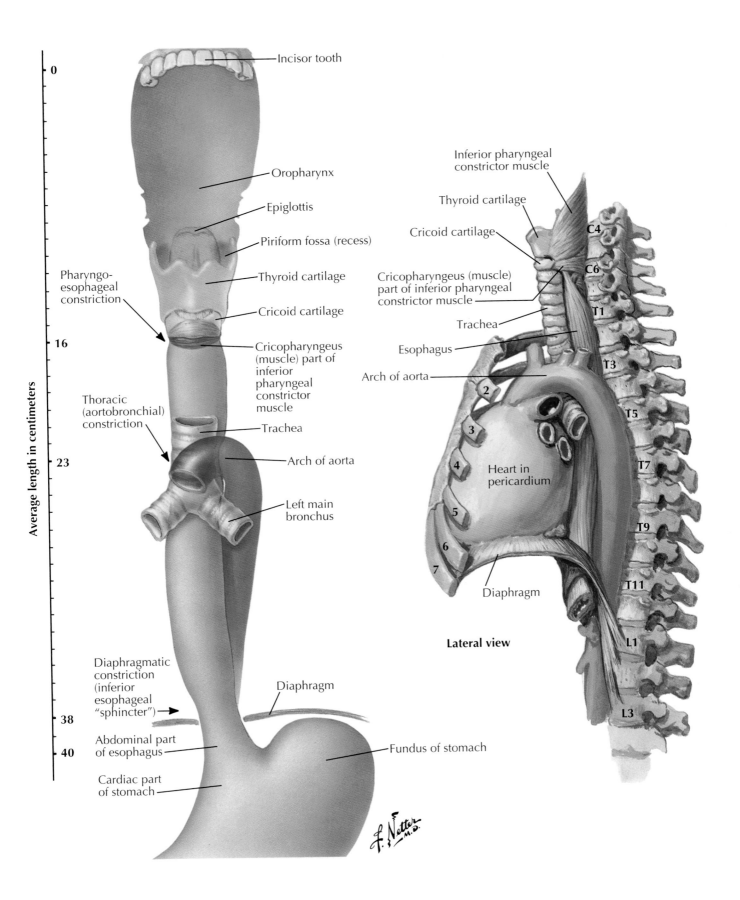

Incisor tooth

Oropharynx

Epiglottis

Piriform fossa (recess)

Pharyngo-esophageal constriction

Thyroid cartilage

Cricoid cartilage

Cricopharyngeus (muscle) part of inferior pharyngeal constrictor muscle

Thoracic (aortobronchial) constriction

Trachea

Arch of aorta

Left main bronchus

Diaphragmatic constriction (inferior esophageal "sphincter")

Abdominal part of esophagus

Cardiac part of stomach

Diaphragm

Fundus of stomach

Average length in centimeters

0

16

23

38

40

Inferior pharyngeal constrictor muscle

Thyroid cartilage

Cricoid cartilage

Cricopharyngeus (muscle) part of inferior pharyngeal constrictor muscle

Trachea

Esophagus

Arch of aorta

Heart in pericardium

Diaphragm

**Lateral view**

C4

C6

T1

T3

T5

T7

T9

T11

L1

L3

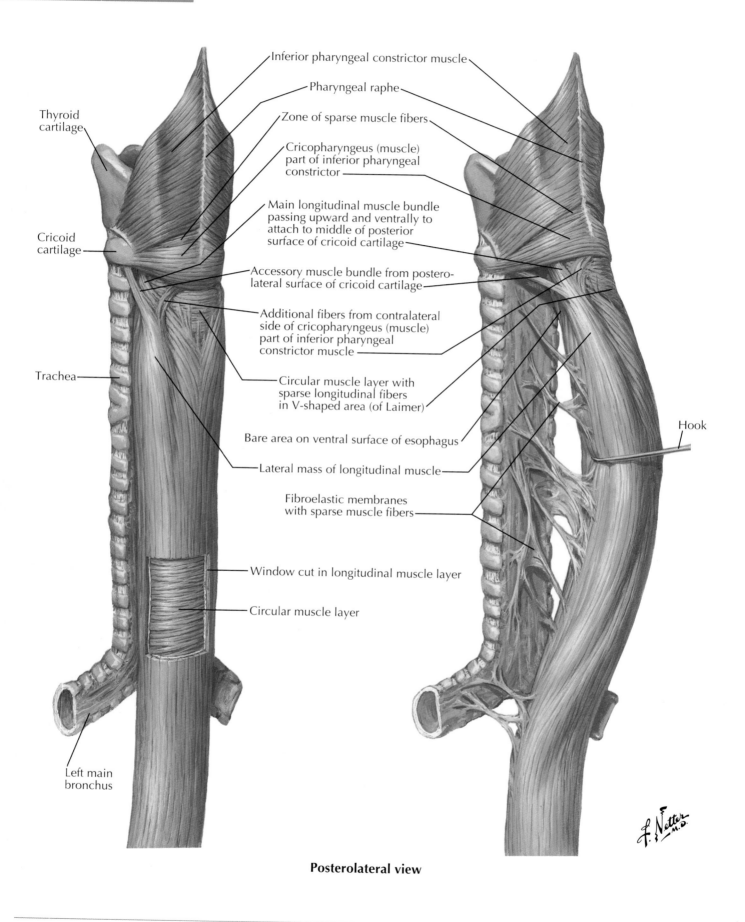

Inferior pharyngeal constrictor muscle

Pharyngeal raphe

Zone of sparse muscle fibers

Thyroid cartilage

Cricopharyngeus (muscle) part of inferior pharyngeal constrictor

Main longitudinal muscle bundle passing upward and ventrally to attach to middle of posterior surface of cricoid cartilage

Cricoid cartilage

Accessory muscle bundle from posterolateral surface of cricoid cartilage

Additional fibers from contralateral side of cricopharyngeus (muscle) part of inferior pharyngeal constrictor muscle

Trachea

Circular muscle layer with sparse longitudinal fibers in V-shaped area (of Laimer)

Bare area on ventral surface of esophagus

Lateral mass of longitudinal muscle

Hook

Fibroelastic membranes with sparse muscle fibers

Window cut in longitudinal muscle layer

Circular muscle layer

Left main bronchus

**Posterolateral view**

**Plate 231**

**Mediastinum**

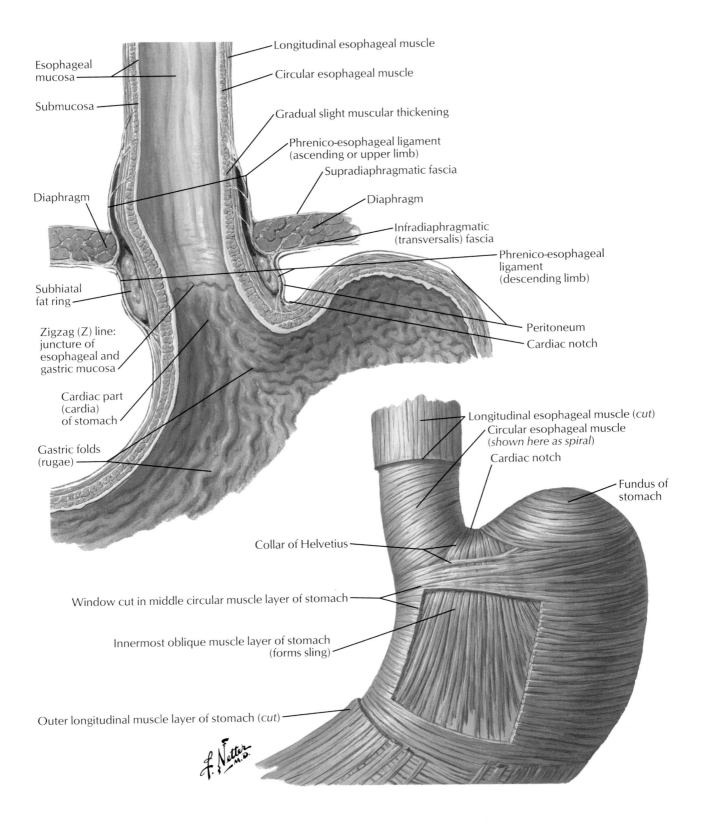

Esophageal mucosa

Longitudinal esophageal muscle

Circular esophageal muscle

Submucosa

Gradual slight muscular thickening

Phrenico-esophageal ligament (ascending or upper limb)

Supradiaphragmatic fascia

Diaphragm

Diaphragm

Infradiaphragmatic (transversalis) fascia

Phrenico-esophageal ligament (descending limb)

Subhiatal fat ring

Peritoneum

Cardiac notch

Zigzag (Z) line: juncture of esophageal and gastric mucosa

Cardiac part (cardia) of stomach

Longitudinal esophageal muscle (cut)

Circular esophageal muscle (shown here as spiral)

Cardiac notch

Fundus of stomach

Gastric folds (rugae)

Collar of Helvetius

Window cut in middle circular muscle layer of stomach

Innermost oblique muscle layer of stomach (forms sling)

Outer longitudinal muscle layer of stomach (cut)

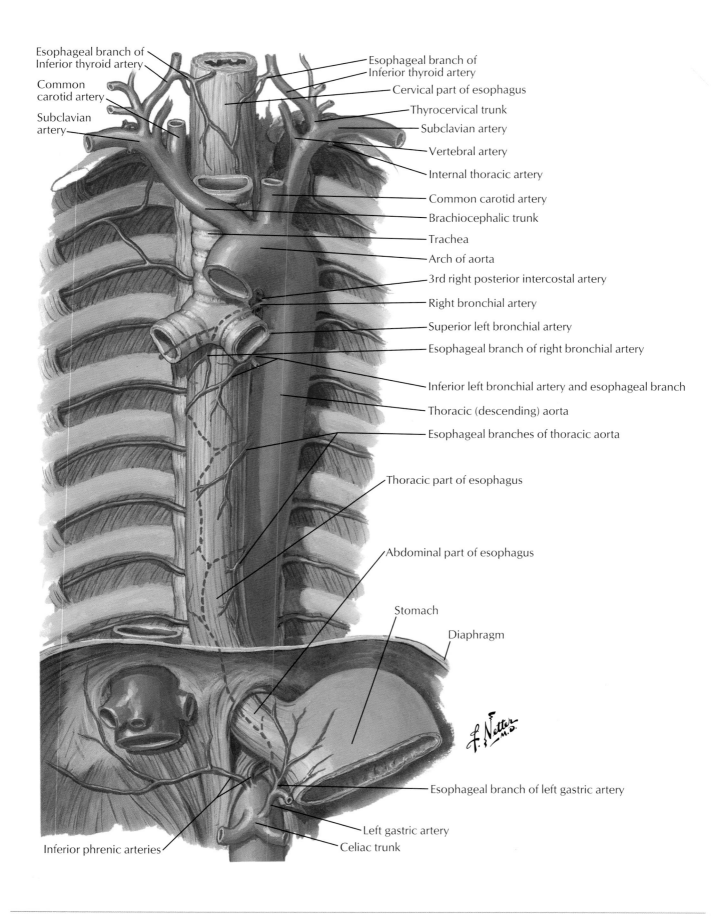

Esophageal branch of
Inferior thyroid artery

Common
carotid artery

Subclavian
artery

Esophageal branch of
Inferior thyroid artery

Cervical part of esophagus

Thyrocervical trunk

Subclavian artery

Vertebral artery

Internal thoracic artery

Common carotid artery

Brachiocephalic trunk

Trachea

Arch of aorta

3rd right posterior intercostal artery

Right bronchial artery

Superior left bronchial artery

Esophageal branch of right bronchial artery

Inferior left bronchial artery and esophageal branch

Thoracic (descending) aorta

Esophageal branches of thoracic aorta

Thoracic part of esophagus

Abdominal part of esophagus

Stomach

Diaphragm

Esophageal branch of left gastric artery

Left gastric artery

Celiac trunk

Inferior phrenic arteries

**Plate 233**

**Mediastinum**

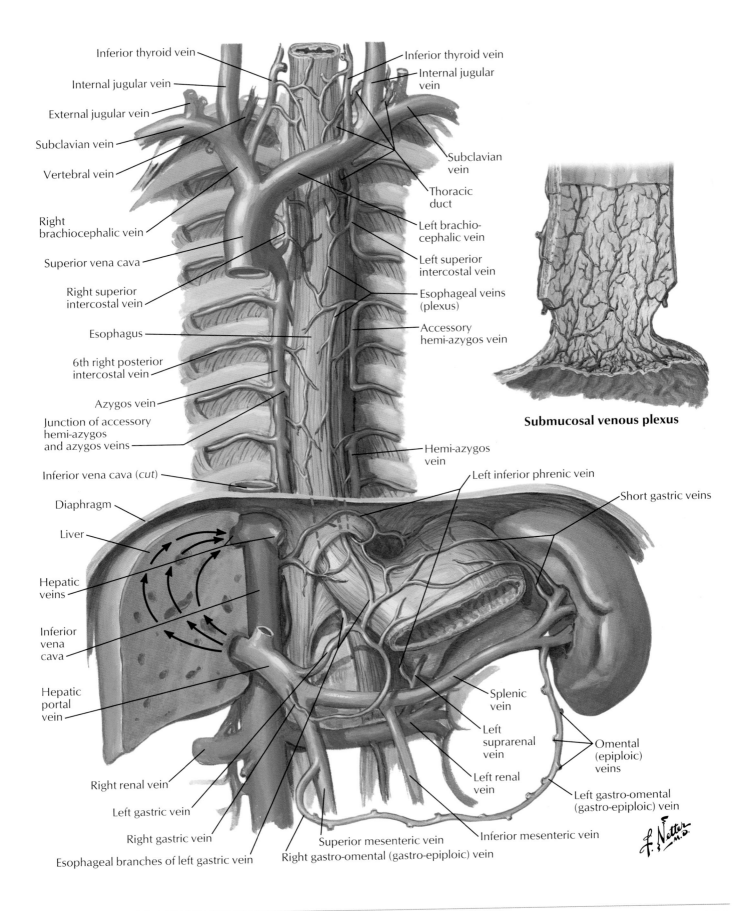

Inferior thyroid vein

Internal jugular vein

External jugular vein

Subclavian vein

Vertebral vein

Right brachiocephalic vein

Superior vena cava

Right superior intercostal vein

Esophagus

6th right posterior intercostal vein

Azygos vein

Junction of accessory hemi-azygos and azygos veins

Inferior vena cava (cut)

Diaphragm

Liver

Hepatic veins

Inferior vena cava

Hepatic portal vein

Right renal vein

Left gastric vein

Right gastric vein

Esophageal branches of left gastric vein

Inferior thyroid vein

Internal jugular vein

Subclavian vein

Thoracic duct

Left brachio-cephalic vein

Left superior intercostal vein

Esophageal veins (plexus)

Accessory hemi-azygos vein

Hemi-azygos vein

Submucosal venous plexus

Left inferior phrenic vein

Short gastric veins

Splenic vein

Left suprarenal vein

Left renal vein

Omental (epiploic) veins

Left gastro-omental (gastro-epiploic) vein

Inferior mesenteric vein

Superior mesenteric vein

Right gastro-omental (gastro-epiploic) vein

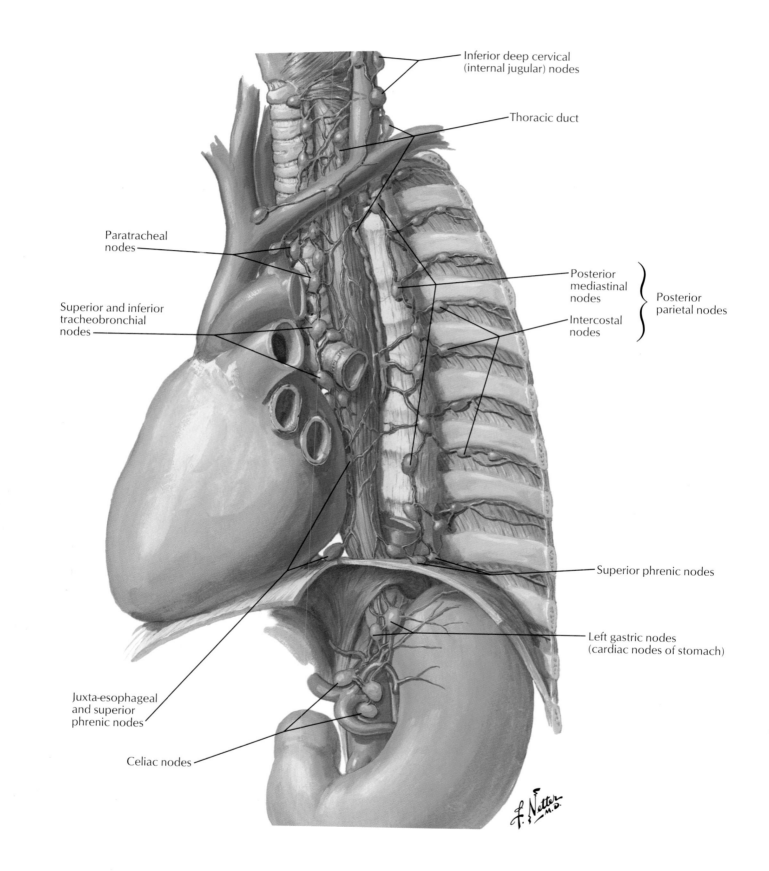

Inferior deep cervical (internal jugular) nodes

Thoracic duct

Paratracheal nodes

Superior and inferior tracheobronchial nodes

Posterior mediastinal nodes

Intercostal nodes

Posterior parietal nodes

Superior phrenic nodes

Left gastric nodes (cardiac nodes of stomach)

Juxta-esophageal and superior phrenic nodes

Celiac nodes

**Plate 235**

**Mediastinum**

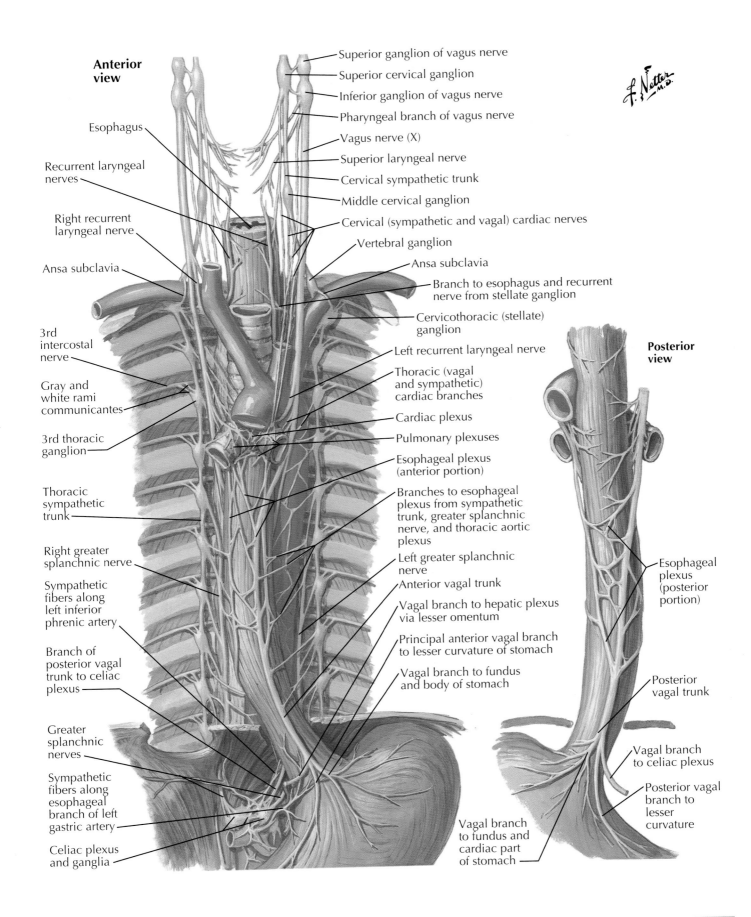

**Anterior view**

Superior ganglion of vagus nerve

Superior cervical ganglion

Inferior ganglion of vagus nerve

Pharyngeal branch of vagus nerve

Vagus nerve (X)

Superior laryngeal nerve

Cervical sympathetic trunk

Middle cervical ganglion

Cervical (sympathetic and vagal) cardiac nerves

Vertebral ganglion

Ansa subclavia

Branch to esophagus and recurrent nerve from stellate ganglion

Cervicothoracic (stellate) ganglion

Left recurrent laryngeal nerve

Thoracic (vagal and sympathetic) cardiac branches

Cardiac plexus

Pulmonary plexuses

Esophageal plexus (anterior portion)

Branches to esophageal plexus from sympathetic trunk, greater splanchnic nerve, and thoracic aortic plexus

Left greater splanchnic nerve

Anterior vagal trunk

Vagal branch to hepatic plexus via lesser omentum

Principal anterior vagal branch to lesser curvature of stomach

Vagal branch to fundus and body of stomach

Esophagus

Recurrent laryngeal nerves

Right recurrent laryngeal nerve

Ansa subclavia

3rd intercostal nerve

Gray and white rami communicantes

3rd thoracic ganglion

Thoracic sympathetic trunk

Right greater splanchnic nerve

Sympathetic fibers along left inferior phrenic artery

Branch of posterior vagal trunk to celiac plexus

Greater splanchnic nerves

Sympathetic fibers along esophageal branch of left gastric artery

Celiac plexus and ganglia

**Posterior view**

Esophageal plexus (posterior portion)

Posterior vagal trunk

Vagal branch to celiac plexus

Posterior vagal branch to lesser curvature

Vagal branch to fundus and cardiac part of stomach

**Series of chest axial CT images from superior (A) to inferior (C)**

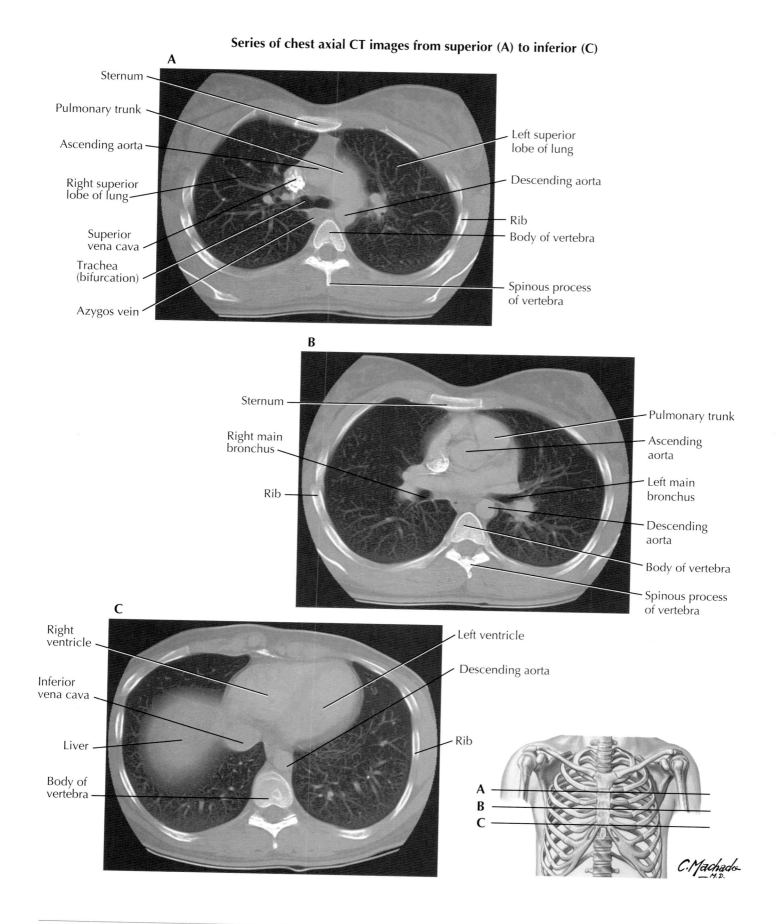

A

Sternum
Pulmonary trunk
Ascending aorta
Right superior lobe of lung
Superior vena cava
Trachea (bifurcation)
Azygos vein

Left superior lobe of lung
Descending aorta
Rib
Body of vertebra
Spinous process of vertebra

B

Sternum
Right main bronchus
Rib

Pulmonary trunk
Ascending aorta
Left main bronchus
Descending aorta
Body of vertebra
Spinous process of vertebra

C

Right ventricle
Inferior vena cava
Liver
Body of vertebra

Left ventricle
Descending aorta
Rib

A
B
C

C. Machado
_M.D._

**Plate 237**

**Regional Scans**

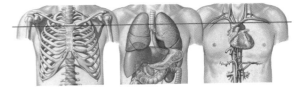

Inferior view

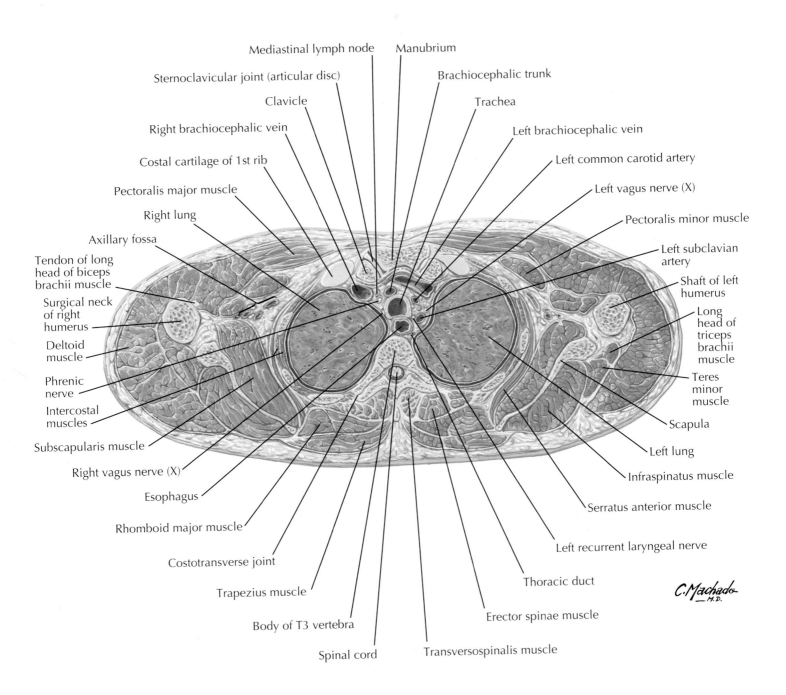

Mediastinal lymph node

Sternoclavicular joint (articular disc)

Clavicle

Right brachiocephalic vein

Costal cartilage of 1st rib

Pectoralis major muscle

Right lung

Axillary fossa

Tendon of long head of biceps brachii muscle

Surgical neck of right humerus

Deltoid muscle

Phrenic nerve

Intercostal muscles

Subscapularis muscle

Right vagus nerve (X)

Esophagus

Rhomboid major muscle

Costotransverse joint

Trapezius muscle

Body of T3 vertebra

Spinal cord

Manubrium

Brachiocephalic trunk

Trachea

Left brachiocephalic vein

Left common carotid artery

Left vagus nerve (X)

Pectoralis minor muscle

Left subclavian artery

Shaft of left humerus

Long head of triceps brachii muscle

Teres minor muscle

Scapula

Left lung

Infraspinatus muscle

Serratus anterior muscle

Left recurrent laryngeal nerve

Thoracic duct

Erector spinae muscle

Transversospinalis muscle

C. Machado
M.D.

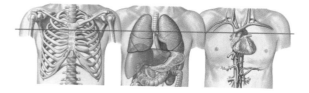

Inferior view

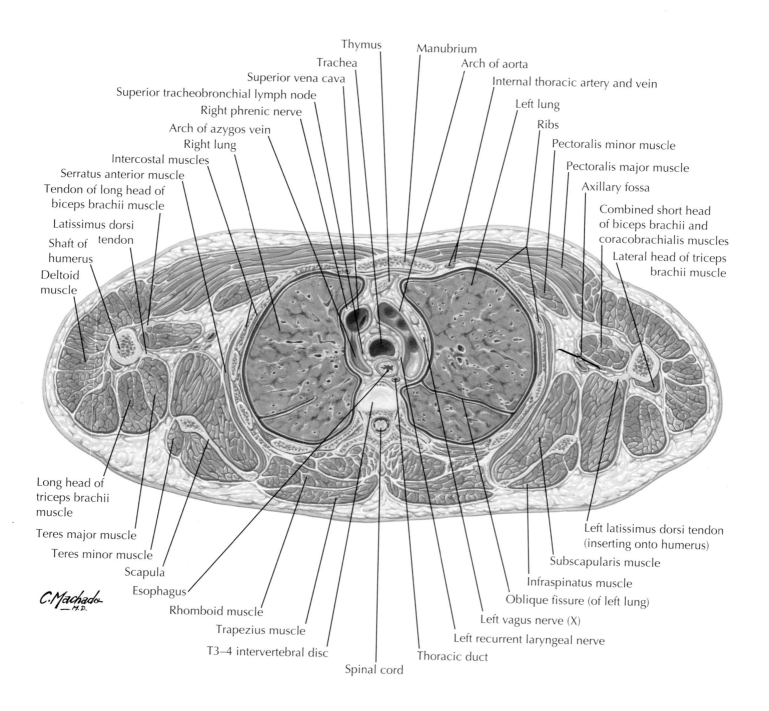

Thymus

Trachea

Superior vena cava

Superior tracheobronchial lymph node

Right phrenic nerve

Arch of azygos vein

Right lung

Intercostal muscles

Serratus anterior muscle

Tendon of long head of biceps brachii muscle

Latissimus dorsi tendon

Shaft of humerus

Deltoid muscle

Manubrium

Arch of aorta

Internal thoracic artery and vein

Left lung

Ribs

Pectoralis minor muscle

Pectoralis major muscle

Axillary fossa

Combined short head of biceps brachii and coracobrachialis muscles

Lateral head of triceps brachii muscle

Long head of triceps brachii muscle

Teres major muscle

Teres minor muscle

Scapula

Esophagus

Rhomboid muscle

Trapezius muscle

T3–4 intervertebral disc

Spinal cord

Left latissimus dorsi tendon (inserting onto humerus)

Subscapularis muscle

Infraspinatus muscle

Oblique fissure (of left lung)

Left vagus nerve (X)

Left recurrent laryngeal nerve

Thoracic duct

C. Machado —M.D.

**Plate 239**

**Cross-Sectional Anatomy**

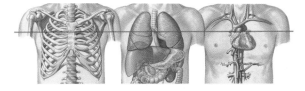

Inferior view

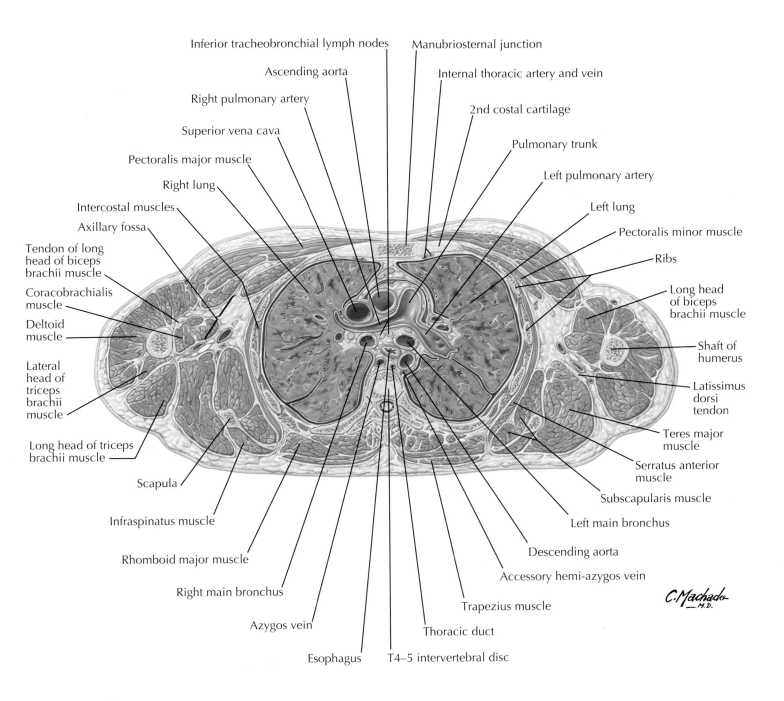

Inferior tracheobronchial lymph nodes

Ascending aorta

Right pulmonary artery

Superior vena cava

Pectoralis major muscle

Right lung

Intercostal muscles

Axillary fossa

Tendon of long head of biceps brachii muscle

Coracobrachialis muscle

Deltoid muscle

Lateral head of triceps brachii muscle

Long head of triceps brachii muscle

Scapula

Infraspinatus muscle

Rhomboid major muscle

Right main bronchus

Azygos vein

Esophagus

T4–5 intervertebral disc

Thoracic duct

Trapezius muscle

Accessory hemi-azygos vein

Descending aorta

Left main bronchus

Subscapularis muscle

Serratus anterior muscle

Teres major muscle

Latissimus dorsi tendon

Shaft of humerus

Long head of biceps brachii muscle

Ribs

Pectoralis minor muscle

Left lung

Left pulmonary artery

Pulmonary trunk

2nd costal cartilage

Internal thoracic artery and vein

Manubriosternal junction

*C. Machado* — *M.D.*

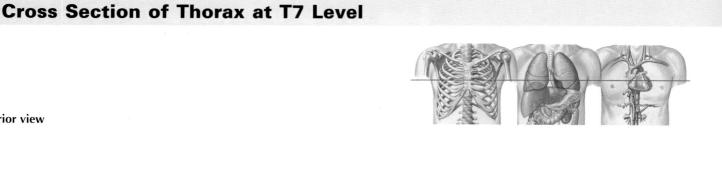

Inferior view

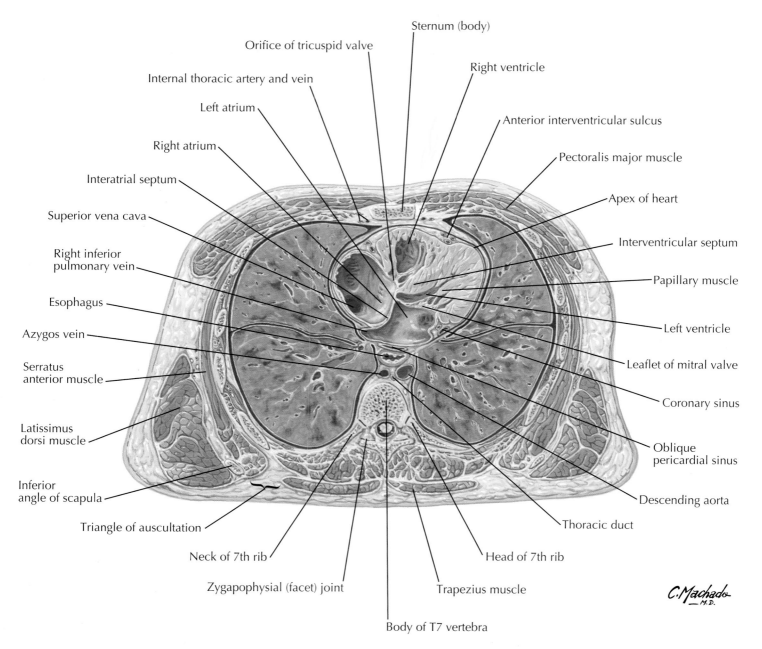

Sternum (body)

Orifice of tricuspid valve

Internal thoracic artery and vein

Right ventricle

Left atrium

Anterior interventricular sulcus

Right atrium

Pectoralis major muscle

Interatrial septum

Apex of heart

Superior vena cava

Interventricular septum

Right inferior pulmonary vein

Papillary muscle

Esophagus

Left ventricle

Azygos vein

Leaflet of mitral valve

Serratus anterior muscle

Coronary sinus

Latissimus dorsi muscle

Oblique pericardial sinus

Inferior angle of scapula

Descending aorta

Triangle of auscultation

Thoracic duct

Neck of 7th rib

Head of 7th rib

Zygapophysial (facet) joint

Trapezius muscle

Body of T7 vertebra

**Plate 241**

**Cross-Sectional Anatomy**

| MUSCLE | PROXIMAL ATTACHMENT (ORIGIN) | DISTAL ATTACHMENT (INSERTION) | INNERVATION | MAIN ACTIONS | BLOOD SUPPLY | MUSCLE GROUP |
|---|---|---|---|---|---|---|
| Diaphragm | Xiphoid process, lower six costal cartilages, L1–L3 vertebrae | Converge into central tendon | Phrenic nerve | Draws central tendon down and forward during inspiration | Pericardiacophrenic, musculophrenic, superior and inferior phrenic arteries | Posterior abdominal wall |
| External intercostal | Lower border of ribs | Upper border of rib below rib of origin | Intercostal nerves | Supports intercostal spaces in inspiration and expiration, elevates ribs in inspiration | Posterior intercostal arteries, collateral branches of posterior intercostal arteries, costocervical trunk, anterior intercostal branches of internal thoracic artery, musculophrenic artery | Thoracic wall |
| Innermost intercostal | Lower border of ribs | Upper border of rib below rib of origin | Intercostal nerves | Elevates ribs | Muscular branches of anterior intercostal arteries, muscular branches of posterior intercostal arteries, intercostal branches of internal thoracic and musculophrenic arteries, costocervical trunk branches | Thoracic wall |
| Internal intercostal | Lower border of ribs | Costal cartilage and edge of costal groove of rib above rib of origin | Intercostal nerves | Prevents pushing out or drawing in of intercostal spaces in inspiration and expiration, lowers ribs in forced expiration | Muscular branches of anterior intercostal arteries, muscular branches of posterior intercostal arteries, intercostal branches of internal thoracic and musculophrenic arteries, costocervical trunk branches | Thoracic wall |
| Levator costarum | Transverse processes of C7 and T1–T11 | Subjacent ribs between tubercle and angle | Dorsal ramus of lower thoracic nerves | Elevates ribs | Posterior intercostal arteries | Thoracic wall |
| Pectoralis major | Sternal half of clavicle, sternum to 7th rib, cartilages of true ribs, aponeurosis of external oblique muscle | Lateral lip of intertubercular sulcus of humerus | Medial and lateral pectoral nerves | Flexes and adducts arm, rotates arm medially | Pectoral branch of thoraco-acromial artery, perforating branches of internal thoracic artery | Pectoral/axilla region |
| Pectoralis minor | Outer surface of upper margin of ribs 3–5 | Coracoid process of scapula | Medial pectoral nerve | Lowers lateral angle of scapula and protracts scapula | Pectoral branch of the thoraco-acromial artery, and superior and lateral thoracic arteries | Pectoral/axilla region |
| Serratus anterior | Lateral surfaces of upper 8–9 ribs | Costal surface of medial border of scapula | Long thoracic nerve | Protracts scapula and holds it against thoracic wall | Lateral thoracic artery | Pectoral/axilla region |
| Serratus posterior inferior | Spinous processes of T11–L2 | Inferior aspect of ribs 9–12 | Ventral rami of lower thoracic nerves | Depresses ribs | Posterior intercostal arteries | Intermediate back |
| Serratus posterior superior | Ligamentum nuchae, spinous processes of C7–T3 | Superior aspect of ribs 2–4 | Ventral rami of upper thoracic nerves | Elevates ribs | Posterior intercostal arteries | Intermediate back |
| Subcostal | Internal surface of lower ribs near their angles | Superior borders of 2nd or 3rd rib below | Intercostal nerves | Depresses ribs | Posterior intercostal artery, musculophrenic artery | Thoracic wall |
| Transversus thoracis | Internal surface of costal cartilages 2–6 | Posterior surface of lower sternum | Intercostal nerves | Depresses ribs and costal cartilages | Anterior intercostal arteries, internal thoracic artery | Thoracic wall |

Variations in spinal nerve contributions to the innervation of muscles, their arterial supply, their attachments, and their actions are common themes in human anatomy. Therefore, expect differences between texts and realize that anatomical variation is normal.

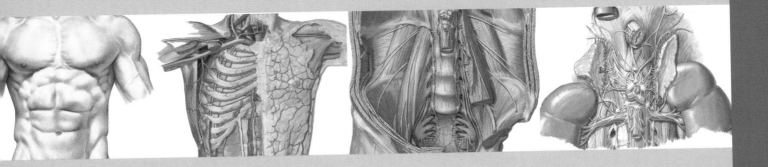

# 4 ABDOMEN

## Topographic Anatomy
**Plate 242**

## Body Wall
**Plates 243–262**

# ABDOMEN

## Sectional Anatomy

## Muscle Table

**Topographic Anatomy**

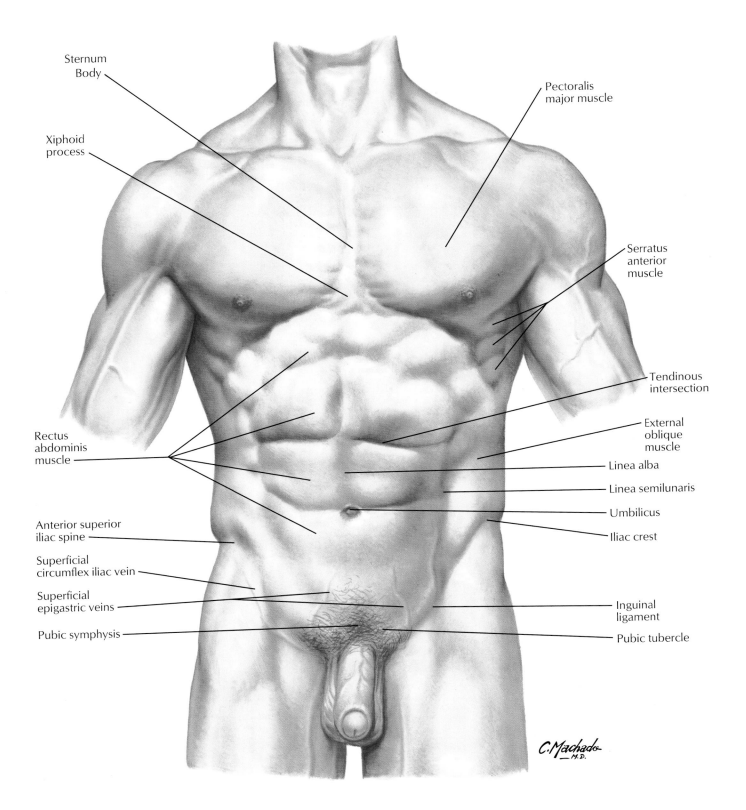

Sternum
Body

Xiphoid
process

Pectoralis
major muscle

Serratus
anterior
muscle

Tendinous
intersection

Rectus
abdominis
muscle

External
oblique
muscle

Linea alba

Linea semilunaris

Umbilicus

Iliac crest

Anterior superior
iliac spine

Superficial
circumflex iliac vein

Superficial
epigastric veins

Pubic symphysis

Inguinal
ligament

Pubic tubercle

C. Machado
_M.D.

**Plate 242**

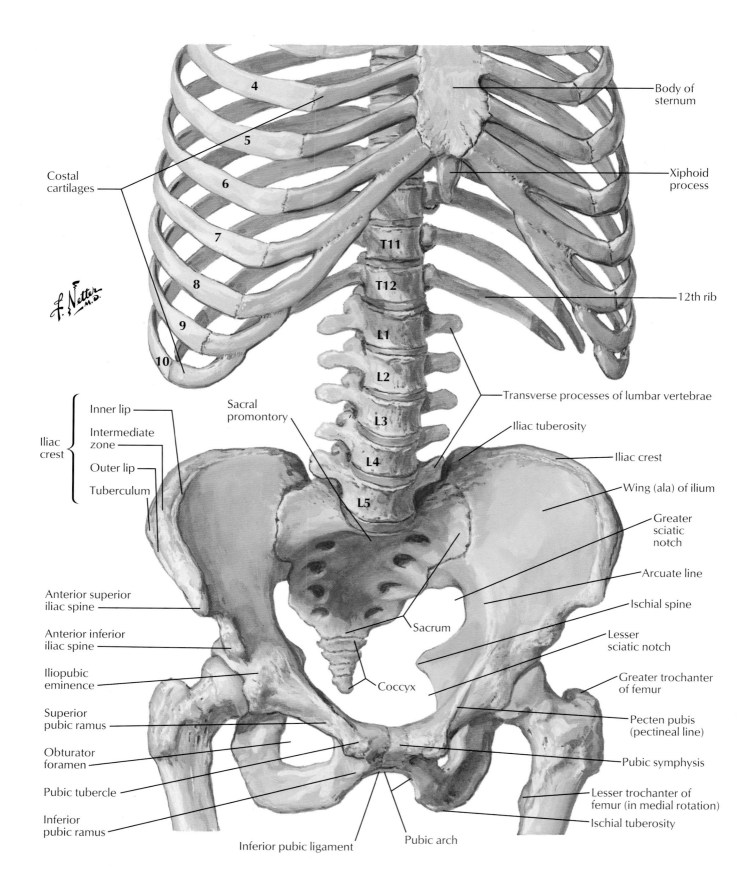

Body of
sternum

Xiphoid
process

Costal
cartilages

4

5

6

7

8

9

10

T11

T12

L1

L2

L3

L4

L5

12th rib

Transverse processes of lumbar vertebrae

Iliac tuberosity

Iliac crest

Wing (ala) of ilium

Greater
sciatic
notch

Arcuate line

Ischial spine

Lesser
sciatic
notch

Greater trochanter
of femur

Pecten pubis
(pectineal line)

Pubic symphysis

Lesser trochanter of
femur (in medial rotation)

Ischial tuberosity

Pubic arch

Iliac
crest

Inner lip

Intermediate
zone

Outer lip

Tuberculum

Sacral
promontory

Sacrum

Coccyx

Anterior superior
iliac spine

Anterior inferior
iliac spine

Iliopubic
eminence

Superior
pubic ramus

Obturator
foramen

Pubic tubercle

Inferior
pubic ramus

Inferior pubic ligament

**Plate 243**

**Body Wall**

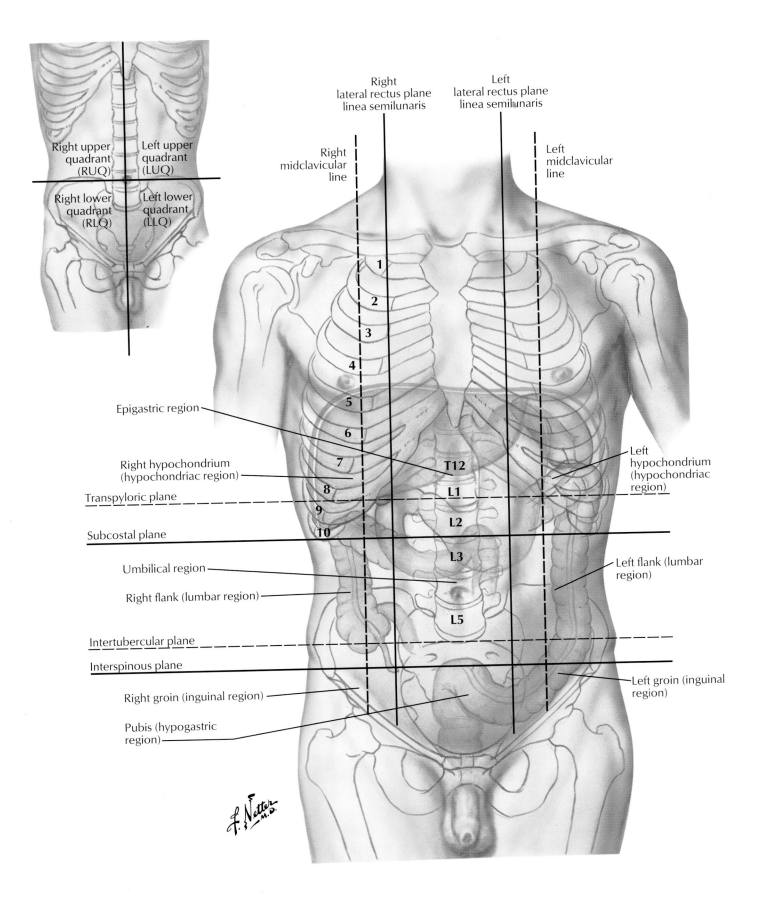

Right upper quadrant (RUQ)

Left upper quadrant (LUQ)

Right lower quadrant (RLQ)

Left lower quadrant (LLQ)

Right lateral rectus plane linea semilunaris

Left lateral rectus plane linea semilunaris

Right midclavicular line

Left midclavicular line

1
2
3
4
5
6
7
8
9
10

T12
L1
L2
L3
L5

Epigastric region

Right hypochondrium (hypochondriac region)

Transpyloric plane

Subcostal plane

Umbilical region

Right flank (lumbar region)

Intertubercular plane

Interspinous plane

Right groin (inguinal region)

Pubis (hypogastric region)

Left hypochondrium (hypochondriac region)

Left flank (lumbar region)

Left groin (inguinal region)

**Plate 244**

**Body Wall**

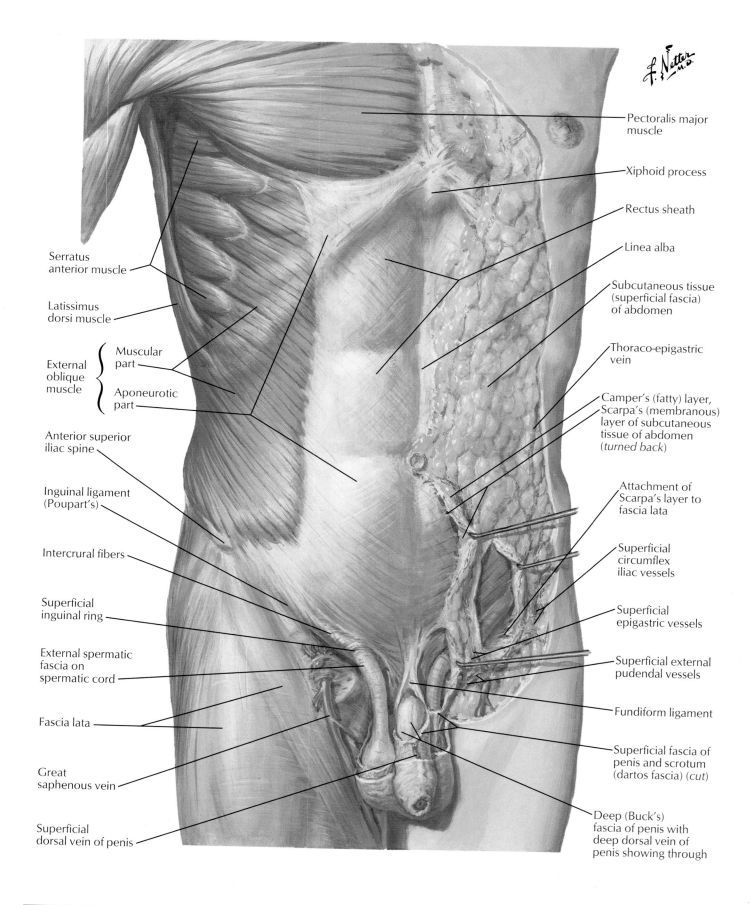

Pectoralis major muscle

Xiphoid process

Rectus sheath

Linea alba

Subcutaneous tissue (superficial fascia) of abdomen

Thoraco-epigastric vein

Camper's (fatty) layer, Scarpa's (membranous) layer of subcutaneous tissue of abdomen (*turned back*)

Attachment of Scarpa's layer to fascia lata

Superficial circumflex iliac vessels

Superficial epigastric vessels

Superficial external pudendal vessels

Fundiform ligament

Superficial fascia of penis and scrotum (dartos fascia) (*cut*)

Deep (Buck's) fascia of penis with deep dorsal vein of penis showing through

Serratus anterior muscle

Latissimus dorsi muscle

External oblique muscle { Muscular part / Aponeurotic part }

Anterior superior iliac spine

Inguinal ligament (Poupart's)

Intercrural fibers

Superficial inguinal ring

External spermatic fascia on spermatic cord

Fascia lata

Great saphenous vein

Superficial dorsal vein of penis

**Plate 245**

**Body Wall**

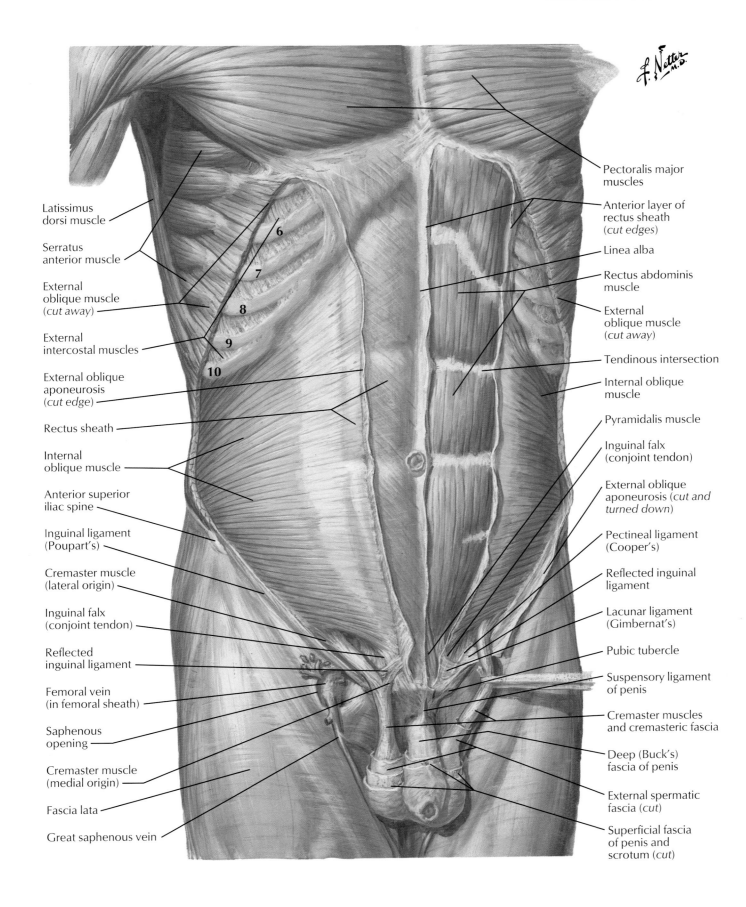

Latissimus
dorsi muscle

Serratus
anterior muscle

External
oblique muscle
(*cut away*)

External
intercostal muscles

External oblique
aponeurosis
(*cut edge*)

Rectus sheath

Internal
oblique muscle

Anterior superior
iliac spine

Inguinal ligament
(Poupart's)

Cremaster muscle
(lateral origin)

Inguinal falx
(conjoint tendon)

Reflected
inguinal ligament

Femoral vein
(in femoral sheath)

Saphenous
opening

Cremaster muscle
(medial origin)

Fascia lata

Great saphenous vein

6

7

8

9

10

Pectoralis major
muscles

Anterior layer of
rectus sheath
(*cut edges*)

Linea alba

Rectus abdominis
muscle

External
oblique muscle
(*cut away*)

Tendinous intersection

Internal oblique
muscle

Pyramidalis muscle

Inguinal falx
(conjoint tendon)

External oblique
aponeurosis (*cut and
turned down*)

Pectineal ligament
(Cooper's)

Reflected inguinal
ligament

Lacunar ligament
(Gimbernat's)

Pubic tubercle

Suspensory ligament
of penis

Cremaster muscles
and cremasteric fascia

Deep (Buck's)
fascia of penis

External spermatic
fascia (*cut*)

Superficial fascia
of penis and
scrotum (*cut*)

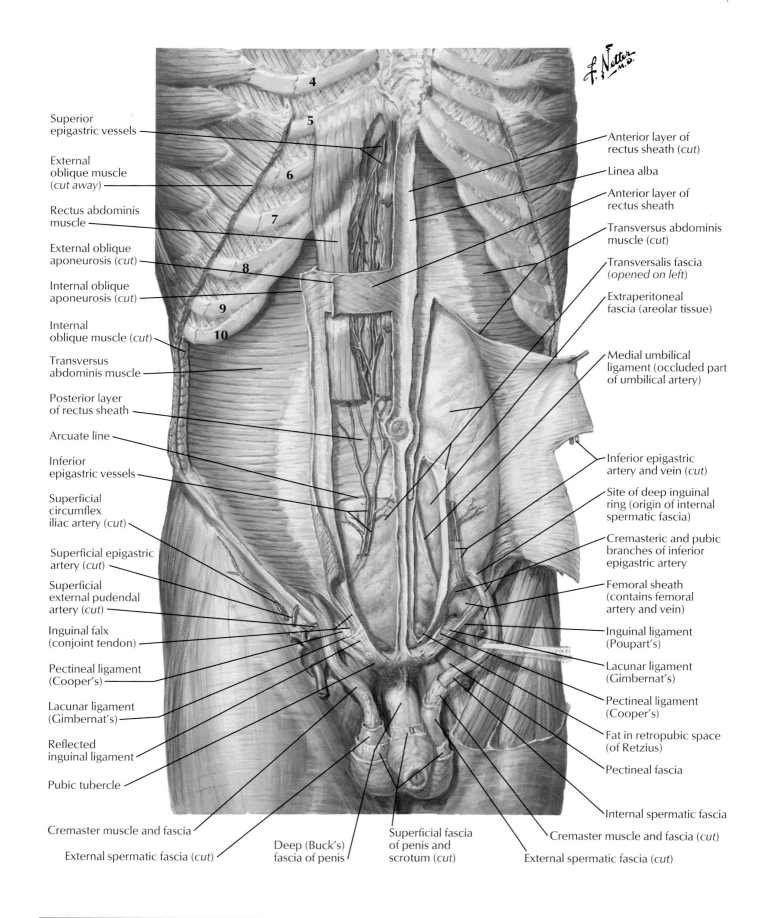

Superior epigastric vessels

External oblique muscle (cut away)

Rectus abdominis muscle

External oblique aponeurosis (cut)

Internal oblique aponeurosis (cut)

Internal oblique muscle (cut)

Transversus abdominis muscle

Posterior layer of rectus sheath

Arcuate line

Inferior epigastric vessels

Superficial circumflex iliac artery (cut)

Superficial epigastric artery (cut)

Superficial external pudendal artery (cut)

Inguinal falx (conjoint tendon)

Pectineal ligament (Cooper's)

Lacunar ligament (Gimbernat's)

Reflected inguinal ligament

Pubic tubercle

Cremaster muscle and fascia

External spermatic fascia (cut)

Deep (Buck's) fascia of penis

Superficial fascia of penis and scrotum (cut)

Anterior layer of rectus sheath (cut)

Linea alba

Anterior layer of rectus sheath

Transversus abdominis muscle (cut)

Transversalis fascia (opened on left)

Extraperitoneal fascia (areolar tissue)

Medial umbilical ligament (occluded part of umbilical artery)

Inferior epigastric artery and vein (cut)

Site of deep inguinal ring (origin of internal spermatic fascia)

Cremasteric and pubic branches of inferior epigastric artery

Femoral sheath (contains femoral artery and vein)

Inguinal ligament (Poupart's)

Lacunar ligament (Gimbernat's)

Pectineal ligament (Cooper's)

Fat in retropubic space (of Retzius)

Pectineal fascia

Internal spermatic fascia

Cremaster muscle and fascia (cut)

External spermatic fascia (cut)

**Plate 247**

**Body Wall**

## Section above arcuate line

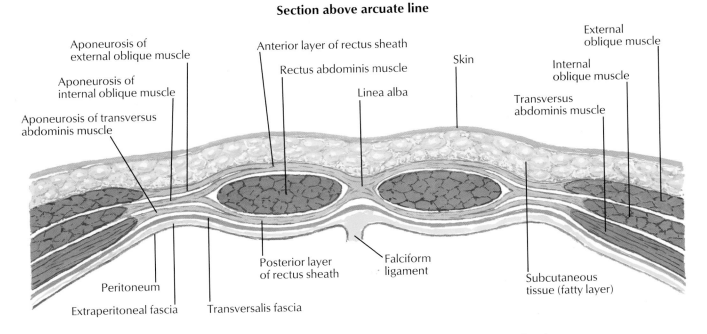

Aponeurosis of external oblique muscle

Aponeurosis of internal oblique muscle

Aponeurosis of transversus abdominis muscle

Anterior layer of rectus sheath

Rectus abdominis muscle

Linea alba

Skin

External oblique muscle

Internal oblique muscle

Transversus abdominis muscle

Peritoneum

Extraperitoneal fascia

Transversalis fascia

Posterior layer of rectus sheath

Falciform ligament

Subcutaneous tissue (fatty layer)

Aponeurosis of internal oblique muscle splits to form anterior and posterior layers of rectus sheath. Aponeurosis of external oblique muscle joins anterior layer of sheath; aponeurosis of transversus abdominis muscle joins posterior layer. Anterior and posterior layers of rectus sheath unite medially to form linea alba.

## Section below arcuate line

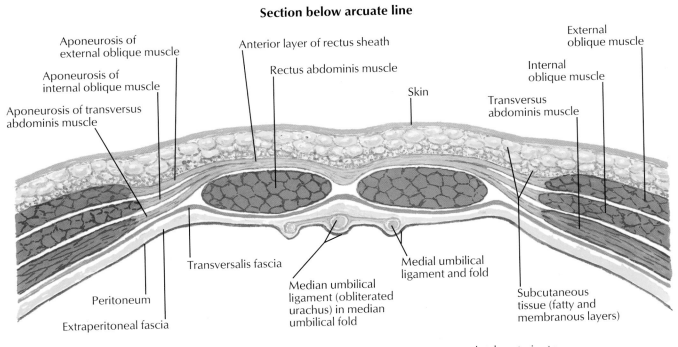

Aponeurosis of external oblique muscle

Aponeurosis of internal oblique muscle

Aponeurosis of transversus abdominis muscle

Anterior layer of rectus sheath

Rectus abdominis muscle

Skin

External oblique muscle

Internal oblique muscle

Transversus abdominis muscle

Transversalis fascia

Median umbilical ligament (obliterated urachus) in median umbilical fold

Medial umbilical ligament and fold

Peritoneum

Extraperitoneal fascia

Subcutaneous tissue (fatty and membranous layers)

Aponeurosis of internal oblique muscle does not split at this level but passes completely anterior to rectus abdominis muscle and is fused there with both aponeurosis of external oblique muscle and that of transversus abdominis muscle. Thus, posterior wall of rectus sheath is absent below arcuate line, leaving only transversalis fascia.

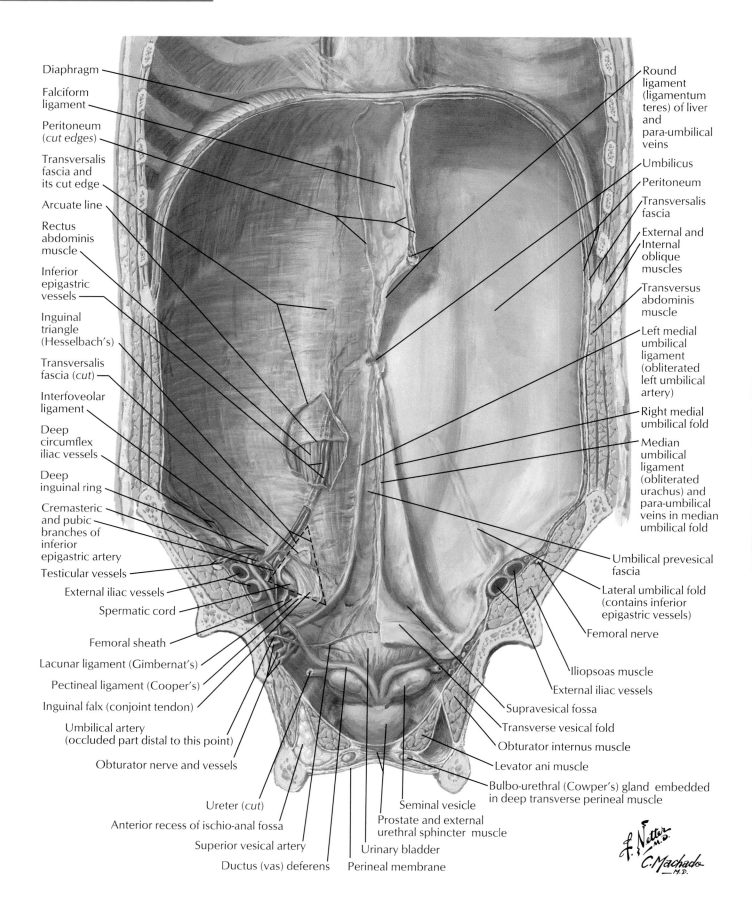

Diaphragm

Falciform ligament

Peritoneum (*cut edges*)

Transversalis fascia and its cut edge

Arcuate line

Rectus abdominis muscle

Inferior epigastric vessels

Inguinal triangle (Hesselbach's)

Transversalis fascia (*cut*)

Interfoveolar ligament

Deep circumflex iliac vessels

Deep inguinal ring

Cremasteric and pubic branches of inferior epigastric artery

Testicular vessels

External iliac vessels

Spermatic cord

Femoral sheath

Lacunar ligament (Gimbernat's)

Pectineal ligament (Cooper's)

Inguinal falx (conjoint tendon)

Umbilical artery (occluded part distal to this point)

Obturator nerve and vessels

Ureter (*cut*)

Anterior recess of ischio-anal fossa

Superior vesical artery

Ductus (vas) deferens

Round ligament (ligamentum teres) of liver and para-umbilical veins

Umbilicus

Peritoneum

Transversalis fascia

External and Internal oblique muscles

Transversus abdominis muscle

Left medial umbilical ligament (obliterated left umbilical artery)

Right medial umbilical fold

Median umbilical ligament (obliterated urachus) and para-umbilical veins in median umbilical fold

Umbilical prevesical fascia

Lateral umbilical fold (contains inferior epigastric vessels)

Femoral nerve

Iliopsoas muscle

External iliac vessels

Supravesical fossa

Transverse vesical fold

Obturator internus muscle

Levator ani muscle

Bulbo-urethral (Cowper's) gland embedded in deep transverse perineal muscle

Seminal vesicle

Prostate and external urethral sphincter muscle

Urinary bladder

Perineal membrane

**Plate 249**

**Body Wall**

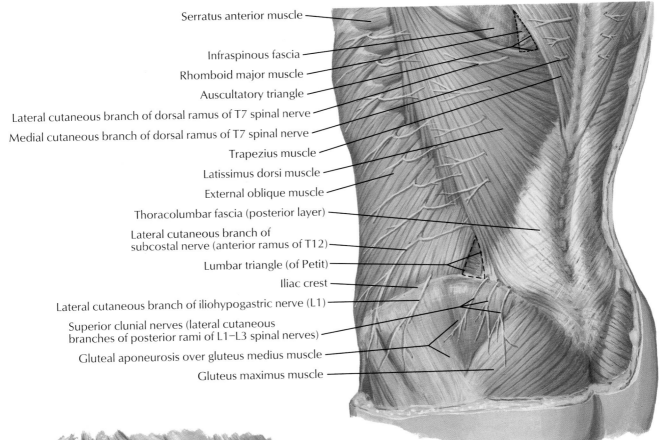

Serratus anterior muscle

Infraspinous fascia

Rhomboid major muscle

Auscultatory triangle

Lateral cutaneous branch of dorsal ramus of T7 spinal nerve

Medial cutaneous branch of dorsal ramus of T7 spinal nerve

Trapezius muscle

Latissimus dorsi muscle

External oblique muscle

Thoracolumbar fascia (posterior layer)

Lateral cutaneous branch of subcostal nerve (anterior ramus of T12)

Lumbar triangle (of Petit)

Iliac crest

Lateral cutaneous branch of iliohypogastric nerve (L1)

Superior clunial nerves (lateral cutaneous branches of posterior rami of L1–L3 spinal nerves)

Gluteal aponeurosis over gluteus medius muscle

Gluteus maximus muscle

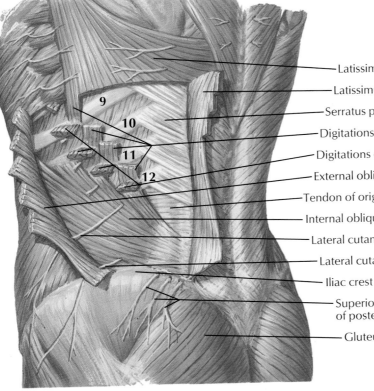

Latissimus dorsi muscle

Latissimus dorsi muscle (*cut and turned back*)

Serratus posterior inferior muscle

Digitations of costal origin of latissimus dorsi muscle

Digitations of costal origin of external oblique muscle

External oblique muscle (*cut and turned back*)

Tendon of origin of transversus abdominis muscle

Internal oblique muscle

Lateral cutaneous branch of subcostal nerve (anterior ramus of T12)

Lateral cutaneous branch of iliohypogastric nerve (L1)

Iliac crest

Superior clunial nerves (lateral cutaneous branches of posterior rami of L1–L3 spinal nerves)

Gluteus maximus muscle

9
10
11
12

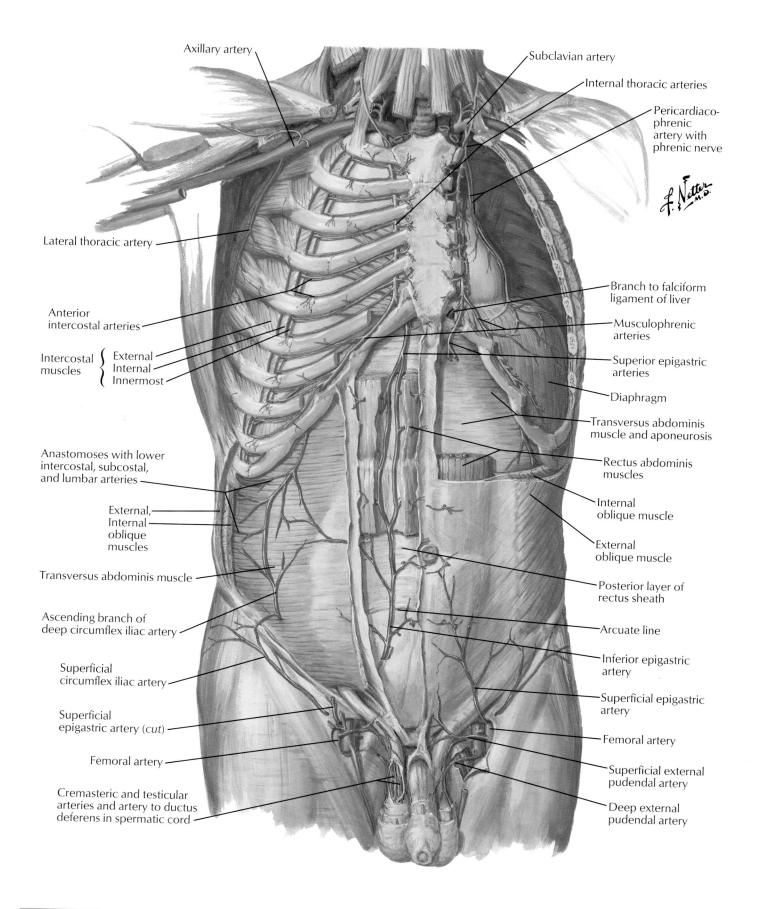

Axillary artery

Subclavian artery

Internal thoracic arteries

Pericardiaco-
phrenic
artery with
phrenic nerve

Lateral thoracic artery

Branch to falciform
ligament of liver

Anterior
intercostal arteries

Musculophrenic
arteries

Intercostal { External
muscles { Internal
{ Innermost

Superior epigastric
arteries

Diaphragm

Transversus abdominis
muscle and aponeurosis

Anastomoses with lower
intercostal, subcostal,
and lumbar arteries

Rectus abdominis
muscles

External,
Internal
oblique
muscles

Internal
oblique muscle

External
oblique muscle

Transversus abdominis muscle

Posterior layer of
rectus sheath

Ascending branch of
deep circumflex iliac artery

Arcuate line

Superficial
circumflex iliac artery

Inferior epigastric
artery

Superficial epigastric
artery

Superficial
epigastric artery (cut)

Femoral artery

Femoral artery

Superficial external
pudendal artery

Cremasteric and testicular
arteries and artery to ductus
deferens in spermatic cord

Deep external
pudendal artery

**Plate 251**

**Body Wall**

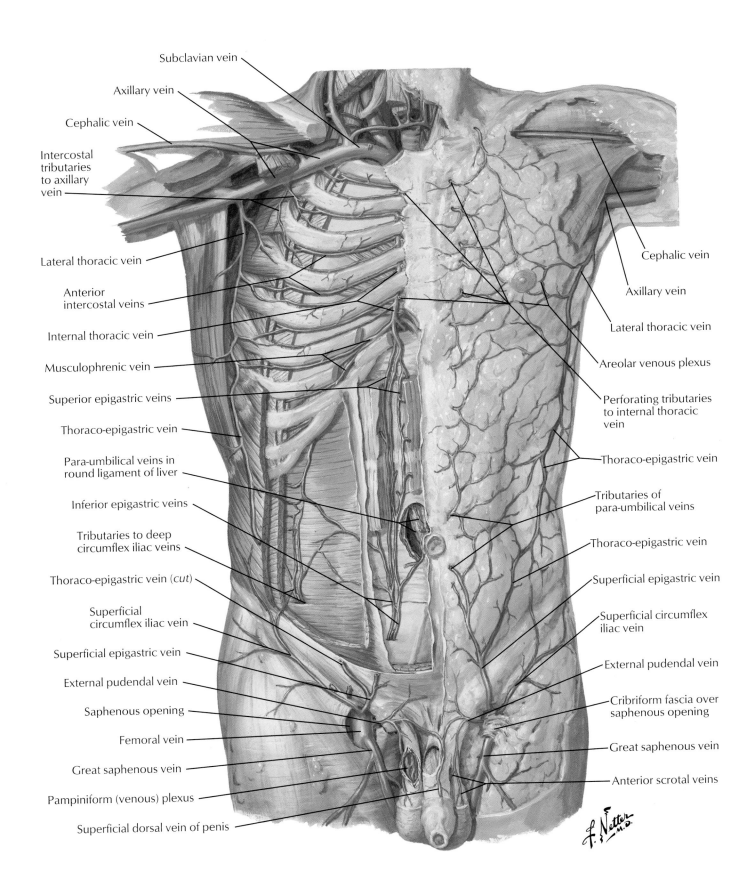

Subclavian vein

Axillary vein

Cephalic vein

Intercostal tributaries to axillary vein

Lateral thoracic vein

Anterior intercostal veins

Internal thoracic vein

Musculophrenic vein

Superior epigastric veins

Thoraco-epigastric vein

Para-umbilical veins in round ligament of liver

Inferior epigastric veins

Tributaries to deep circumflex iliac veins

Thoraco-epigastric vein (*cut*)

Superficial circumflex iliac vein

Superficial epigastric vein

External pudendal vein

Saphenous opening

Femoral vein

Great saphenous vein

Pampiniform (venous) plexus

Superficial dorsal vein of penis

Cephalic vein

Axillary vein

Lateral thoracic vein

Areolar venous plexus

Perforating tributaries to internal thoracic vein

Thoraco-epigastric vein

Tributaries of para-umbilical veins

Thoraco-epigastric vein

Superficial epigastric vein

Superficial circumflex iliac vein

External pudendal vein

Cribriform fascia over saphenous opening

Great saphenous vein

Anterior scrotal veins

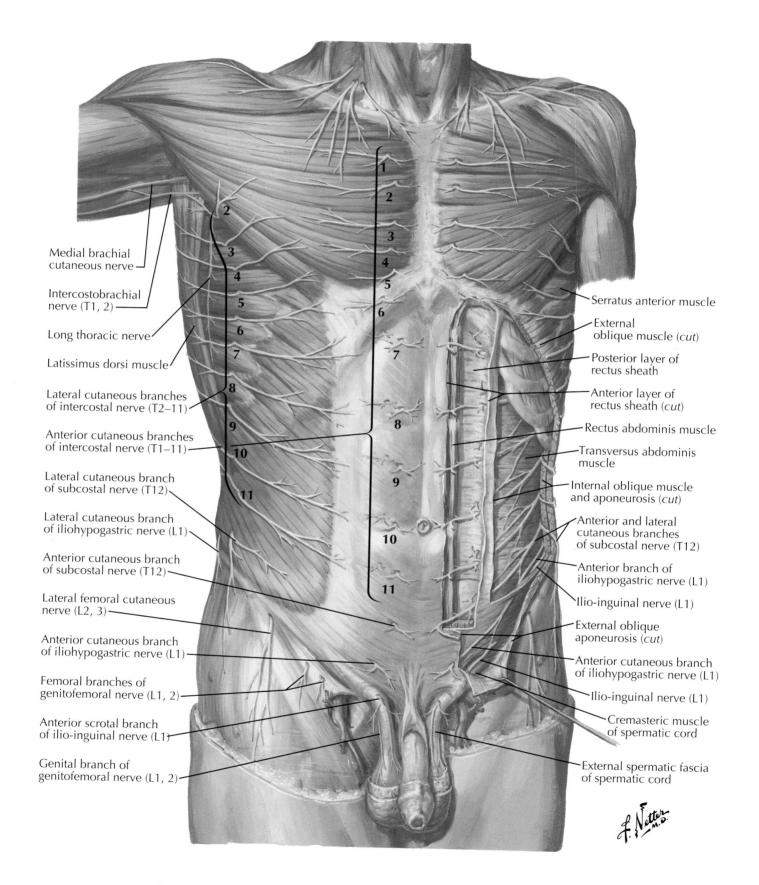

Medial brachial cutaneous nerve

Intercostobrachial nerve (T1, 2)

Long thoracic nerve

Latissimus dorsi muscle

Lateral cutaneous branches of intercostal nerve (T2–11)

Anterior cutaneous branches of intercostal nerve (T1–11)

Lateral cutaneous branch of subcostal nerve (T12)

Lateral cutaneous branch of iliohypogastric nerve (L1)

Anterior cutaneous branch of subcostal nerve (T12)

Lateral femoral cutaneous nerve (L2, 3)

Anterior cutaneous branch of iliohypogastric nerve (L1)

Femoral branches of genitofemoral nerve (L1, 2)

Anterior scrotal branch of ilio-inguinal nerve (L1)

Genital branch of genitofemoral nerve (L1, 2)

Serratus anterior muscle

External oblique muscle (cut)

Posterior layer of rectus sheath

Anterior layer of rectus sheath (cut)

Rectus abdominis muscle

Transversus abdominis muscle

Internal oblique muscle and aponeurosis (cut)

Anterior and lateral cutaneous branches of subcostal nerve (T12)

Anterior branch of iliohypogastric nerve (L1)

Ilio-inguinal nerve (L1)

External oblique aponeurosis (cut)

Anterior cutaneous branch of iliohypogastric nerve (L1)

Ilio-inguinal nerve (L1)

Cremasteric muscle of spermatic cord

External spermatic fascia of spermatic cord

**Plate 253**

**Body Wall**

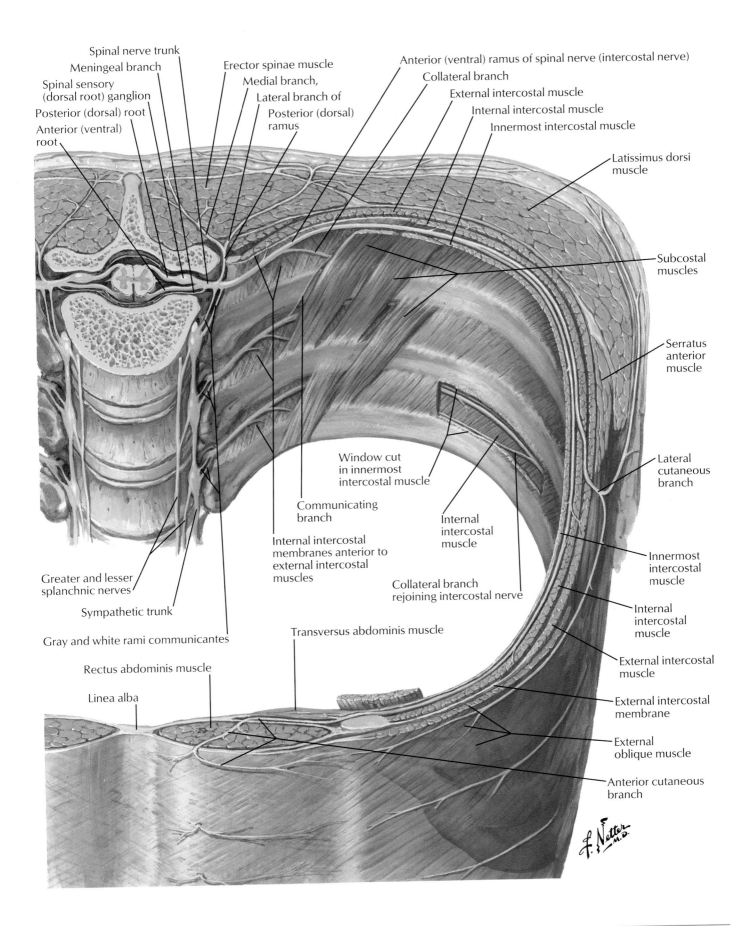

Spinal nerve trunk

Meningeal branch

Spinal sensory (dorsal root) ganglion

Posterior (dorsal) root

Anterior (ventral) root

Erector spinae muscle

Medial branch,

Lateral branch of Posterior (dorsal) ramus

Anterior (ventral) ramus of spinal nerve (intercostal nerve)

Collateral branch

External intercostal muscle

Internal intercostal muscle

Innermost intercostal muscle

Latissimus dorsi muscle

Subcostal muscles

Serratus anterior muscle

Lateral cutaneous branch

Innermost intercostal muscle

Internal intercostal muscle

External intercostal muscle

External intercostal membrane

External oblique muscle

Anterior cutaneous branch

Window cut in innermost intercostal muscle

Internal intercostal muscle

Collateral branch rejoining intercostal nerve

Communicating branch

Internal intercostal membranes anterior to external intercostal muscles

Greater and lesser splanchnic nerves

Sympathetic trunk

Gray and white rami communicantes

Rectus abdominis muscle

Linea alba

Transversus abdominis muscle

*F. Netter M.D.*

**Body Wall**

**Plate 254**

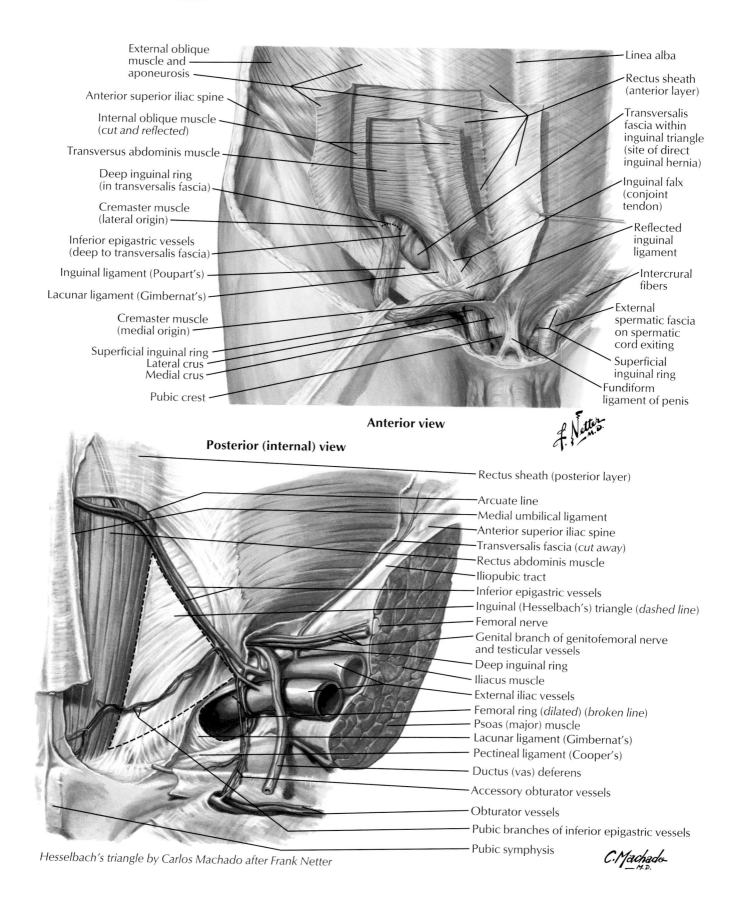

External oblique muscle and aponeurosis

Anterior superior iliac spine

Internal oblique muscle (*cut and reflected*)

Transversus abdominis muscle

Deep inguinal ring (in transversalis fascia)

Cremaster muscle (lateral origin)

Inferior epigastric vessels (deep to transversalis fascia)

Inguinal ligament (Poupart's)

Lacunar ligament (Gimbernat's)

Cremaster muscle (medial origin)

Superficial inguinal ring
Lateral crus
Medial crus

Pubic crest

Linea alba

Rectus sheath (anterior layer)

Transversalis fascia within inguinal triangle (site of direct inguinal hernia)

Inguinal falx (conjoint tendon)

Reflected inguinal ligament

Intercrural fibers

External spermatic fascia on spermatic cord exiting

Superficial inguinal ring

Fundiform ligament of penis

**Anterior view**

**Posterior (internal) view**

Rectus sheath (posterior layer)

Arcuate line

Medial umbilical ligament

Anterior superior iliac spine

Transversalis fascia (*cut away*)

Rectus abdominis muscle

Iliopubic tract

Inferior epigastric vessels

Inguinal (Hesselbach's) triangle (*dashed line*)

Femoral nerve

Genital branch of genitofemoral nerve and testicular vessels

Deep inguinal ring

Iliacus muscle

External iliac vessels

Femoral ring (*dilated*) (*broken line*)

Psoas (major) muscle

Lacunar ligament (Gimbernat's)

Pectineal ligament (Cooper's)

Ductus (vas) deferens

Accessory obturator vessels

Obturator vessels

Pubic branches of inferior epigastric vessels

Pubic symphysis

*Hesselbach's triangle by Carlos Machado after Frank Netter*

**Plate 255**

**Body Wall**

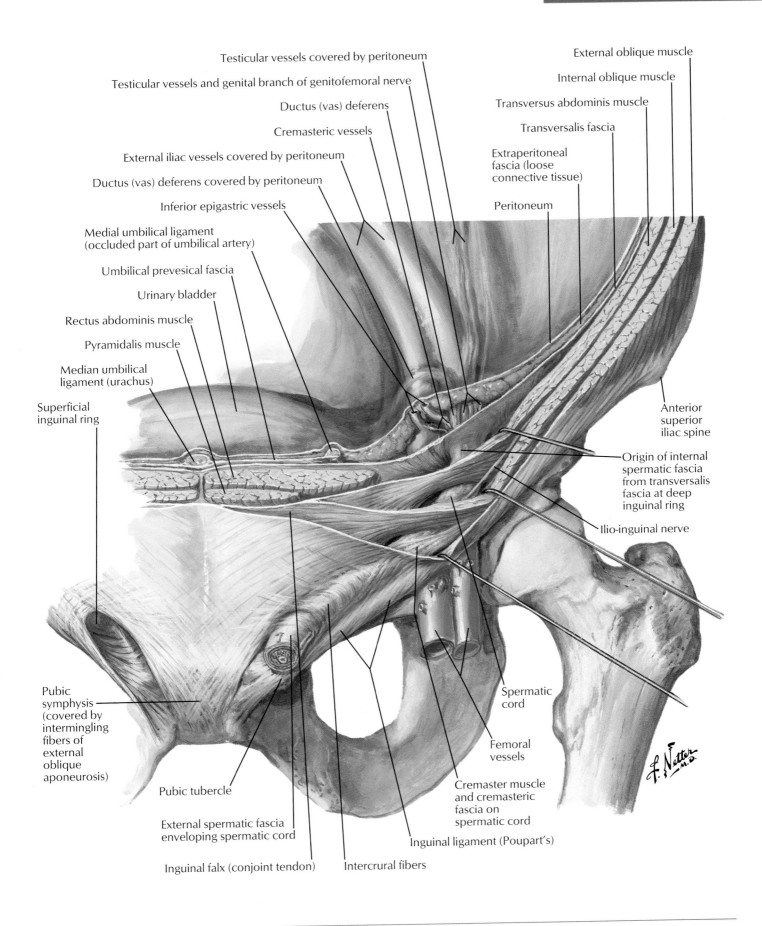

Testicular vessels covered by peritoneum

Testicular vessels and genital branch of genitofemoral nerve

Ductus (vas) deferens

Cremasteric vessels

External iliac vessels covered by peritoneum

Ductus (vas) deferens covered by peritoneum

Inferior epigastric vessels

Medial umbilical ligament (occluded part of umbilical artery)

Umbilical prevesical fascia

Urinary bladder

Rectus abdominis muscle

Pyramidalis muscle

Median umbilical ligament (urachus)

Superficial inguinal ring

Pubic symphysis (covered by intermingling fibers of external oblique aponeurosis)

External oblique muscle

Internal oblique muscle

Transversus abdominis muscle

Transversalis fascia

Extraperitoneal fascia (loose connective tissue)

Peritoneum

Anterior superior iliac spine

Origin of internal spermatic fascia from transversalis fascia at deep inguinal ring

Ilio-inguinal nerve

Spermatic cord

Femoral vessels

Cremaster muscle and cremasteric fascia on spermatic cord

Inguinal ligament (Poupart's)

Pubic tubercle

External spermatic fascia enveloping spermatic cord

Inguinal falx (conjoint tendon)

Intercrural fibers

Transversalis fascia (*cut edge*)

Extraperitoneal fascia

Parietal peritoneum

Median umbilical ligament (urachus)

Medial umbilical ligament (occluded part of umbilical artery)

Inferior epigastric vessels

Deep circumflex iliac vessels

Testicular vessels

Cremasteric artery

Ductus (vas) deferens

External iliac vessels

Accessory obturator vessels

External oblique aponeurosis (*cut*)

Internal spermatic fascia on spermatic cord

Femoral nerve (deep to iliopsoas fascia)

Femoral vessels in femoral sheath

Falciform margin of saphenous opening (*cut and reflected*)

Urinary bladder

Pectineal ligament (Cooper's)

Lacunar ligament (Gimbernat's)

Inguinal ligament (Poupart's)

Transversalis fascia forms anterior wall of femoral sheath (posterior wall formed by iliopsoas fascia)

Ureter

Genitofemoral nerve

Lateral femoral cutaneous nerve

Iliac fascia

Genital branch of genitofemoral nerve

Femoral branch of genitofemoral nerve

Testicular vessels

External iliac vessels

Inferior epigastric vessels

Ductus (vas) deferens and cremasteric artery

Pectineal ligament (Cooper's)

Femoral ring

Transversalis fascia forms anterior wall of femoral sheath

Lacunar ligament (Gimbernat's)

Inguinal ligament (Poupart's)

Lymph node (Cloquet's) in femoral canal

Femoral sheath (*cut open*)

**Plate 257**

**Body Wall**

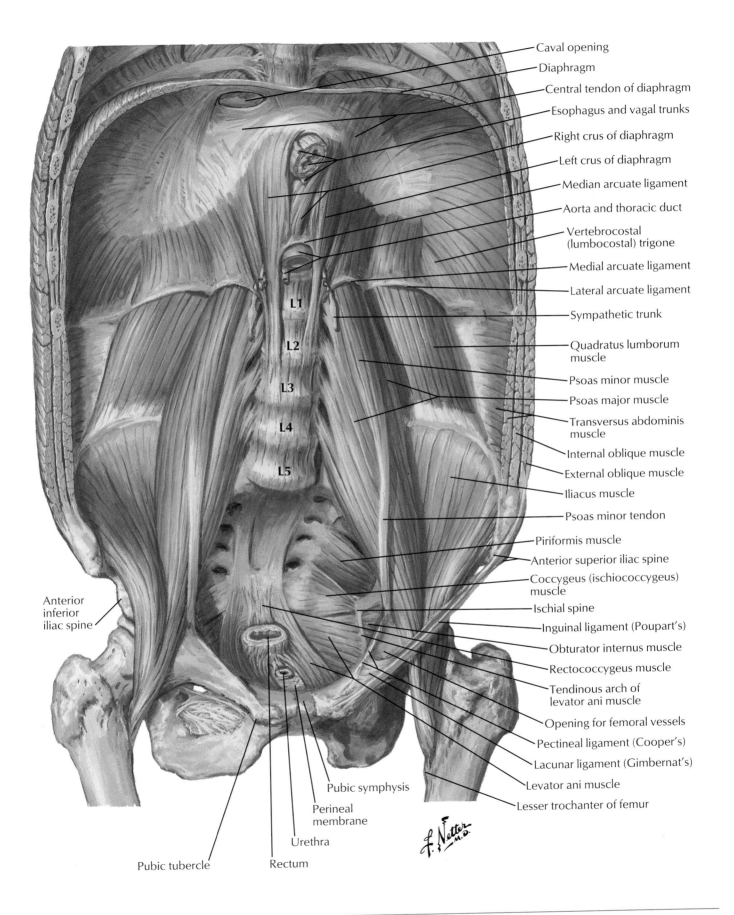

Caval opening

Diaphragm

Central tendon of diaphragm

Esophagus and vagal trunks

Right crus of diaphragm

Left crus of diaphragm

Median arcuate ligament

Aorta and thoracic duct

Vertebrocostal (lumbocostal) trigone

Medial arcuate ligament

Lateral arcuate ligament

Sympathetic trunk

Quadratus lumborum muscle

Psoas minor muscle

Psoas major muscle

Transversus abdominis muscle

Internal oblique muscle

External oblique muscle

Iliacus muscle

Psoas minor tendon

Piriformis muscle

Anterior superior iliac spine

Coccygeus (ischiococcygeus) muscle

Ischial spine

Inguinal ligament (Poupart's)

Obturator internus muscle

Rectococcygeus muscle

Tendinous arch of levator ani muscle

Opening for femoral vessels

Pectineal ligament (Cooper's)

Lacunar ligament (Gimbernat's)

Levator ani muscle

Lesser trochanter of femur

L1

L2

L3

L4

L5

Anterior inferior iliac spine

Pubic symphysis

Perineal membrane

Urethra

Rectum

Pubic tubercle

**Body Wall**

**Plate 258**

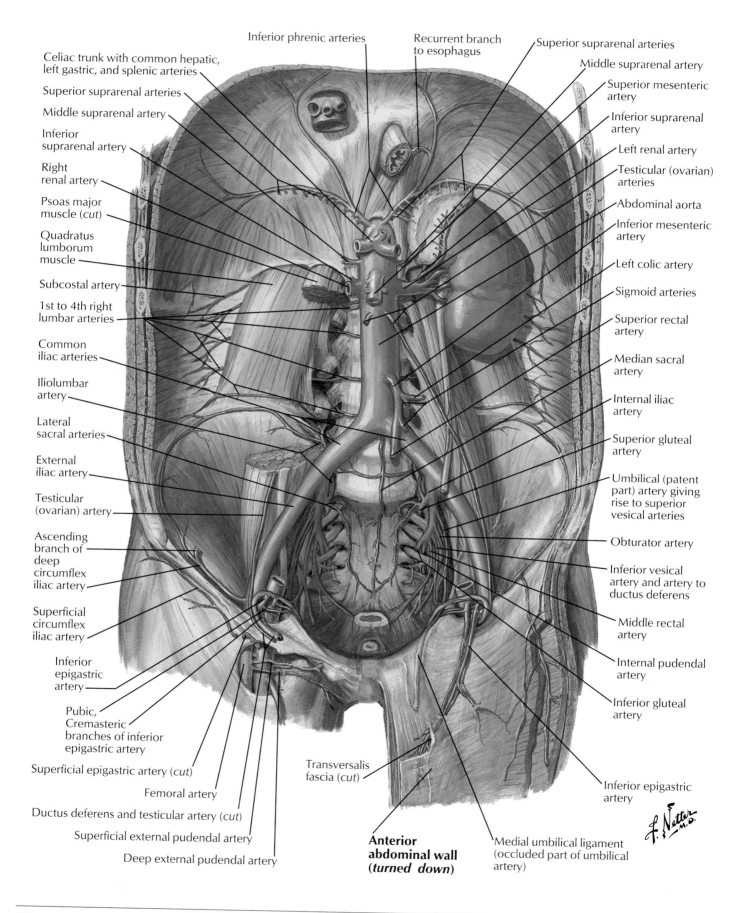

Inferior phrenic arteries

Recurrent branch to esophagus

Superior suprarenal arteries

Celiac trunk with common hepatic, left gastric, and splenic arteries

Superior suprarenal arteries

Middle suprarenal artery

Inferior suprarenal artery

Right renal artery

Psoas major muscle (*cut*)

Quadratus lumborum muscle

Subcostal artery

1st to 4th right lumbar arteries

Common iliac arteries

Iliolumbar artery

Lateral sacral arteries

External iliac artery

Testicular (ovarian) artery

Ascending branch of deep circumflex iliac artery

Superficial circumflex iliac artery

Inferior epigastric artery

Pubic, Cremasteric branches of inferior epigastric artery

Superficial epigastric artery (*cut*)

Femoral artery

Ductus deferens and testicular artery (*cut*)

Superficial external pudendal artery

Deep external pudendal artery

Middle suprarenal artery

Superior mesenteric artery

Inferior suprarenal artery

Left renal artery

Testicular (ovarian) arteries

Abdominal aorta

Inferior mesenteric artery

Left colic artery

Sigmoid arteries

Superior rectal artery

Median sacral artery

Internal iliac artery

Superior gluteal artery

Umbilical (patent part) artery giving rise to superior vesical arteries

Obturator artery

Inferior vesical artery and artery to ductus deferens

Middle rectal artery

Internal pudendal artery

Inferior gluteal artery

Inferior epigastric artery

Transversalis fascia (*cut*)

**Anterior abdominal wall (*turned down*)**

Medial umbilical ligament (occluded part of umbilical artery)

**Plate 259**

**Body Wall**

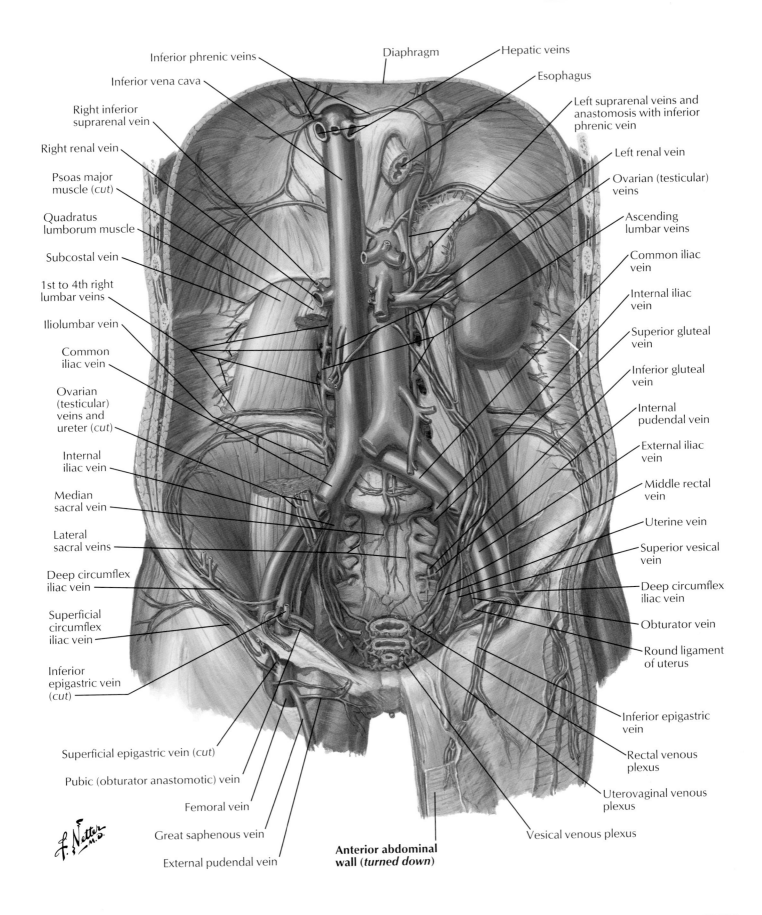

Inferior phrenic veins

Diaphragm

Hepatic veins

Inferior vena cava

Esophagus

Right inferior suprarenal vein

Left suprarenal veins and anastomosis with inferior phrenic vein

Right renal vein

Left renal vein

Psoas major muscle (*cut*)

Ovarian (testicular) veins

Quadratus lumborum muscle

Ascending lumbar veins

Subcostal vein

Common iliac vein

1st to 4th right lumbar veins

Internal iliac vein

Iliolumbar vein

Superior gluteal vein

Common iliac vein

Inferior gluteal vein

Ovarian (testicular) veins and ureter (*cut*)

Internal pudendal vein

Internal iliac vein

External iliac vein

Median sacral vein

Middle rectal vein

Lateral sacral veins

Uterine vein

Deep circumflex iliac vein

Superior vesical vein

Superficial circumflex iliac vein

Deep circumflex iliac vein

Inferior epigastric vein (*cut*)

Obturator vein

Round ligament of uterus

Superficial epigastric vein (*cut*)

Inferior epigastric vein

Pubic (obturator anastomotic) vein

Rectal venous plexus

Femoral vein

Uterovaginal venous plexus

Great saphenous vein

**Anterior abdominal wall (*turned down*)**

Vesical venous plexus

External pudendal vein

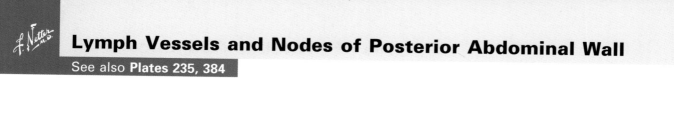

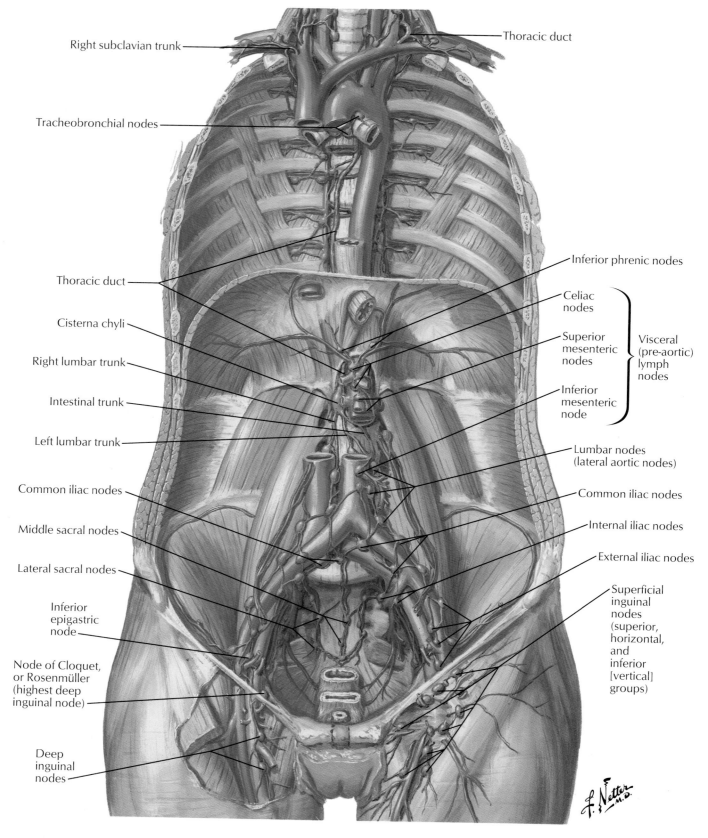

Right subclavian trunk

Thoracic duct

Tracheobronchial nodes

Thoracic duct

Cisterna chyli

Right lumbar trunk

Intestinal trunk

Left lumbar trunk

Common iliac nodes

Middle sacral nodes

Lateral sacral nodes

Inferior epigastric node

Node of Cloquet, or Rosenmüller (highest deep inguinal node)

Deep inguinal nodes

Inferior phrenic nodes

Celiac nodes

Superior mesenteric nodes

Inferior mesenteric node

Visceral (pre-aortic) lymph nodes

Lumbar nodes (lateral aortic nodes)

Common iliac nodes

Internal iliac nodes

External iliac nodes

Superficial inguinal nodes (superior, horizontal, and inferior [vertical] groups)

**Plate 261**

**Body Wall**

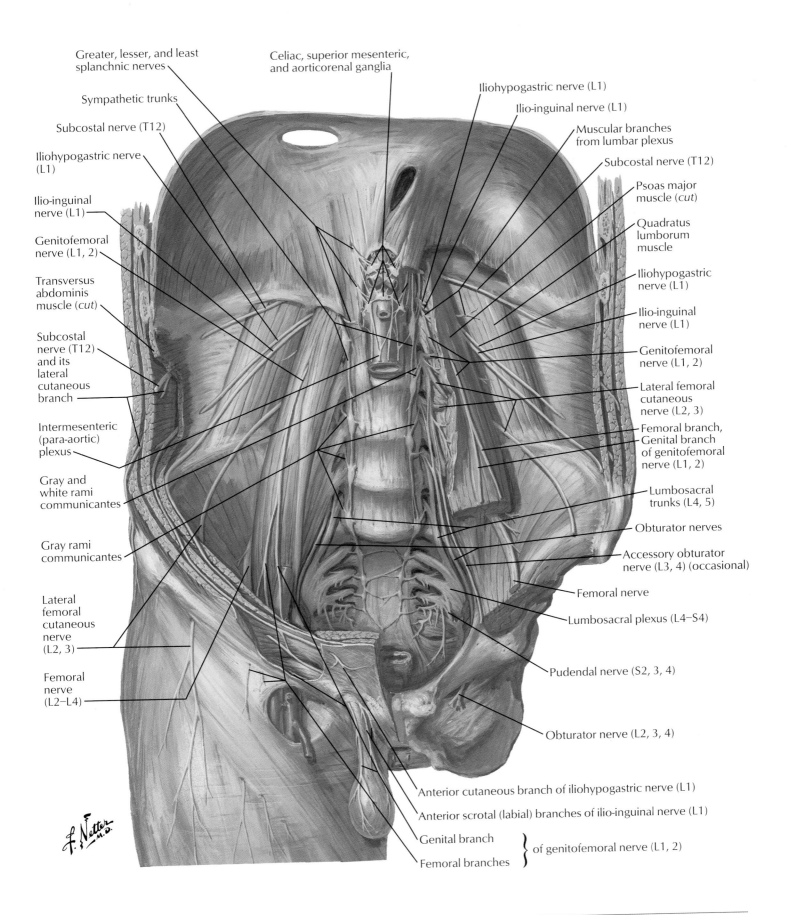

Greater, lesser, and least splanchnic nerves

Celiac, superior mesenteric, and aorticorenal ganglia

Iliohypogastric nerve (L1)

Ilio-inguinal nerve (L1)

Sympathetic trunks

Muscular branches from lumbar plexus

Subcostal nerve (T12)

Subcostal nerve (T12)

Iliohypogastric nerve (L1)

Psoas major muscle (cut)

Ilio-inguinal nerve (L1)

Quadratus lumborum muscle

Genitofemoral nerve (L1, 2)

Iliohypogastric nerve (L1)

Transversus abdominis muscle (cut)

Ilio-inguinal nerve (L1)

Subcostal nerve (T12) and its lateral cutaneous branch

Genitofemoral nerve (L1, 2)

Lateral femoral cutaneous nerve (L2, 3)

Intermesenteric (para-aortic) plexus

Femoral branch, Genital branch of genitofemoral nerve (L1, 2)

Gray and white rami communicantes

Lumbosacral trunks (L4, 5)

Obturator nerves

Gray rami communicantes

Accessory obturator nerve (L3, 4) (occasional)

Femoral nerve

Lateral femoral cutaneous nerve (L2, 3)

Lumbosacral plexus (L4–S4)

Femoral nerve (L2–L4)

Pudendal nerve (S2, 3, 4)

Obturator nerve (L2, 3, 4)

Anterior cutaneous branch of iliohypogastric nerve (L1)

Anterior scrotal (labial) branches of ilio-inguinal nerve (L1)

Genital branch } of genitofemoral nerve (L1, 2)

Femoral branches

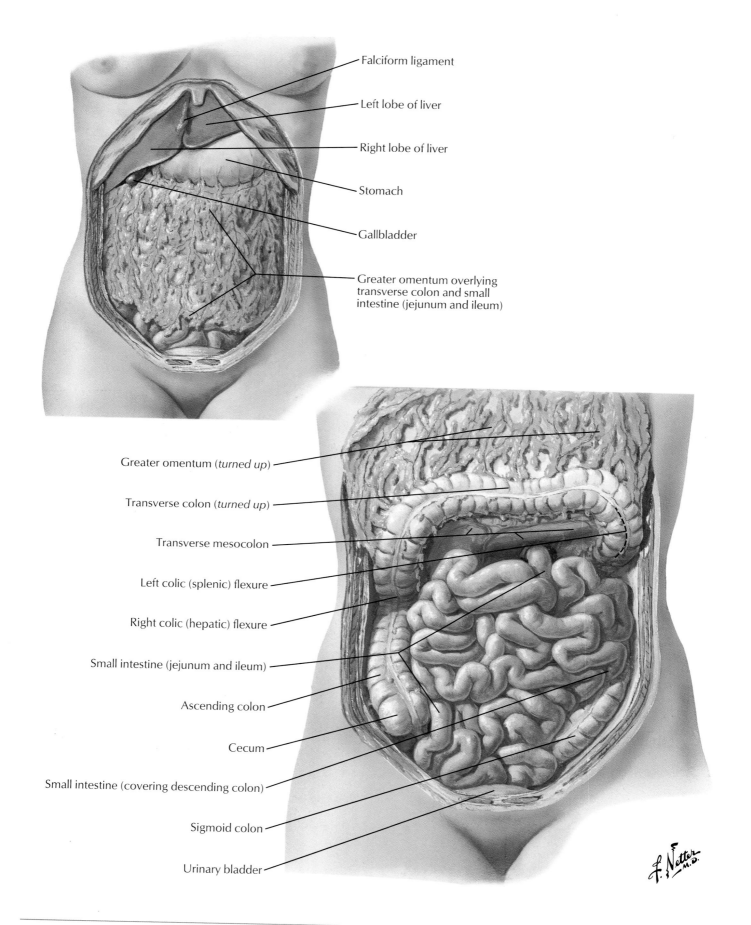

Falciform ligament

Left lobe of liver

Right lobe of liver

Stomach

Gallbladder

Greater omentum overlying transverse colon and small intestine (jejunum and ileum)

Greater omentum (*turned up*)

Transverse colon (*turned up*)

Transverse mesocolon

Left colic (splenic) flexure

Right colic (hepatic) flexure

Small intestine (jejunum and ileum)

Ascending colon

Cecum

Small intestine (covering descending colon)

Sigmoid colon

Urinary bladder

**Plate 263**

**Peritoneal Cavity**

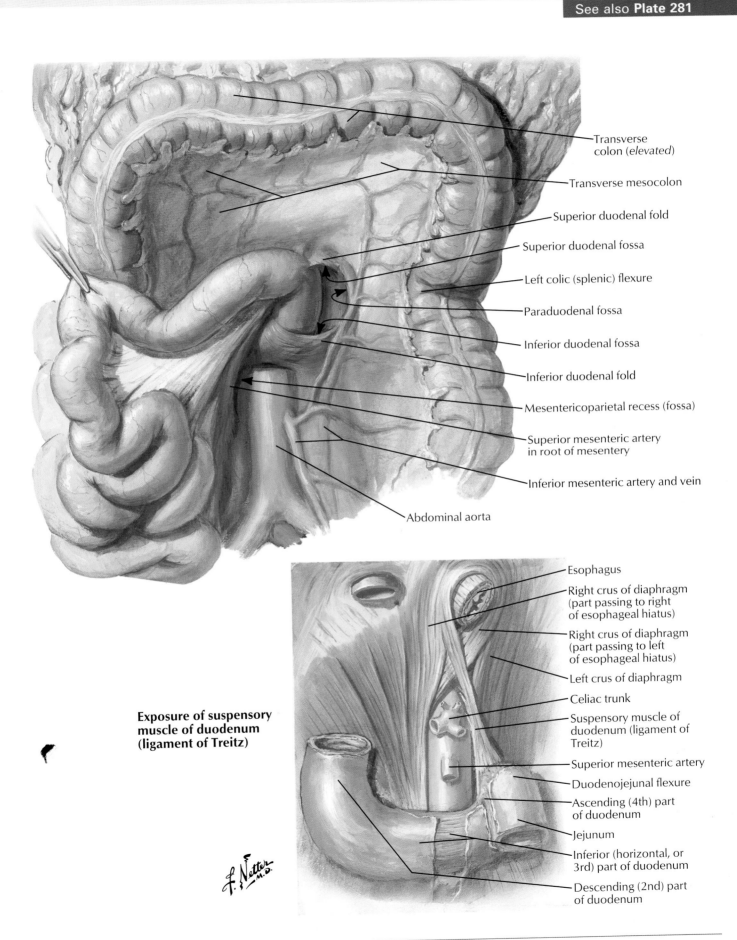

Transverse colon (*elevated*)

Transverse mesocolon

Superior duodenal fold

Superior duodenal fossa

Left colic (splenic) flexure

Paraduodenal fossa

Inferior duodenal fossa

Inferior duodenal fold

Mesentericoparietal recess (fossa)

Superior mesenteric artery in root of mesentery

Inferior mesenteric artery and vein

Abdominal aorta

Esophagus

Right crus of diaphragm (part passing to right of esophageal hiatus)

Right crus of diaphragm (part passing to left of esophageal hiatus)

Left crus of diaphragm

Celiac trunk

Suspensory muscle of duodenum (ligament of Treitz)

Superior mesenteric artery

Duodenojejunal flexure

Ascending (4th) part of duodenum

Jejunum

Inferior (horizontal, or 3rd) part of duodenum

Descending (2nd) part of duodenum

**Exposure of suspensory muscle of duodenum (ligament of Treitz)**

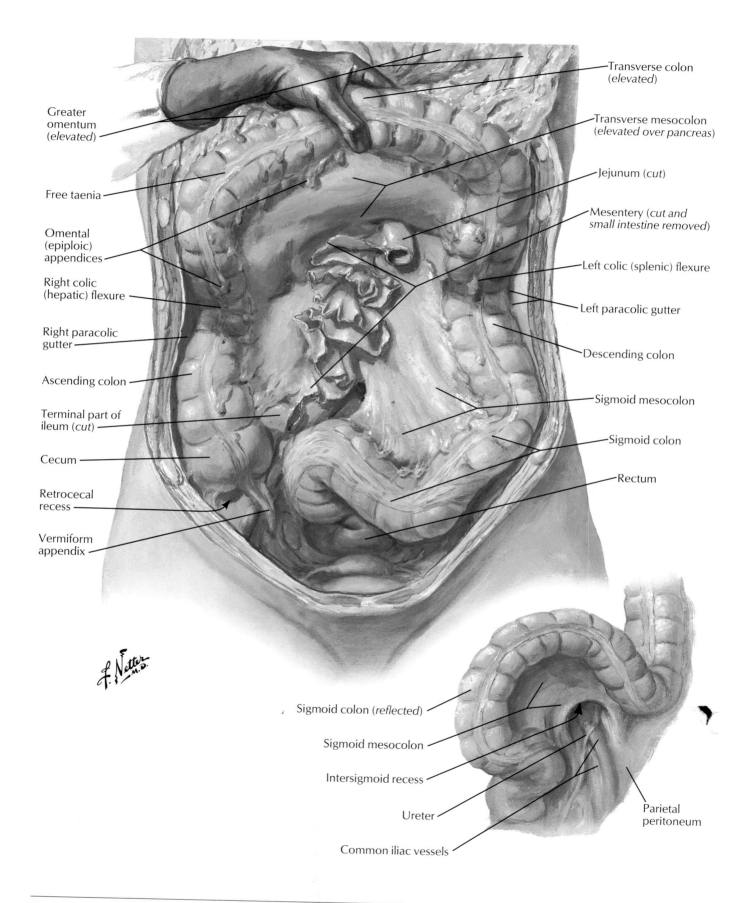

Greater omentum (*elevated*)

Free taenia

Omental (epiploic) appendices

Right colic (hepatic) flexure

Right paracolic gutter

Ascending colon

Terminal part of ileum (*cut*)

Cecum

Retrocecal recess

Vermiform appendix

Transverse colon (*elevated*)

Transverse mesocolon (*elevated over pancreas*)

Jejunum (*cut*)

Mesentery (*cut and small intestine removed*)

Left colic (splenic) flexure

Left paracolic gutter

Descending colon

Sigmoid mesocolon

Sigmoid colon

Rectum

Sigmoid colon (*reflected*)

Sigmoid mesocolon

Intersigmoid recess

Ureter

Common iliac vessels

Parietal peritoneum

**Plate 265**

**Peritoneal Cavity**

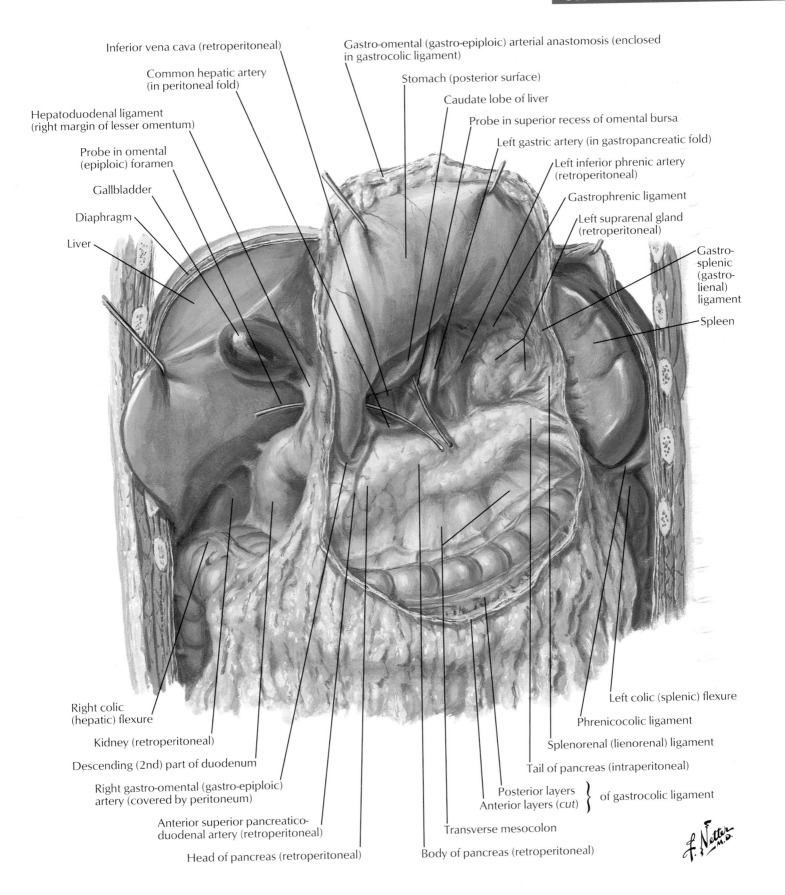

Inferior vena cava (retroperitoneal)

Common hepatic artery (in peritoneal fold)

Hepatoduodenal ligament (right margin of lesser omentum)

Probe in omental (epiploic) foramen

Gallbladder

Diaphragm

Liver

Gastro-omental (gastro-epiploic) arterial anastomosis (enclosed in gastrocolic ligament)

Stomach (posterior surface)

Caudate lobe of liver

Probe in superior recess of omental bursa

Left gastric artery (in gastropancreatic fold)

Left inferior phrenic artery (retroperitoneal)

Gastrophrenic ligament

Left suprarenal gland (retroperitoneal)

Gastro-splenic (gastro-lienal) ligament

Spleen

Right colic (hepatic) flexure

Kidney (retroperitoneal)

Descending (2nd) part of duodenum

Right gastro-omental (gastro-epiploic) artery (covered by peritoneum)

Anterior superior pancreatico-duodenal artery (retroperitoneal)

Head of pancreas (retroperitoneal)

Transverse mesocolon

Body of pancreas (retroperitoneal)

Posterior layers } of gastrocolic ligament
Anterior layers (cut)

Tail of pancreas (intraperitoneal)

Splenorenal (lienorenal) ligament

Phrenicocolic ligament

Left colic (splenic) flexure

*f. Netter*
*M.D.*

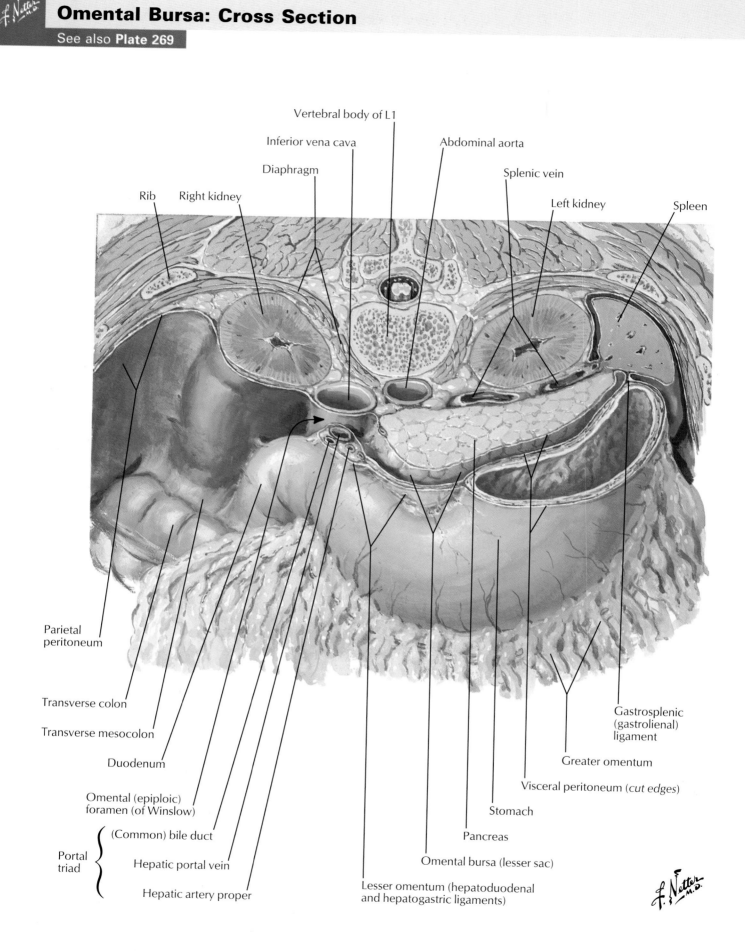

Vertebral body of L1

Inferior vena cava

Diaphragm

Abdominal aorta

Splenic vein

Rib    Right kidney

Left kidney

Spleen

Parietal
peritoneum

Transverse colon

Transverse mesocolon

Duodenum

Omental (epiploic)
foramen (of Winslow)

(Common) bile duct

Portal
triad

Hepatic portal vein

Hepatic artery proper

Lesser omentum (hepatoduodenal
and hepatogastric ligaments)

Omental bursa (lesser sac)

Pancreas

Stomach

Visceral peritoneum (*cut edges*)

Greater omentum

Gastrosplenic
(gastrolienal)
ligament

**Plate 267**

**Peritoneal Cavity**

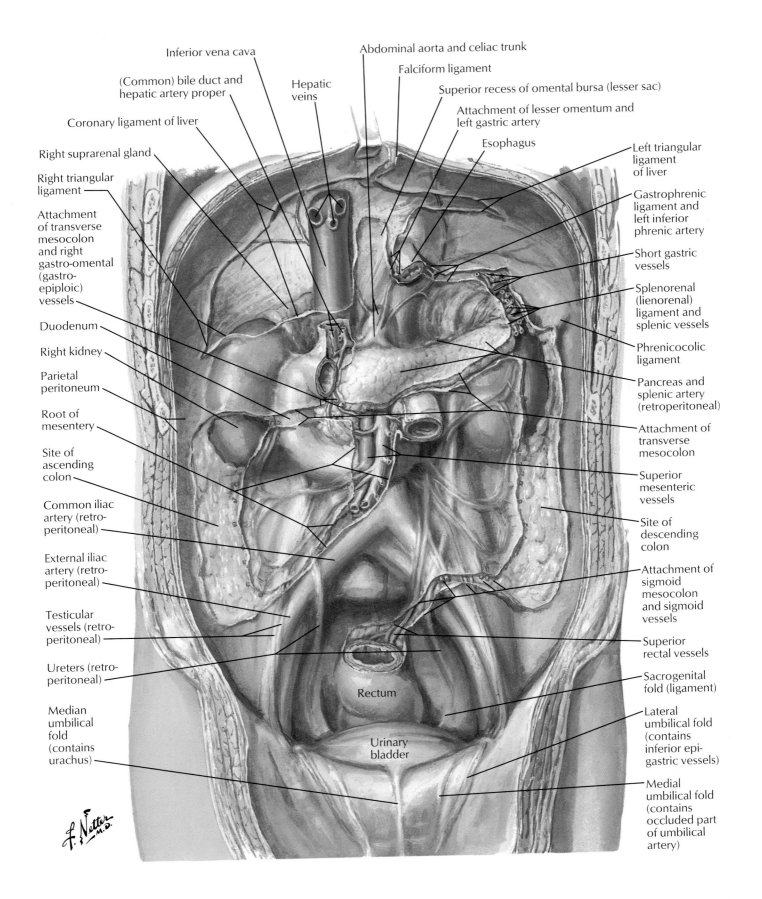

Inferior vena cava

Abdominal aorta and celiac trunk

(Common) bile duct and hepatic artery proper

Hepatic veins

Falciform ligament

Superior recess of omental bursa (lesser sac)

Coronary ligament of liver

Attachment of lesser omentum and left gastric artery

Esophagus

Right suprarenal gland

Left triangular ligament of liver

Right triangular ligament

Gastrophrenic ligament and left inferior phrenic artery

Attachment of transverse mesocolon and right gastro-omental (gastro-epiploic) vessels

Short gastric vessels

Splenorenal (lienorenal) ligament and splenic vessels

Duodenum

Phrenicocolic ligament

Right kidney

Pancreas and splenic artery (retroperitoneal)

Parietal peritoneum

Attachment of transverse mesocolon

Root of mesentery

Superior mesenteric vessels

Site of ascending colon

Site of descending colon

Common iliac artery (retroperitoneal)

External iliac artery (retroperitoneal)

Attachment of sigmoid mesocolon and sigmoid vessels

Testicular vessels (retroperitoneal)

Superior rectal vessels

Ureters (retroperitoneal)

Sacrogenital fold (ligament)

Median umbilical fold (contains urachus)

Rectum

Lateral umbilical fold (contains inferior epigastric vessels)

Urinary bladder

Medial umbilical fold (contains occluded part of umbilical artery)

**Peritoneal Cavity**

**Plate 268**

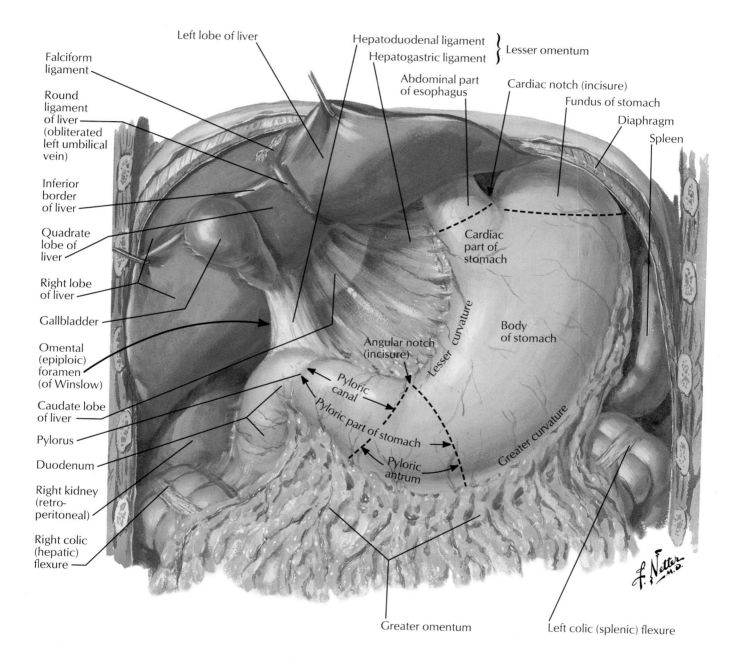

Falciform ligament

Round ligament of liver (obliterated left umbilical vein)

Inferior border of liver

Quadrate lobe of liver

Right lobe of liver

Gallbladder

Omental (epiploic) foramen (of Winslow)

Caudate lobe of liver

Pylorus

Duodenum

Right kidney (retroperitoneal)

Right colic (hepatic) flexure

Left lobe of liver

Hepatoduodenal ligament
Hepatogastric ligament
} Lesser omentum

Abdominal part of esophagus

Cardiac notch (incisure)

Fundus of stomach

Diaphragm

Spleen

Cardiac part of stomach

Lesser curvature

Body of stomach

Angular notch (incisure)

Pyloric canal

Pyloric part of stomach

Pyloric antrum

Greater curvature

Greater omentum

Left colic (splenic) flexure

**Plate 269**

**Viscera (Gut)**

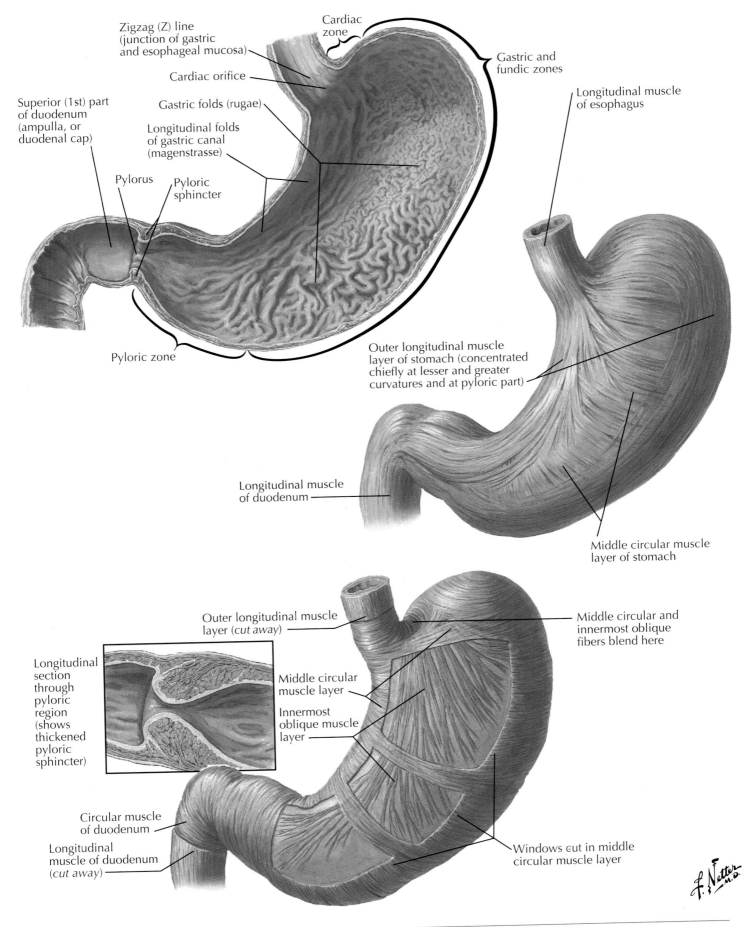

Zigzag (Z) line (junction of gastric and esophageal mucosa)

Cardiac zone

Cardiac orifice

Gastric and fundic zones

Longitudinal muscle of esophagus

Superior (1st) part of duodenum (ampulla, or duodenal cap)

Gastric folds (rugae)

Longitudinal folds of gastric canal (magenstrasse)

Pylorus

Pyloric sphincter

Pyloric zone

Outer longitudinal muscle layer of stomach (concentrated chiefly at lesser and greater curvatures and at pyloric part)

Longitudinal muscle of duodenum

Middle circular muscle layer of stomach

Outer longitudinal muscle layer (cut away)

Middle circular and innermost oblique fibers blend here

Longitudinal section through pyloric region (shows thickened pyloric sphincter)

Middle circular muscle layer

Innermost oblique muscle layer

Circular muscle of duodenum

Longitudinal muscle of duodenum (cut away)

Windows cut in middle circular muscle layer

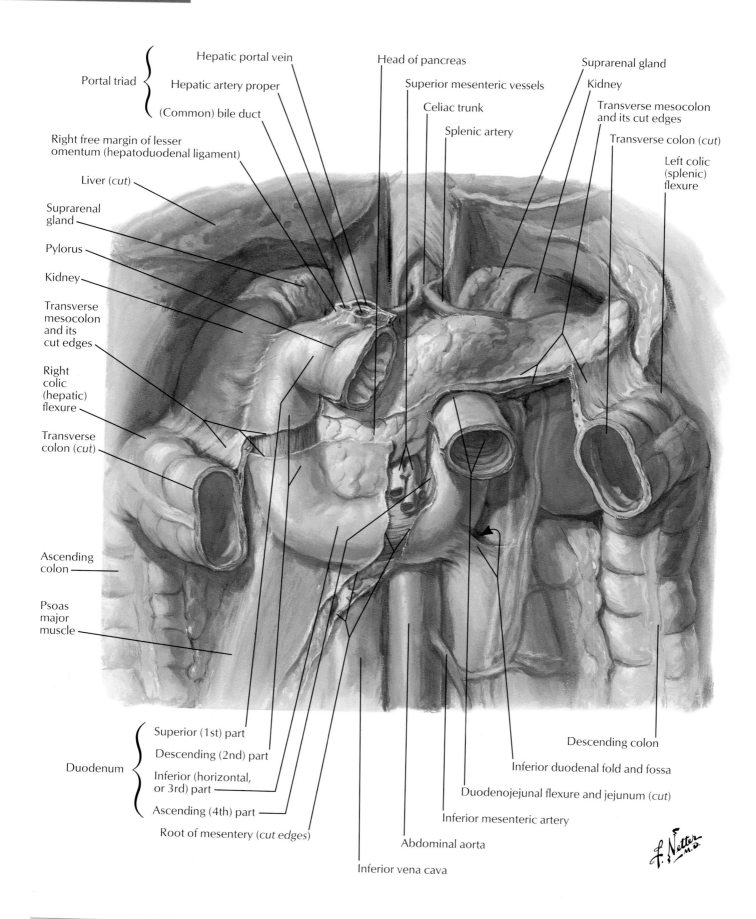

Portal triad { Hepatic portal vein

Hepatic artery proper

(Common) bile duct

Right free margin of lesser omentum (hepatoduodenal ligament)

Liver (*cut*)

Suprarenal gland

Pylorus

Kidney

Transverse mesocolon and its cut edges

Right colic (hepatic) flexure

Transverse colon (*cut*)

Ascending colon

Psoas major muscle

Duodenum {
Superior (1st) part

Descending (2nd) part

Inferior (horizontal, or 3rd) part

Ascending (4th) part

Root of mesentery (*cut edges*)

Head of pancreas

Superior mesenteric vessels

Celiac trunk

Splenic artery

Suprarenal gland

Kidney

Transverse mesocolon and its cut edges

Transverse colon (*cut*)

Left colic (splenic) flexure

Descending colon

Inferior duodenal fold and fossa

Duodenojejunal flexure and jejunum (*cut*)

Inferior mesenteric artery

Abdominal aorta

Inferior vena cava

**Plate 271**

**Viscera (Gut)**

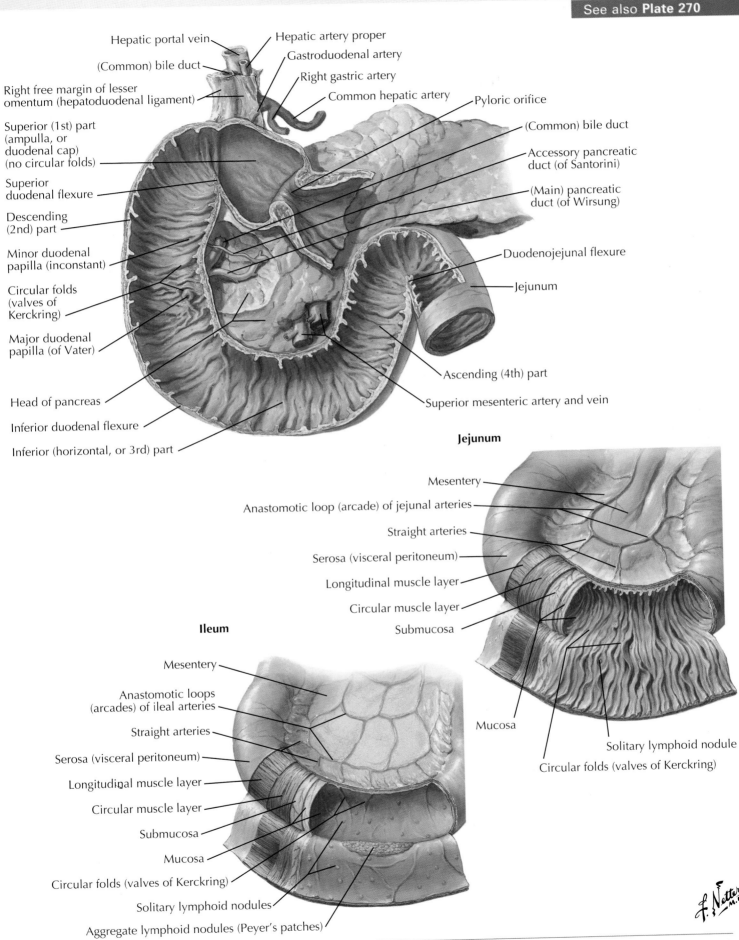

Hepatic portal vein

(Common) bile duct

Right free margin of lesser omentum (hepatoduodenal ligament)

Superior (1st) part (ampulla, or duodenal cap) (no circular folds)

Superior duodenal flexure

Descending (2nd) part

Minor duodenal papilla (inconstant)

Circular folds (valves of Kerckring)

Major duodenal papilla (of Vater)

Head of pancreas

Inferior duodenal flexure

Inferior (horizontal, or 3rd) part

Hepatic artery proper

Gastroduodenal artery

Right gastric artery

Common hepatic artery

Pyloric orifice

(Common) bile duct

Accessory pancreatic duct (of Santorini)

(Main) pancreatic duct (of Wirsung)

Duodenojejunal flexure

Jejunum

Ascending (4th) part

Superior mesenteric artery and vein

**Jejunum**

Mesentery

Anastomotic loop (arcade) of jejunal arteries

Straight arteries

Serosa (visceral peritoneum)

Longitudinal muscle layer

Circular muscle layer

Submucosa

Mucosa

Solitary lymphoid nodule

Circular folds (valves of Kerckring)

**Ileum**

Mesentery

Anastomotic loops (arcades) of ileal arteries

Straight arteries

Serosa (visceral peritoneum)

Longitudinal muscle layer

Circular muscle layer

Submucosa

Mucosa

Circular folds (valves of Kerckring)

Solitary lymphoid nodules

Aggregate lymphoid nodules (Peyer's patches)

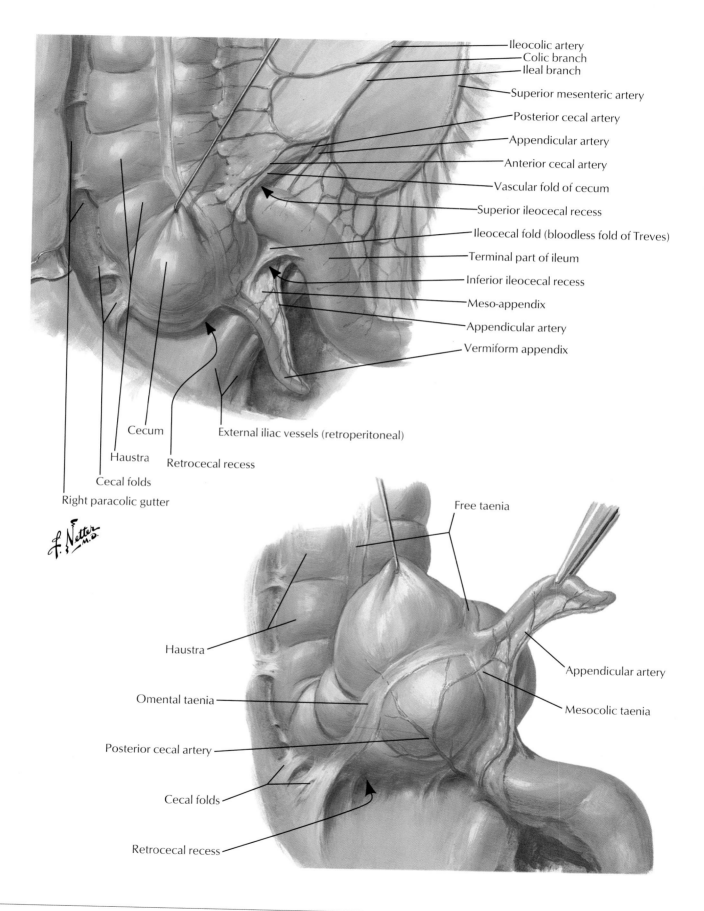

Ileocolic artery
Colic branch
Ileal branch
Superior mesenteric artery
Posterior cecal artery
Appendicular artery
Anterior cecal artery
Vascular fold of cecum
Superior ileocecal recess
Ileocecal fold (bloodless fold of Treves)
Terminal part of ileum
Inferior ileocecal recess
Meso-appendix
Appendicular artery
Vermiform appendix

External iliac vessels (retroperitoneal)
Cecum
Retrocecal recess
Haustra
Cecal folds
Right paracolic gutter

Free taenia
Haustra
Appendicular artery
Omental taenia
Mesocolic taenia
Posterior cecal artery
Cecal folds
Retrocecal recess

**Plate 273**

**Viscera (Gut)**

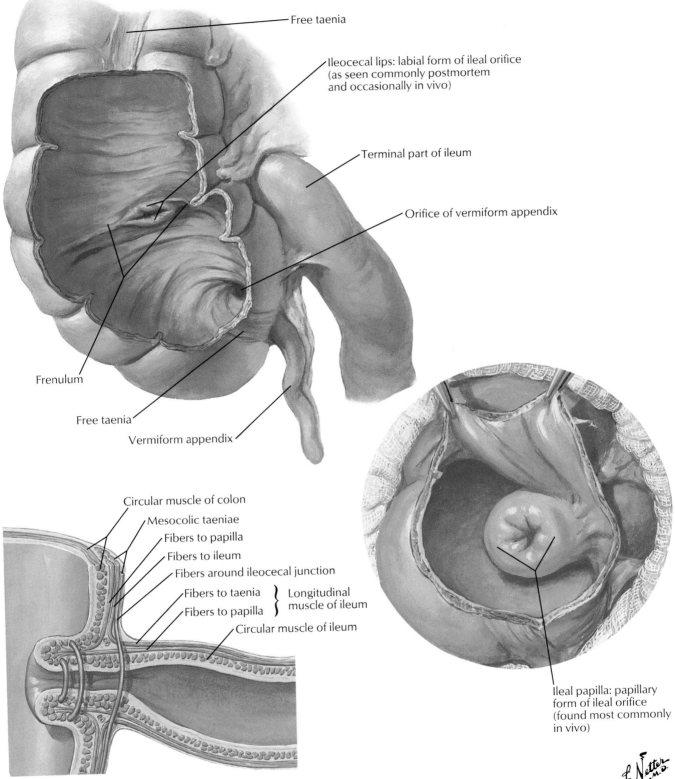

Free taenia

Ileocecal lips: labial form of ileal orifice (as seen commonly postmortem and occasionally in vivo)

Terminal part of ileum

Orifice of vermiform appendix

Frenulum

Free taenia

Vermiform appendix

Circular muscle of colon

Mesocolic taeniae

Fibers to papilla

Fibers to ileum

Fibers around ileocecal junction

Fibers to taenia

Fibers to papilla } Longitudinal muscle of ileum

Circular muscle of ileum

Ileal papilla: papillary form of ileal orifice (found most commonly in vivo)

**Schema of muscle fibers at ileal orifice**

# (Vermiform) Appendix

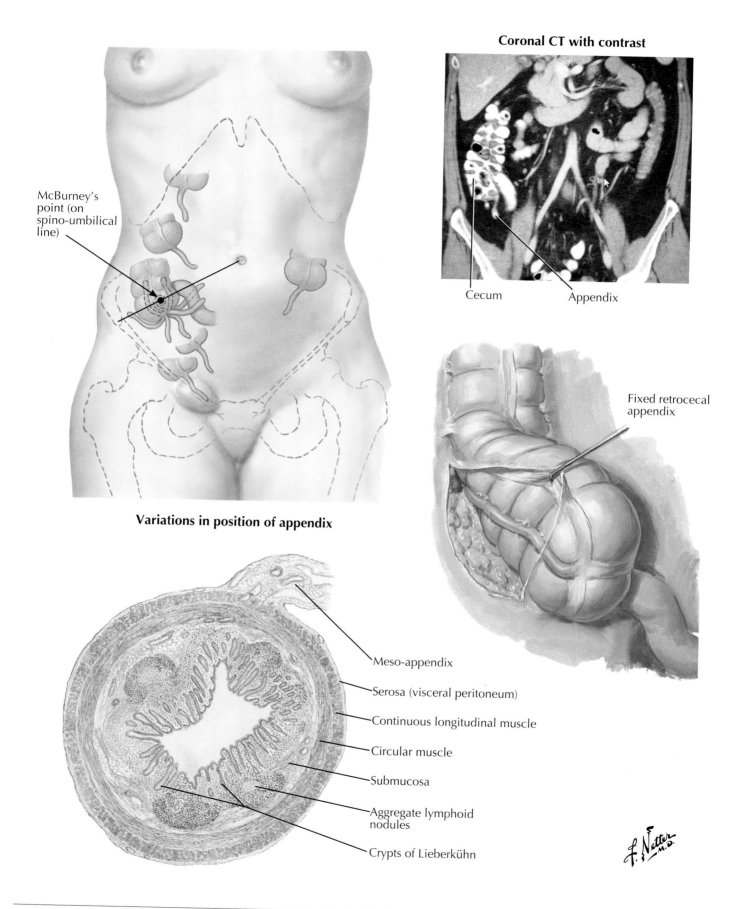

**Coronal CT with contrast**

Cecum

Appendix

McBurney's point (on spino-umbilical line)

**Variations in position of appendix**

Fixed retrocecal appendix

Meso-appendix

Serosa (visceral peritoneum)

Continuous longitudinal muscle

Circular muscle

Submucosa

Aggregate lymphoid nodules

Crypts of Lieberkühn

**Plate 275**

**Viscera (Gut)**

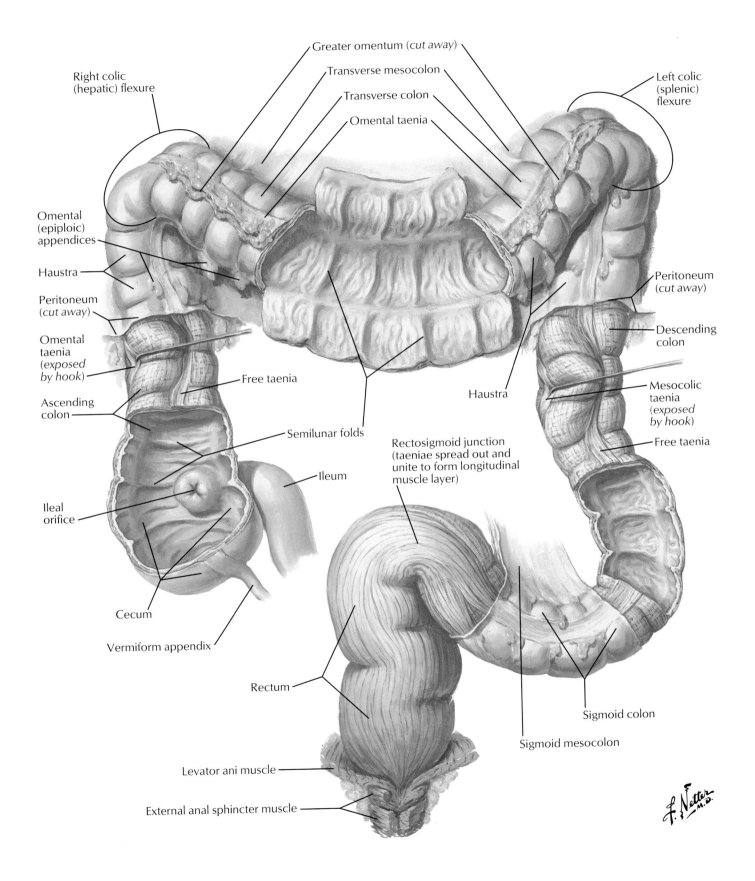

Right colic (hepatic) flexure

Greater omentum (*cut away*)

Transverse mesocolon

Transverse colon

Omental taenia

Left colic (splenic) flexure

Omental (epiploic) appendices

Haustra

Peritoneum (*cut away*)

Omental taenia (*exposed by hook*)

Ascending colon

Ileal orifice

Cecum

Vermiform appendix

Free taenia

Semilunar folds

Ileum

Rectosigmoid junction (taeniae spread out and unite to form longitudinal muscle layer)

Peritoneum (*cut away*)

Descending colon

Mesocolic taenia (*exposed by hook*)

Free taenia

Haustra

Rectum

Levator ani muscle

External anal sphincter muscle

Sigmoid colon

Sigmoid mesocolon

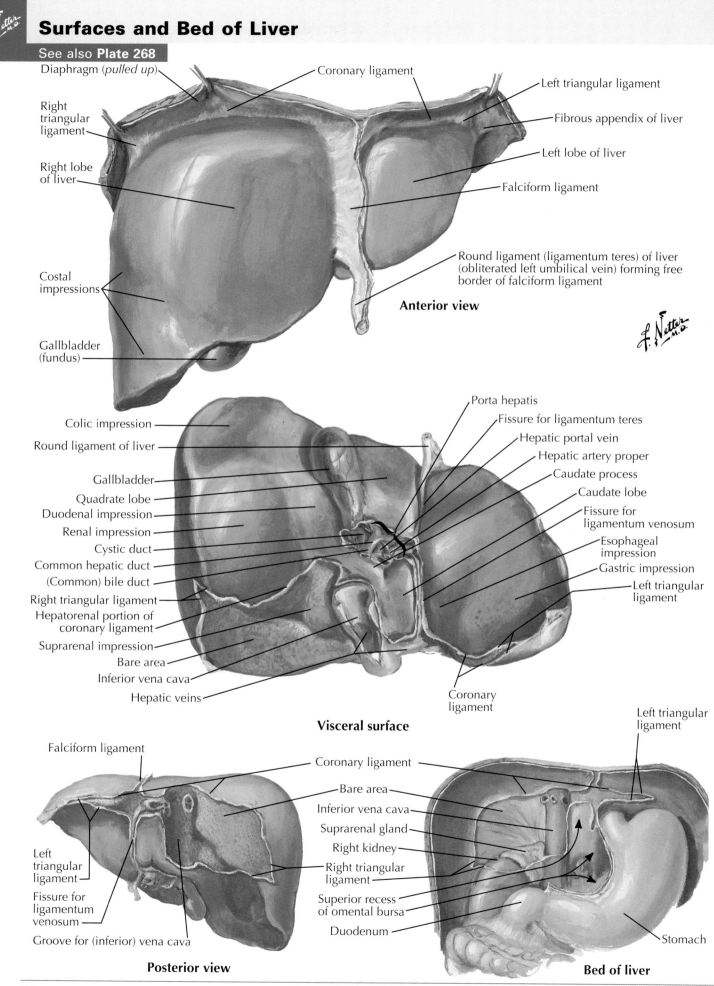

Diaphragm (*pulled up*)

Coronary ligament

Left triangular ligament

Fibrous appendix of liver

Right triangular ligament

Left lobe of liver

Right lobe of liver

Falciform ligament

Costal impressions

Round ligament (ligamentum teres) of liver (obliterated left umbilical vein) forming free border of falciform ligament

Gallbladder (fundus)

**Anterior view**

Colic impression

Porta hepatis

Fissure for ligamentum teres

Round ligament of liver

Hepatic portal vein

Hepatic artery proper

Gallbladder

Caudate process

Quadrate lobe

Caudate lobe

Duodenal impression

Fissure for ligamentum venosum

Renal impression

Cystic duct

Esophageal impression

Common hepatic duct

Gastric impression

(Common) bile duct

Left triangular ligament

Right triangular ligament

Hepatorenal portion of coronary ligament

Suprarenal impression

Bare area

Inferior vena cava

Hepatic veins

Coronary ligament

**Visceral surface**

Falciform ligament

Left triangular ligament

Coronary ligament

Bare area

Inferior vena cava

Suprarenal gland

Left triangular ligament

Right kidney

Fissure for ligamentum venosum

Right triangular ligament

Superior recess of omental bursa

Groove for (inferior) vena cava

Duodenum

Stomach

**Posterior view**

**Bed of liver**

**Plate 277**

**Viscera (Accessory Organs)**

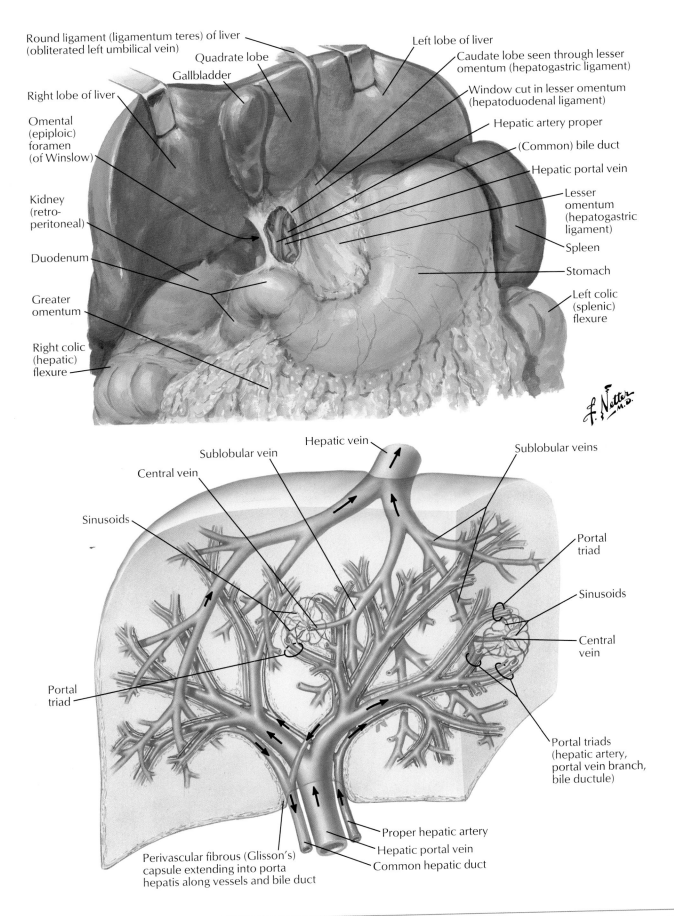

Round ligament (ligamentum teres) of liver (obliterated left umbilical vein)

Quadrate lobe

Gallbladder

Right lobe of liver

Omental (epiploic) foramen (of Winslow)

Kidney (retro-peritoneal)

Duodenum

Greater omentum

Right colic (hepatic) flexure

Left lobe of liver

Caudate lobe seen through lesser omentum (hepatogastric ligament)

Window cut in lesser omentum (hepatoduodenal ligament)

Hepatic artery proper

(Common) bile duct

Hepatic portal vein

Lesser omentum (hepatogastric ligament)

Spleen

Stomach

Left colic (splenic) flexure

Hepatic vein

Sublobular vein

Central vein

Sinusoids

Portal triad

Sublobular veins

Portal triad

Sinusoids

Central vein

Portal triads (hepatic artery, portal vein branch, bile ductule)

Proper hepatic artery

Hepatic portal vein

Common hepatic duct

Perivascular fibrous (Glisson's) capsule extending into porta hepatis along vessels and bile duct

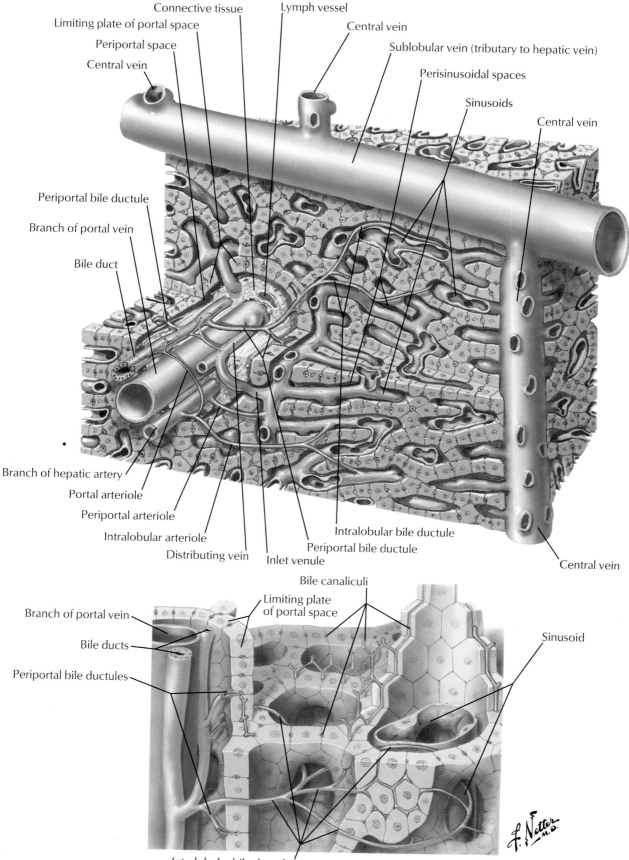

Connective tissue

Limiting plate of portal space

Periportal space

Central vein

Lymph vessel

Central vein

Sublobular vein (tributary to hepatic vein)

Perisinusoidal spaces

Sinusoids

Central vein

Periportal bile ductule

Branch of portal vein

Bile duct

Central vein

Branch of hepatic artery

Portal arteriole

Periportal arteriole

Intralobular arteriole

Distributing vein

Inlet venule

Periportal bile ductule

Intralobular bile ductule

Central vein

Bile canaliculi

Limiting plate of portal space

Branch of portal vein

Bile ducts

Periportal bile ductules

Sinusoid

Intralobular bile ductules

**Plate 279**

**Viscera (Accessory Organs)**

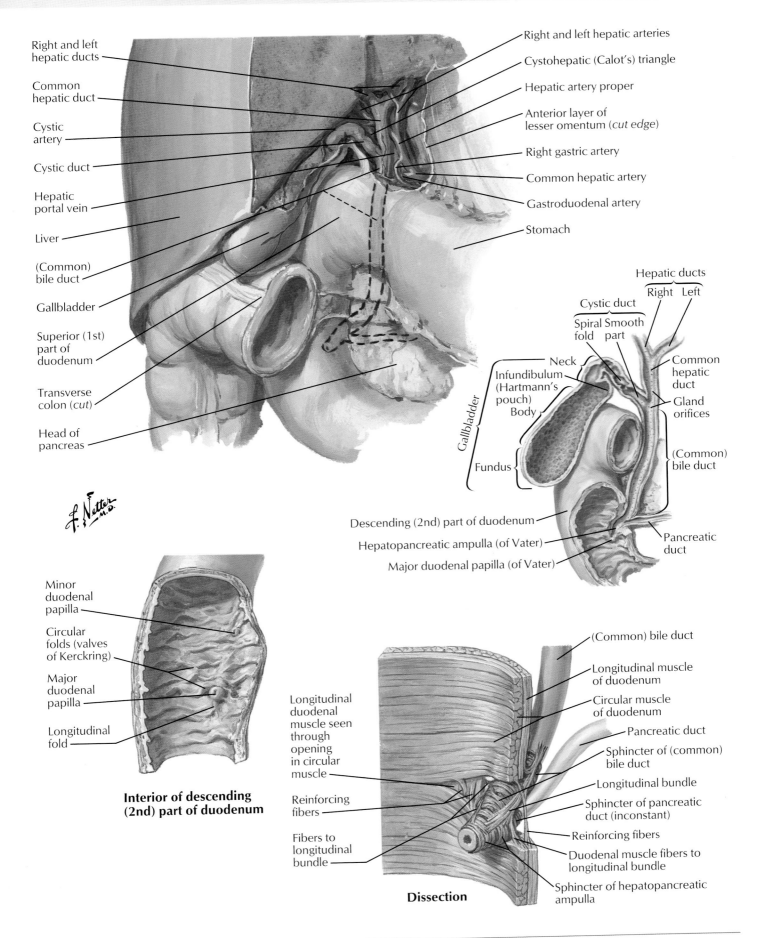

Right and left hepatic ducts

Common hepatic duct

Cystic artery

Cystic duct

Hepatic portal vein

Liver

(Common) bile duct

Gallbladder

Superior (1st) part of duodenum

Transverse colon (cut)

Head of pancreas

Right and left hepatic arteries

Cystohepatic (Calot's) triangle

Hepatic artery proper

Anterior layer of lesser omentum (cut edge)

Right gastric artery

Common hepatic artery

Gastroduodenal artery

Stomach

Hepatic ducts
Right  Left

Cystic duct

Spiral Smooth fold  part

Neck

Infundibulum (Hartmann's pouch)

Body

Gallbladder

Fundus

Common hepatic duct

Gland orifices

(Common) bile duct

Descending (2nd) part of duodenum

Hepatopancreatic ampulla (of Vater)

Major duodenal papilla (of Vater)

Pancreatic duct

Minor duodenal papilla

Circular folds (valves of Kerckring)

Major duodenal papilla

Longitudinal fold

**Interior of descending (2nd) part of duodenum**

Longitudinal duodenal muscle seen through opening in circular muscle

Reinforcing fibers

Fibers to longitudinal bundle

(Common) bile duct

Longitudinal muscle of duodenum

Circular muscle of duodenum

Pancreatic duct

Sphincter of (common) bile duct

Longitudinal bundle

Sphincter of pancreatic duct (inconstant)

Reinforcing fibers

Duodenal muscle fibers to longitudinal bundle

Sphincter of hepatopancreatic ampulla

**Dissection**

**Viscera (Accessory Organs)**

**Plate 280**

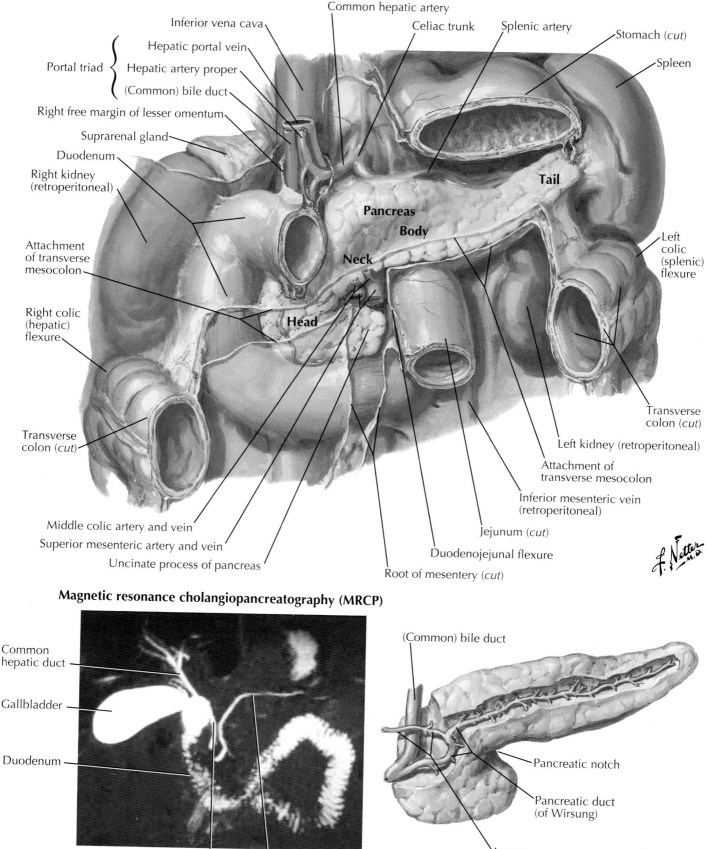

Common hepatic artery

Celiac trunk

Splenic artery

Stomach (*cut*)

Inferior vena cava

Spleen

Portal triad
- Hepatic portal vein
- Hepatic artery proper
- (Common) bile duct

Right free margin of lesser omentum

Suprarenal gland

Duodenum

Right kidney (retroperitoneal)

Attachment of transverse mesocolon

Right colic (hepatic) flexure

Transverse colon (*cut*)

Middle colic artery and vein

Superior mesenteric artery and vein

Uncinate process of pancreas

Tail

Pancreas

Body

Neck

Head

Left colic (splenic) flexure

Transverse colon (*cut*)

Left kidney (retroperitoneal)

Attachment of transverse mesocolon

Inferior mesenteric vein (retroperitoneal)

Jejunum (*cut*)

Duodenojejunal flexure

Root of mesentery (*cut*)

### Magnetic resonance cholangiopancreatography (MRCP)

Common hepatic duct

Gallbladder

Duodenum

(Common) bile duct

Pancreatic duct (of Wirsung)

(Common) bile duct

Pancreatic notch

Pancreatic duct (of Wirsung)

Accessory pancreatic duct (of Santorini)

**Plate 281**

**Viscera (Accessory Organs)**

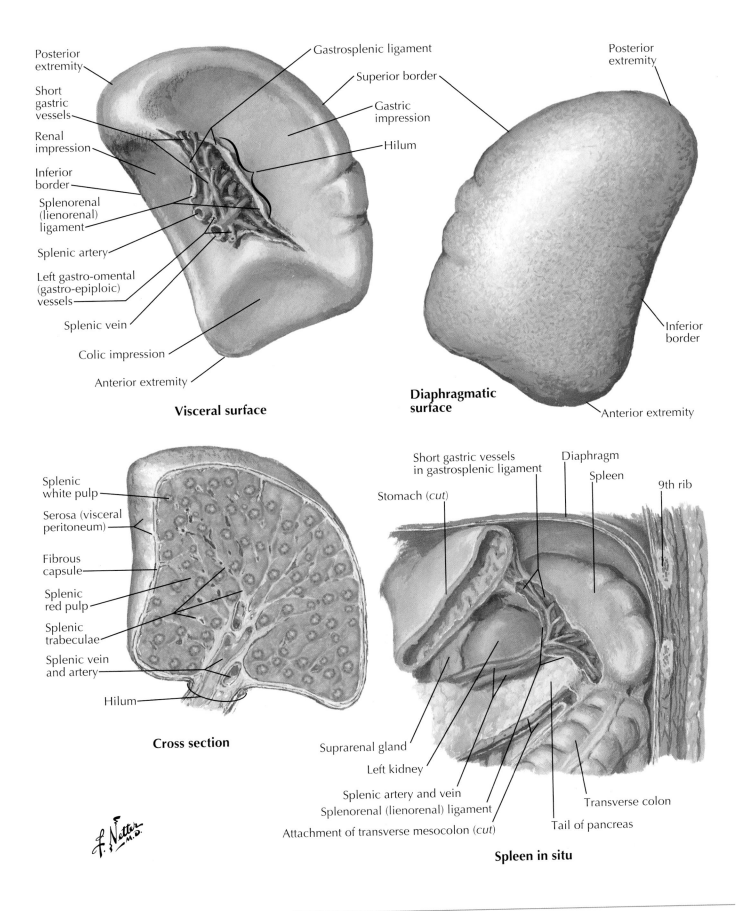

Posterior extremity

Short gastric vessels

Renal impression

Inferior border

Splenorenal (lienorenal) ligament

Splenic artery

Left gastro-omental (gastro-epiploic) vessels

Splenic vein

Colic impression

Anterior extremity

Gastrosplenic ligament

Superior border

Gastric impression

Hilum

**Visceral surface**

Posterior extremity

Inferior border

Anterior extremity

**Diaphragmatic surface**

Splenic white pulp

Serosa (visceral peritoneum)

Fibrous capsule

Splenic red pulp

Splenic trabeculae

Splenic vein and artery

Hilum

**Cross section**

Short gastric vessels in gastrosplenic ligament

Diaphragm

Spleen

9th rib

Stomach (cut)

Suprarenal gland

Left kidney

Splenic artery and vein

Splenorenal (lienorenal) ligament

Attachment of transverse mesocolon (cut)

Transverse colon

Tail of pancreas

**Spleen in situ**

**Viscera (Accessory Organs)**

**Plate 282**

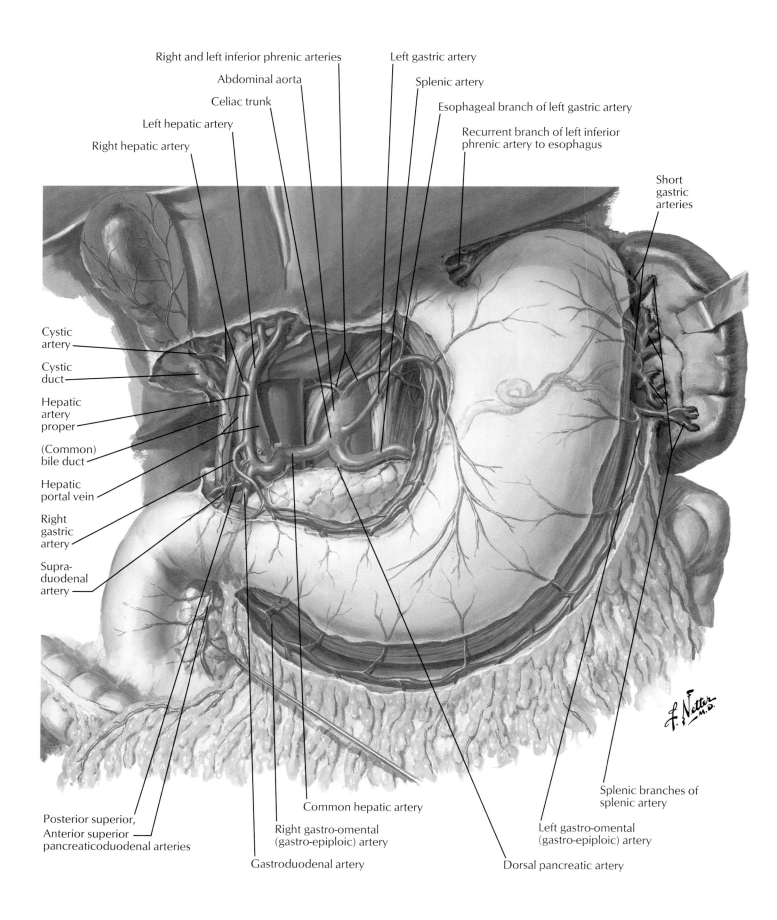

Right and left inferior phrenic arteries

Abdominal aorta

Celiac trunk

Left hepatic artery

Right hepatic artery

Left gastric artery

Splenic artery

Esophageal branch of left gastric artery

Recurrent branch of left inferior phrenic artery to esophagus

Short gastric arteries

Cystic artery

Cystic duct

Hepatic artery proper

(Common) bile duct

Hepatic portal vein

Right gastric artery

Supra-duodenal artery

Posterior superior, Anterior superior pancreaticoduodenal arteries

Gastroduodenal artery

Right gastro-omental (gastro-epiploic) artery

Common hepatic artery

Dorsal pancreatic artery

Left gastro-omental (gastro-epiploic) artery

Splenic branches of splenic artery

**Plate 283**

**Visceral Vasculature**

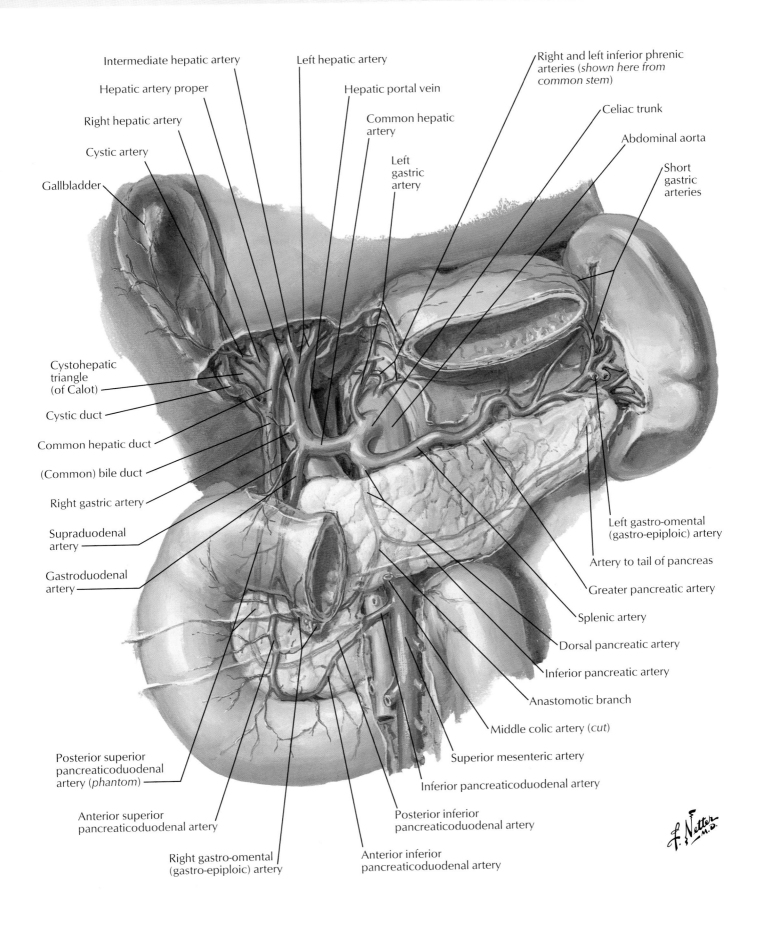

Intermediate hepatic artery

Hepatic artery proper

Right hepatic artery

Cystic artery

Gallbladder

Left hepatic artery

Hepatic portal vein

Common hepatic artery

Left gastric artery

Right and left inferior phrenic arteries (*shown here from common stem*)

Celiac trunk

Abdominal aorta

Short gastric arteries

Cystohepatic triangle (of Calot)

Cystic duct

Common hepatic duct

(Common) bile duct

Right gastric artery

Supraduodenal artery

Gastroduodenal artery

Posterior superior pancreaticoduodenal artery (*phantom*)

Anterior superior pancreaticoduodenal artery

Right gastro-omental (gastro-epiploic) artery

Anterior inferior pancreaticoduodenal artery

Posterior inferior pancreaticoduodenal artery

Inferior pancreaticoduodenal artery

Superior mesenteric artery

Middle colic artery (*cut*)

Anastomotic branch

Inferior pancreatic artery

Dorsal pancreatic artery

Splenic artery

Greater pancreatic artery

Artery to tail of pancreas

Left gastro-omental (gastro-epiploic) artery

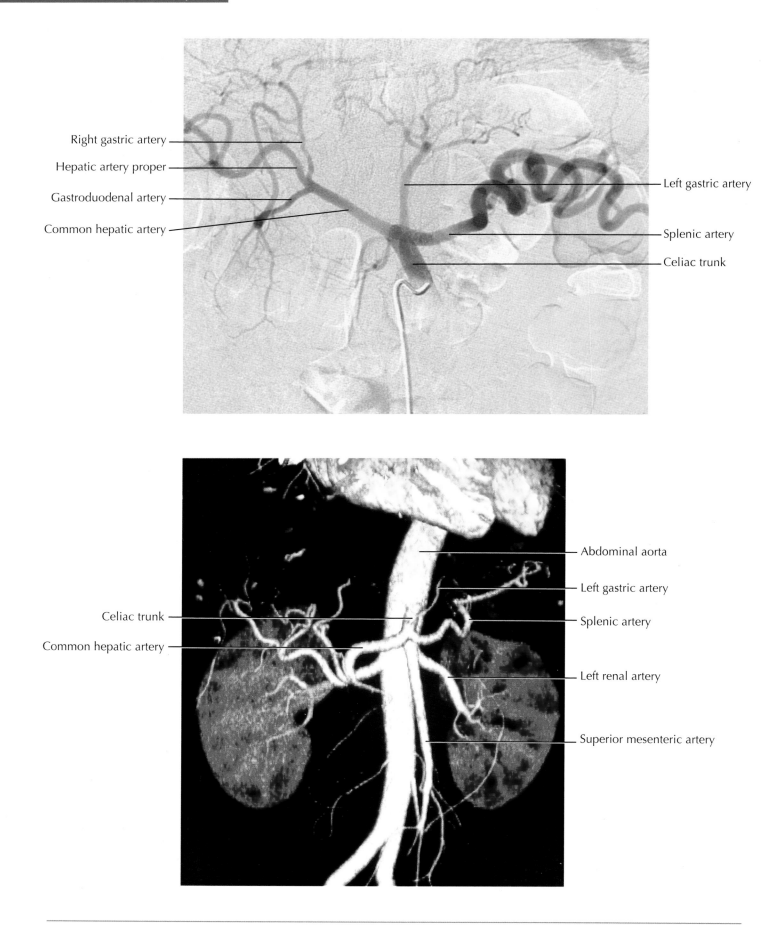

Right gastric artery

Hepatic artery proper

Gastroduodenal artery

Common hepatic artery

Left gastric artery

Splenic artery

Celiac trunk

Celiac trunk

Common hepatic artery

Abdominal aorta

Left gastric artery

Splenic artery

Left renal artery

Superior mesenteric artery

**Plate 285**

**Visceral Vasculature**

**Duodenum and head of pancreas reflected to left**

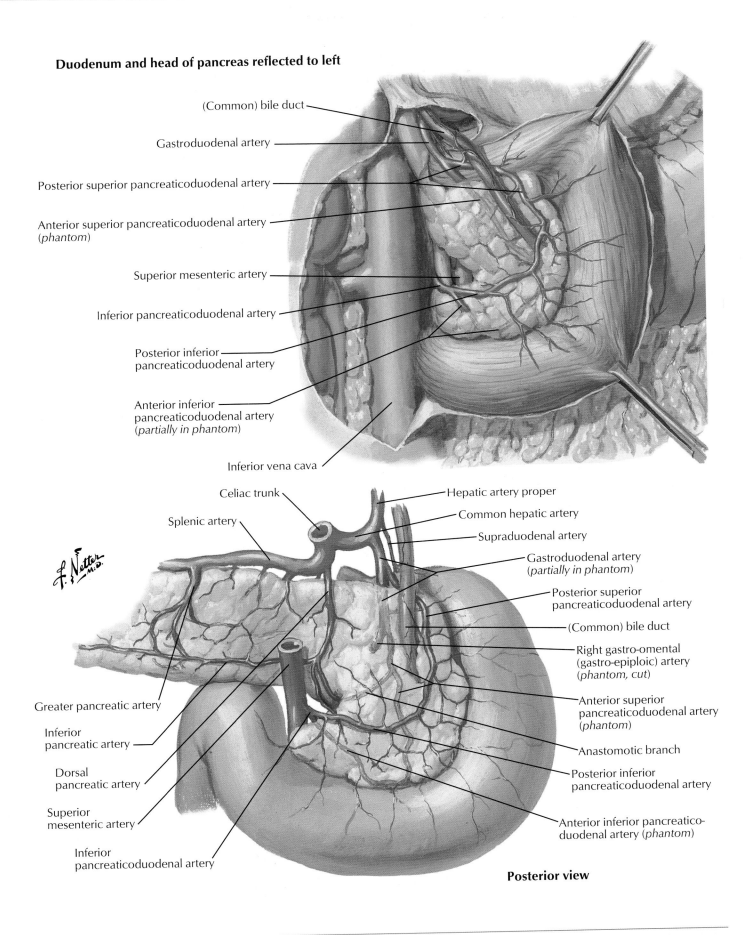

(Common) bile duct

Gastroduodenal artery

Posterior superior pancreaticoduodenal artery

Anterior superior pancreaticoduodenal artery (*phantom*)

Superior mesenteric artery

Inferior pancreaticoduodenal artery

Posterior inferior pancreaticoduodenal artery

Anterior inferior pancreaticoduodenal artery (*partially in phantom*)

Inferior vena cava

Celiac trunk

Splenic artery

Hepatic artery proper

Common hepatic artery

Supraduodenal artery

Gastroduodenal artery (*partially in phantom*)

Posterior superior pancreaticoduodenal artery

(Common) bile duct

Right gastro-omental (gastro-epiploic) artery (*phantom, cut*)

Anterior superior pancreaticoduodenal artery (*phantom*)

Anastomotic branch

Posterior inferior pancreaticoduodenal artery

Anterior inferior pancreatico-duodenal artery (*phantom*)

Greater pancreatic artery

Inferior pancreatic artery

Dorsal pancreatic artery

Superior mesenteric artery

Inferior pancreaticoduodenal artery

**Posterior view**

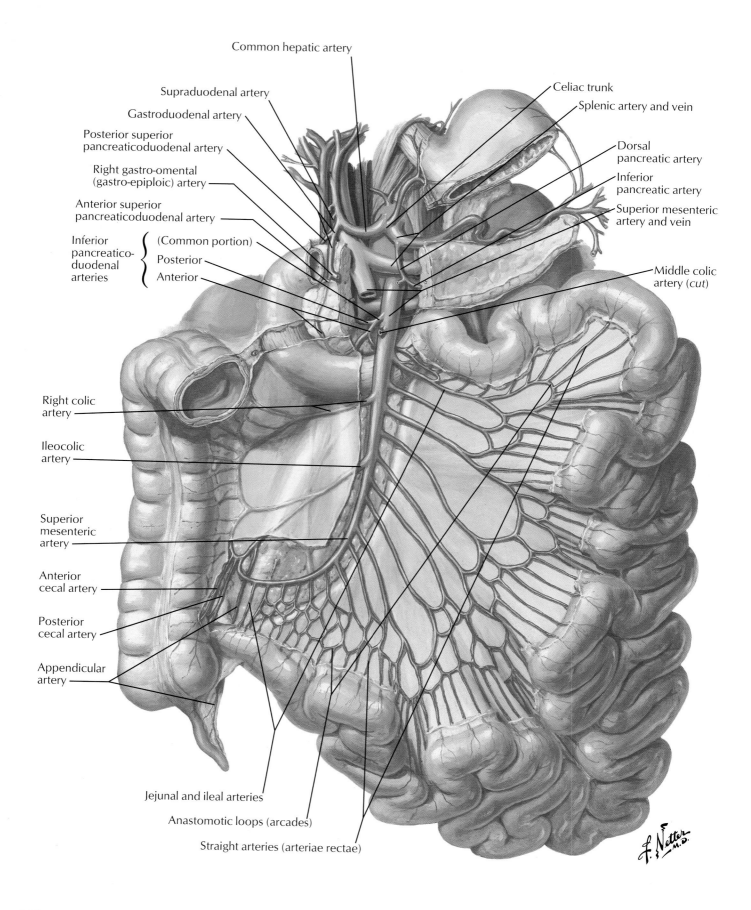

Common hepatic artery

Supraduodenal artery

Gastroduodenal artery

Posterior superior
pancreaticoduodenal artery

Right gastro-omental
(gastro-epiploic) artery

Anterior superior
pancreaticoduodenal artery

Inferior
pancreatico-
duodenal
arteries

(Common portion)

Posterior

Anterior

Celiac trunk

Splenic artery and vein

Dorsal
pancreatic artery

Inferior
pancreatic artery

Superior mesenteric
artery and vein

Middle colic
artery (cut)

Right colic
artery

Ileocolic
artery

Superior
mesenteric
artery

Anterior
cecal artery

Posterior
cecal artery

Appendicular
artery

Jejunal and ileal arteries

Anastomotic loops (arcades)

Straight arteries (arteriae rectae)

**Plate 287**

**Visceral Vasculature**

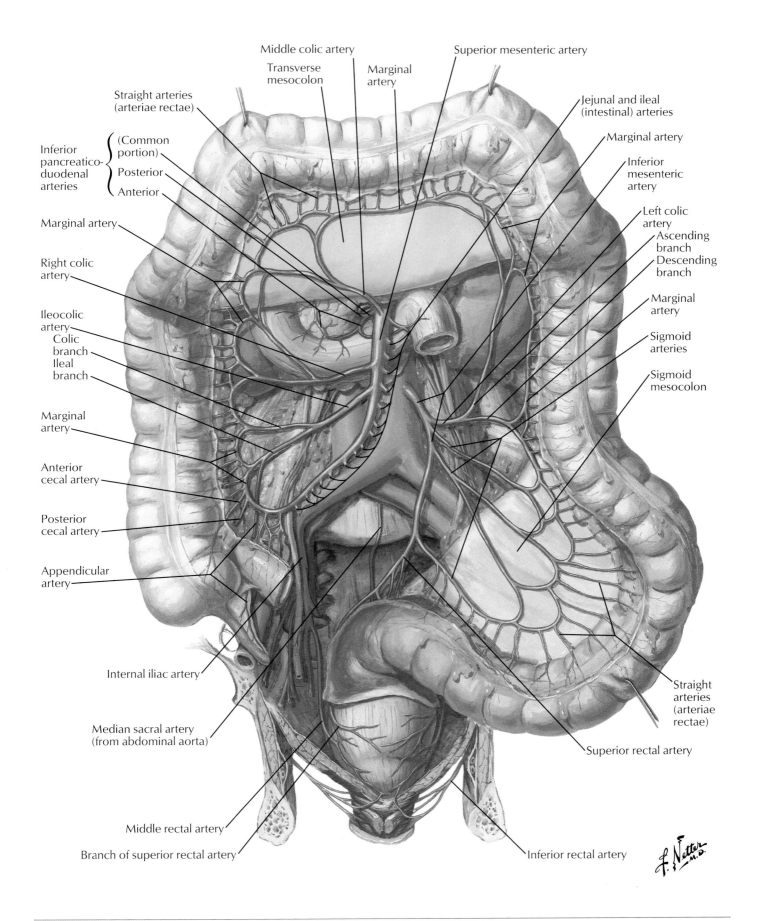

Middle colic artery

Transverse mesocolon

Marginal artery

Superior mesenteric artery

Straight arteries (arteriae rectae)

Jejunal and ileal (intestinal) arteries

Inferior pancreatico-duodenal arteries

(Common portion)

Posterior

Anterior

Marginal artery

Inferior mesenteric artery

Left colic artery

Ascending branch

Descending branch

Marginal artery

Right colic artery

Ileocolic artery

Colic branch

Ileal branch

Sigmoid arteries

Sigmoid mesocolon

Marginal artery

Anterior cecal artery

Posterior cecal artery

Appendicular artery

Internal iliac artery

Median sacral artery (from abdominal aorta)

Straight arteries (arteriae rectae)

Superior rectal artery

Middle rectal artery

Branch of superior rectal artery

Inferior rectal artery

*f. Netter*
M.D.

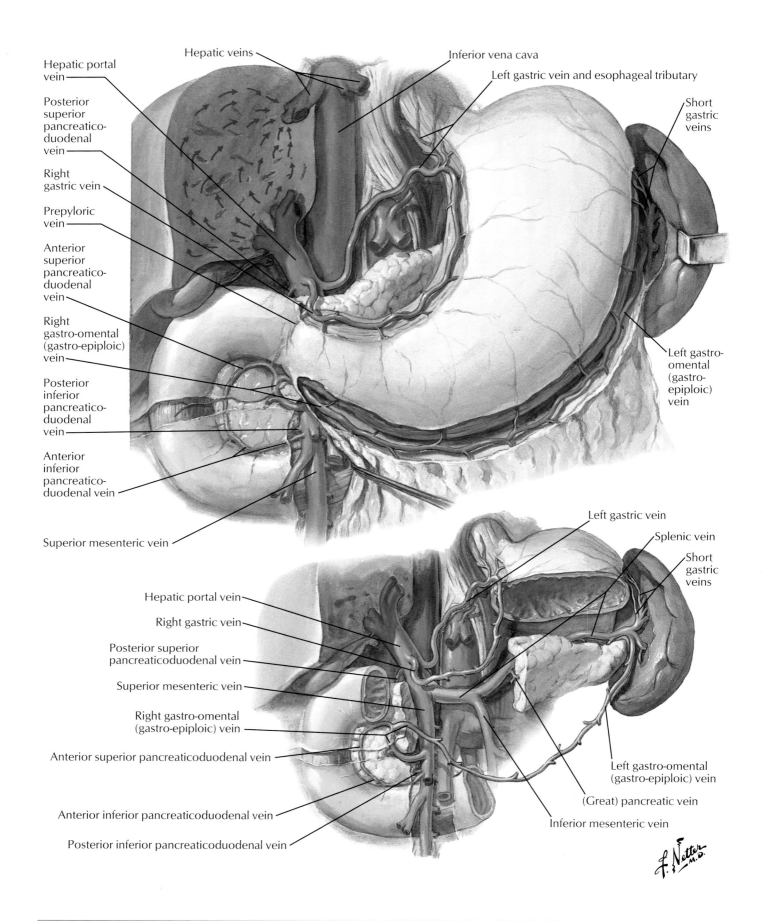

Hepatic veins

Inferior vena cava

Hepatic portal vein

Left gastric vein and esophageal tributary

Posterior superior pancreatico-duodenal vein

Short gastric veins

Right gastric vein

Prepyloric vein

Anterior superior pancreatico-duodenal vein

Right gastro-omental (gastro-epiploic) vein

Posterior inferior pancreatico-duodenal vein

Left gastro-omental (gastro-epiploic) vein

Anterior inferior pancreatico-duodenal vein

Superior mesenteric vein

Left gastric vein

Hepatic portal vein

Splenic vein

Right gastric vein

Short gastric veins

Posterior superior pancreaticoduodenal vein

Superior mesenteric vein

Right gastro-omental (gastro-epiploic) vein

Anterior superior pancreaticoduodenal vein

Left gastro-omental (gastro-epiploic) vein

Anterior inferior pancreaticoduodenal vein

(Great) pancreatic vein

Posterior inferior pancreaticoduodenal vein

Inferior mesenteric vein

**Plate 289**

**Visceral Vasculature**

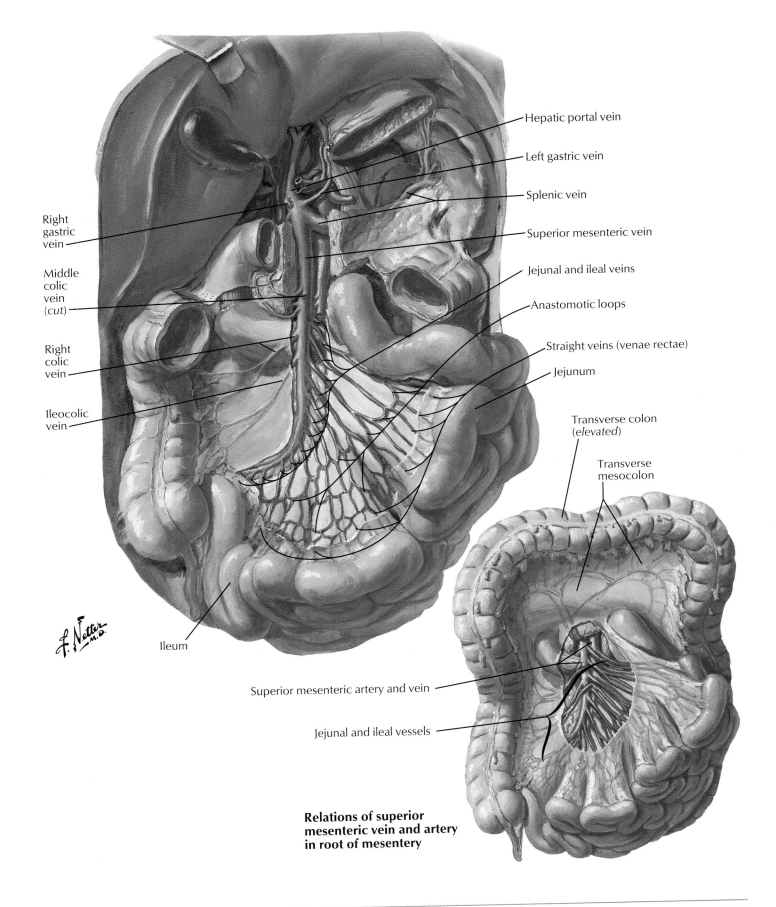

Right gastric vein

Middle colic vein (*cut*)

Right colic vein

Ileocolic vein

Ileum

Hepatic portal vein

Left gastric vein

Splenic vein

Superior mesenteric vein

Jejunal and ileal veins

Anastomotic loops

Straight veins (venae rectae)

Jejunum

Transverse colon (*elevated*)

Transverse mesocolon

Superior mesenteric artery and vein

Jejunal and ileal vessels

**Relations of superior mesenteric vein and artery in root of mesentery**

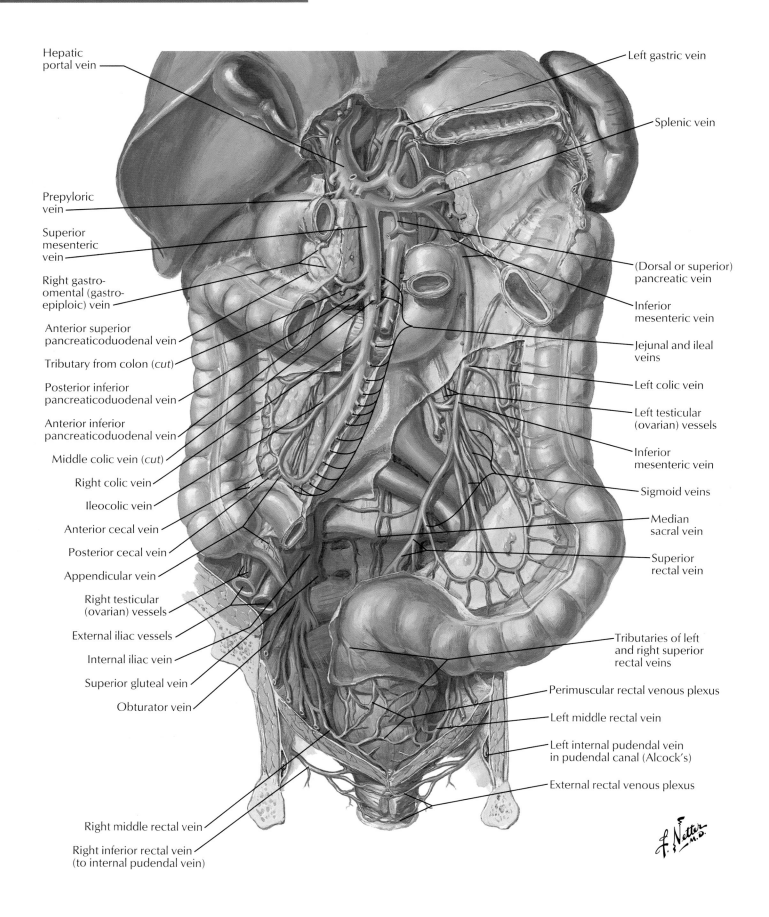

Hepatic portal vein

Prepyloric vein

Superior mesenteric vein

Right gastro-omental (gastro-epiploic) vein

Anterior superior pancreaticoduodenal vein

Tributary from colon (*cut*)

Posterior inferior pancreaticoduodenal vein

Anterior inferior pancreaticoduodenal vein

Middle colic vein (*cut*)

Right colic vein

Ileocolic vein

Anterior cecal vein

Posterior cecal vein

Appendicular vein

Right testicular (ovarian) vessels

External iliac vessels

Internal iliac vein

Superior gluteal vein

Obturator vein

Right middle rectal vein

Right inferior rectal vein (to internal pudendal vein)

Left gastric vein

Splenic vein

(Dorsal or superior) pancreatic vein

Inferior mesenteric vein

Jejunal and ileal veins

Left colic vein

Left testicular (ovarian) vessels

Inferior mesenteric vein

Sigmoid veins

Median sacral vein

Superior rectal vein

Tributaries of left and right superior rectal veins

Perimuscular rectal venous plexus

Left middle rectal vein

Left internal pudendal vein in pudendal canal (Alcock's)

External rectal venous plexus

**Plate 291**

**Visceral Vasculature**

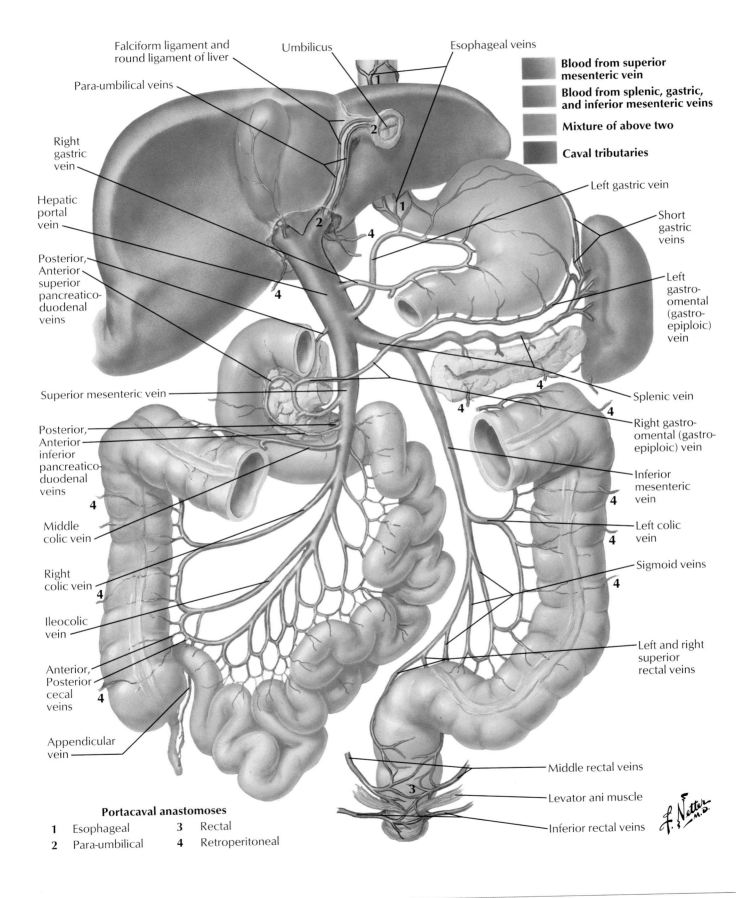

Falciform ligament and round ligament of liver

Umbilicus

Esophageal veins

Blood from superior mesenteric vein

Blood from splenic, gastric, and inferior mesenteric veins

Mixture of above two

Caval tributaries

Para-umbilical veins

Right gastric vein

Hepatic portal vein

Posterior, Anterior superior pancreatico-duodenal veins

Left gastric vein

Short gastric veins

Left gastro-omental (gastro-epiploic) vein

Superior mesenteric vein

Posterior, Anterior inferior pancreatico-duodenal veins

Splenic vein

Right gastro-omental (gastro-epiploic) vein

Inferior mesenteric vein

Middle colic vein

Right colic vein

Ileocolic vein

Left colic vein

Sigmoid veins

Left and right superior rectal veins

Anterior, Posterior cecal veins

Appendicular vein

Middle rectal veins

Levator ani muscle

Inferior rectal veins

**Portacaval anastomoses**

| | | | |
|---|---|---|---|
| 1 | Esophageal | 3 | Rectal |
| 2 | Para-umbilical | 4 | Retroperitoneal |

**Visceral Vasculature**

**Plate 292**

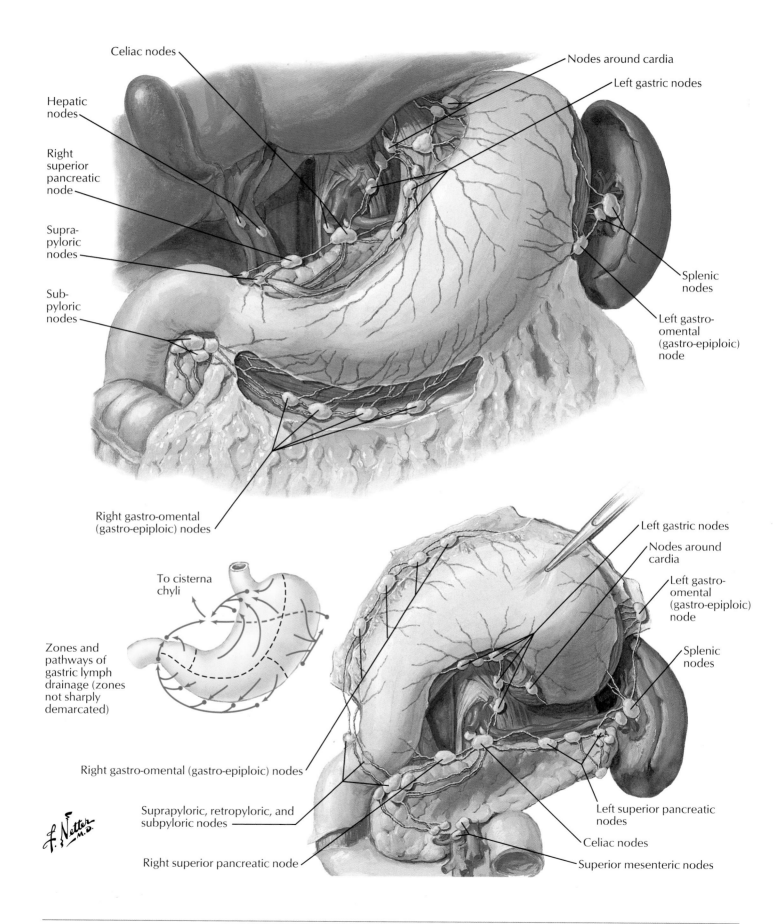

Celiac nodes

Hepatic nodes

Right superior pancreatic node

Supra-pyloric nodes

Sub-pyloric nodes

Nodes around cardia

Left gastric nodes

Splenic nodes

Left gastro-omental (gastro-epiploic) node

Right gastro-omental (gastro-epiploic) nodes

To cisterna chyli

Zones and pathways of gastric lymph drainage (zones not sharply demarcated)

Left gastric nodes

Nodes around cardia

Left gastro-omental (gastro-epiploic) node

Splenic nodes

Left superior pancreatic nodes

Celiac nodes

Superior mesenteric nodes

Right gastro-omental (gastro-epiploic) nodes

Suprapyloric, retropyloric, and subpyloric nodes

Right superior pancreatic node

**Plate 293**                                          **Visceral Vasculature**

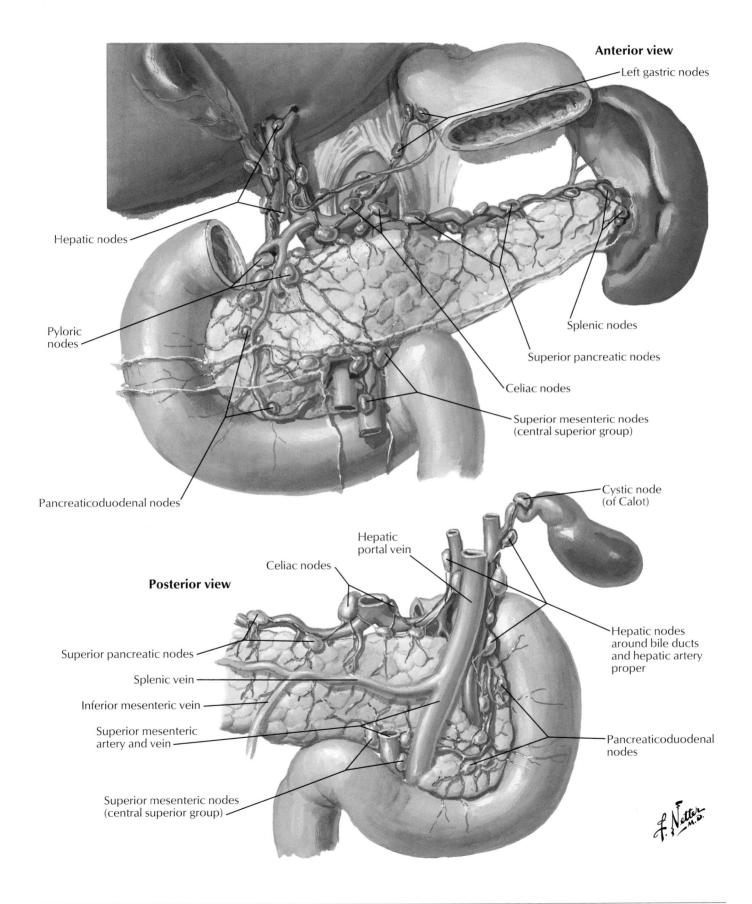

**Anterior view**

Left gastric nodes

Hepatic nodes

Pyloric nodes

Splenic nodes

Superior pancreatic nodes

Celiac nodes

Superior mesenteric nodes (central superior group)

Pancreaticoduodenal nodes

Cystic node (of Calot)

Hepatic portal vein

Celiac nodes

**Posterior view**

Superior pancreatic nodes

Splenic vein

Inferior mesenteric vein

Superior mesenteric artery and vein

Hepatic nodes around bile ducts and hepatic artery proper

Pancreaticoduodenal nodes

Superior mesenteric nodes (central superior group)

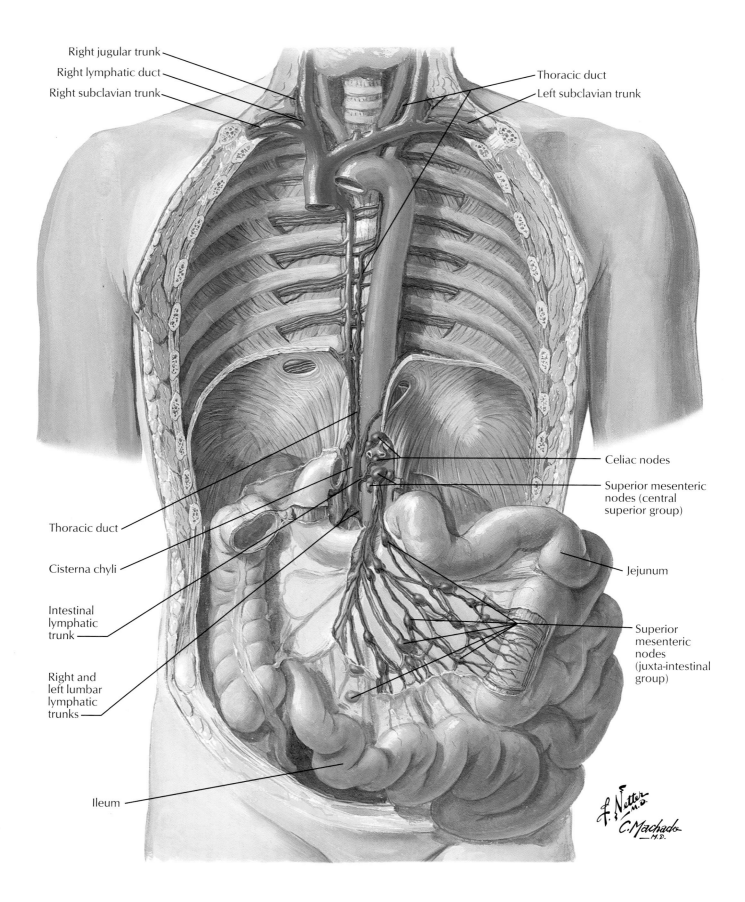

Right jugular trunk

Right lymphatic duct

Right subclavian trunk

Thoracic duct

Left subclavian trunk

Celiac nodes

Superior mesenteric nodes (central superior group)

Thoracic duct

Jejunum

Cisterna chyli

Intestinal lymphatic trunk

Superior mesenteric nodes (juxta-intestinal group)

Right and left lumbar lymphatic trunks

Ileum

**Plate 295**

**Visceral Vasculature**

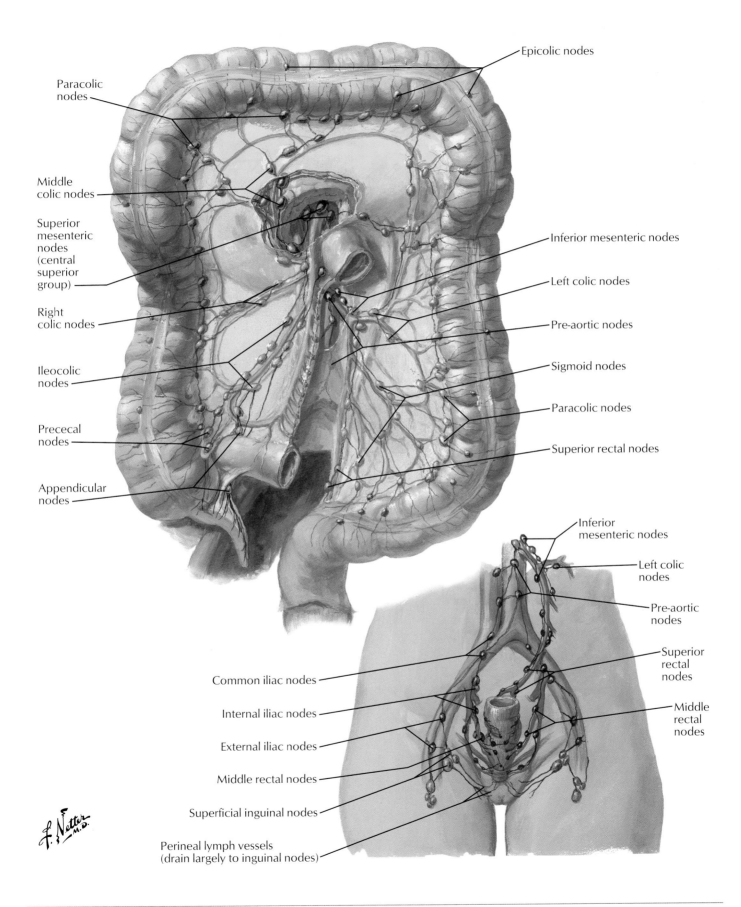

Epicolic nodes

Paracolic nodes

Middle colic nodes

Superior mesenteric nodes (central superior group)

Right colic nodes

Ileocolic nodes

Prececal nodes

Appendicular nodes

Inferior mesenteric nodes

Left colic nodes

Pre-aortic nodes

Sigmoid nodes

Paracolic nodes

Superior rectal nodes

Inferior mesenteric nodes

Left colic nodes

Pre-aortic nodes

Superior rectal nodes

Middle rectal nodes

Common iliac nodes

Internal iliac nodes

External iliac nodes

Middle rectal nodes

Superficial inguinal nodes

Perineal lymph vessels (drain largely to inguinal nodes)

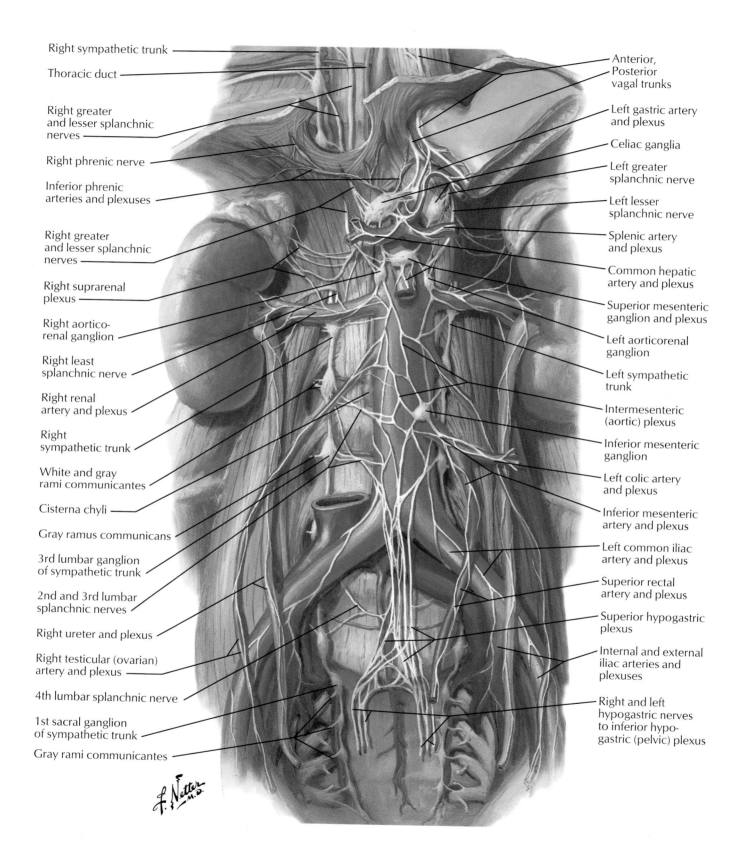

Right sympathetic trunk

Thoracic duct

Right greater and lesser splanchnic nerves

Right phrenic nerve

Inferior phrenic arteries and plexuses

Right greater and lesser splanchnic nerves

Right suprarenal plexus

Right aortico-renal ganglion

Right least splanchnic nerve

Right renal artery and plexus

Right sympathetic trunk

White and gray rami communicantes

Cisterna chyli

Gray ramus communicans

3rd lumbar ganglion of sympathetic trunk

2nd and 3rd lumbar splanchnic nerves

Right ureter and plexus

Right testicular (ovarian) artery and plexus

4th lumbar splanchnic nerve

1st sacral ganglion of sympathetic trunk

Gray rami communicantes

Anterior, Posterior vagal trunks

Left gastric artery and plexus

Celiac ganglia

Left greater splanchnic nerve

Left lesser splanchnic nerve

Splenic artery and plexus

Common hepatic artery and plexus

Superior mesenteric ganglion and plexus

Left aorticorenal ganglion

Left sympathetic trunk

Intermesenteric (aortic) plexus

Inferior mesenteric ganglion

Left colic artery and plexus

Inferior mesenteric artery and plexus

Left common iliac artery and plexus

Superior rectal artery and plexus

Superior hypogastric plexus

Internal and external iliac arteries and plexuses

Right and left hypogastric nerves to inferior hypo-gastric (pelvic) plexus

**Plate 297**

**Innervation**

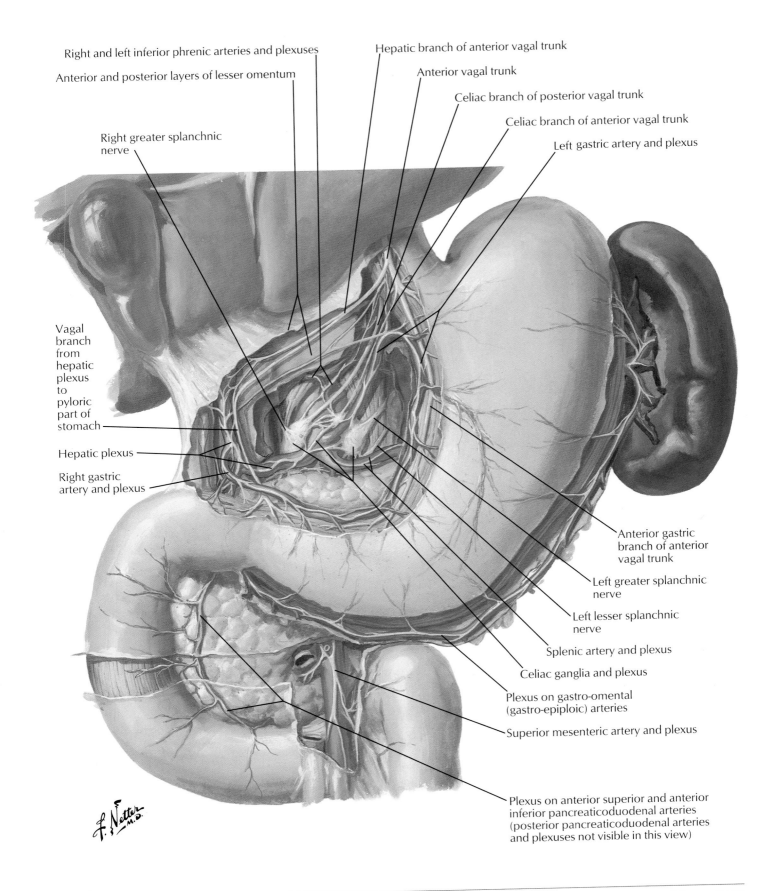

Right and left inferior phrenic arteries and plexuses

Anterior and posterior layers of lesser omentum

Right greater splanchnic nerve

Hepatic branch of anterior vagal trunk

Anterior vagal trunk

Celiac branch of posterior vagal trunk

Celiac branch of anterior vagal trunk

Left gastric artery and plexus

Vagal branch from hepatic plexus to pyloric part of stomach

Hepatic plexus

Right gastric artery and plexus

Anterior gastric branch of anterior vagal trunk

Left greater splanchnic nerve

Left lesser splanchnic nerve

Splenic artery and plexus

Celiac ganglia and plexus

Plexus on gastro-omental (gastro-epiploic) arteries

Superior mesenteric artery and plexus

Plexus on anterior superior and anterior inferior pancreaticoduodenal arteries (posterior pancreaticoduodenal arteries and plexuses not visible in this view)

**Plate 298**

**Innervation**

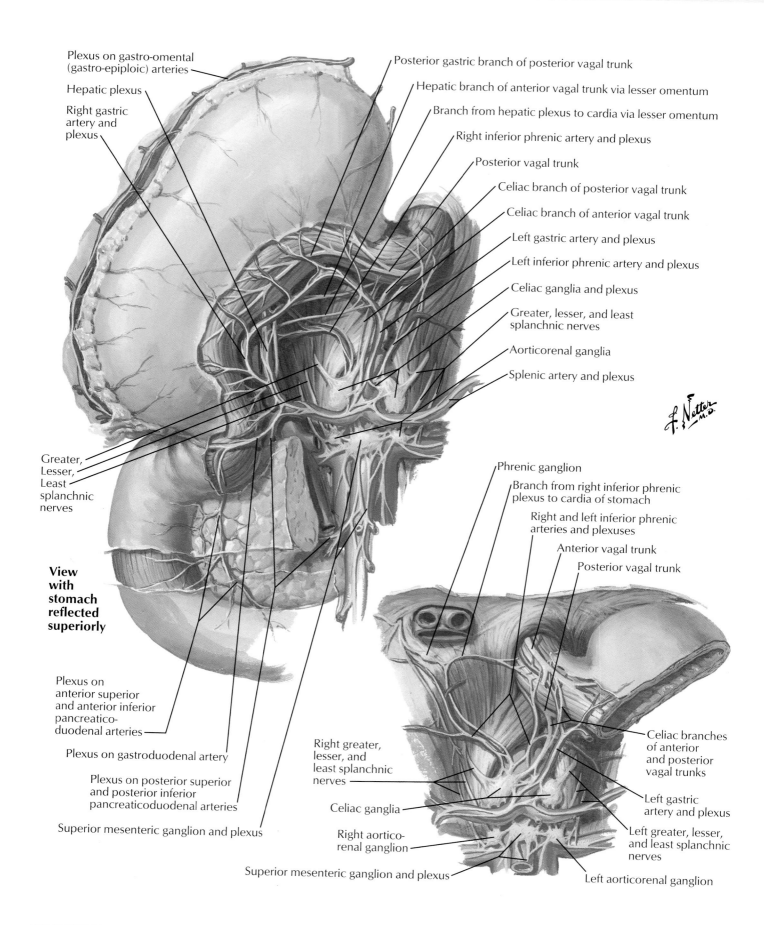

Plexus on gastro-omental (gastro-epiploic) arteries

Hepatic plexus

Right gastric artery and plexus

Posterior gastric branch of posterior vagal trunk

Hepatic branch of anterior vagal trunk via lesser omentum

Branch from hepatic plexus to cardia via lesser omentum

Right inferior phrenic artery and plexus

Posterior vagal trunk

Celiac branch of posterior vagal trunk

Celiac branch of anterior vagal trunk

Left gastric artery and plexus

Left inferior phrenic artery and plexus

Celiac ganglia and plexus

Greater, lesser, and least splanchnic nerves

Aorticorenal ganglia

Splenic artery and plexus

Greater, Lesser, Least splanchnic nerves

Phrenic ganglion

Branch from right inferior phrenic plexus to cardia of stomach

Right and left inferior phrenic arteries and plexuses

Anterior vagal trunk

Posterior vagal trunk

**View with stomach reflected superiorly**

Plexus on anterior superior and anterior inferior pancreaticoduodenal arteries

Plexus on gastroduodenal artery

Plexus on posterior superior and posterior inferior pancreaticoduodenal arteries

Superior mesenteric ganglion and plexus

Right greater, lesser, and least splanchnic nerves

Celiac ganglia

Right aorticorenal ganglion

Superior mesenteric ganglion and plexus

Celiac branches of anterior and posterior vagal trunks

Left gastric artery and plexus

Left greater, lesser, and least splanchnic nerves

Left aorticorenal ganglion

**Plate 299**

**Innervation**

Right 6th thoracic ganglion of sympathetic trunk

Gray, White rami communicantes

Spinal sensory (dorsal root) ganglion

Anterior (ventral) root of spinal nerve

Right greater splanchnic nerve

Right lesser splanchnic nerve

Celiac ganglia

Least splanchnic nerve

Common hepatic artery

Hepatic artery proper

Superior mesenteric ganglion

Aorticorenal ganglia

Right gastric artery

Right renal artery

Gastroduodenal artery

Posterior and anterior superior pancreatico-duodenal arteries

Superior mesenteric artery

Posterior and anterior inferior pancreatico-duodenal arteries

Esophageal plexus

Left greater splanchnic nerve

Aortic plexus

Left 9th thoracic ganglion of sympathetic trunk

Posterior vagal trunk and celiac branch

Anterior vagal trunk and celiac branch of vagus nerve (X)

Left gastric artery

Celiac trunk

Splenic artery

Short gastric arteries

Left, Right gastro-omental (gastro-epiploic) arteries

**Sympathetic fibers**
Preganglionic ———
Postganglionic - - - -

**Parasympathetic fibers**
Preganglionic ———
Postganglionic - - - -

Afferent fibers ———

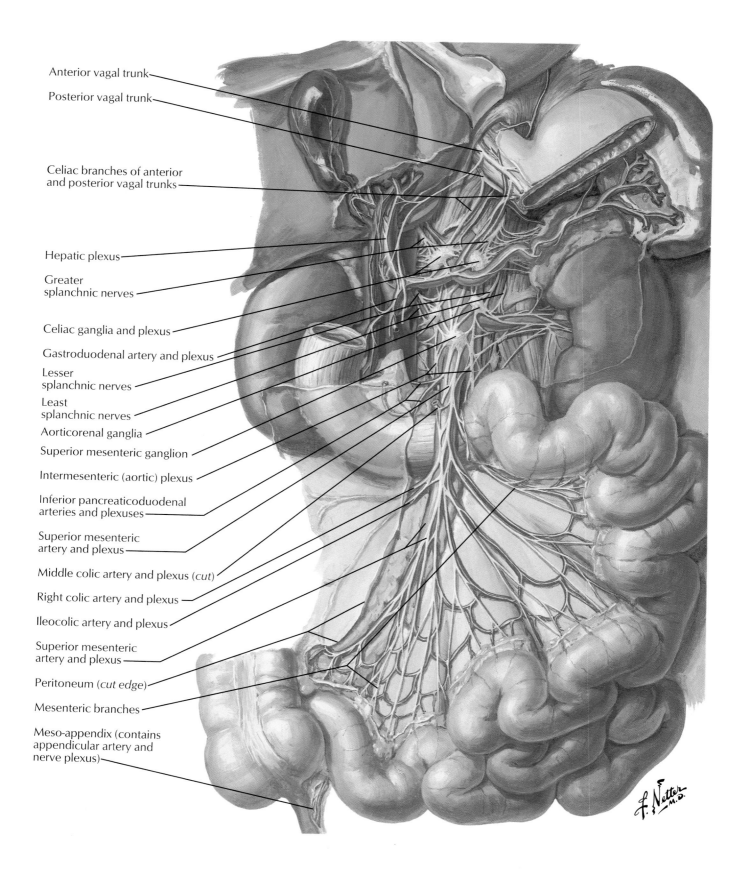

Anterior vagal trunk

Posterior vagal trunk

Celiac branches of anterior and posterior vagal trunks

Hepatic plexus

Greater splanchnic nerves

Celiac ganglia and plexus

Gastroduodenal artery and plexus

Lesser splanchnic nerves

Least splanchnic nerves

Aorticorenal ganglia

Superior mesenteric ganglion

Intermesenteric (aortic) plexus

Inferior pancreaticoduodenal arteries and plexuses

Superior mesenteric artery and plexus

Middle colic artery and plexus (cut)

Right colic artery and plexus

Ileocolic artery and plexus

Superior mesenteric artery and plexus

Peritoneum (cut edge)

Mesenteric branches

Meso-appendix (contains appendicular artery and nerve plexus)

**Plate 301**

**Innervation**

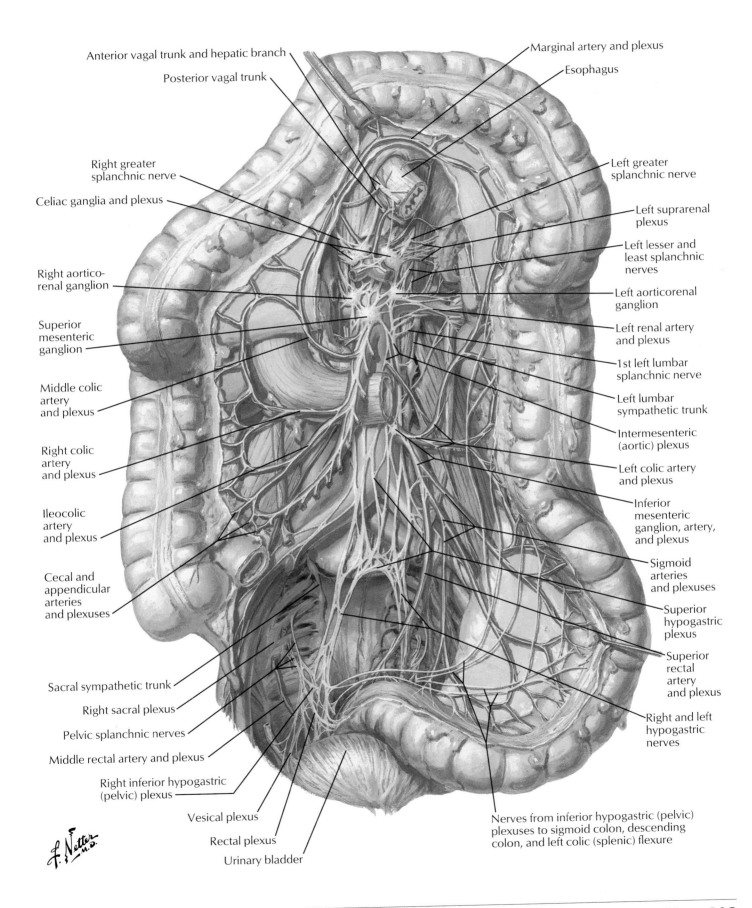

Anterior vagal trunk and hepatic branch

Posterior vagal trunk

Right greater splanchnic nerve

Celiac ganglia and plexus

Right aortico-renal ganglion

Superior mesenteric ganglion

Middle colic artery and plexus

Right colic artery and plexus

Ileocolic artery and plexus

Cecal and appendicular arteries and plexuses

Sacral sympathetic trunk

Right sacral plexus

Pelvic splanchnic nerves

Middle rectal artery and plexus

Right inferior hypogastric (pelvic) plexus

Vesical plexus

Rectal plexus

Urinary bladder

Marginal artery and plexus

Esophagus

Left greater splanchnic nerve

Left suprarenal plexus

Left lesser and least splanchnic nerves

Left aorticorenal ganglion

Left renal artery and plexus

1st left lumbar splanchnic nerve

Left lumbar sympathetic trunk

Intermesenteric (aortic) plexus

Left colic artery and plexus

Inferior mesenteric ganglion, artery, and plexus

Sigmoid arteries and plexuses

Superior hypogastric plexus

Superior rectal artery and plexus

Right and left hypogastric nerves

Nerves from inferior hypogastric (pelvic) plexuses to sigmoid colon, descending colon, and left colic (splenic) flexure

**Innervation**

**Plate 302**

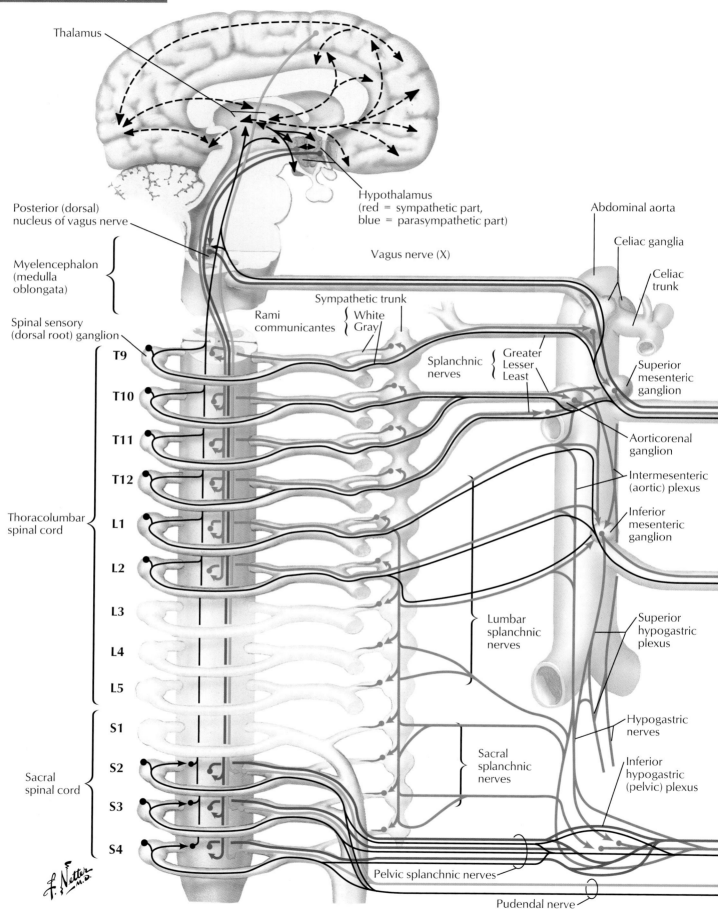

Thalamus

Hypothalamus
(red = sympathetic part,
blue = parasympathetic part)

Posterior (dorsal)
nucleus of vagus nerve

Vagus nerve (X)

Abdominal aorta

Celiac ganglia

Celiac trunk

Myelencephalon
(medulla
oblongata)

Sympathetic trunk

Rami
communicantes { White
Gray

Splanchnic
nerves { Greater
Lesser
Least

Spinal sensory
(dorsal root) ganglion

T9

Superior
mesenteric
ganglion

T10

T11

Aorticorenal
ganglion

T12

Intermesenteric
(aortic) plexus

Thoracolumbar
spinal cord

L1

Inferior
mesenteric
ganglion

L2

L3

Lumbar
splanchnic
nerves

Superior
hypogastric
plexus

L4

L5

S1

Hypogastric
nerves

Sacral
spinal cord

S2

Sacral
splanchnic
nerves

Inferior
hypogastric
(pelvic) plexus

S3

S4

Pelvic splanchnic nerves

Pudendal nerve

**Plate 303**

**Innervation**

Sympathetic efferents ——————
Parasympathetic efferents ——————
Somatic efferents ——————
Afferents and CNS connections ——————
Indefinite paths – – – – –

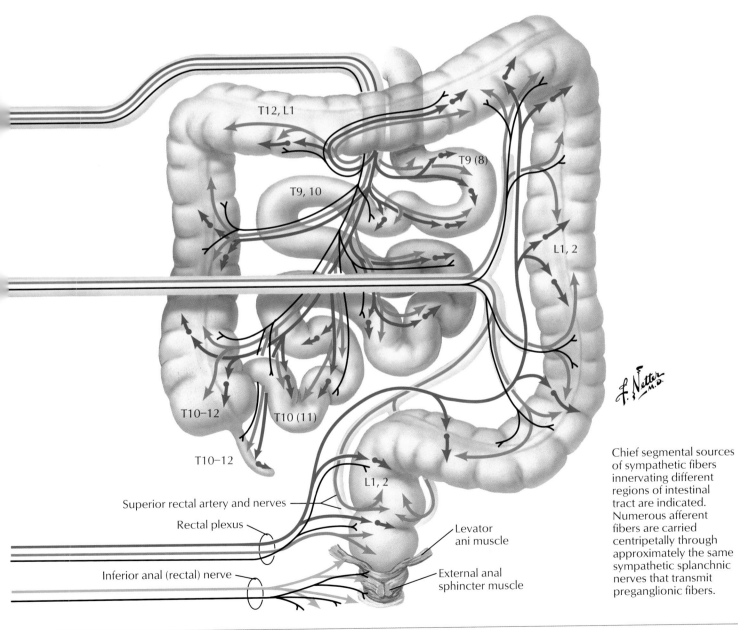

T12, L1

T9 (8)

T9, 10

L1, 2

T10–12

T10 (11)

T10–12

L1, 2

Superior rectal artery and nerves

Rectal plexus

Levator ani muscle

Inferior anal (rectal) nerve

External anal sphincter muscle

Chief segmental sources of sympathetic fibers innervating different regions of intestinal tract are indicated. Numerous afferent fibers are carried centripetally through approximately the same sympathetic splanchnic nerves that transmit preganglionic fibers.

**Innervation**

**Plate 303**

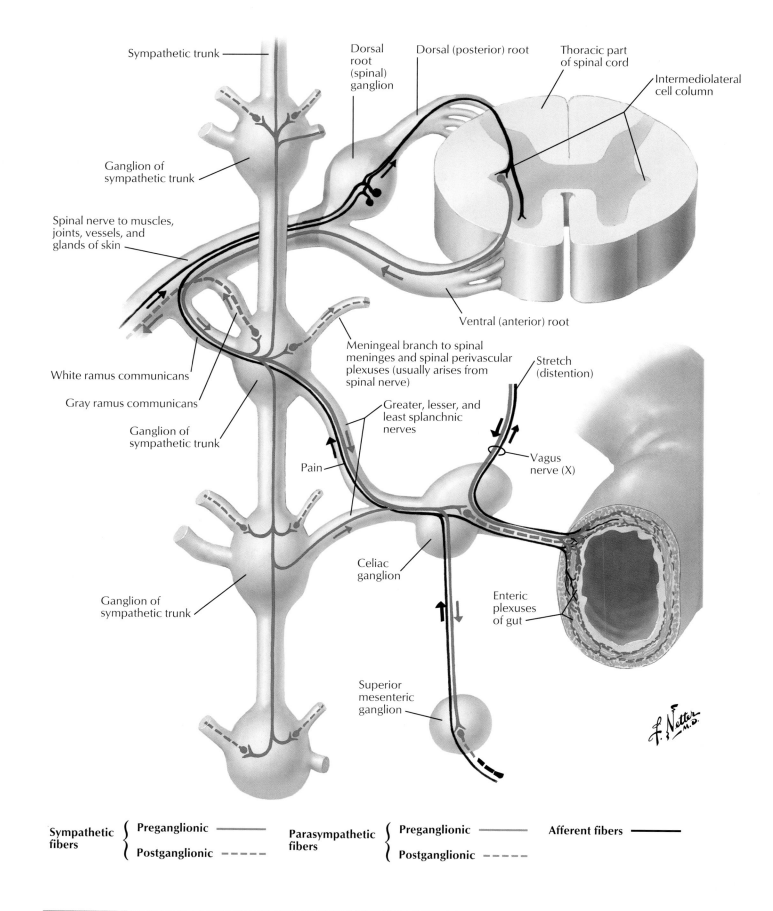

Sympathetic trunk

Dorsal root (spinal) ganglion

Dorsal (posterior) root

Thoracic part of spinal cord

Intermediolateral cell column

Ganglion of sympathetic trunk

Spinal nerve to muscles, joints, vessels, and glands of skin

White ramus communicans

Gray ramus communicans

Ganglion of sympathetic trunk

Ventral (anterior) root

Meningeal branch to spinal meninges and spinal perivascular plexuses (usually arises from spinal nerve)

Greater, lesser, and least splanchnic nerves

Stretch (distention)

Pain

Vagus nerve (X)

Ganglion of sympathetic trunk

Celiac ganglion

Enteric plexuses of gut

Superior mesenteric ganglion

| Sympathetic fibers | Preganglionic ——— | Parasympathetic fibers | Preganglionic ——— | Afferent fibers ——— |
|---|---|---|---|---|
| | Postganglionic - - - - | | Postganglionic - - - - | |

**Plate 304**

**Innervation**

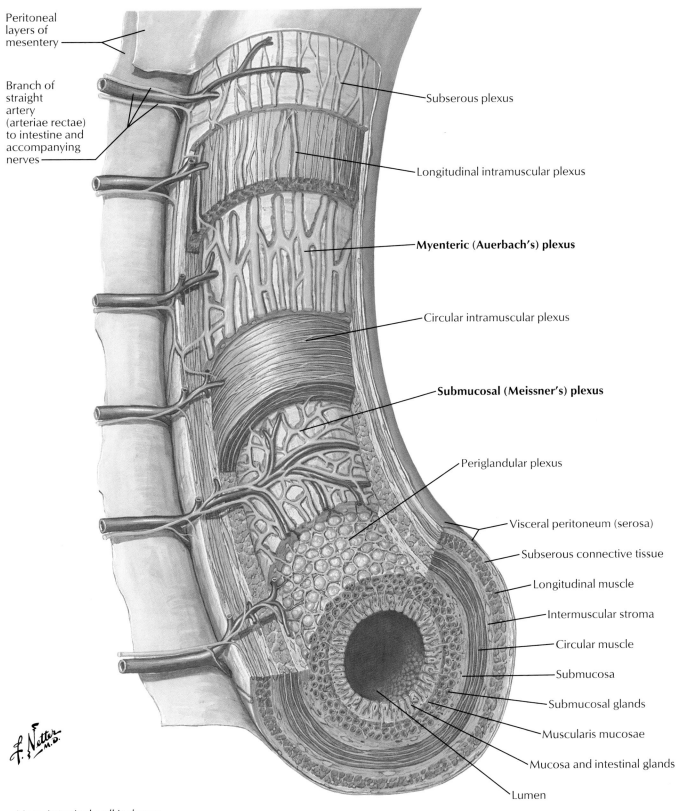

Peritoneal layers of mesentery

Branch of straight artery (arteriae rectae) to intestine and accompanying nerves

Subserous plexus

Longitudinal intramuscular plexus

**Myenteric (Auerbach's) plexus**

Circular intramuscular plexus

**Submucosal (Meissner's) plexus**

Periglandular plexus

Visceral peritoneum (serosa)

Subserous connective tissue

Longitudinal muscle

Intermuscular stroma

Circular muscle

Submucosa

Submucosal glands

Muscularis mucosae

Mucosa and intestinal glands

Lumen

*Note: Intestinal wall is shown much thicker than in actuality.*

**Innervation**

**Plate 305**

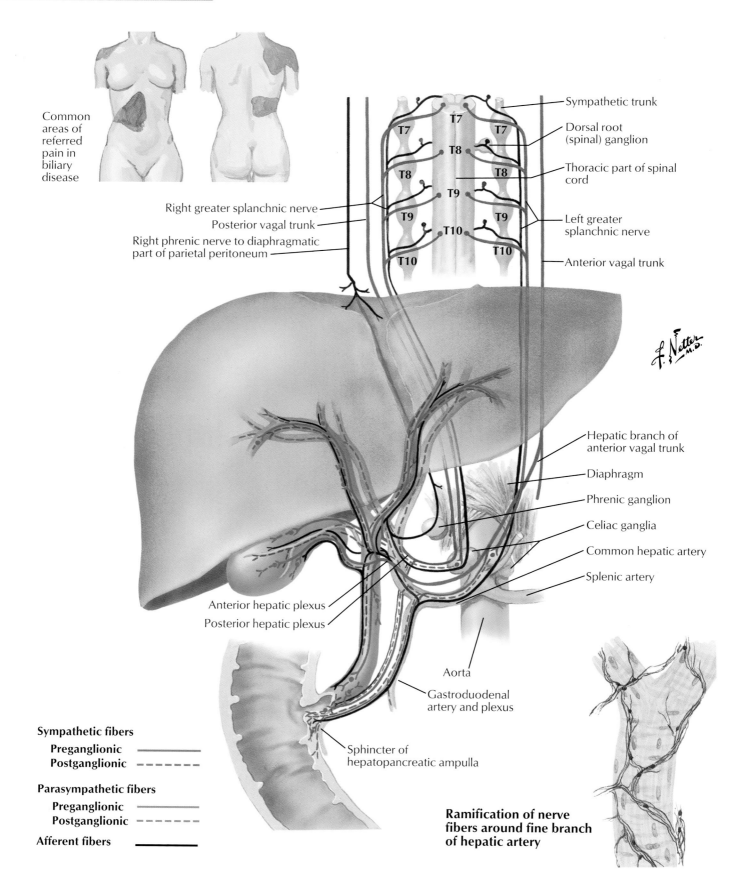

Common areas of referred pain in biliary disease

Sympathetic trunk

Dorsal root (spinal) ganglion

Thoracic part of spinal cord

Right greater splanchnic nerve

Posterior vagal trunk

Right phrenic nerve to diaphragmatic part of parietal peritoneum

Left greater splanchnic nerve

Anterior vagal trunk

Hepatic branch of anterior vagal trunk

Diaphragm

Phrenic ganglion

Celiac ganglia

Common hepatic artery

Splenic artery

Anterior hepatic plexus

Posterior hepatic plexus

Aorta

Gastroduodenal artery and plexus

Sphincter of hepatopancreatic ampulla

**Sympathetic fibers**

Preganglionic

Postganglionic

**Parasympathetic fibers**

Preganglionic

Postganglionic

**Afferent fibers**

**Ramification of nerve fibers around fine branch of hepatic artery**

**Plate 306**

**Innervation**

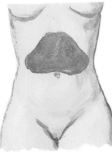

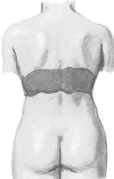

Common areas of
pancreatic pain

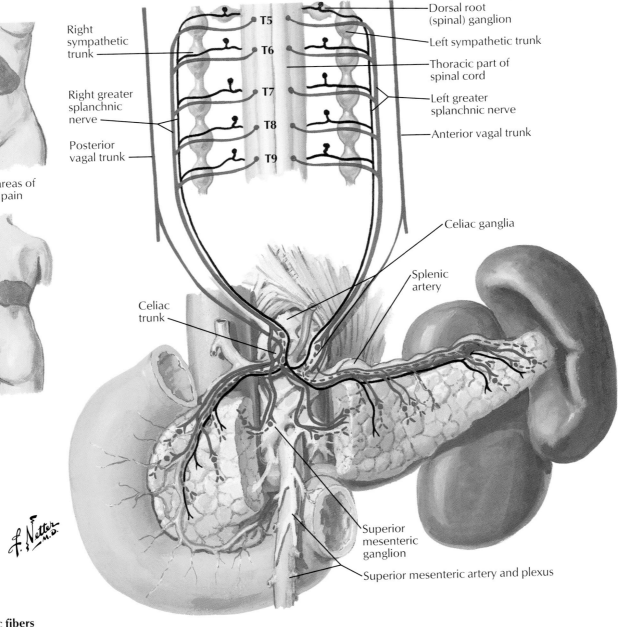

Right
sympathetic
trunk

Right greater
splanchnic
nerve

Posterior
vagal trunk

T5
T6
T7
T8
T9

Dorsal root
(spinal) ganglion

Left sympathetic trunk

Thoracic part of
spinal cord

Left greater
splanchnic nerve

Anterior vagal trunk

Celiac ganglia

Splenic
artery

Celiac
trunk

Superior
mesenteric
ganglion

Superior mesenteric artery and plexus

**Sympathetic fibers**

Preganglionic ———————

Postganglionic - - - - - - - -

**Parasympathetic fibers**

Preganglionic ———————

Postganglionic - - - - - - - -

**Afferent fibers** ———————

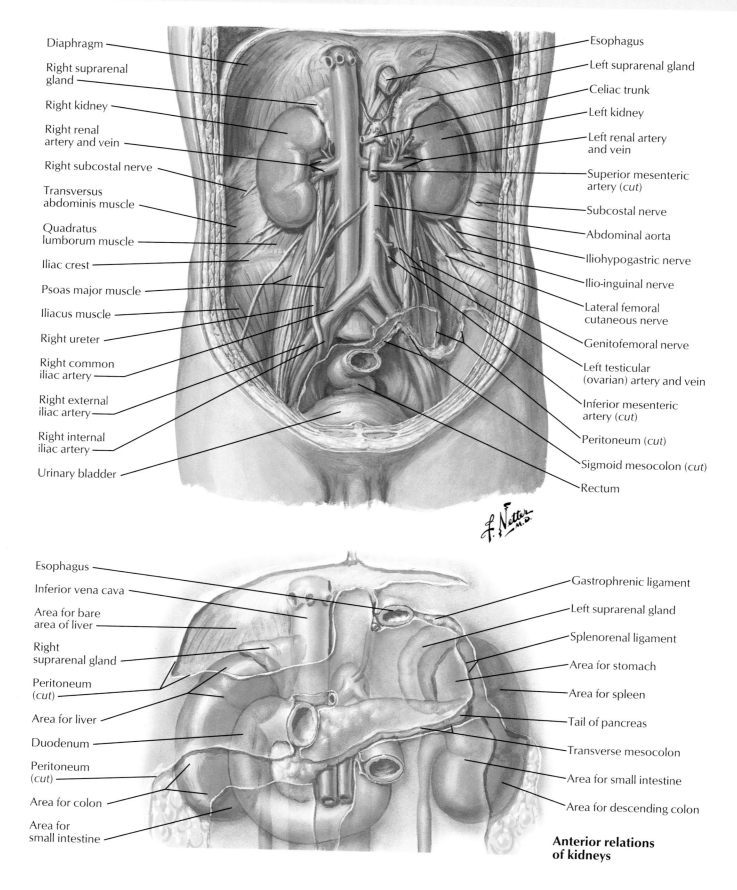

Diaphragm

Right suprarenal gland

Right kidney

Right renal artery and vein

Right subcostal nerve

Transversus abdominis muscle

Quadratus lumborum muscle

Iliac crest

Psoas major muscle

Iliacus muscle

Right ureter

Right common iliac artery

Right external iliac artery

Right internal iliac artery

Urinary bladder

Esophagus

Left suprarenal gland

Celiac trunk

Left kidney

Left renal artery and vein

Superior mesenteric artery (cut)

Subcostal nerve

Abdominal aorta

Iliohypogastric nerve

Ilio-inguinal nerve

Lateral femoral cutaneous nerve

Genitofemoral nerve

Left testicular (ovarian) artery and vein

Inferior mesenteric artery (cut)

Peritoneum (cut)

Sigmoid mesocolon (cut)

Rectum

Esophagus

Inferior vena cava

Area for bare area of liver

Right suprarenal gland

Peritoneum (cut)

Area for liver

Duodenum

Peritoneum (cut)

Area for colon

Area for small intestine

Gastrophrenic ligament

Left suprarenal gland

Splenorenal ligament

Area for stomach

Area for spleen

Tail of pancreas

Transverse mesocolon

Area for small intestine

Area for descending colon

**Anterior relations of kidneys**

**Plate 308**

**Kidneys and Suprarenal Glands**

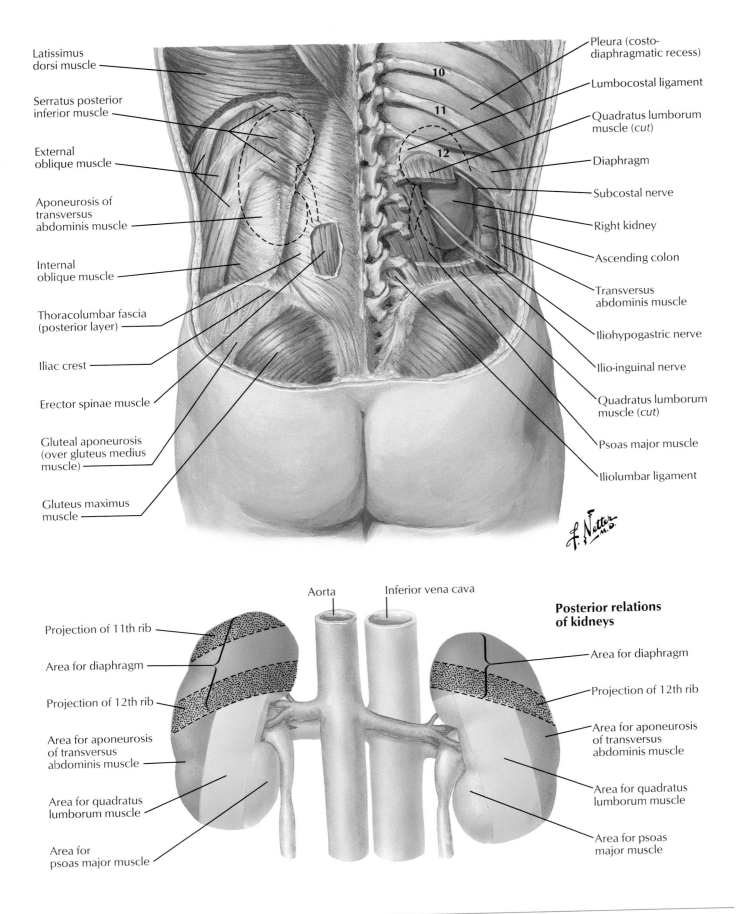

Latissimus dorsi muscle

Serratus posterior inferior muscle

External oblique muscle

Aponeurosis of transversus abdominis muscle

Internal oblique muscle

Thoracolumbar fascia (posterior layer)

Iliac crest

Erector spinae muscle

Gluteal aponeurosis (over gluteus medius muscle)

Gluteus maximus muscle

Pleura (costo-diaphragmatic recess)

Lumbocostal ligament

Quadratus lumborum muscle (cut)

Diaphragm

Subcostal nerve

Right kidney

Ascending colon

Transversus abdominis muscle

Iliohypogastric nerve

Ilio-inguinal nerve

Quadratus lumborum muscle (cut)

Psoas major muscle

Iliolumbar ligament

10

11

12

Aorta

Inferior vena cava

**Posterior relations of kidneys**

Projection of 11th rib

Area for diaphragm

Projection of 12th rib

Area for aponeurosis of transversus abdominis muscle

Area for quadratus lumborum muscle

Area for psoas major muscle

Area for diaphragm

Projection of 12th rib

Area for aponeurosis of transversus abdominis muscle

Area for quadratus lumborum muscle

Area for psoas major muscle

**Kidneys and Suprarenal Glands**

**Plate 309**

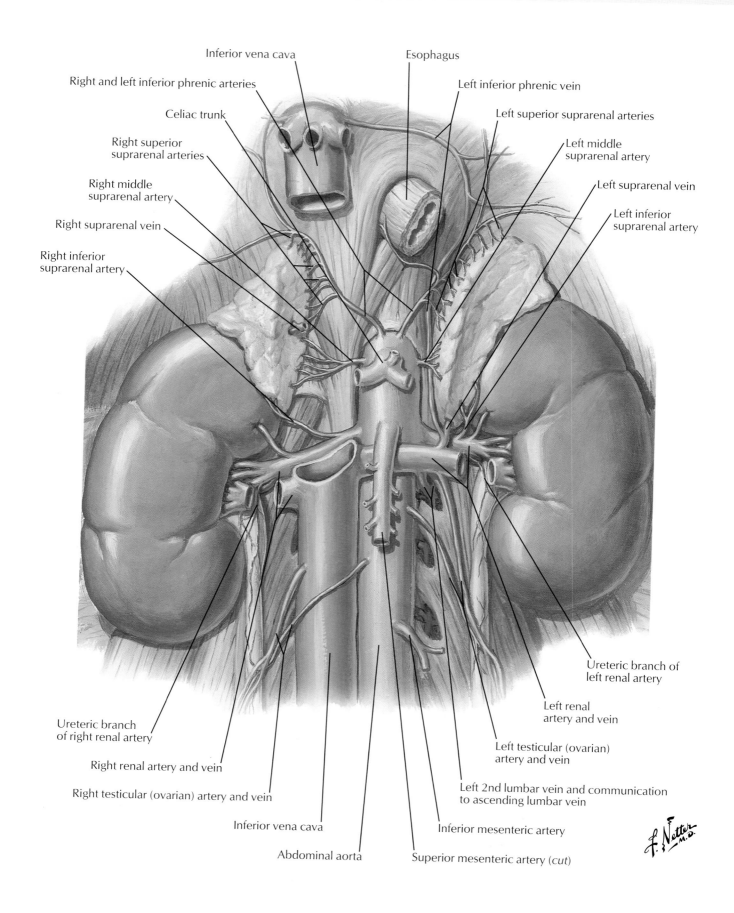

Inferior vena cava

Esophagus

Right and left inferior phrenic arteries

Left inferior phrenic vein

Celiac trunk

Left superior suprarenal arteries

Right superior suprarenal arteries

Left middle suprarenal artery

Right middle suprarenal artery

Left suprarenal vein

Right suprarenal vein

Left inferior suprarenal artery

Right inferior suprarenal artery

Ureteric branch of left renal artery

Left renal artery and vein

Left testicular (ovarian) artery and vein

Ureteric branch of right renal artery

Left 2nd lumbar vein and communication to ascending lumbar vein

Right renal artery and vein

Right testicular (ovarian) artery and vein

Inferior vena cava

Inferior mesenteric artery

Abdominal aorta

Superior mesenteric artery (cut)

**Plate 310**

**Kidneys and Suprarenal Glands**

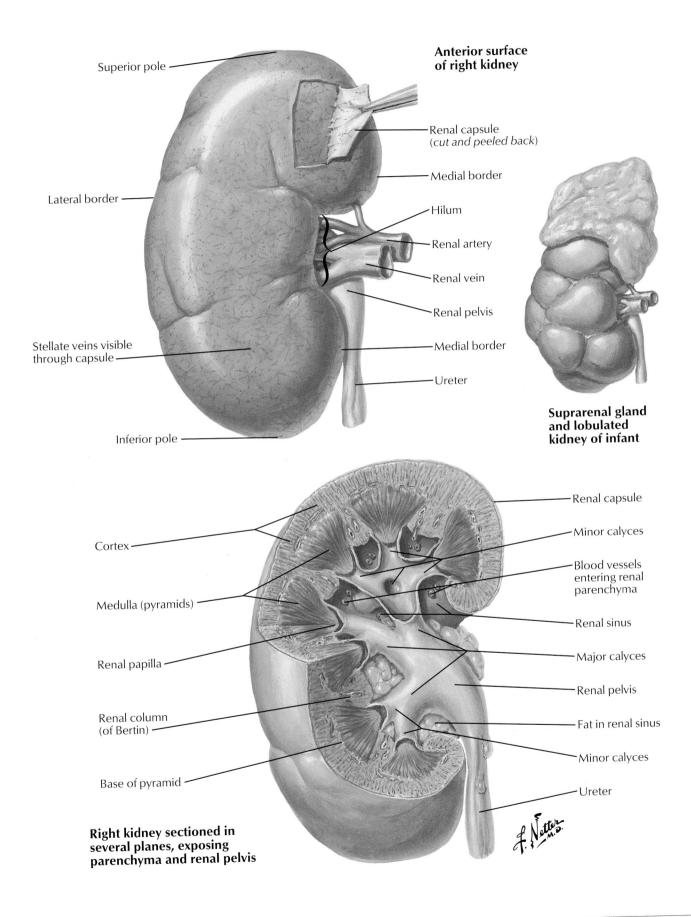

**Anterior surface
of right kidney**

Superior pole

Renal capsule
(*cut and peeled back*)

Lateral border

Medial border

Hilum

Renal artery

Renal vein

Renal pelvis

Stellate veins visible
through capsule

Medial border

Ureter

Inferior pole

**Suprarenal gland
and lobulated
kidney of infant**

Renal capsule

Minor calyces

Cortex

Blood vessels
entering renal
parenchyma

Medulla (pyramids)

Renal sinus

Major calyces

Renal papilla

Renal pelvis

Fat in renal sinus

Renal column
(of Bertin)

Minor calyces

Base of pyramid

Ureter

**Right kidney sectioned in
several planes, exposing
parenchyma and renal pelvis**

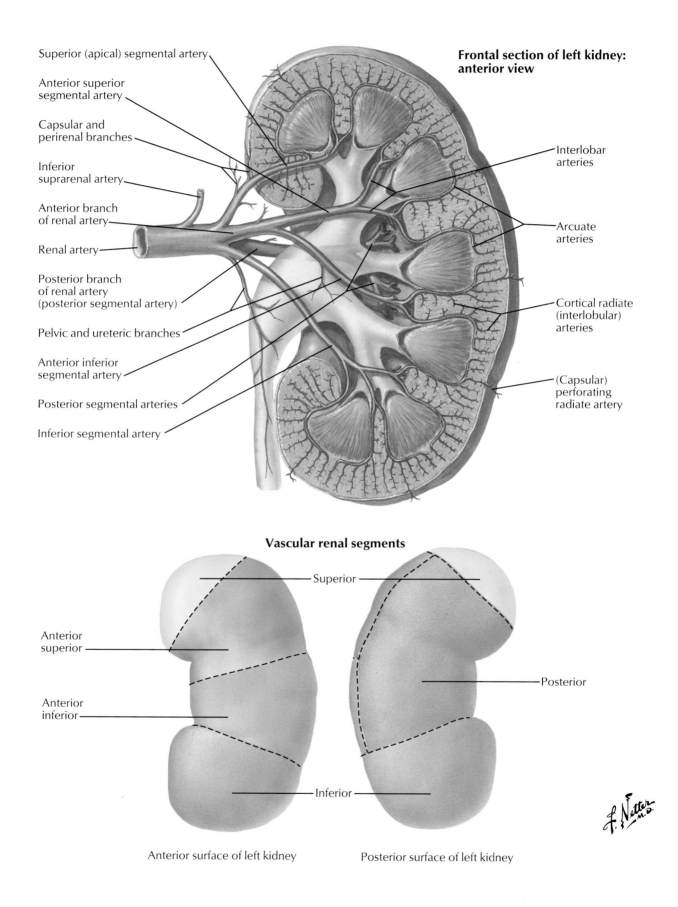

Superior (apical) segmental artery

Anterior superior segmental artery

Capsular and perirenal branches

Inferior suprarenal artery

Anterior branch of renal artery

Renal artery

Posterior branch of renal artery (posterior segmental artery)

Pelvic and ureteric branches

Anterior inferior segmental artery

Posterior segmental arteries

Inferior segmental artery

**Frontal section of left kidney: anterior view**

Interlobar arteries

Arcuate arteries

Cortical radiate (interlobular) arteries

(Capsular) perforating radiate artery

**Vascular renal segments**

Superior

Anterior superior

Anterior inferior

Posterior

Inferior

Anterior surface of left kidney

Posterior surface of left kidney

**Plate 312**

**Kidneys and Suprarenal Glands**

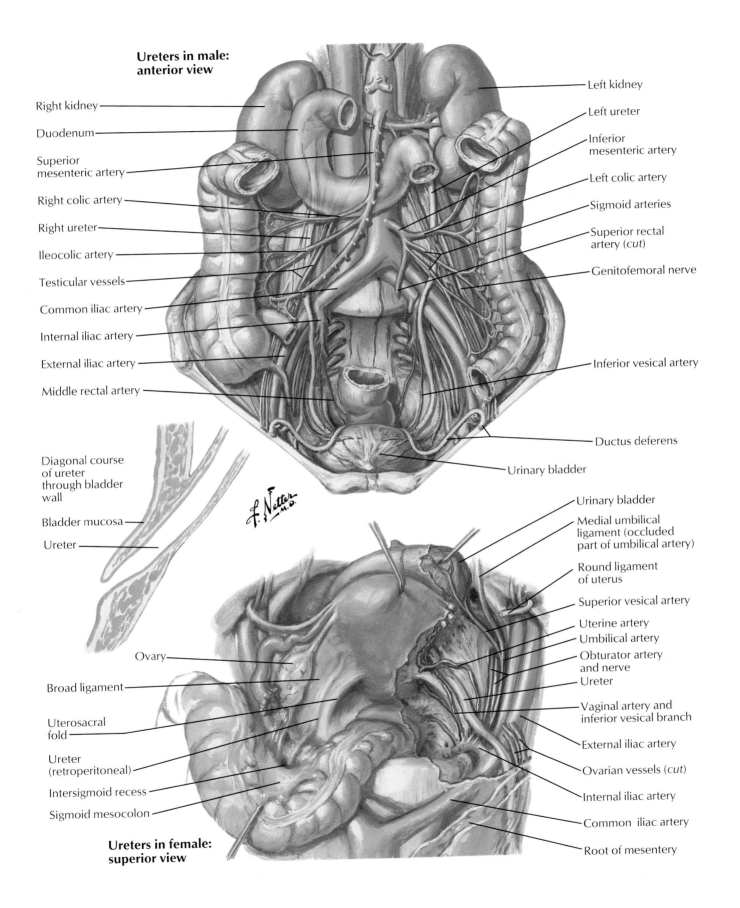

**Ureters in male: anterior view**

Right kidney

Duodenum

Superior mesenteric artery

Right colic artery

Right ureter

Ileocolic artery

Testicular vessels

Common iliac artery

Internal iliac artery

External iliac artery

Middle rectal artery

Left kidney

Left ureter

Inferior mesenteric artery

Left colic artery

Sigmoid arteries

Superior rectal artery (cut)

Genitofemoral nerve

Inferior vesical artery

Ductus deferens

Urinary bladder

Diagonal course of ureter through bladder wall

Bladder mucosa

Ureter

Urinary bladder

Medial umbilical ligament (occluded part of umbilical artery)

Round ligament of uterus

Superior vesical artery

Uterine artery

Umbilical artery

Obturator artery and nerve

Ureter

Vaginal artery and inferior vesical branch

External iliac artery

Ovarian vessels (cut)

Internal iliac artery

Common iliac artery

Root of mesentery

Ovary

Broad ligament

Uterosacral fold

Ureter (retroperitoneal)

Intersigmoid recess

Sigmoid mesocolon

**Ureters in female: superior view**

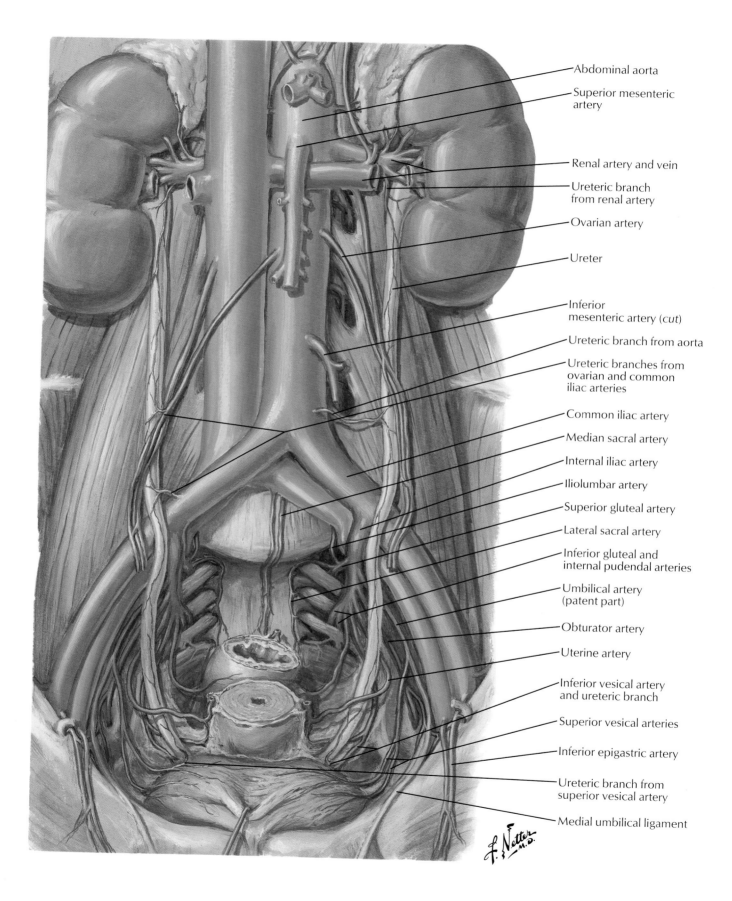

Abdominal aorta

Superior mesenteric artery

Renal artery and vein

Ureteric branch from renal artery

Ovarian artery

Ureter

Inferior mesenteric artery (*cut*)

Ureteric branch from aorta

Ureteric branches from ovarian and common iliac arteries

Common iliac artery

Median sacral artery

Internal iliac artery

Iliolumbar artery

Superior gluteal artery

Lateral sacral artery

Inferior gluteal and internal pudendal arteries

Umbilical artery (patent part)

Obturator artery

Uterine artery

Inferior vesical artery and ureteric branch

Superior vesical arteries

Inferior epigastric artery

Ureteric branch from superior vesical artery

Medial umbilical ligament

**Plate 314**

**Kidneys and Suprarenal Glands**

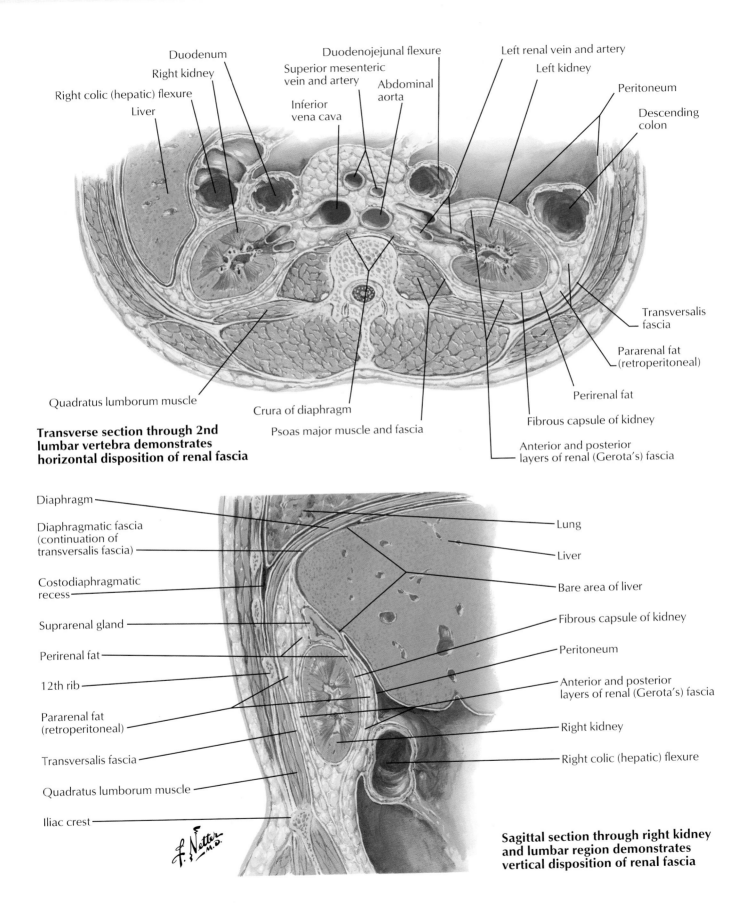

Duodenum
Right kidney
Right colic (hepatic) flexure
Liver
Duodenojejunal flexure
Superior mesenteric vein and artery
Inferior vena cava
Abdominal aorta
Left renal vein and artery
Left kidney
Peritoneum
Descending colon

Transversalis fascia
Pararenal fat (retroperitoneal)
Perirenal fat
Fibrous capsule of kidney
Anterior and posterior layers of renal (Gerota's) fascia

Quadratus lumborum muscle
Crura of diaphragm
Psoas major muscle and fascia

**Transverse section through 2nd lumbar vertebra demonstrates horizontal disposition of renal fascia**

Diaphragm
Diaphragmatic fascia (continuation of transversalis fascia)
Costodiaphragmatic recess
Suprarenal gland
Perirenal fat
12th rib
Pararenal fat (retroperitoneal)
Transversalis fascia
Quadratus lumborum muscle
Iliac crest

Lung
Liver
Bare area of liver
Fibrous capsule of kidney
Peritoneum
Anterior and posterior layers of renal (Gerota's) fascia
Right kidney
Right colic (hepatic) flexure

**Sagittal section through right kidney and lumbar region demonstrates vertical disposition of renal fascia**

**Kidneys and Suprarenal Glands**

**Plate 315**

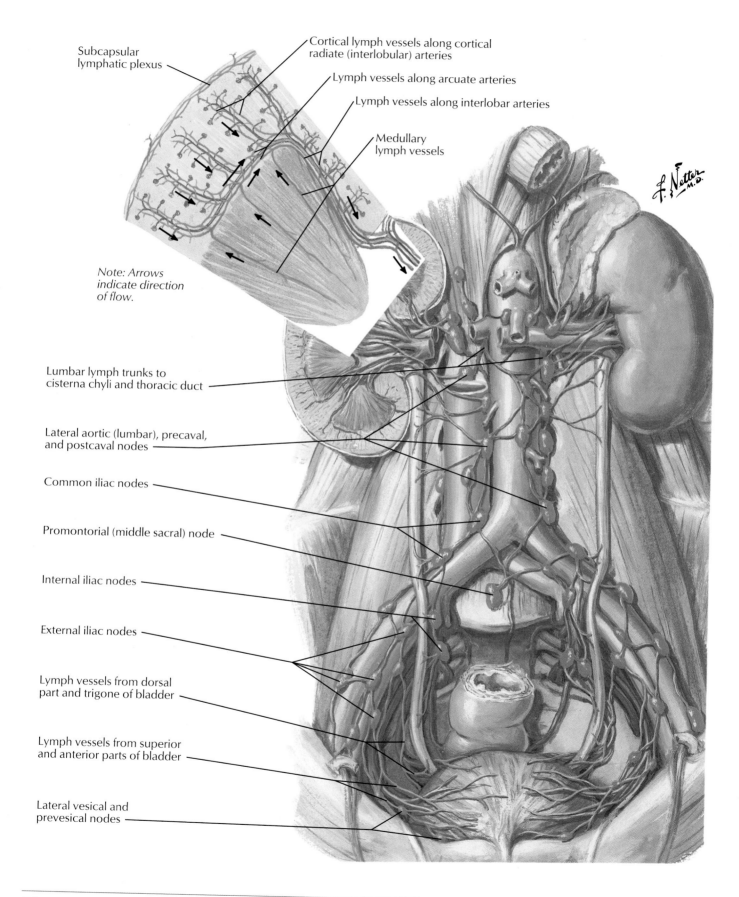

Subcapsular lymphatic plexus

Cortical lymph vessels along cortical radiate (interlobular) arteries

Lymph vessels along arcuate arteries

Lymph vessels along interlobar arteries

Medullary lymph vessels

*Note: Arrows indicate direction of flow.*

Lumbar lymph trunks to cisterna chyli and thoracic duct

Lateral aortic (lumbar), precaval, and postcaval nodes

Common iliac nodes

Promontorial (middle sacral) node

Internal iliac nodes

External iliac nodes

Lymph vessels from dorsal part and trigone of bladder

Lymph vessels from superior and anterior parts of bladder

Lateral vesical and prevesical nodes

**Plate 316**

**Kidneys and Suprarenal Glands**

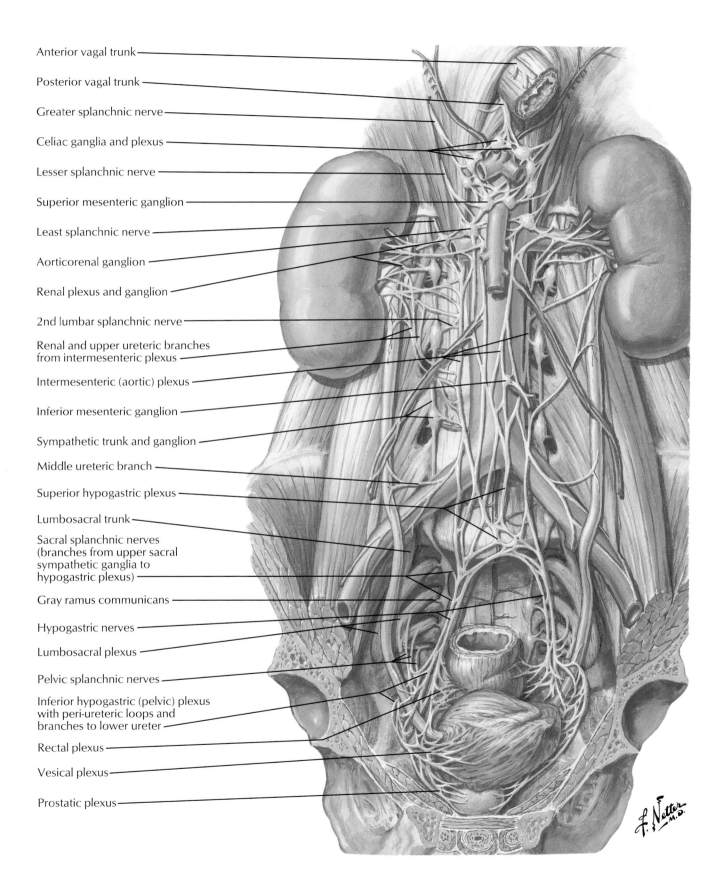

Anterior vagal trunk

Posterior vagal trunk

Greater splanchnic nerve

Celiac ganglia and plexus

Lesser splanchnic nerve

Superior mesenteric ganglion

Least splanchnic nerve

Aorticorenal ganglion

Renal plexus and ganglion

2nd lumbar splanchnic nerve

Renal and upper ureteric branches from intermesenteric plexus

Intermesenteric (aortic) plexus

Inferior mesenteric ganglion

Sympathetic trunk and ganglion

Middle ureteric branch

Superior hypogastric plexus

Lumbosacral trunk

Sacral splanchnic nerves (branches from upper sacral sympathetic ganglia to hypogastric plexus)

Gray ramus communicans

Hypogastric nerves

Lumbosacral plexus

Pelvic splanchnic nerves

Inferior hypogastric (pelvic) plexus with peri-ureteric loops and branches to lower ureter

Rectal plexus

Vesical plexus

Prostatic plexus

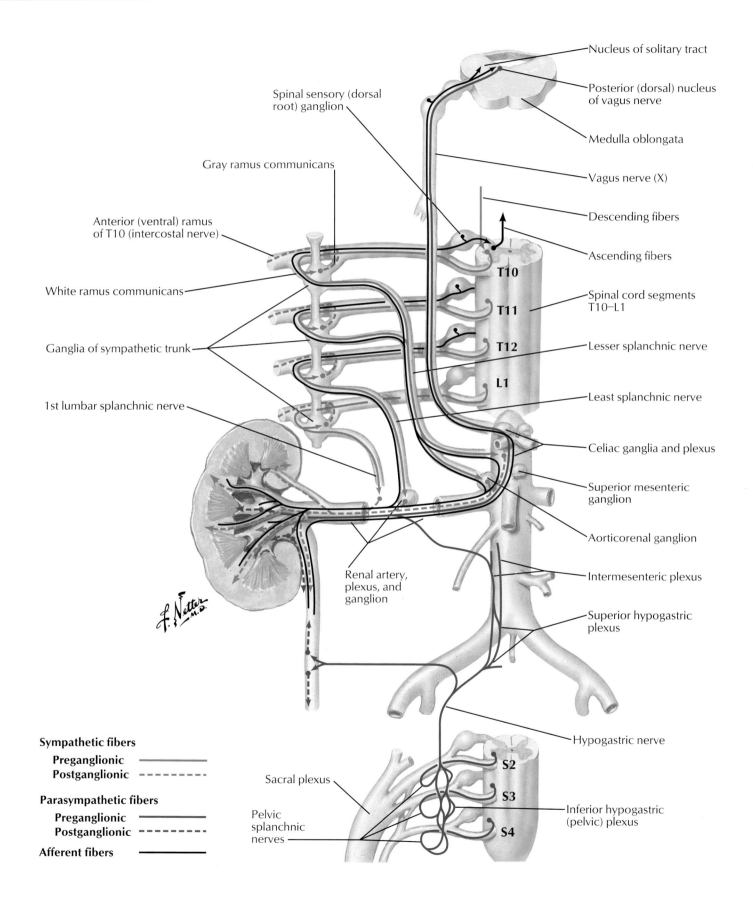

Nucleus of solitary tract

Spinal sensory (dorsal root) ganglion

Posterior (dorsal) nucleus of vagus nerve

Medulla oblongata

Gray ramus communicans

Vagus nerve (X)

Anterior (ventral) ramus of T10 (intercostal nerve)

Descending fibers

Ascending fibers

White ramus communicans

T10

T11

Spinal cord segments T10–L1

Ganglia of sympathetic trunk

T12

Lesser splanchnic nerve

L1

Least splanchnic nerve

1st lumbar splanchnic nerve

Celiac ganglia and plexus

Superior mesenteric ganglion

Aorticorenal ganglion

Renal artery, plexus, and ganglion

Intermesenteric plexus

Superior hypogastric plexus

Hypogastric nerve

**Sympathetic fibers**
 **Preganglionic** ———
 **Postganglionic** ------

**Parasympathetic fibers**
 **Preganglionic** ———
 **Postganglionic** ------

**Afferent fibers** ———

Sacral plexus

Pelvic splanchnic nerves

S2

S3

S4

Inferior hypogastric (pelvic) plexus

**Plate 318**

**Kidneys and Suprarenal Glands**

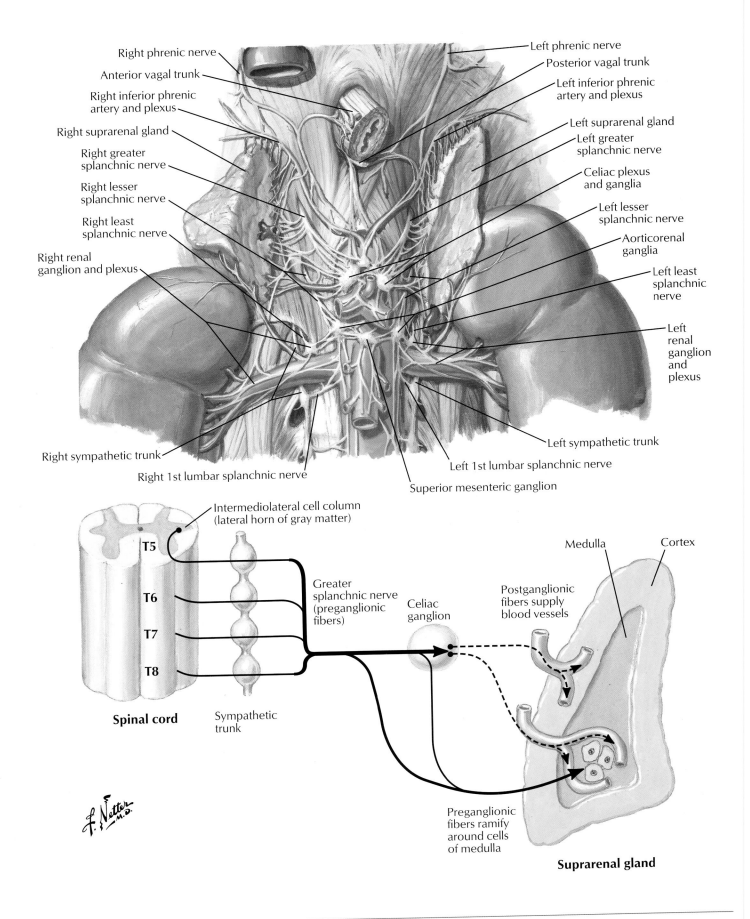

Right phrenic nerve

Anterior vagal trunk

Right inferior phrenic artery and plexus

Right suprarenal gland

Right greater splanchnic nerve

Right lesser splanchnic nerve

Right least splanchnic nerve

Right renal ganglion and plexus

Right sympathetic trunk

Right 1st lumbar splanchnic nerve

Left phrenic nerve

Posterior vagal trunk

Left inferior phrenic artery and plexus

Left suprarenal gland

Left greater splanchnic nerve

Celiac plexus and ganglia

Left lesser splanchnic nerve

Aorticorenal ganglia

Left least splanchnic nerve

Left renal ganglion and plexus

Left sympathetic trunk

Left 1st lumbar splanchnic nerve

Superior mesenteric ganglion

Intermediolateral cell column (lateral horn of gray matter)

Medulla

Cortex

**T5**

**T6**

**T7**

**T8**

Greater splanchnic nerve (preganglionic fibers)

Celiac ganglion

Postganglionic fibers supply blood vessels

**Spinal cord**

Sympathetic trunk

Preganglionic fibers ramify around cells of medulla

**Suprarenal gland**

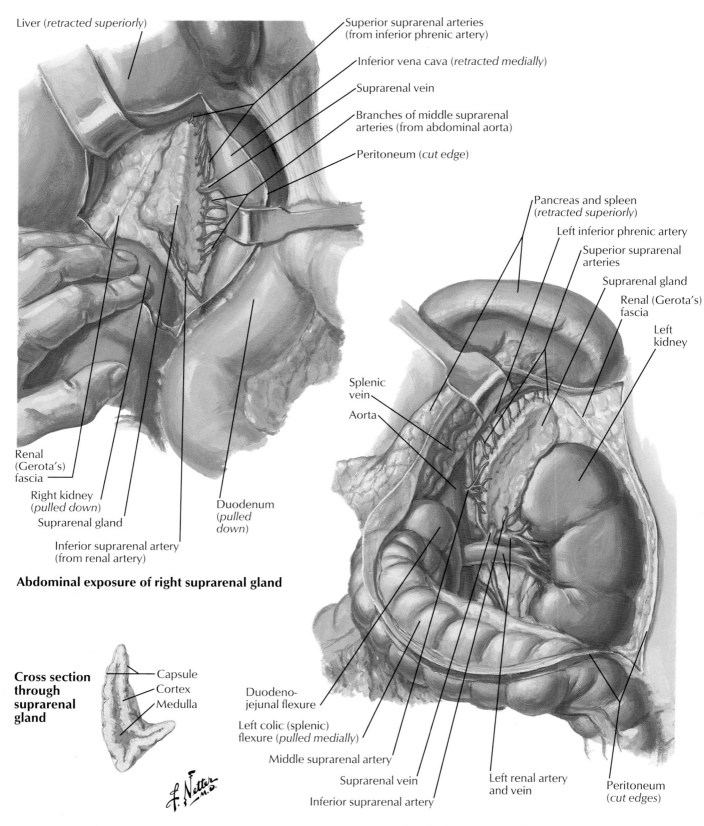

Liver (retracted superiorly)

Superior suprarenal arteries (from inferior phrenic artery)

Inferior vena cava (retracted medially)

Suprarenal vein

Branches of middle suprarenal arteries (from abdominal aorta)

Peritoneum (cut edge)

Pancreas and spleen (retracted superiorly)

Left inferior phrenic artery

Superior suprarenal arteries

Suprarenal gland

Renal (Gerota's) fascia

Left kidney

Splenic vein

Aorta

Renal (Gerota's) fascia

Right kidney (pulled down)

Suprarenal gland

Inferior suprarenal artery (from renal artery)

Duodenum (pulled down)

**Abdominal exposure of right suprarenal gland**

**Cross section through suprarenal gland**

Capsule

Cortex

Medulla

Duodeno-jejunal flexure

Left colic (splenic) flexure (pulled medially)

Middle suprarenal artery

Suprarenal vein

Inferior suprarenal artery

Left renal artery and vein

Peritoneum (cut edges)

**Abdominal exposure of left suprarenal gland**

**Plate 320**

**Kidneys and Suprarenal Glands**

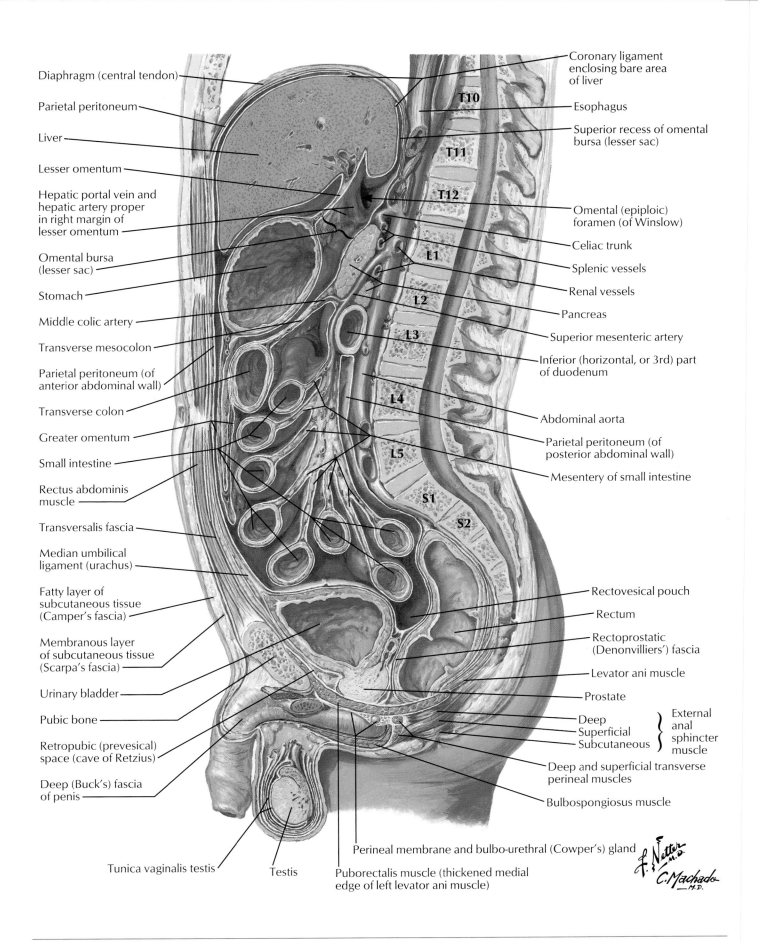

Diaphragm (central tendon)

Parietal peritoneum

Liver

Lesser omentum

Hepatic portal vein and hepatic artery proper in right margin of lesser omentum

Omental bursa (lesser sac)

Stomach

Middle colic artery

Transverse mesocolon

Parietal peritoneum (of anterior abdominal wall)

Transverse colon

Greater omentum

Small intestine

Rectus abdominis muscle

Transversalis fascia

Median umbilical ligament (urachus)

Fatty layer of subcutaneous tissue (Camper's fascia)

Membranous layer of subcutaneous tissue (Scarpa's fascia)

Urinary bladder

Pubic bone

Retropubic (prevesical) space (cave of Retzius)

Deep (Buck's) fascia of penis

Tunica vaginalis testis

Testis

Coronary ligament enclosing bare area of liver

Esophagus

Superior recess of omental bursa (lesser sac)

T10

T11

T12

Omental (epiploic) foramen (of Winslow)

L1

Celiac trunk

Splenic vessels

Renal vessels

L2

Pancreas

Superior mesenteric artery

L3

Inferior (horizontal, or 3rd) part of duodenum

L4

Abdominal aorta

Parietal peritoneum (of posterior abdominal wall)

L5

Mesentery of small intestine

S1

S2

Rectovesical pouch

Rectum

Rectoprostatic (Denonvilliers') fascia

Levator ani muscle

Prostate

Deep
Superficial
Subcutaneous

} External anal sphincter muscle

Deep and superficial transverse perineal muscles

Bulbospongiosus muscle

Perineal membrane and bulbo-urethral (Cowper's) gland

Puborectalis muscle (thickened medial edge of left levator ani muscle)

**Series of abdominal axial CT images from superior (A) to inferior (C)**

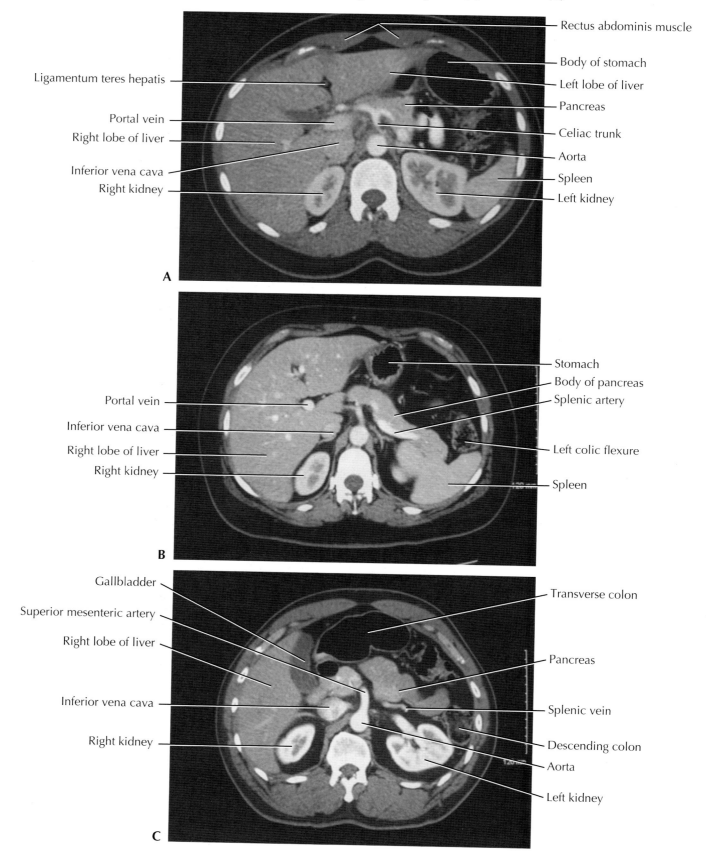

A

Rectus abdominis muscle

Body of stomach

Ligamentum teres hepatis — Left lobe of liver

Pancreas

Portal vein — Celiac trunk

Right lobe of liver — Aorta

Inferior vena cava — Spleen

Right kidney — Left kidney

B

Stomach

Body of pancreas

Portal vein — Splenic artery

Inferior vena cava —

Right lobe of liver — Left colic flexure

Right kidney —

Spleen

C

Gallbladder — Transverse colon

Superior mesenteric artery —

Right lobe of liver —

Pancreas

Inferior vena cava —

Splenic vein

Right kidney —

Descending colon

Aorta

Left kidney

**Plate 322**

**Sectional Anatomy**

Series of abdominal axial CT images from superior (D) to inferior (E)

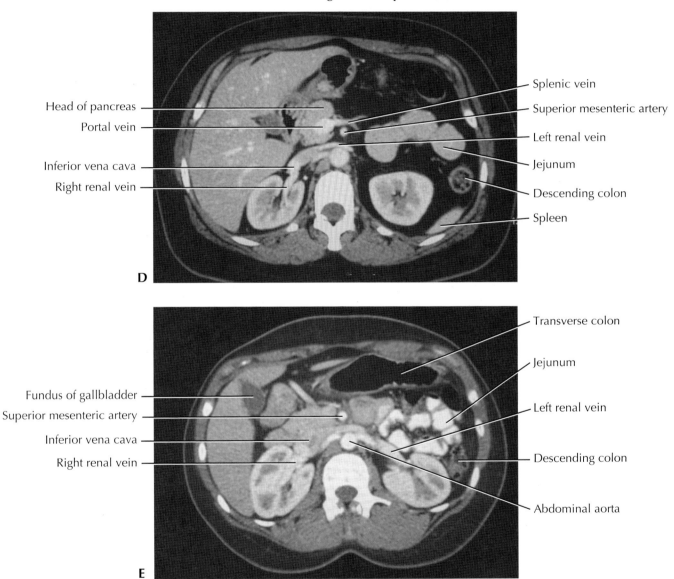

**D**

Head of pancreas

Portal vein

Inferior vena cava

Right renal vein

Splenic vein

Superior mesenteric artery

Left renal vein

Jejunum

Descending colon

Spleen

**E**

Fundus of gallbladder

Superior mesenteric artery

Inferior vena cava

Right renal vein

Transverse colon

Jejunum

Left renal vein

Descending colon

Abdominal aorta

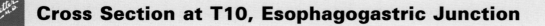

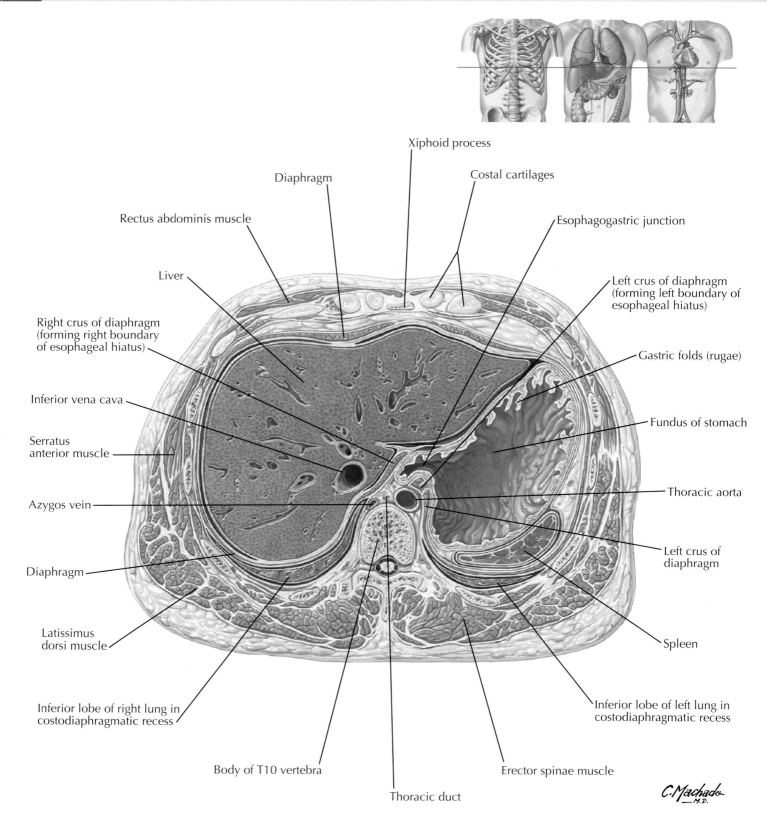

Xiphoid process

Diaphragm

Costal cartilages

Rectus abdominis muscle

Esophagogastric junction

Liver

Left crus of diaphragm (forming left boundary of esophageal hiatus)

Right crus of diaphragm (forming right boundary of esophageal hiatus)

Gastric folds (rugae)

Inferior vena cava

Fundus of stomach

Serratus anterior muscle

Thoracic aorta

Azygos vein

Left crus of diaphragm

Diaphragm

Latissimus dorsi muscle

Spleen

Inferior lobe of right lung in costodiaphragmatic recess

Inferior lobe of left lung in costodiaphragmatic recess

Body of T10 vertebra

Erector spinae muscle

Thoracic duct

C. Machado
—M.D.

**Plate 324**

**Cross-Sectional Anatomy**

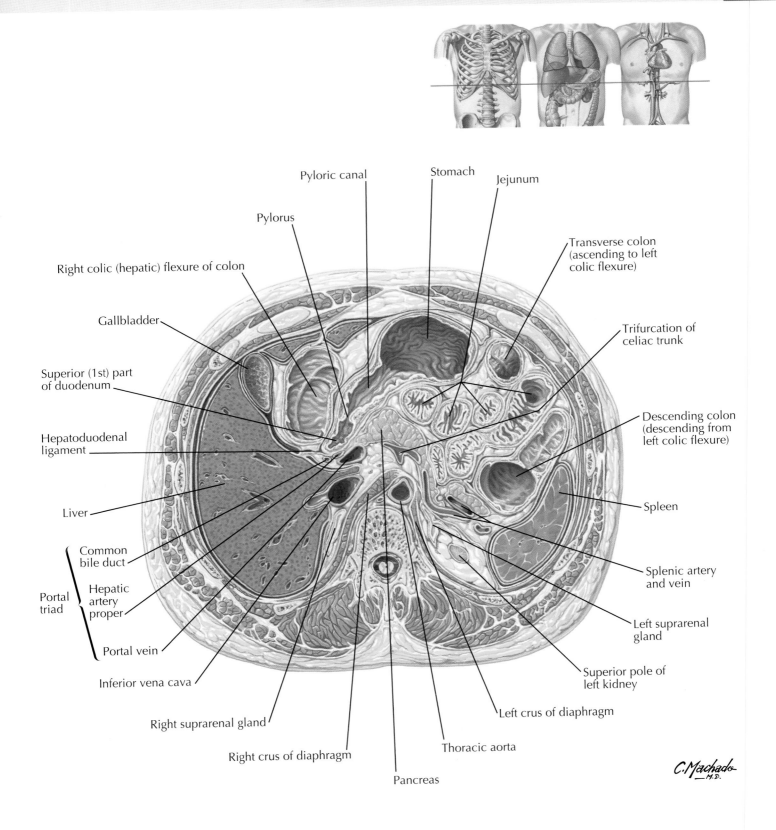

Pyloric canal

Stomach

Jejunum

Pylorus

Transverse colon
(ascending to left
colic flexure)

Right colic (hepatic) flexure of colon

Gallbladder

Trifurcation of
celiac trunk

Superior (1st) part
of duodenum

Descending colon
(descending from
left colic flexure)

Hepatoduodenal
ligament

Liver

Spleen

Common
bile duct

Hepatic
artery
proper

Portal
triad

Splenic artery
and vein

Left suprarenal
gland

Portal vein

Inferior vena cava

Superior pole of
left kidney

Right suprarenal gland

Left crus of diaphragm

Right crus of diaphragm

Thoracic aorta

Pancreas

*C. Machado*
_M.D._

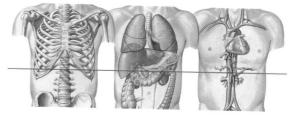

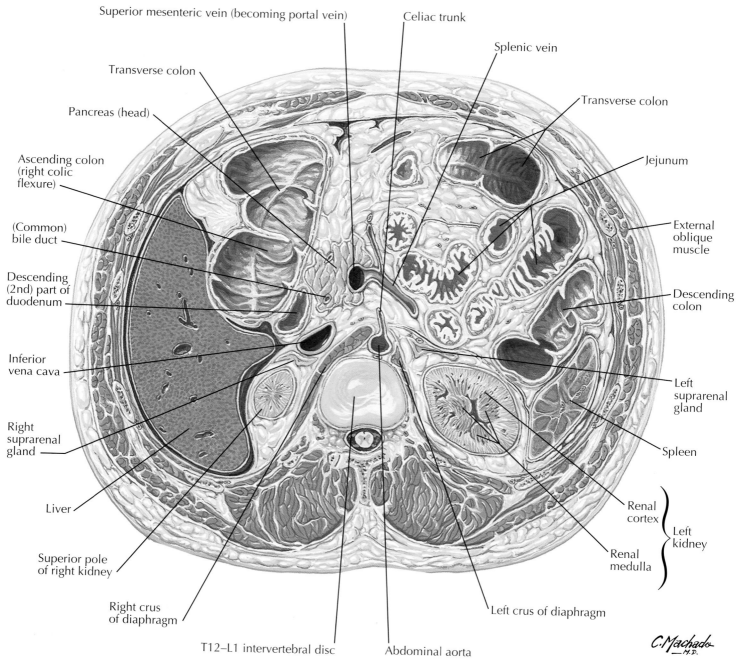

Superior mesenteric vein (becoming portal vein)

Celiac trunk

Splenic vein

Transverse colon

Transverse colon

Pancreas (head)

Jejunum

Ascending colon (right colic flexure)

(Common) bile duct

External oblique muscle

Descending (2nd) part of duodenum

Descending colon

Inferior vena cava

Left suprarenal gland

Right suprarenal gland

Spleen

Liver

Renal cortex

Left kidney

Superior pole of right kidney

Renal medulla

Right crus of diaphragm

Left crus of diaphragm

T12–L1 intervertebral disc

Abdominal aorta

C. Machado
—M.D.

**Plate 326**

**Cross-Sectional Anatomy**

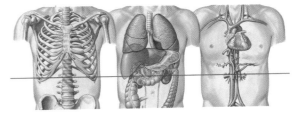

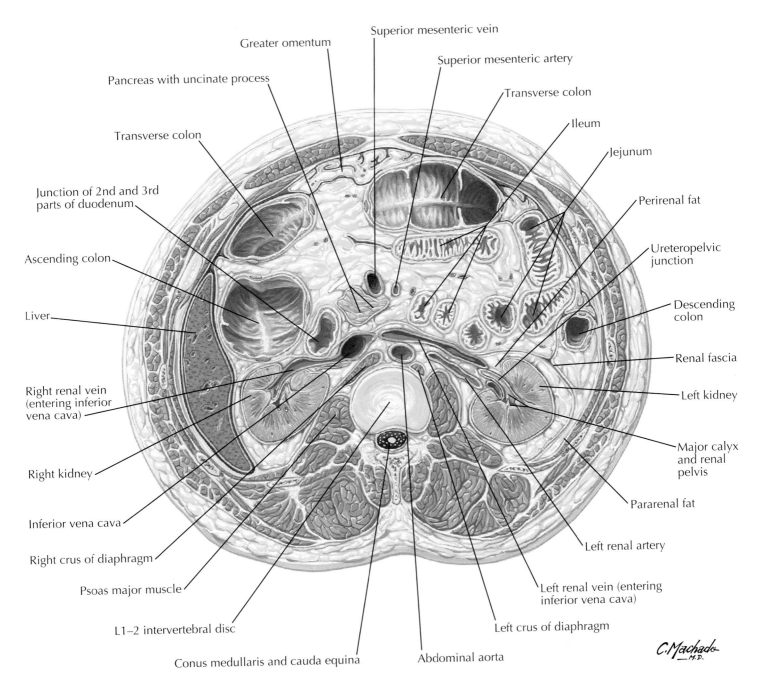

Greater omentum

Superior mesenteric vein

Superior mesenteric artery

Pancreas with uncinate process

Transverse colon

Ileum

Transverse colon

Jejunum

Junction of 2nd and 3rd parts of duodenum

Perirenal fat

Ascending colon

Ureteropelvic junction

Liver

Descending colon

Right renal vein (entering inferior vena cava)

Renal fascia

Left kidney

Right kidney

Major calyx and renal pelvis

Inferior vena cava

Pararenal fat

Right crus of diaphragm

Left renal artery

Psoas major muscle

Left renal vein (entering inferior vena cava)

L1–2 intervertebral disc

Left crus of diaphragm

Conus medullaris and cauda equina

Abdominal aorta

*C.Machado*
_M.D._

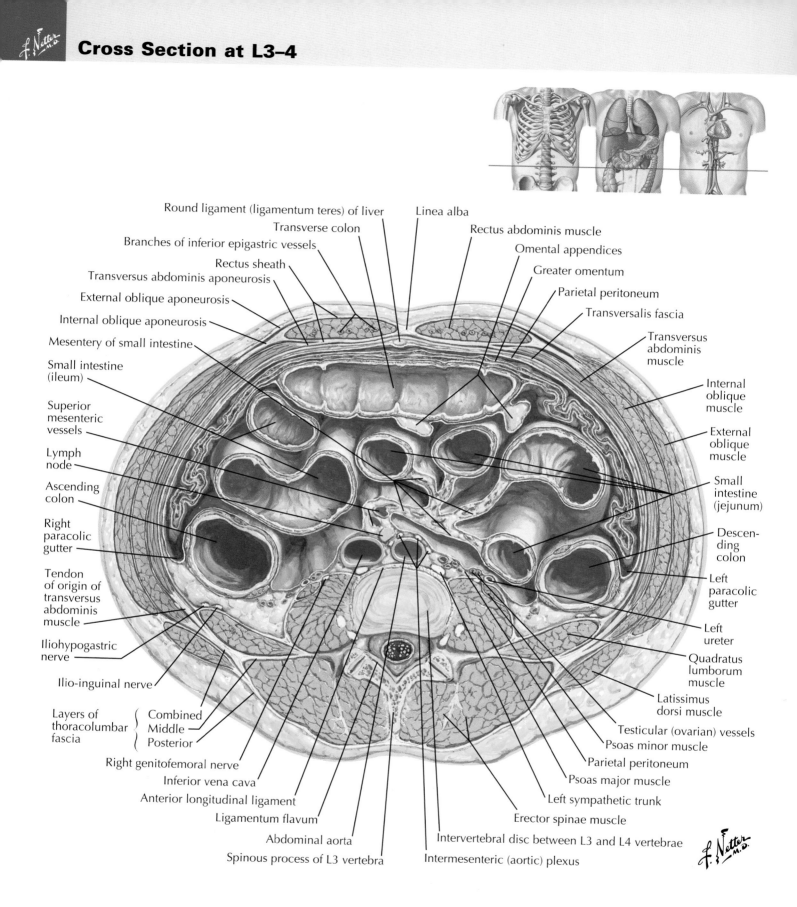

Round ligament (ligamentum teres) of liver

Transverse colon

Branches of inferior epigastric vessels

Rectus sheath

Transversus abdominis aponeurosis

External oblique aponeurosis

Internal oblique aponeurosis

Mesentery of small intestine

Small intestine (ileum)

Superior mesenteric vessels

Lymph node

Ascending colon

Right paracolic gutter

Tendon of origin of transversus abdominis muscle

Iliohypogastric nerve

Ilio-inguinal nerve

Layers of thoracolumbar fascia { Combined / Middle / Posterior }

Right genitofemoral nerve

Inferior vena cava

Anterior longitudinal ligament

Ligamentum flavum

Abdominal aorta

Spinous process of L3 vertebra

Linea alba

Rectus abdominis muscle

Omental appendices

Greater omentum

Parietal peritoneum

Transversalis fascia

Transversus abdominis muscle

Internal oblique muscle

External oblique muscle

Small intestine (jejunum)

Descending colon

Left paracolic gutter

Left ureter

Quadratus lumborum muscle

Latissimus dorsi muscle

Testicular (ovarian) vessels

Psoas minor muscle

Parietal peritoneum

Psoas major muscle

Left sympathetic trunk

Erector spinae muscle

Intervertebral disc between L3 and L4 vertebrae

Intermesenteric (aortic) plexus

**Plate 328**

**Cross-Sectional Anatomy**

| MUSCLE | PROXIMAL ATTACHMENT (ORIGIN) | DISTAL ATTACHMENT (INSERTION) | INNERVATION | MAIN ACTIONS | BLOOD SUPPLY | MUSCLE GROUP |
|---|---|---|---|---|---|---|
| Diaphragm | Xiphoid process, lower six costal cartilages, L1–L3 vertebrae | Converges into central tendon | Phrenic nerve | Draws central tendon down and forward during inspiration | Pericardiacophrenic, musculophrenic, superior and inferior phrenic arteries | Posterior abdominal wall |
| External oblique | External surfaces of ribs 5–12 | Linea alba, pubic tubercle, anterior half of iliac crest | Ventral rami of six inferior thoracic nerves | Compresses and supports abdominal viscera, flexes and rotates trunk | Superior and inferior epigastric arteries | Abdominal wall |
| Iliacus | Superior 2/3 iliac fossa, ala of sacrum, anterior sacro-iliac ligaments | Lesser trochanter of femur and shaft inferior to it, and to psoas major tendon | Femoral nerve | Flexes hip and stabilizes hip joint; acts with psoas major | Iliac branches of iliolumbar artery | Posterior abdominal wall |
| Internal oblique | Thoracolumbar fascia, anterior 2/3 of iliac crest, lateral half of inguinal ligament | Inferior borders of ribs 10–12, linea alba, pubis via conjoint tendon | Ventral rami of six inferior thoracic and first lumbar nerves | Compresses and supports abdominal viscera, flexes and rotates trunk | Superior and inferior epigastric and deep circumflex iliac arteries | Abdominal wall |
| Psoas major | Transverse processes of lumbar vertebrae, sides of bodies of T12–L5 vertebrae, intervening intervertebral discs | Lesser trochanter of femur | Ventral rami of first four lumbar nerves | Acting superiorly with iliacus, flexes hip; acting inferiorly, flexes vertebral column laterally; used to balance trunk in sitting position; acting inferiorly with iliacus, flexes trunk | Lumbar branches of iliolumbar artery | Posterior abdominal wall |
| Psoas minor | Vertebral margins of T12–L1 vertebrae, corresponding intervertebral disc | Pectineal line, iliopectineal eminence | Ventral rami of first lumbar nerve | Flexes pelvis on vertebral column | Lumbar branch of iliolumbar artery | Posterior abdominal wall |
| Pyramidalis | Body of pubis, anterior to rectus abdominis | Linea alba | Iliohypogastric nerve | Tenses linea alba | Inferior epigastric artery | Abdominal wall |
| Quadratus lumborum | Medial half of inferior border of 12th rib, tips of lumbar transverse processes | Iliolumbar ligament, internal lip of iliac crest | Ventral rami of T12 and first four lumbar nerves | Extends and laterally flexes vertebral column, fixes 12th rib during inspiration | Iliolumbar artery | Posterior abdominal wall |
| Rectus abdominis | Pubic symphysis, pubic crest | Xiphoid process, costal cartilages 5–7 | Ventral rami of six inferior thoracic nerves | Flexes trunk, compresses abdominal viscera | Superior and inferior epigastric arteries | Abdominal wall |
| Transversus abdominis | Internal surfaces of costal cartilages 7–12, thoracolumbar fascia, iliac crest, lateral third of inguinal ligament | Linea alba with aponeurosis of internal oblique, pubic crest, and pecten pubis via conjoint tendon | Ventral rami of six inferior thoracic and first lumbar nerves | Compresses and supports abdominal viscera | Deep circumflex iliac and inferior epigastric arteries | Abdominal wall |

Variations in spinal nerve contributions to the innervation of muscles, their arterial supply, their attachments, and their actions are common themes in human anatomy. Therefore, expect differences between texts and realize that anatomical variation is normal.

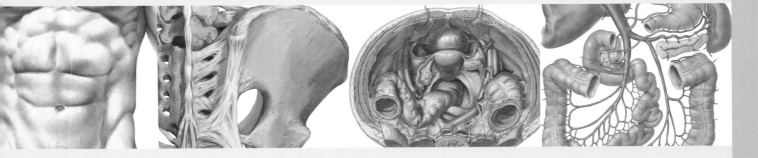

# 5 PELVIS AND PERINEUM

## Topographic Anatomy
**Plate 329**

## Bones and Ligaments
**Plates 330–334**

## Pelvic Floor and Contents
**Plates 335–345**

# PELVIS AND PERINEUM

## Innervation
**Plates 387–395**

## Cross-Sectional Anatomy
**Plates 396–397**

## Muscle Tables

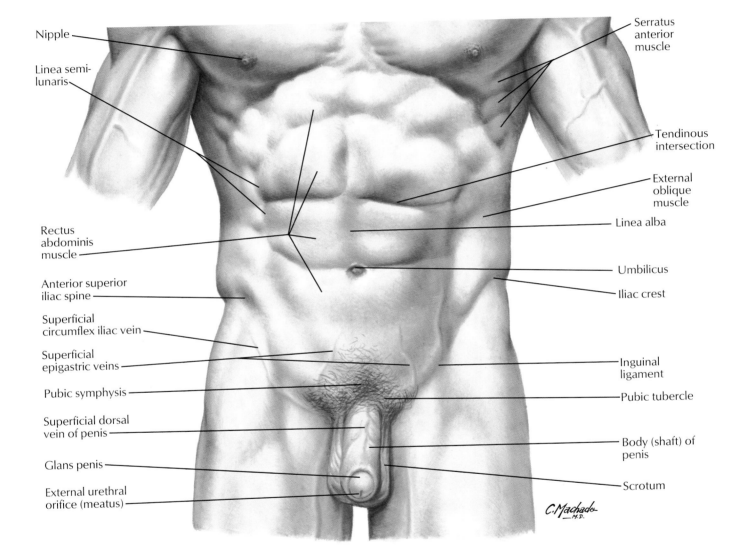

Nipple

Linea semi-lunaris

Rectus abdominis muscle

Anterior superior iliac spine

Superficial circumflex iliac vein

Superficial epigastric veins

Pubic symphysis

Superficial dorsal vein of penis

Glans penis

External urethral orifice (meatus)

Serratus anterior muscle

Tendinous intersection

External oblique muscle

Linea alba

Umbilicus

Iliac crest

Inguinal ligament

Pubic tubercle

Body (shaft) of penis

Scrotum

*C.Machado*
_M.D._

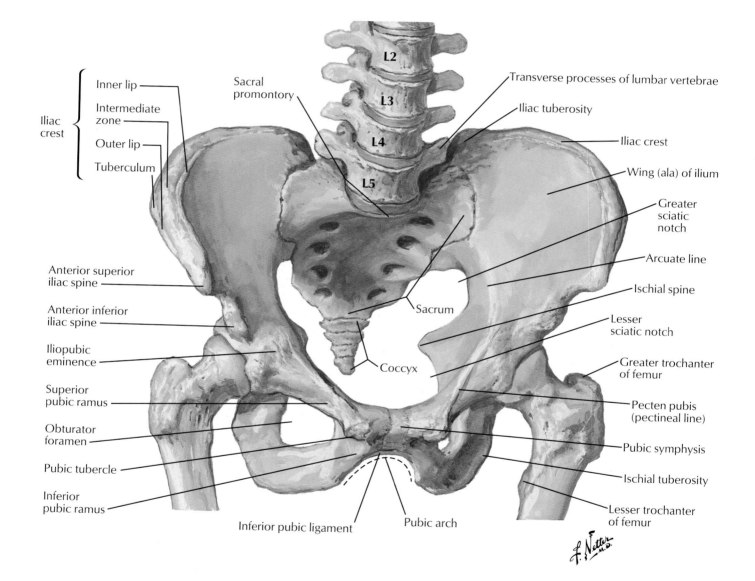

Iliac crest
- Inner lip
- Intermediate zone
- Outer lip
- Tuberculum

Sacral promontory

L2

L3

L4

L5

Transverse processes of lumbar vertebrae

Iliac tuberosity

Iliac crest

Wing (ala) of ilium

Greater sciatic notch

Arcuate line

Ischial spine

Sacrum

Anterior superior iliac spine

Anterior inferior iliac spine

Iliopubic eminence

Superior pubic ramus

Obturator foramen

Pubic tubercle

Inferior pubic ramus

Coccyx

Lesser sciatic notch

Greater trochanter of femur

Pecten pubis (pectineal line)

Pubic symphysis

Ischial tuberosity

Lesser trochanter of femur

Inferior pubic ligament

Pubic arch

**Plate 330**

**Bones and Ligaments**

## Bones and Ligaments

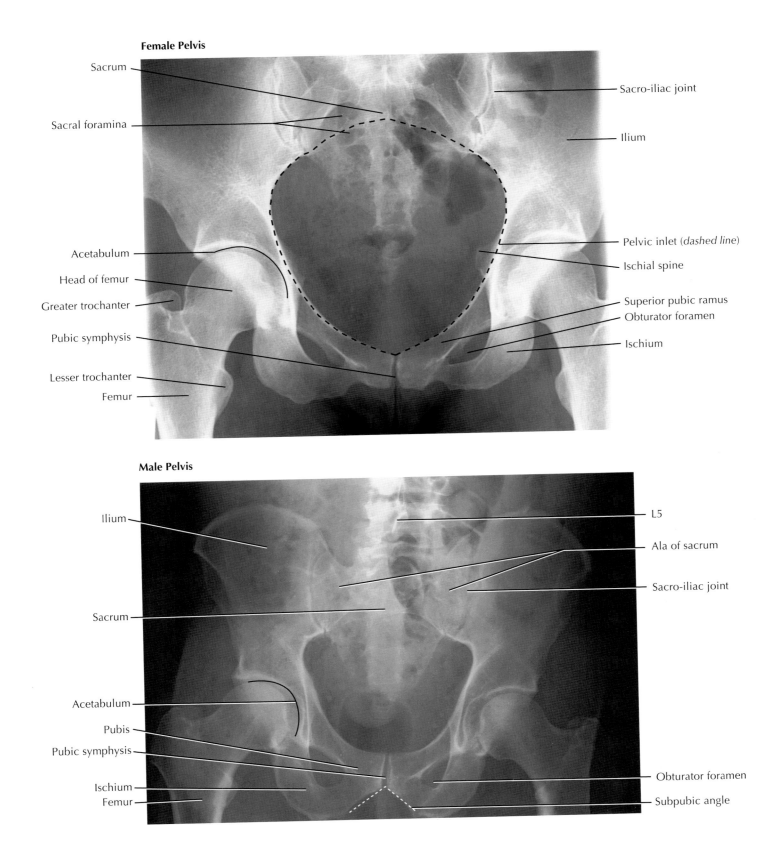

**Female Pelvis**

Sacrum

Sacral foramina

Acetabulum

Head of femur

Greater trochanter

Pubic symphysis

Lesser trochanter

Femur

Sacro-iliac joint

Ilium

Pelvic inlet (*dashed line*)

Ischial spine

Superior pubic ramus

Obturator foramen

Ischium

**Male Pelvis**

Ilium

Sacrum

Acetabulum

Pubis

Pubic symphysis

Ischium

Femur

L5

Ala of sacrum

Sacro-iliac joint

Obturator foramen

Subpubic angle

**Plate 331**

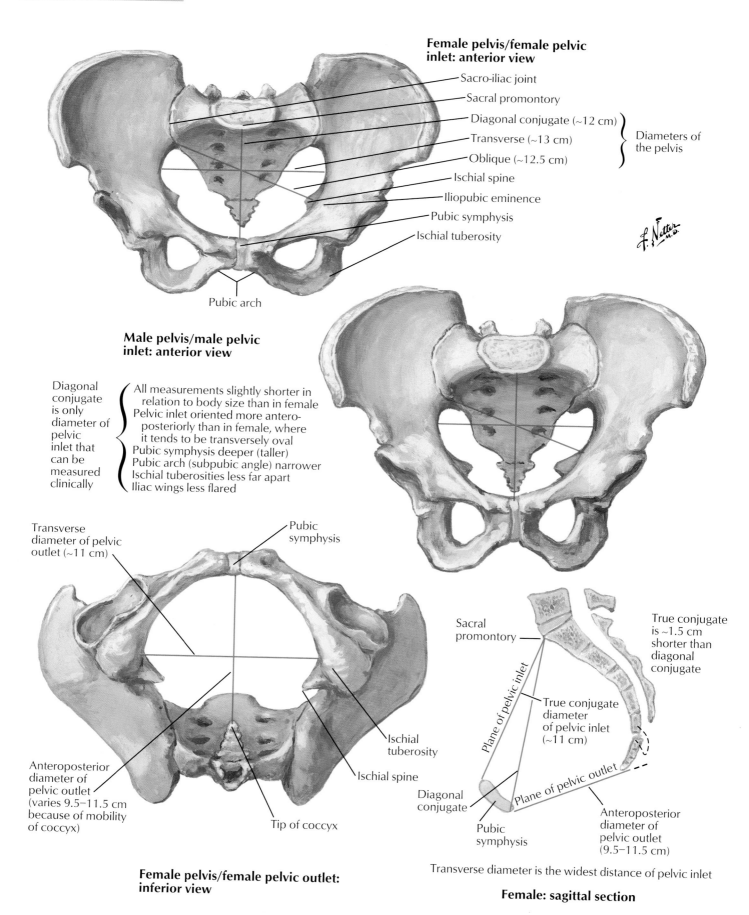

**Female pelvis/female pelvic inlet: anterior view**

Sacro-iliac joint
Sacral promontory
Diagonal conjugate (~12 cm)
Transverse (~13 cm)
Oblique (~12.5 cm)
— Diameters of the pelvis
Ischial spine
Iliopubic eminence
Pubic symphysis
Ischial tuberosity

Pubic arch

**Male pelvis/male pelvic inlet: anterior view**

Diagonal conjugate is only diameter of pelvic inlet that can be measured clinically

All measurements slightly shorter in relation to body size than in female
Pelvic inlet oriented more antero-posteriorly than in female, where it tends to be transversely oval
Pubic symphysis deeper (taller)
Pubic arch (subpubic angle) narrower
Ischial tuberosities less far apart
Iliac wings less flared

Transverse diameter of pelvic outlet (~11 cm)

Pubic symphysis

Anteroposterior diameter of pelvic outlet (varies 9.5–11.5 cm because of mobility of coccyx)

Ischial tuberosity

Ischial spine

Tip of coccyx

**Female pelvis/female pelvic outlet: inferior view**

Sacral promontory

True conjugate is ~1.5 cm shorter than diagonal conjugate

Plane of pelvic inlet

True conjugate diameter of pelvic inlet (~11 cm)

Diagonal conjugate

Pubic symphysis

Plane of pelvic outlet

Anteroposterior diameter of pelvic outlet (9.5–11.5 cm)

Transverse diameter is the widest distance of pelvic inlet

**Female: sagittal section**

**Plate 332**

**Bones and Ligaments**

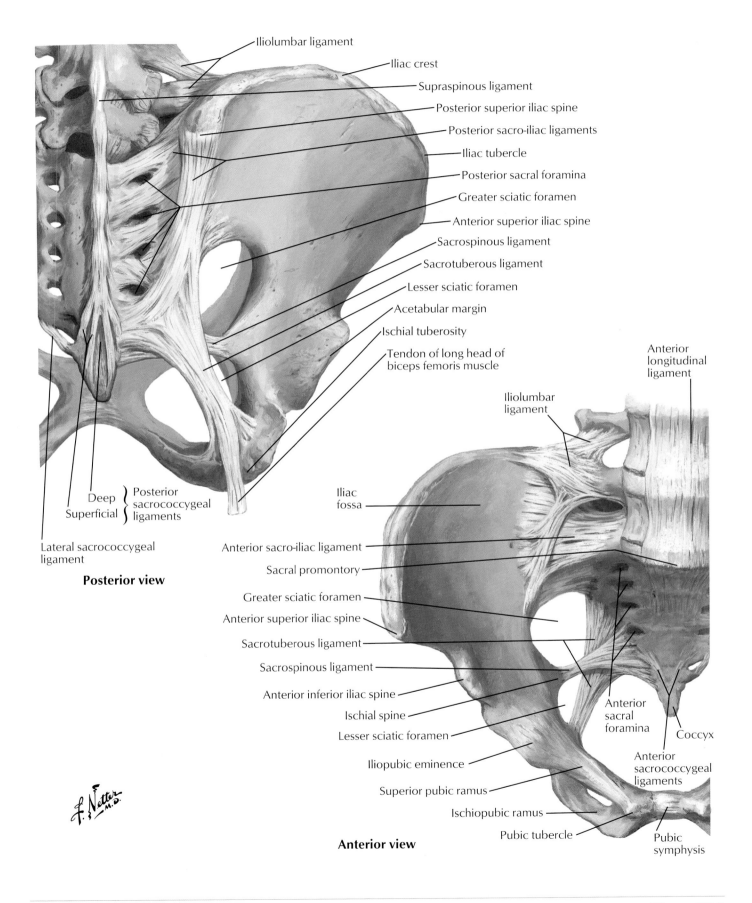

Iliolumbar ligament

Iliac crest

Supraspinous ligament

Posterior superior iliac spine

Posterior sacro-iliac ligaments

Iliac tubercle

Posterior sacral foramina

Greater sciatic foramen

Anterior superior iliac spine

Sacrospinous ligament

Sacrotuberous ligament

Lesser sciatic foramen

Acetabular margin

Ischial tuberosity

Tendon of long head of biceps femoris muscle

Deep
Superficial } Posterior sacrococcygeal ligaments

Lateral sacrococcygeal ligament

**Posterior view**

Anterior longitudinal ligament

Iliolumbar ligament

Iliac fossa

Anterior sacro-iliac ligament

Sacral promontory

Greater sciatic foramen

Anterior superior iliac spine

Sacrotuberous ligament

Sacrospinous ligament

Anterior inferior iliac spine

Ischial spine

Lesser sciatic foramen

Iliopubic eminence

Superior pubic ramus

Ischiopubic ramus

Pubic tubercle

Anterior sacral foramina

Coccyx

Anterior sacrococcygeal ligaments

Pubic symphysis

**Anterior view**

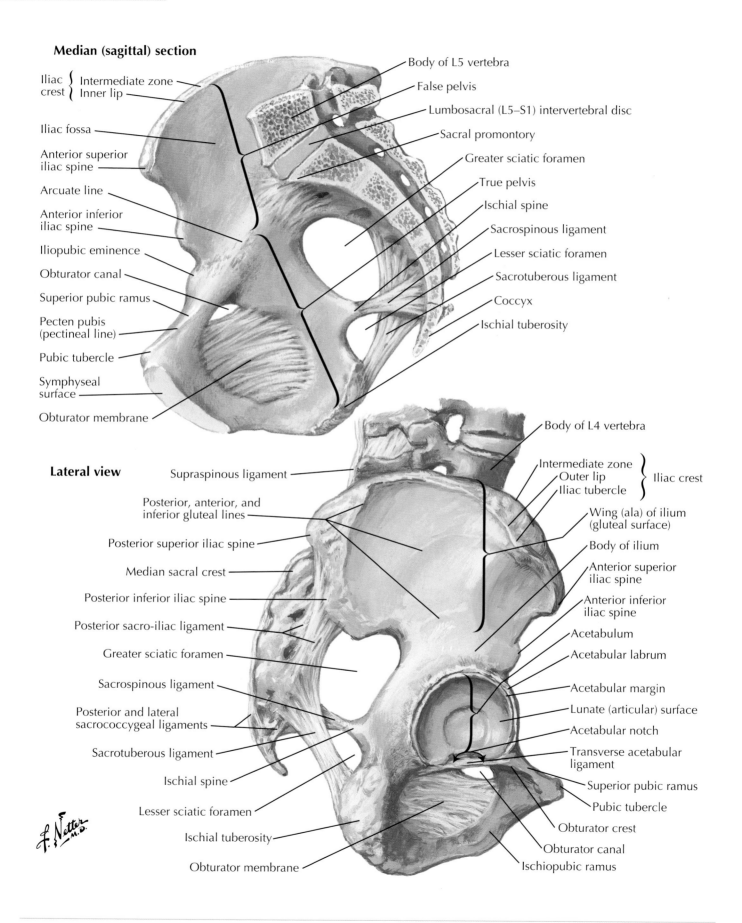

**Median (sagittal) section**

Iliac crest { Intermediate zone / Inner lip

Iliac fossa

Anterior superior iliac spine

Arcuate line

Anterior inferior iliac spine

Iliopubic eminence

Obturator canal

Superior pubic ramus

Pecten pubis (pectineal line)

Pubic tubercle

Symphyseal surface

Obturator membrane

Body of L5 vertebra

False pelvis

Lumbosacral (L5–S1) intervertebral disc

Sacral promontory

Greater sciatic foramen

True pelvis

Ischial spine

Sacrospinous ligament

Lesser sciatic foramen

Sacrotuberous ligament

Coccyx

Ischial tuberosity

**Lateral view**

Supraspinous ligament

Posterior, anterior, and inferior gluteal lines

Posterior superior iliac spine

Median sacral crest

Posterior inferior iliac spine

Posterior sacro-iliac ligament

Greater sciatic foramen

Sacrospinous ligament

Posterior and lateral sacrococcygeal ligaments

Sacrotuberous ligament

Ischial spine

Lesser sciatic foramen

Ischial tuberosity

Obturator membrane

Body of L4 vertebra

Intermediate zone / Outer lip / Iliac tubercle } Iliac crest

Wing (ala) of ilium (gluteal surface)

Body of ilium

Anterior superior iliac spine

Anterior inferior iliac spine

Acetabulum

Acetabular labrum

Acetabular margin

Lunate (articular) surface

Acetabular notch

Transverse acetabular ligament

Superior pubic ramus

Pubic tubercle

Obturator crest

Obturator canal

Ischiopubic ramus

**Plate 334**

**Bones and Ligaments**

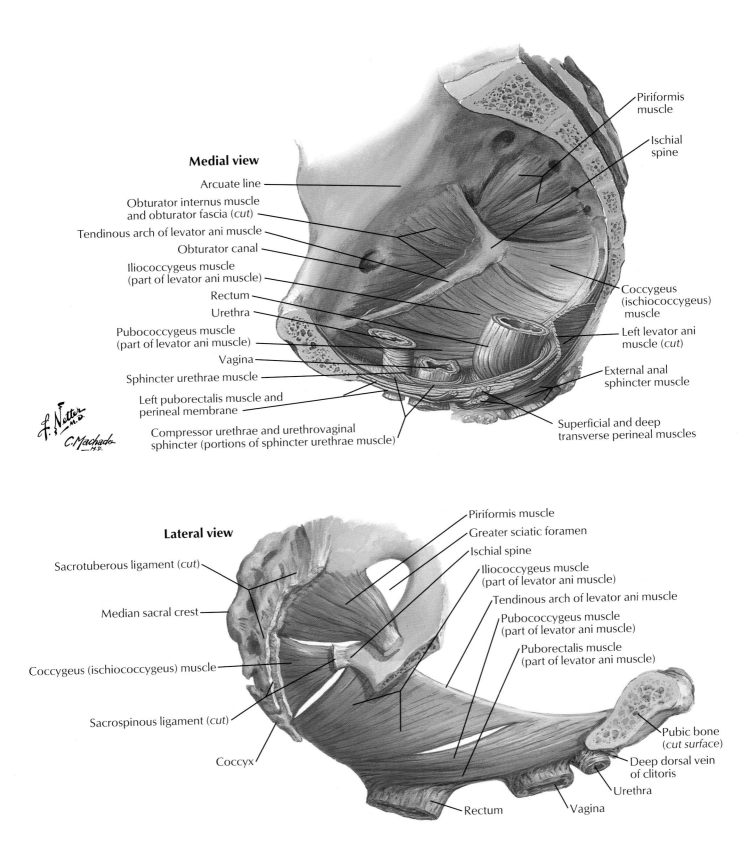

**Medial view**

Arcuate line

Obturator internus muscle and obturator fascia (cut)

Tendinous arch of levator ani muscle

Obturator canal

Iliococcygeus muscle (part of levator ani muscle)

Rectum

Urethra

Pubococcygeus muscle (part of levator ani muscle)

Vagina

Sphincter urethrae muscle

Left puborectalis muscle and perineal membrane

Compressor urethrae and urethrovaginal sphincter (portions of sphincter urethrae muscle)

Piriformis muscle

Ischial spine

Coccygeus (ischiococcygeus) muscle

Left levator ani muscle (cut)

External anal sphincter muscle

Superficial and deep transverse perineal muscles

**Lateral view**

Sacrotuberous ligament (cut)

Median sacral crest

Coccygeus (ischiococcygeus) muscle

Sacrospinous ligament (cut)

Coccyx

Piriformis muscle

Greater sciatic foramen

Ischial spine

Iliococcygeus muscle (part of levator ani muscle)

Tendinous arch of levator ani muscle

Pubococcygeus muscle (part of levator ani muscle)

Puborectalis muscle (part of levator ani muscle)

Pubic bone (cut surface)

Deep dorsal vein of clitoris

Urethra

Rectum

Vagina

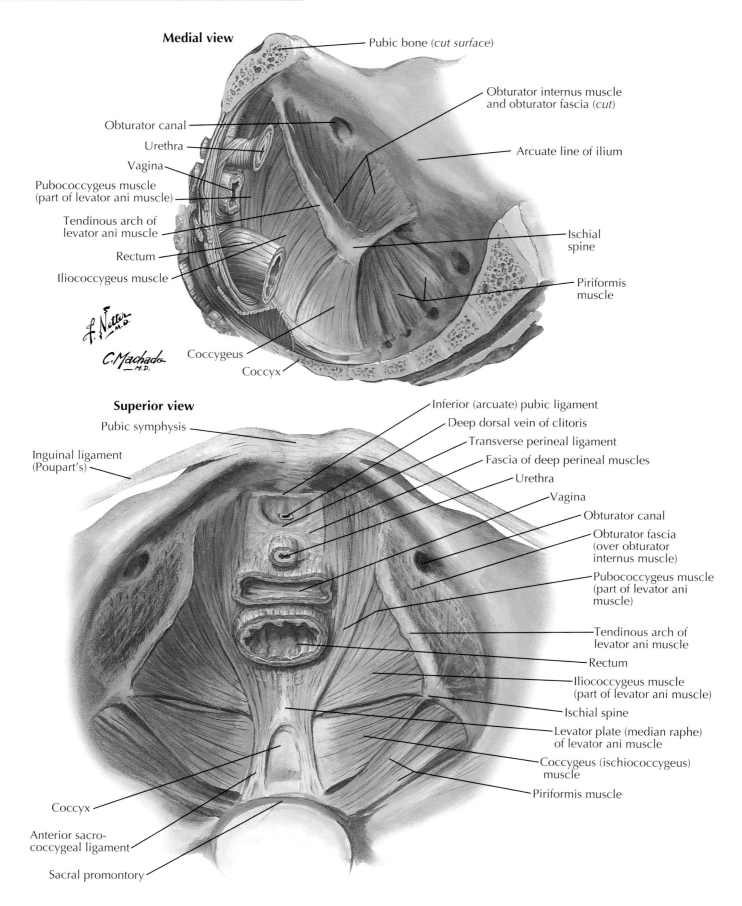

**Medial view**

Pubic bone (*cut surface*)

Obturator internus muscle and obturator fascia (*cut*)

Obturator canal

Urethra

Arcuate line of ilium

Vagina

Pubococcygeus muscle (part of levator ani muscle)

Tendinous arch of levator ani muscle

Ischial spine

Rectum

Iliococcygeus muscle

Piriformis muscle

Coccygeus

Coccyx

**Superior view**

Pubic symphysis

Inferior (arcuate) pubic ligament

Deep dorsal vein of clitoris

Transverse perineal ligament

Fascia of deep perineal muscles

Urethra

Vagina

Inguinal ligament (Poupart's)

Obturator canal

Obturator fascia (over obturator internus muscle)

Pubococcygeus muscle (part of levator ani muscle)

Tendinous arch of levator ani muscle

Rectum

Iliococcygeus muscle (part of levator ani muscle)

Ischial spine

Levator plate (median raphe) of levator ani muscle

Coccygeus (ischiococcygeus) muscle

Piriformis muscle

Coccyx

Anterior sacro-coccygeal ligament

Sacral promontory

**Plate 336**

**Pelvic Floor and Contents**

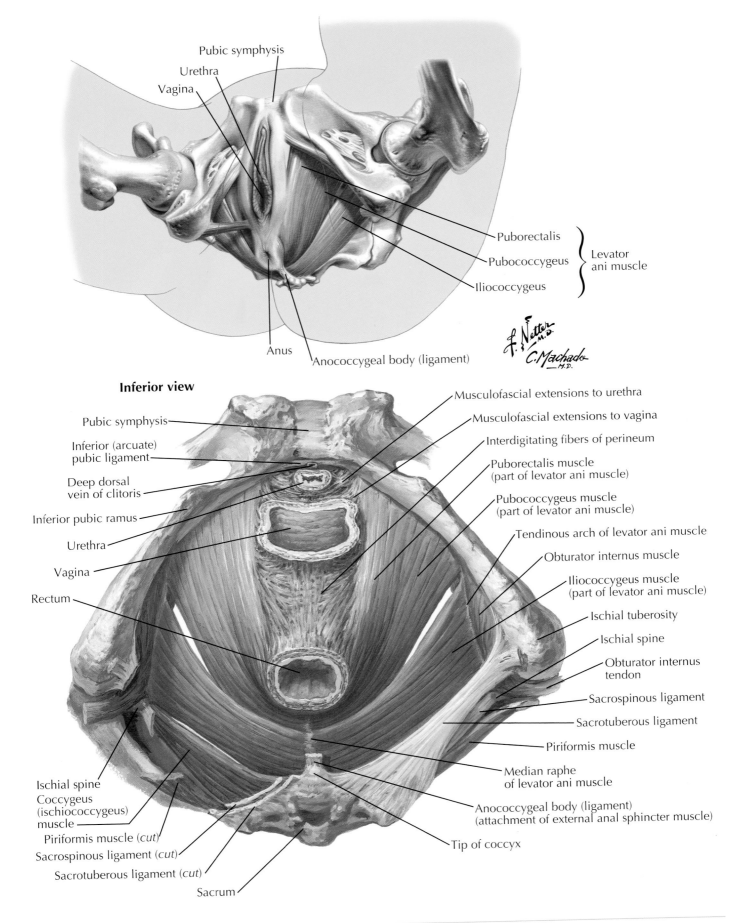

Pubic symphysis

Urethra

Vagina

Puborectalis

Pubococcygeus

Iliococcygeus

} Levator ani muscle

Anus

Anococcygeal body (ligament)

**Inferior view**

Pubic symphysis

Inferior (arcuate) pubic ligament

Deep dorsal vein of clitoris

Inferior pubic ramus

Urethra

Vagina

Rectum

Ischial spine

Coccygeus (ischiococcygeus) muscle

Piriformis muscle (*cut*)

Sacrospinous ligament (*cut*)

Sacrotuberous ligament (*cut*)

Sacrum

Musculofascial extensions to urethra

Musculofascial extensions to vagina

Interdigitating fibers of perineum

Puborectalis muscle (part of levator ani muscle)

Pubococcygeus muscle (part of levator ani muscle)

Tendinous arch of levator ani muscle

Obturator internus muscle

Iliococcygeus muscle (part of levator ani muscle)

Ischial tuberosity

Ischial spine

Obturator internus tendon

Sacrospinous ligament

Sacrotuberous ligament

Piriformis muscle

Median raphe of levator ani muscle

Anococcygeal body (ligament) (attachment of external anal sphincter muscle)

Tip of coccyx

**Superior view**
(*viscera removed*)

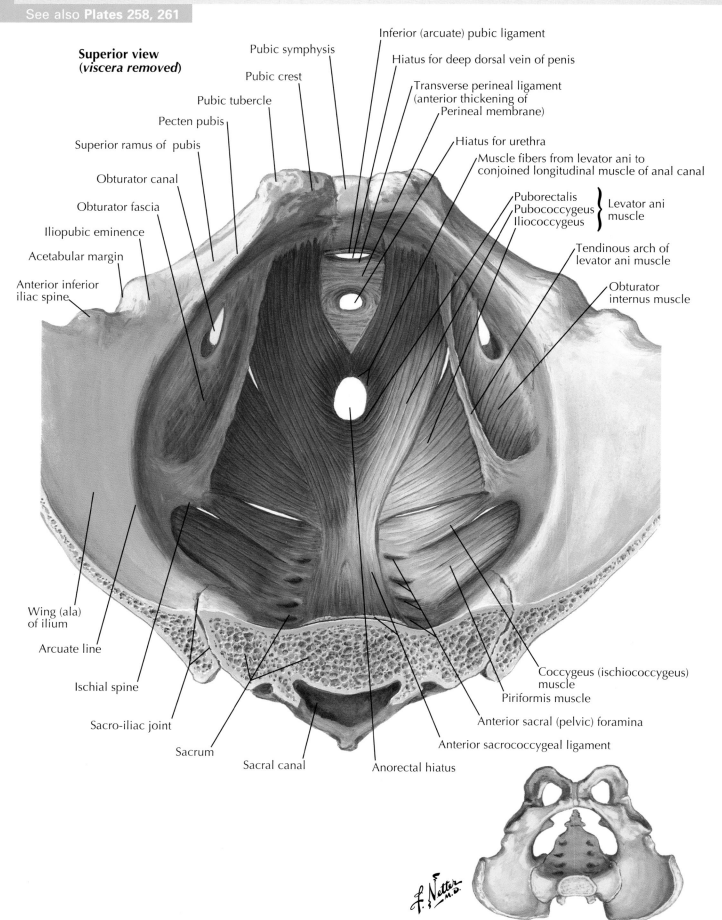

Pubic symphysis

Pubic crest

Pubic tubercle

Pecten pubis

Superior ramus of pubis

Obturator canal

Obturator fascia

Iliopubic eminence

Acetabular margin

Anterior inferior iliac spine

Inferior (arcuate) pubic ligament

Hiatus for deep dorsal vein of penis

Transverse perineal ligament (anterior thickening of Perineal membrane)

Hiatus for urethra

Muscle fibers from levator ani to conjoined longitudinal muscle of anal canal

Puborectalis
Pubococcygeus    } Levator ani muscle
Iliococcygeus

Tendinous arch of levator ani muscle

Obturator internus muscle

Wing (ala) of ilium

Arcuate line

Ischial spine

Sacro-iliac joint

Sacrum

Sacral canal

Anorectal hiatus

Coccygeus (ischiococcygeus) muscle

Piriformis muscle

Anterior sacral (pelvic) foramina

Anterior sacrococcygeal ligament

**Plate 338**

**Pelvic Floor and Contents**

**Inferior view**

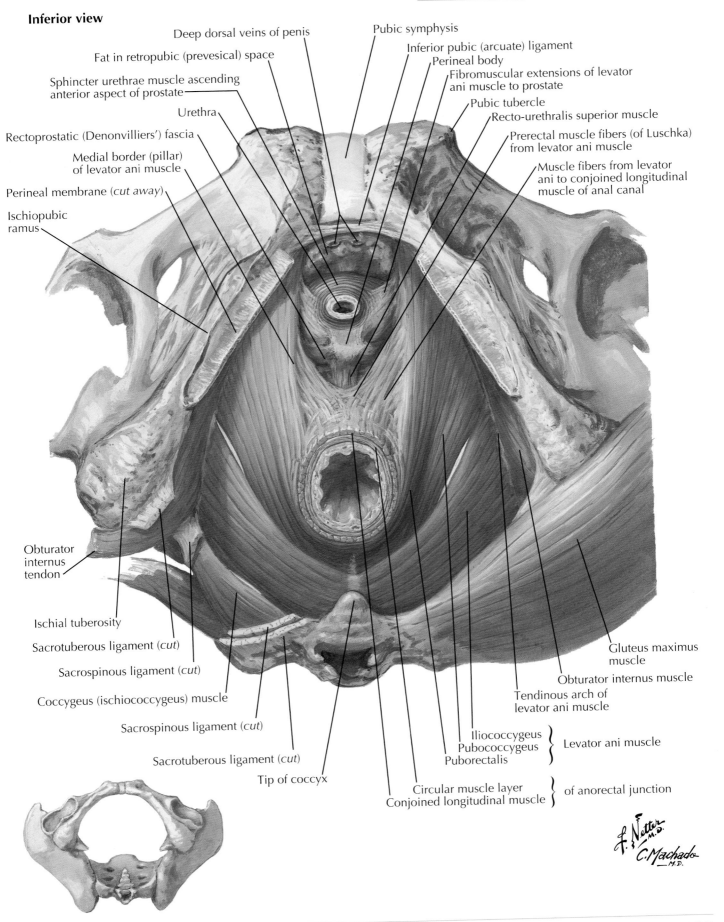

Deep dorsal veins of penis

Fat in retropubic (prevesical) space

Sphincter urethrae muscle ascending
anterior aspect of prostate

Urethra

Rectoprostatic (Denonvilliers') fascia

Medial border (pillar)
of levator ani muscle

Perineal membrane (*cut away*)

Ischiopubic
ramus

Obturator
internus
tendon

Ischial tuberosity

Sacrotuberous ligament (*cut*)

Sacrospinous ligament (*cut*)

Coccygeus (ischiococcygeus) muscle

Sacrospinous ligament (*cut*)

Sacrotuberous ligament (*cut*)

Tip of coccyx

Pubic symphysis

Inferior pubic (arcuate) ligament

Perineal body

Fibromuscular extensions of levator
ani muscle to prostate

Pubic tubercle

Recto-urethralis superior muscle

Prerectal muscle fibers (of Luschka)
from levator ani muscle

Muscle fibers from levator
ani to conjoined longitudinal
muscle of anal canal

Gluteus maximus
muscle

Obturator internus muscle

Tendinous arch of
levator ani muscle

Iliococcygeus  }
Pubococcygeus  } Levator ani muscle
Puborectalis  }

Circular muscle layer  } of anorectal junction
Conjoined longitudinal muscle  }

*f. Netter M.D.*
*C. Machado M.D.*

**Pelvic Floor and Contents**

**Plate 339**

## Paramedian (sagittal) dissection

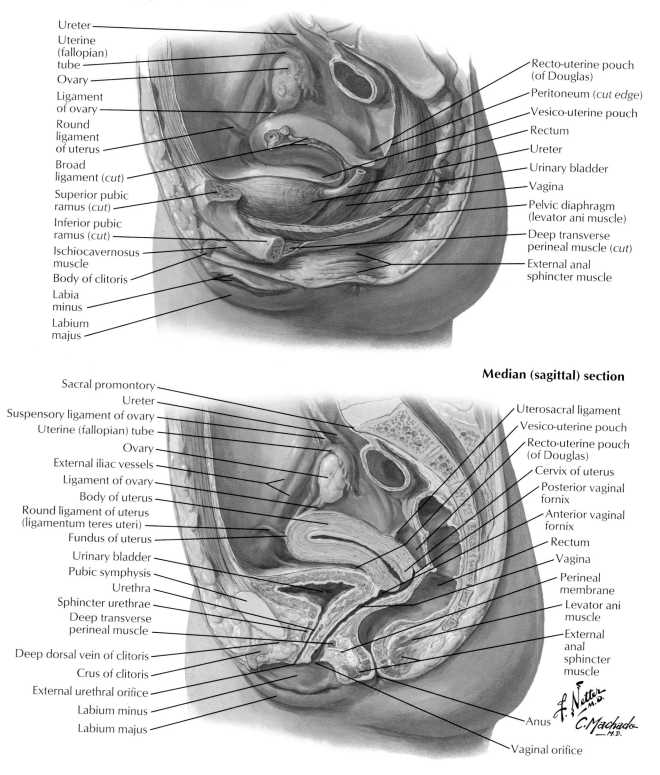

Ureter

Uterine (fallopian) tube

Ovary

Ligament of ovary

Round ligament of uterus

Broad ligament (*cut*)

Superior pubic ramus (*cut*)

Inferior pubic ramus (*cut*)

Ischiocavernosus muscle

Body of clitoris

Labia minus

Labium majus

Recto-uterine pouch (of Douglas)

Peritoneum (*cut edge*)

Vesico-uterine pouch

Rectum

Ureter

Urinary bladder

Vagina

Pelvic diaphragm (levator ani muscle)

Deep transverse perineal muscle (*cut*)

External anal sphincter muscle

## Median (sagittal) section

Sacral promontory

Ureter

Suspensory ligament of ovary

Uterine (fallopian) tube

Ovary

External iliac vessels

Ligament of ovary

Body of uterus

Round ligament of uterus (ligamentum teres uteri)

Fundus of uterus

Urinary bladder

Pubic symphysis

Urethra

Sphincter urethrae

Deep transverse perineal muscle

Deep dorsal vein of clitoris

Crus of clitoris

External urethral orifice

Labium minus

Labium majus

Uterosacral ligament

Vesico-uterine pouch

Recto-uterine pouch (of Douglas)

Cervix of uterus

Posterior vaginal fornix

Anterior vaginal fornix

Rectum

Vagina

Perineal membrane

Levator ani muscle

External anal sphincter muscle

Anus

Vaginal orifice

**Plate 340**

**Pelvic Floor and Contents**

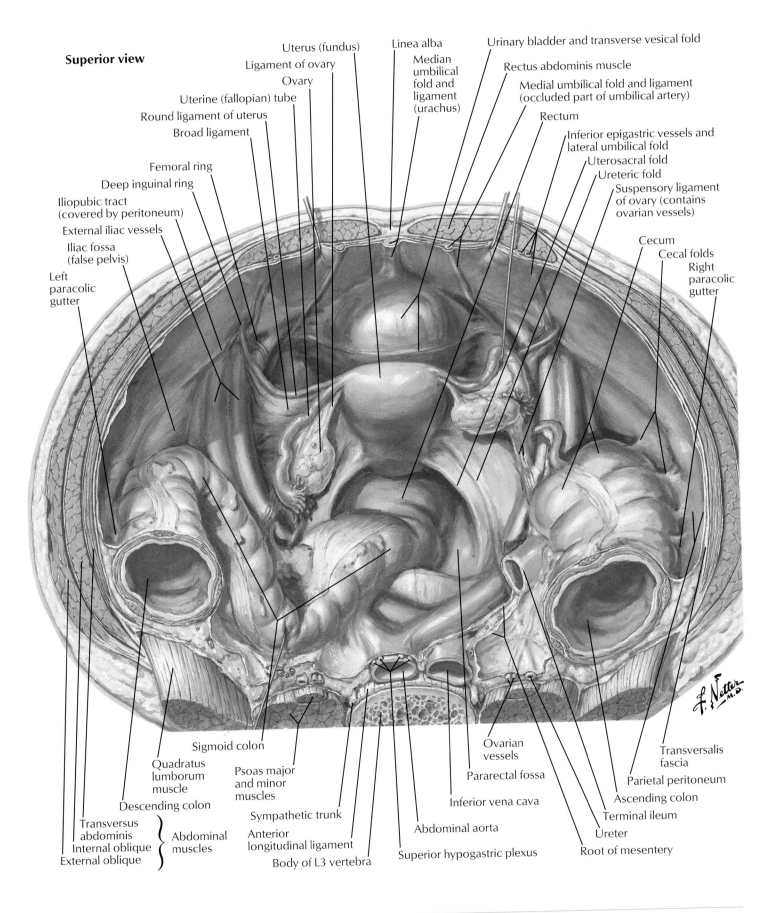

**Superior view**

Uterus (fundus)
Ligament of ovary
Ovary
Uterine (fallopian) tube
Round ligament of uterus
Broad ligament
Femoral ring
Deep inguinal ring
Iliopubic tract (covered by peritoneum)
External iliac vessels
Iliac fossa (false pelvis)
Left paracolic gutter

Linea alba
Median umbilical fold and ligament (urachus)

Urinary bladder and transverse vesical fold
Rectus abdominis muscle
Medial umbilical fold and ligament (occluded part of umbilical artery)
Rectum
Inferior epigastric vessels and lateral umbilical fold
Uterosacral fold
Ureteric fold
Suspensory ligament of ovary (contains ovarian vessels)
Cecum
Cecal folds
Right paracolic gutter

Sigmoid colon
Quadratus lumborum muscle
Psoas major and minor muscles
Descending colon
Transversus abdominis
Internal oblique
External oblique
} Abdominal muscles
Sympathetic trunk
Anterior longitudinal ligament
Body of L3 vertebra
Superior hypogastric plexus
Abdominal aorta
Inferior vena cava
Pararectal fossa
Ovarian vessels
Ascending colon
Terminal ileum
Ureter
Root of mesentery
Parietal peritoneum
Transversalis fascia

**Superior view with peritoneum intact**

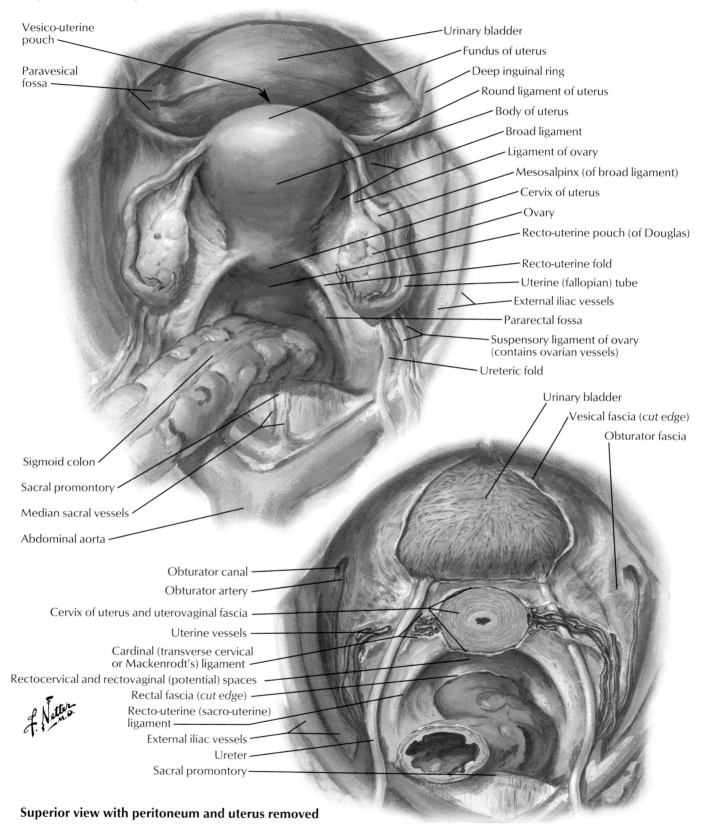

Vesico-uterine pouch

Paravesical fossa

Urinary bladder

Fundus of uterus

Deep inguinal ring

Round ligament of uterus

Body of uterus

Broad ligament

Ligament of ovary

Mesosalpinx (of broad ligament)

Cervix of uterus

Ovary

Recto-uterine pouch (of Douglas)

Recto-uterine fold

Uterine (fallopian) tube

External iliac vessels

Pararectal fossa

Suspensory ligament of ovary (contains ovarian vessels)

Ureteric fold

Urinary bladder

Vesical fascia (cut edge)

Obturator fascia

Sigmoid colon

Sacral promontory

Median sacral vessels

Abdominal aorta

Obturator canal

Obturator artery

Cervix of uterus and uterovaginal fascia

Uterine vessels

Cardinal (transverse cervical or Mackenrodt's) ligament

Rectocervical and rectovaginal (potential) spaces

Rectal fascia (cut edge)

Recto-uterine (sacro-uterine) ligament

External iliac vessels

Ureter

Sacral promontory

**Superior view with peritoneum and uterus removed**

**Plate 342**

**Pelvic Floor and Contents**

**Female: superior view (peritoneum and loose areolar tissue removed)**

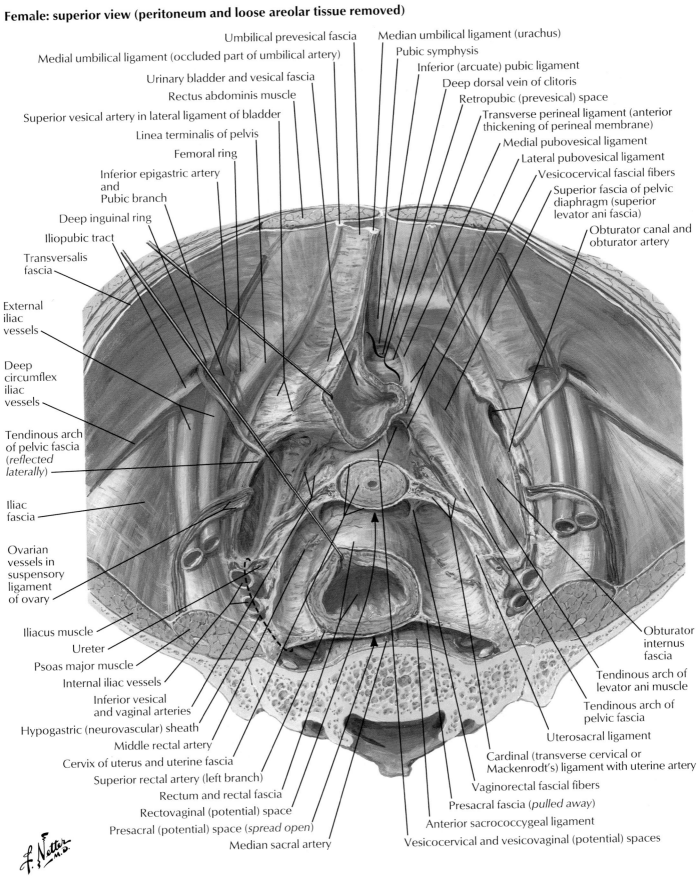

Umbilical prevesical fascia

Median umbilical ligament (urachus)

Medial umbilical ligament (occluded part of umbilical artery)

Pubic symphysis

Urinary bladder and vesical fascia

Inferior (arcuate) pubic ligament

Rectus abdominis muscle

Deep dorsal vein of clitoris

Superior vesical artery in lateral ligament of bladder

Retropubic (prevesical) space

Linea terminalis of pelvis

Transverse perineal ligament (anterior thickening of perineal membrane)

Femoral ring

Medial pubovesical ligament

Inferior epigastric artery and Pubic branch

Lateral pubovesical ligament

Vesicocervical fascial fibers

Deep inguinal ring

Superior fascia of pelvic diaphragm (superior levator ani fascia)

Iliopubic tract

Obturator canal and obturator artery

Transversalis fascia

External iliac vessels

Deep circumflex iliac vessels

Tendinous arch of pelvic fascia (*reflected laterally*)

Iliac fascia

Ovarian vessels in suspensory ligament of ovary

Iliacus muscle

Obturator internus fascia

Ureter

Psoas major muscle

Tendinous arch of levator ani muscle

Internal iliac vessels

Tendinous arch of pelvic fascia

Inferior vesical and vaginal arteries

Hypogastric (neurovascular) sheath

Uterosacral ligament

Middle rectal artery

Cardinal (transverse cervical or Mackenrodt's) ligament with uterine artery

Cervix of uterus and uterine fascia

Superior rectal artery (left branch)

Vaginorectal fascial fibers

Rectum and rectal fascia

Presacral fascia (*pulled away*)

Rectovaginal (potential) space

Anterior sacrococcygeal ligament

Presacral (potential) space (*spread open*)

Vesicocervical and vesicovaginal (potential) spaces

Median sacral artery

*f. Netter M.D.*

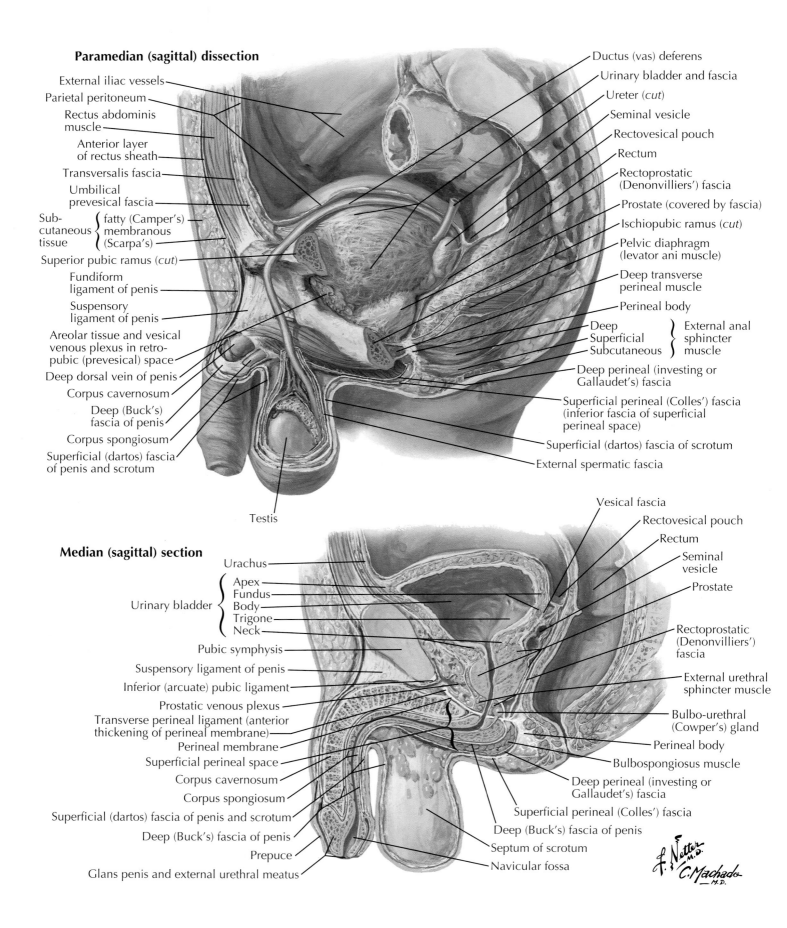

**Paramedian (sagittal) dissection**

External iliac vessels
Parietal peritoneum
Rectus abdominis muscle
Anterior layer of rectus sheath
Transversalis fascia
Umbilical prevesical fascia
Subcutaneous tissue { fatty (Camper's) / membranous (Scarpa's)
Superior pubic ramus (cut)
Fundiform ligament of penis
Suspensory ligament of penis
Areolar tissue and vesical venous plexus in retropubic (prevesical) space
Deep dorsal vein of penis
Corpus cavernosum
Deep (Buck's) fascia of penis
Corpus spongiosum
Superficial (dartos) fascia of penis and scrotum

Ductus (vas) deferens
Urinary bladder and fascia
Ureter (cut)
Seminal vesicle
Rectovesical pouch
Rectum
Rectoprostatic (Denonvilliers') fascia
Prostate (covered by fascia)
Ischiopubic ramus (cut)
Pelvic diaphragm (levator ani muscle)
Deep transverse perineal muscle
Perineal body
Deep / Superficial / Subcutaneous } External anal sphincter muscle
Deep perineal (investing or Gallaudet's) fascia
Superficial perineal (Colles') fascia (inferior fascia of superficial perineal space)
Superficial (dartos) fascia of scrotum
External spermatic fascia

Testis

**Median (sagittal) section**

Urachus
Urinary bladder { Apex / Fundus / Body / Trigone / Neck
Pubic symphysis
Suspensory ligament of penis
Inferior (arcuate) pubic ligament
Prostatic venous plexus
Transverse perineal ligament (anterior thickening of perineal membrane)
Perineal membrane
Superficial perineal space
Corpus cavernosum
Corpus spongiosum
Superficial (dartos) fascia of penis and scrotum
Deep (Buck's) fascia of penis
Prepuce
Glans penis and external urethral meatus

Vesical fascia
Rectovesical pouch
Rectum
Seminal vesicle
Prostate
Rectoprostatic (Denonvilliers') fascia
External urethral sphincter muscle
Bulbo-urethral (Cowper's) gland
Perineal body
Bulbospongiosus muscle
Deep perineal (investing or Gallaudet's) fascia
Superficial perineal (Colles') fascia
Deep (Buck's) fascia of penis
Septum of scrotum
Navicular fossa

**Plate 344**     **Pelvic Floor and Contents**

Superior view

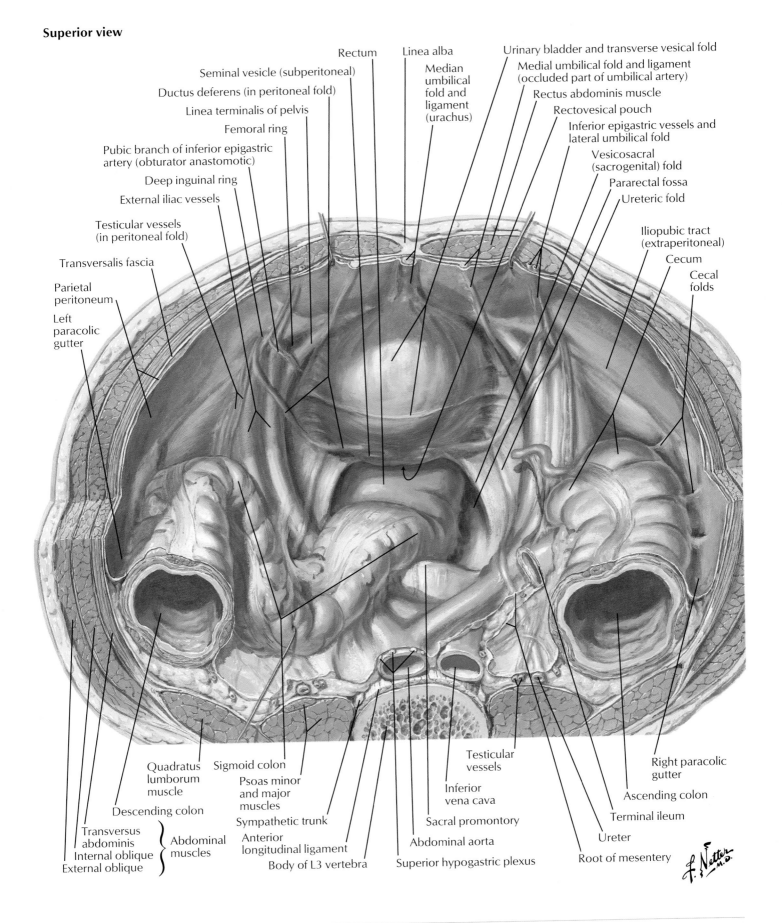

Rectum

Linea alba

Urinary bladder and transverse vesical fold

Seminal vesicle (subperitoneal)

Median umbilical fold and ligament (urachus)

Medial umbilical fold and ligament (occluded part of umbilical artery)

Ductus deferens (in peritoneal fold)

Rectus abdominis muscle

Linea terminalis of pelvis

Rectovesical pouch

Femoral ring

Inferior epigastric vessels and lateral umbilical fold

Pubic branch of inferior epigastric artery (obturator anastomotic)

Vesicosacral (sacrogenital) fold

Deep inguinal ring

Pararectal fossa

External iliac vessels

Ureteric fold

Testicular vessels (in peritoneal fold)

Iliopubic tract (extraperitoneal)

Transversalis fascia

Cecum

Parietal peritoneum

Cecal folds

Left paracolic gutter

Quadratus lumborum muscle

Sigmoid colon

Testicular vessels

Right paracolic gutter

Psoas minor and major muscles

Inferior vena cava

Descending colon

Ascending colon

Sympathetic trunk

Terminal ileum

Transversus abdominis

Anterior longitudinal ligament

Sacral promontory

Internal oblique

Abdominal muscles

Abdominal aorta

Ureter

External oblique

Body of L3 vertebra

Superior hypogastric plexus

Root of mesentery

**Female: midsagittal section**

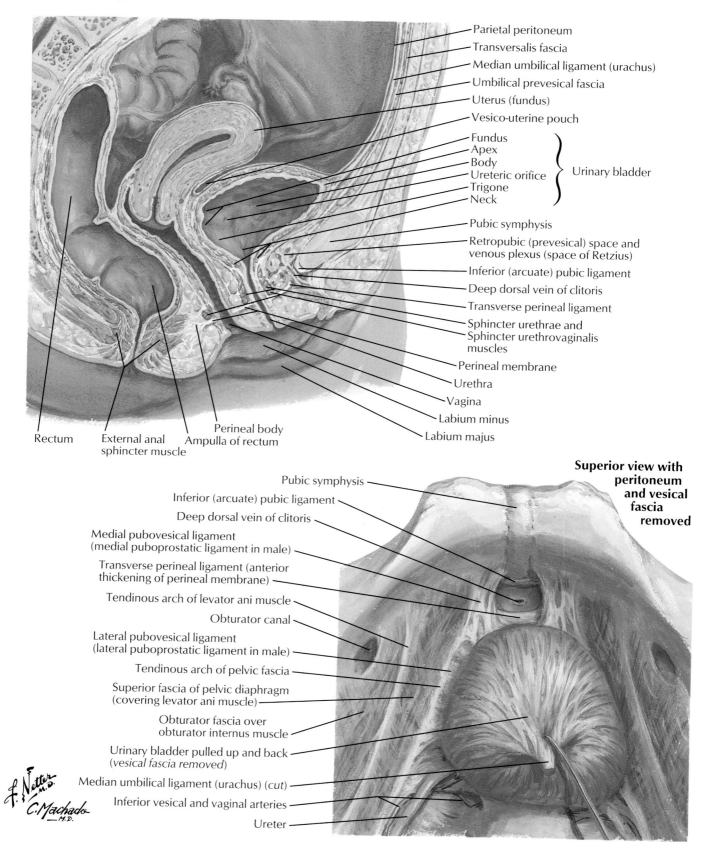

Parietal peritoneum

Transversalis fascia

Median umbilical ligament (urachus)

Umbilical prevesical fascia

Uterus (fundus)

Vesico-uterine pouch

Fundus
Apex
Body
Ureteric orifice
Trigone
Neck
} Urinary bladder

Pubic symphysis

Retropubic (prevesical) space and venous plexus (space of Retzius)

Inferior (arcuate) pubic ligament

Deep dorsal vein of clitoris

Transverse perineal ligament

Sphincter urethrae and Sphincter urethrovaginalis muscles

Perineal membrane

Urethra

Vagina

Labium minus

Labium majus

Rectum

External anal sphincter muscle

Ampulla of rectum

Perineal body

**Superior view with peritoneum and vesical fascia removed**

Pubic symphysis

Inferior (arcuate) pubic ligament

Deep dorsal vein of clitoris

Medial pubovesical ligament (medial puboprostatic ligament in male)

Transverse perineal ligament (anterior thickening of perineal membrane)

Tendinous arch of levator ani muscle

Obturator canal

Lateral pubovesical ligament (lateral puboprostatic ligament in male)

Tendinous arch of pelvic fascia

Superior fascia of pelvic diaphragm (covering levator ani muscle)

Obturator fascia over obturator internus muscle

Urinary bladder pulled up and back (vesical fascia removed)

Median umbilical ligament (urachus) (cut)

Inferior vesical and vaginal arteries

Ureter

**Plate 346**

**Urinary Bladder**

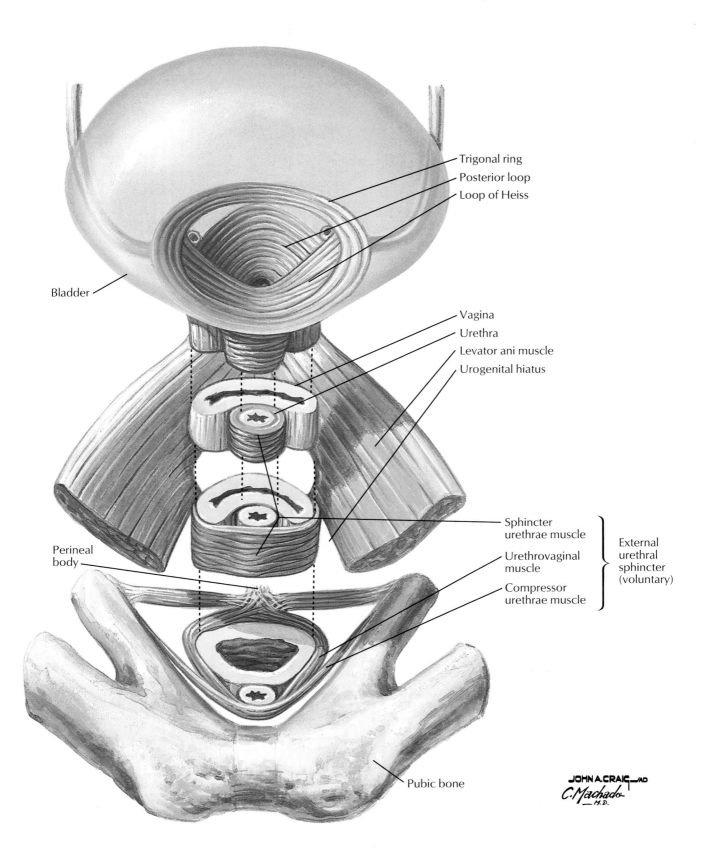

Trigonal ring

Posterior loop

Loop of Heiss

Bladder

Vagina

Urethra

Levator ani muscle

Urogenital hiatus

Sphincter
urethrae muscle

Urethrovaginal
muscle

Compressor
urethrae muscle

External
urethral
sphincter
(voluntary)

Perineal
body

Pubic bone

JOHN A. CRAIG—MD
C. Machado—M.D.

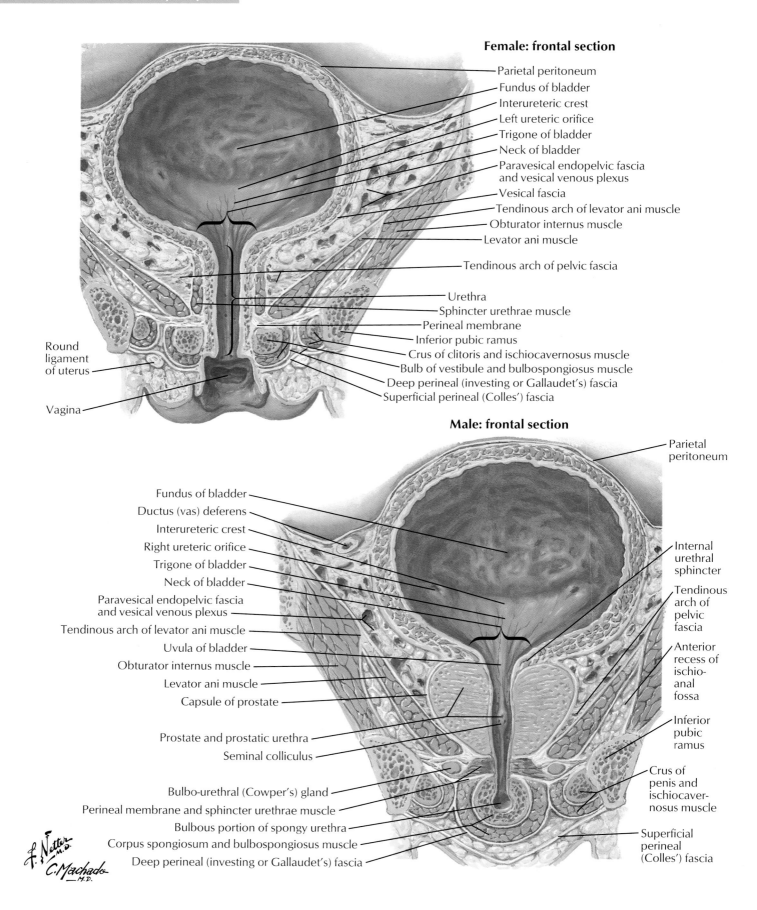

**Female: frontal section**

- Parietal peritoneum
- Fundus of bladder
- Interureteric crest
- Left ureteric orifice
- Trigone of bladder
- Neck of bladder
- Paravesical endopelvic fascia and vesical venous plexus
- Vesical fascia
- Tendinous arch of levator ani muscle
- Obturator internus muscle
- Levator ani muscle
- Tendinous arch of pelvic fascia
- Urethra
- Sphincter urethrae muscle
- Perineal membrane
- Inferior pubic ramus
- Crus of clitoris and ischiocavernosus muscle
- Bulb of vestibule and bulbospongiosus muscle
- Deep perineal (investing or Gallaudet's) fascia
- Superficial perineal (Colles') fascia

Round ligament of uterus

Vagina

**Male: frontal section**

- Parietal peritoneum
- Fundus of bladder
- Ductus (vas) deferens
- Interureteric crest
- Right ureteric orifice
- Trigone of bladder
- Neck of bladder
- Paravesical endopelvic fascia and vesical venous plexus
- Tendinous arch of levator ani muscle
- Uvula of bladder
- Obturator internus muscle
- Levator ani muscle
- Capsule of prostate
- Prostate and prostatic urethra
- Seminal colliculus
- Bulbo-urethral (Cowper's) gland
- Perineal membrane and sphincter urethrae muscle
- Bulbous portion of spongy urethra
- Corpus spongiosum and bulbospongiosus muscle
- Deep perineal (investing or Gallaudet's) fascia
- Internal urethral sphincter
- Tendinous arch of pelvic fascia
- Anterior recess of ischio-anal fossa
- Inferior pubic ramus
- Crus of penis and ischiocavernosus muscle
- Superficial perineal (Colles') fascia

**Plate 348**

**Urinary Bladder**

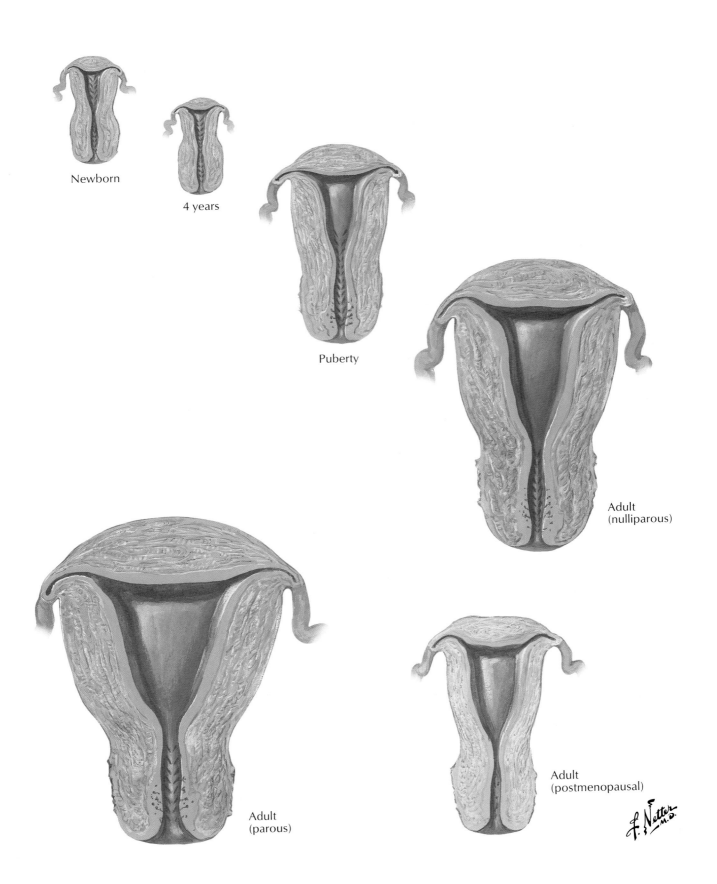

Newborn

4 years

Puberty

Adult
(nulliparous)

Adult
(parous)

Adult
(postmenopausal)

*f. Netter*
M.D.

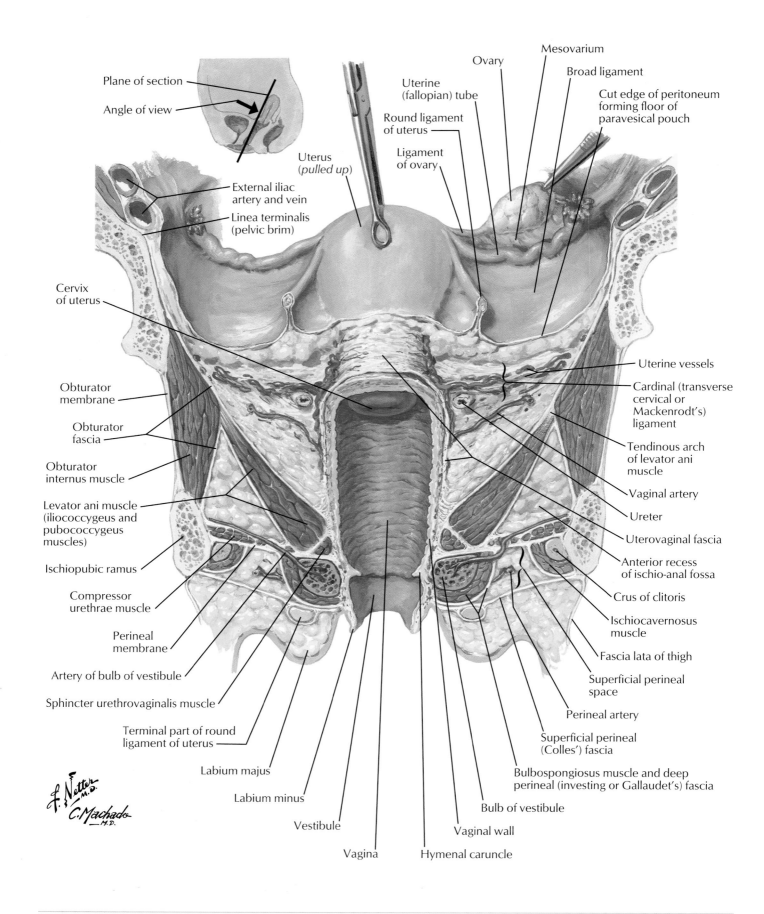

Plane of section

Angle of view

Ovary

Mesovarium

Broad ligament

Uterine (fallopian) tube

Cut edge of peritoneum forming floor of paravesical pouch

Round ligament of uterus

Ligament of ovary

Uterus (*pulled up*)

External iliac artery and vein

Linea terminalis (pelvic brim)

Cervix of uterus

Uterine vessels

Cardinal (transverse cervical or Mackenrodt's) ligament

Obturator membrane

Obturator fascia

Tendinous arch of levator ani muscle

Vaginal artery

Obturator internus muscle

Ureter

Levator ani muscle (iliococcygeus and pubococcygeus muscles)

Uterovaginal fascia

Anterior recess of ischio-anal fossa

Ischiopubic ramus

Crus of clitoris

Compressor urethrae muscle

Ischiocavernosus muscle

Perineal membrane

Fascia lata of thigh

Artery of bulb of vestibule

Superficial perineal space

Sphincter urethrovaginalis muscle

Perineal artery

Terminal part of round ligament of uterus

Superficial perineal (Colles') fascia

Labium majus

Bulbospongiosus muscle and deep perineal (investing or Gallaudet's) fascia

Labium minus

Bulb of vestibule

Vestibule

Vaginal wall

Vagina

Hymenal caruncle

**Plate 350**

**Uterus, Vagina, and Supporting Structures**

**Fascial ligaments of uterus**

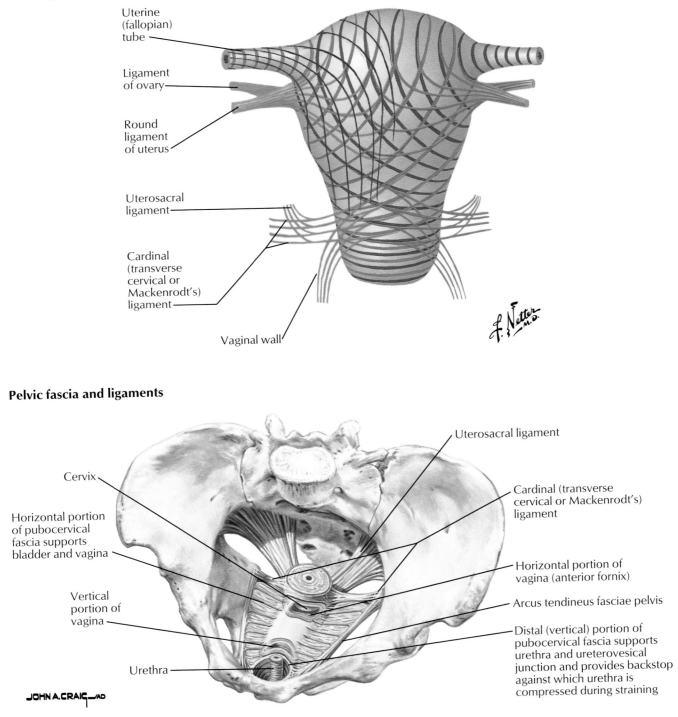

Uterine (fallopian) tube

Ligament of ovary

Round ligament of uterus

Uterosacral ligament

Cardinal (transverse cervical or Mackenrodt's) ligament

Vaginal wall

**Pelvic fascia and ligaments**

Cervix

Horizontal portion of pubocervical fascia supports bladder and vagina

Vertical portion of vagina

Urethra

Uterosacral ligament

Cardinal (transverse cervical or Mackenrodt's) ligament

Horizontal portion of vagina (anterior fornix)

Arcus tendineus fasciae pelvis

Distal (vertical) portion of pubocervical fascia supports urethra and ureterovesical junction and provides backstop against which urethra is compressed during straining

JOHN A. CRAIG—AD

**Uterus, Vagina, and Supporting Structures**

**Plate 351**

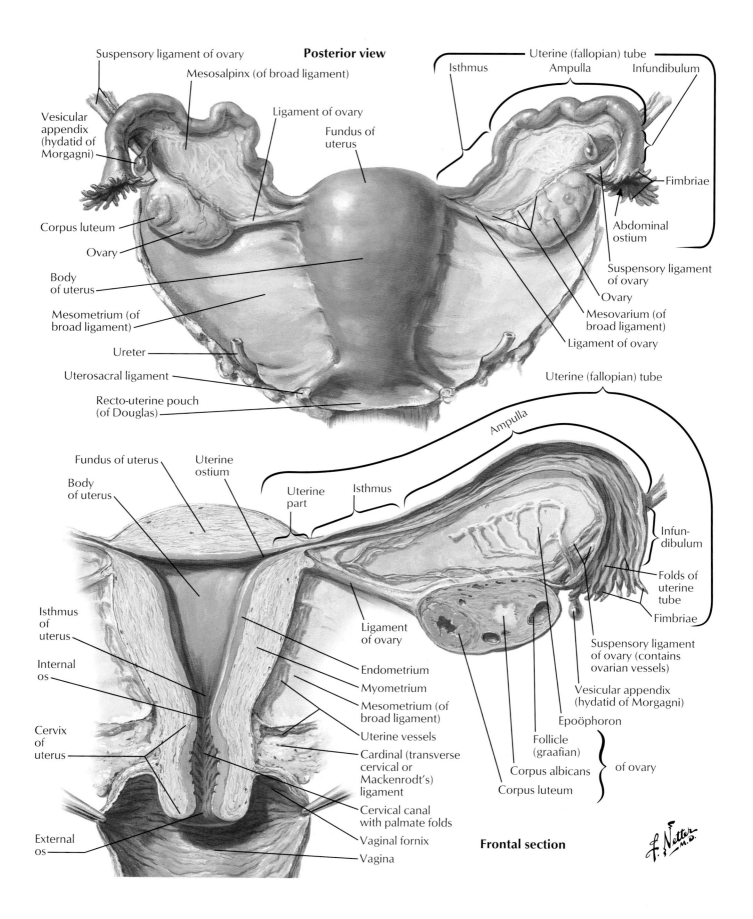

**Posterior view**

Suspensory ligament of ovary

Mesosalpinx (of broad ligament)

Vesicular appendix (hydatid of Morgagni)

Ligament of ovary

Fundus of uterus

Corpus luteum

Ovary

Body of uterus

Mesometrium (of broad ligament)

Ureter

Uterosacral ligament

Recto-uterine pouch (of Douglas)

Uterine (fallopian) tube

Isthmus

Ampulla

Infundibulum

Fimbriae

Abdominal ostium

Suspensory ligament of ovary

Ovary

Mesovarium (of broad ligament)

Ligament of ovary

Uterine (fallopian) tube

Ampulla

Fundus of uterus

Uterine ostium

Body of uterus

Uterine part

Isthmus

Infundibulum

Folds of uterine tube

Fimbriae

Suspensory ligament of ovary (contains ovarian vessels)

Vesicular appendix (hydatid of Morgagni)

Epoöphoron

Follicle (graafian)

Corpus albicans

Corpus luteum

of ovary

Isthmus of uterus

Internal os

Cervix of uterus

External os

Ligament of ovary

Endometrium

Myometrium

Mesometrium (of broad ligament)

Uterine vessels

Cardinal (transverse cervical or Mackenrodt's) ligament

Cervical canal with palmate folds

Vaginal fornix

Vagina

**Frontal section**

**Plate 352**

**Uterus, Vagina, and Supporting Structures**

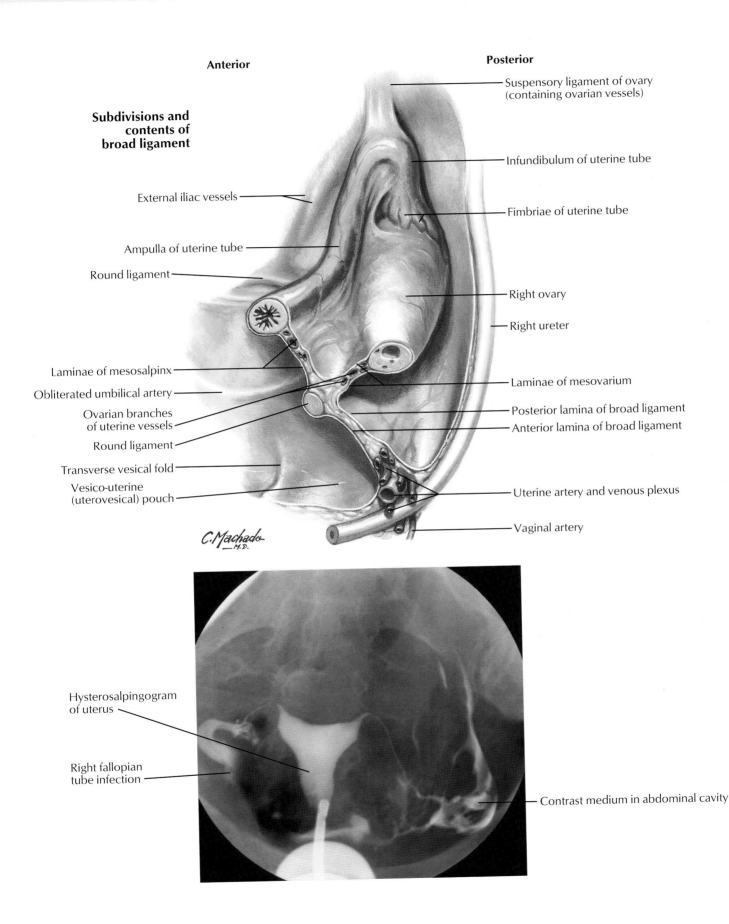

Anterior
Posterior

Suspensory ligament of ovary
(containing ovarian vessels)

**Subdivisions and
contents of
broad ligament**

Infundibulum of uterine tube

External iliac vessels

Fimbriae of uterine tube

Ampulla of uterine tube

Round ligament

Right ovary

Right ureter

Laminae of mesosalpinx

Laminae of mesovarium

Obliterated umbilical artery

Posterior lamina of broad ligament

Ovarian branches
of uterine vessels

Anterior lamina of broad ligament

Round ligament

Transverse vesical fold

Vesico-uterine
(uterovesical) pouch

Uterine artery and venous plexus

Vaginal artery

C. Machado
_M.D._

Hysterosalpingogram
of uterus

Right fallopian
tube infection

Contrast medium in abdominal cavity

**Uterus, Vagina, and Supporting Structures**

**Plate 353**

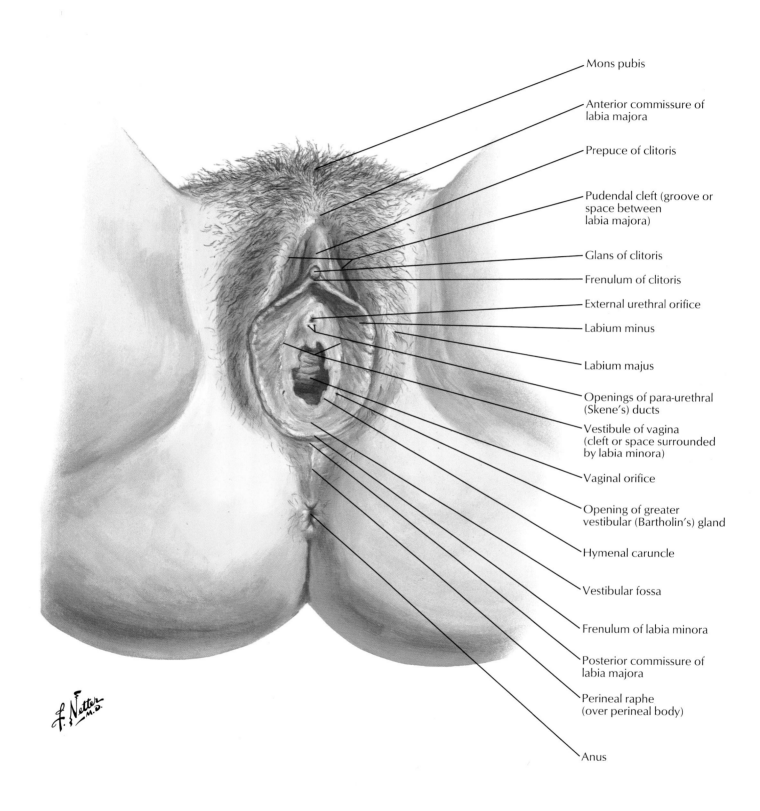

Mons pubis

Anterior commissure of labia majora

Prepuce of clitoris

Pudendal cleft (groove or space between labia majora)

Glans of clitoris

Frenulum of clitoris

External urethral orifice

Labium minus

Labium majus

Openings of para-urethral (Skene's) ducts

Vestibule of vagina (cleft or space surrounded by labia minora)

Vaginal orifice

Opening of greater vestibular (Bartholin's) gland

Hymenal caruncle

Vestibular fossa

Frenulum of labia minora

Posterior commissure of labia majora

Perineal raphe (over perineal body)

Anus

**Plate 354**

**Perineum and External Genitalia: Female**

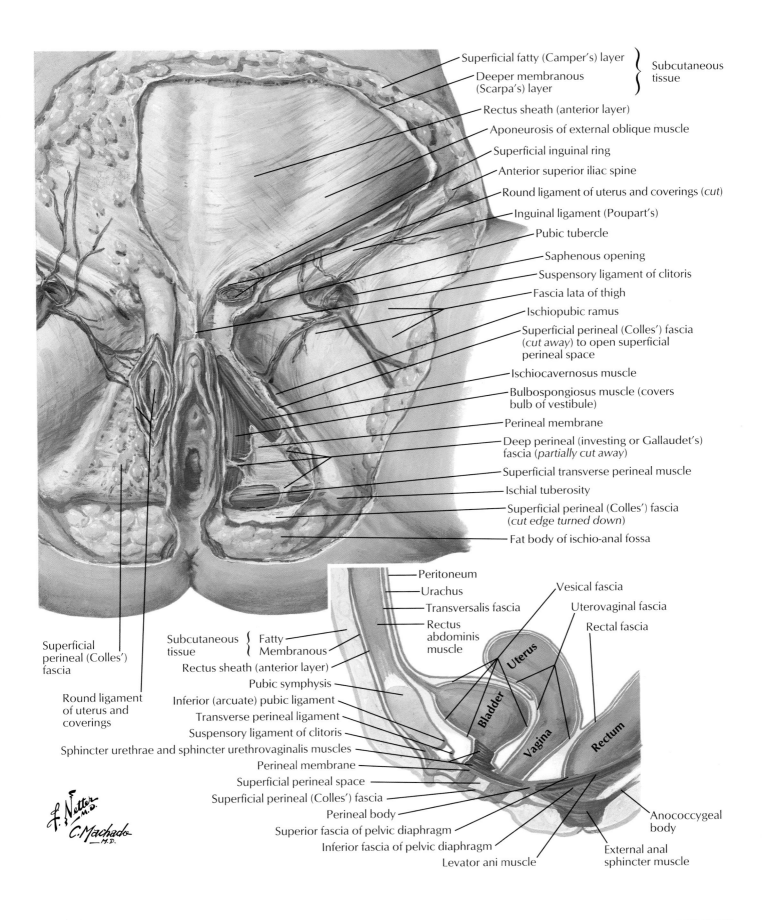

Superficial fatty (Camper's) layer ⎫
Deeper membranous (Scarpa's) layer ⎬ Subcutaneous tissue

Rectus sheath (anterior layer)

Aponeurosis of external oblique muscle

Superficial inguinal ring

Anterior superior iliac spine

Round ligament of uterus and coverings (*cut*)

Inguinal ligament (Poupart's)

Pubic tubercle

Saphenous opening

Suspensory ligament of clitoris

Fascia lata of thigh

Ischiopubic ramus

Superficial perineal (Colles') fascia (*cut away*) to open superficial perineal space

Ischiocavernosus muscle

Bulbospongiosus muscle (covers bulb of vestibule)

Perineal membrane

Deep perineal (investing or Gallaudet's) fascia (*partially cut away*)

Superficial transverse perineal muscle

Ischial tuberosity

Superficial perineal (Colles') fascia (*cut edge turned down*)

Fat body of ischio-anal fossa

Superficial perineal (Colles') fascia

Round ligament of uterus and coverings

Subcutaneous tissue ⎧ Fatty
⎨
⎩ Membranous

Rectus sheath (anterior layer)

Pubic symphysis

Inferior (arcuate) pubic ligament

Transverse perineal ligament

Suspensory ligament of clitoris

Sphincter urethrae and sphincter urethrovaginalis muscles

Perineal membrane

Superficial perineal space

Superficial perineal (Colles') fascia

Perineal body

Superior fascia of pelvic diaphragm

Inferior fascia of pelvic diaphragm

Levator ani muscle

Peritoneum

Urachus

Transversalis fascia

Rectus abdominis muscle

Vesical fascia

Uterovaginal fascia

Rectal fascia

Uterus

Bladder

Vagina

Rectum

Anococcygeal body

External anal sphincter muscle

**Perineum and External Genitalia: Female**

**Plate 355**

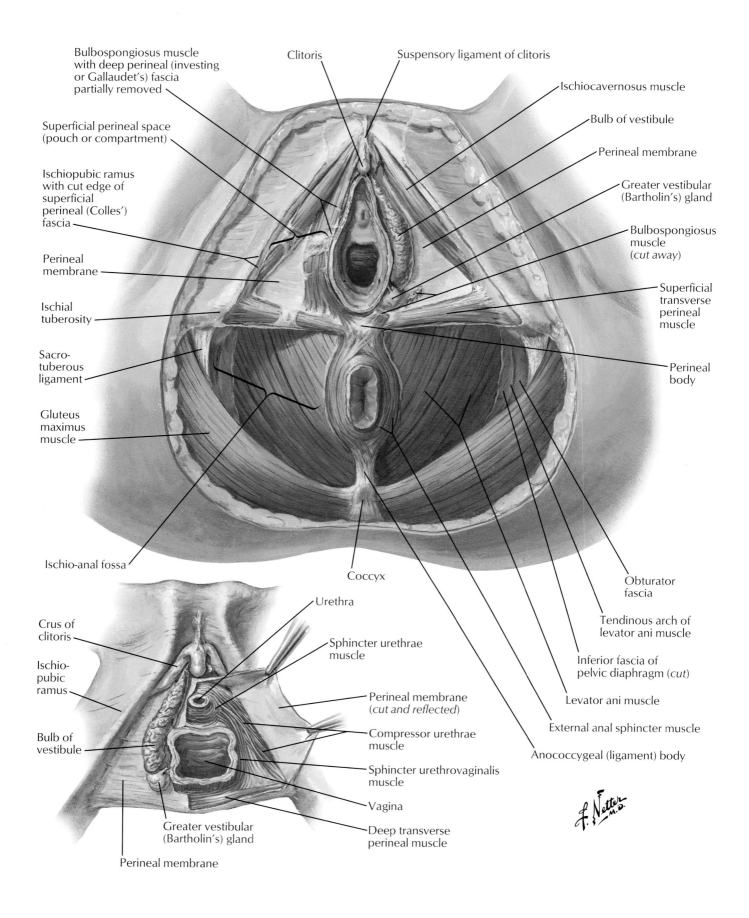

Bulbospongiosus muscle with deep perineal (investing or Gallaudet's) fascia partially removed

Superficial perineal space (pouch or compartment)

Ischiopubic ramus with cut edge of superficial perineal (Colles') fascia

Perineal membrane

Ischial tuberosity

Sacro-tuberous ligament

Gluteus maximus muscle

Ischio-anal fossa

Clitoris

Suspensory ligament of clitoris

Ischiocavernosus muscle

Bulb of vestibule

Perineal membrane

Greater vestibular (Bartholin's) gland

Bulbospongiosus muscle (cut away)

Superficial transverse perineal muscle

Perineal body

Obturator fascia

Tendinous arch of levator ani muscle

Inferior fascia of pelvic diaphragm (cut)

Levator ani muscle

External anal sphincter muscle

Anococcygeal (ligament) body

Coccyx

Crus of clitoris

Ischio-pubic ramus

Bulb of vestibule

Urethra

Sphincter urethrae muscle

Perineal membrane (cut and reflected)

Compressor urethrae muscle

Sphincter urethrovaginalis muscle

Vagina

Deep transverse perineal muscle

Greater vestibular (Bartholin's) gland

Perineal membrane

**Plate 356**

**Perineum and External Genitalia: Female**

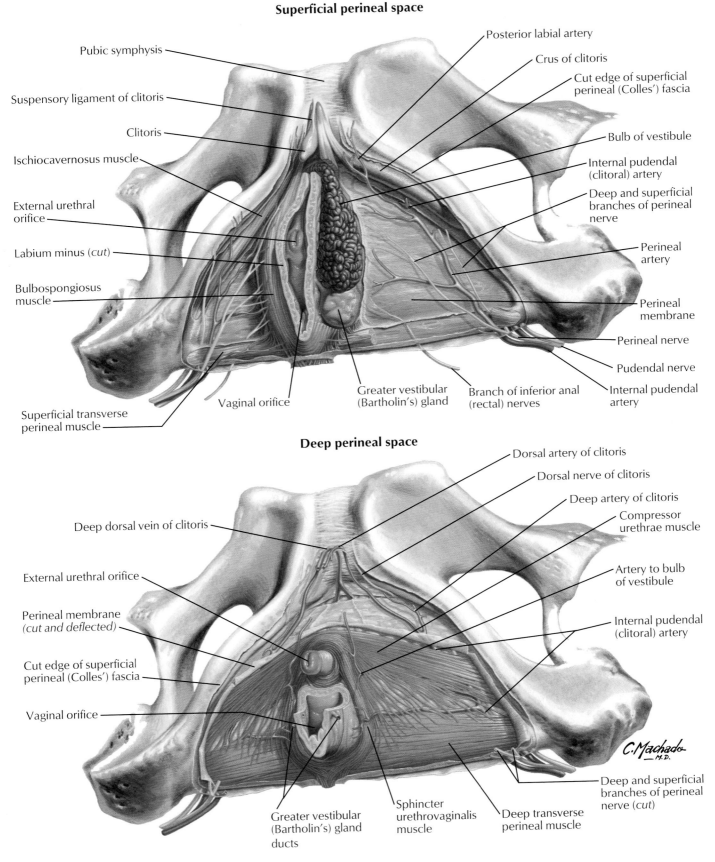

**Superficial perineal space**

Pubic symphysis

Suspensory ligament of clitoris

Clitoris

Ischiocavernosus muscle

External urethral orifice

Labium minus (cut)

Bulbospongiosus muscle

Superficial transverse perineal muscle

Posterior labial artery

Crus of clitoris

Cut edge of superficial perineal (Colles') fascia

Bulb of vestibule

Internal pudendal (clitoral) artery

Deep and superficial branches of perineal nerve

Perineal artery

Perineal membrane

Perineal nerve

Pudendal nerve

Internal pudendal artery

Vaginal orifice

Greater vestibular (Bartholin's) gland

Branch of inferior anal (rectal) nerves

**Deep perineal space**

Deep dorsal vein of clitoris

External urethral orifice

Perineal membrane (cut and deflected)

Cut edge of superficial perineal (Colles') fascia

Vaginal orifice

Dorsal artery of clitoris

Dorsal nerve of clitoris

Deep artery of clitoris

Compressor urethrae muscle

Artery to bulb of vestibule

Internal pudendal (clitoral) artery

Deep and superficial branches of perineal nerve (cut)

Greater vestibular (Bartholin's) gland ducts

Sphincter urethrovaginalis muscle

Deep transverse perineal muscle

C. Machado M.D.

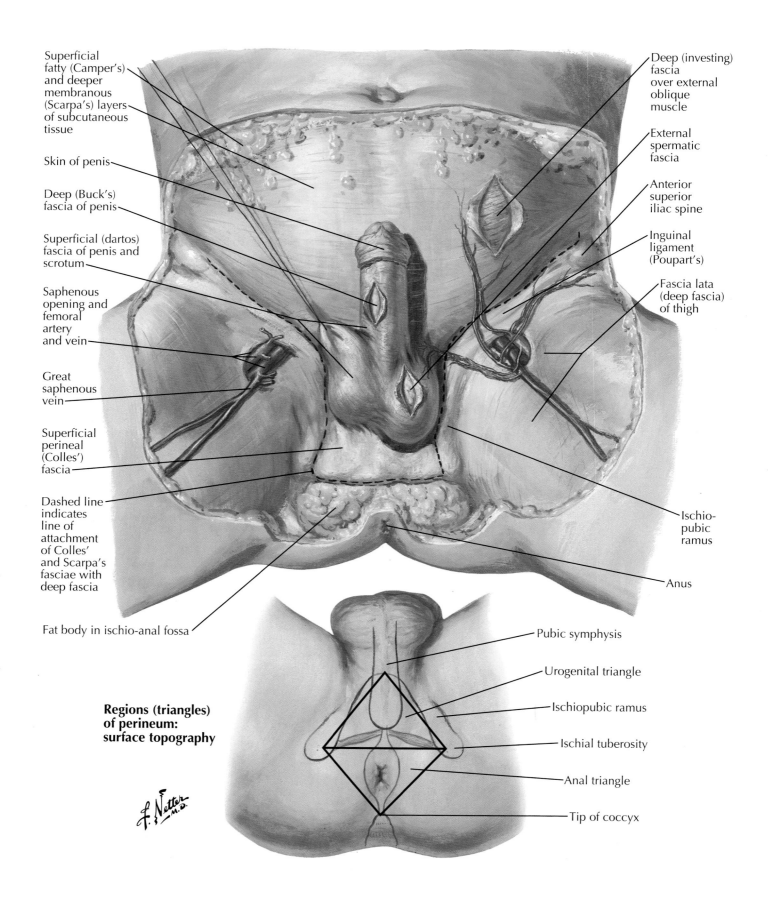

Superficial fatty (Camper's) and deeper membranous (Scarpa's) layers of subcutaneous tissue

Skin of penis

Deep (Buck's) fascia of penis

Superficial (dartos) fascia of penis and scrotum

Saphenous opening and femoral artery and vein

Great saphenous vein

Superficial perineal (Colles') fascia

Dashed line indicates line of attachment of Colles' and Scarpa's fasciae with deep fascia

Fat body in ischio-anal fossa

Deep (investing) fascia over external oblique muscle

External spermatic fascia

Anterior superior iliac spine

Inguinal ligament (Poupart's)

Fascia lata (deep fascia) of thigh

Ischio-pubic ramus

Anus

**Regions (triangles) of perineum: surface topography**

Pubic symphysis

Urogenital triangle

Ischiopubic ramus

Ischial tuberosity

Anal triangle

Tip of coccyx

# Male Perineum and External Genitalia (Deeper Dissection)

See also Plates 378, 380, 383

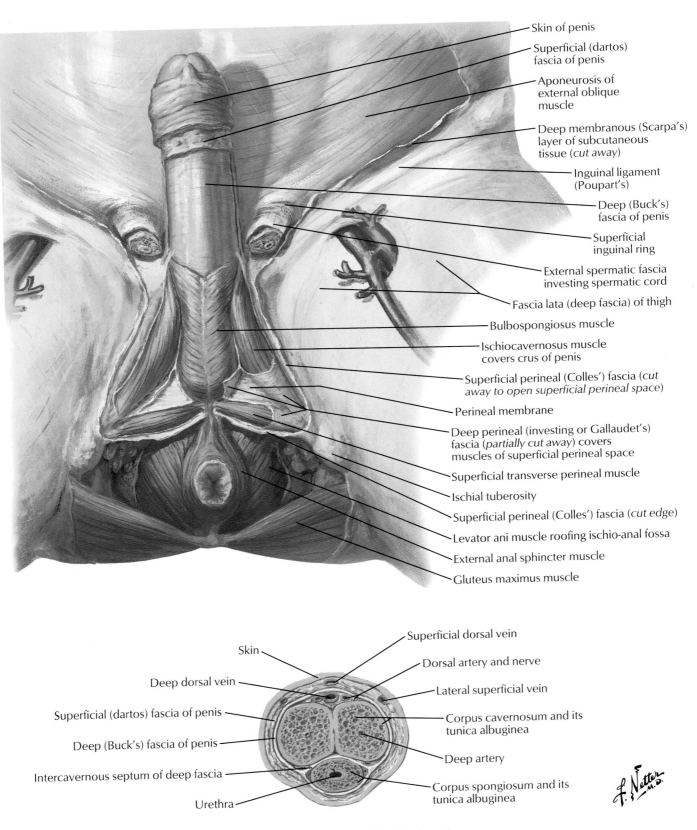

- Skin of penis
- Superficial (dartos) fascia of penis
- Aponeurosis of external oblique muscle
- Deep membranous (Scarpa's) layer of subcutaneous tissue (*cut away*)
- Inguinal ligament (Poupart's)
- Deep (Buck's) fascia of penis
- Superficial inguinal ring
- External spermatic fascia investing spermatic cord
- Fascia lata (deep fascia) of thigh
- Bulbospongiosus muscle
- Ischiocavernosus muscle covers crus of penis
- Superficial perineal (Colles') fascia (*cut away to open superficial perineal space*)
- Perineal membrane
- Deep perineal (investing or Gallaudet's) fascia (*partially cut away*) covers muscles of superficial perineal space
- Superficial transverse perineal muscle
- Ischial tuberosity
- Superficial perineal (Colles') fascia (*cut edge*)
- Levator ani muscle roofing ischio-anal fossa
- External anal sphincter muscle
- Gluteus maximus muscle

Skin —
Deep dorsal vein —
Superficial (dartos) fascia of penis —
Deep (Buck's) fascia of penis —
Intercavernous septum of deep fascia —
Urethra —

Superficial dorsal vein
Dorsal artery and nerve
Lateral superficial vein
Corpus cavernosum and its tunica albuginea
Deep artery
Corpus spongiosum and its tunica albuginea

**Transverse section through body of penis**

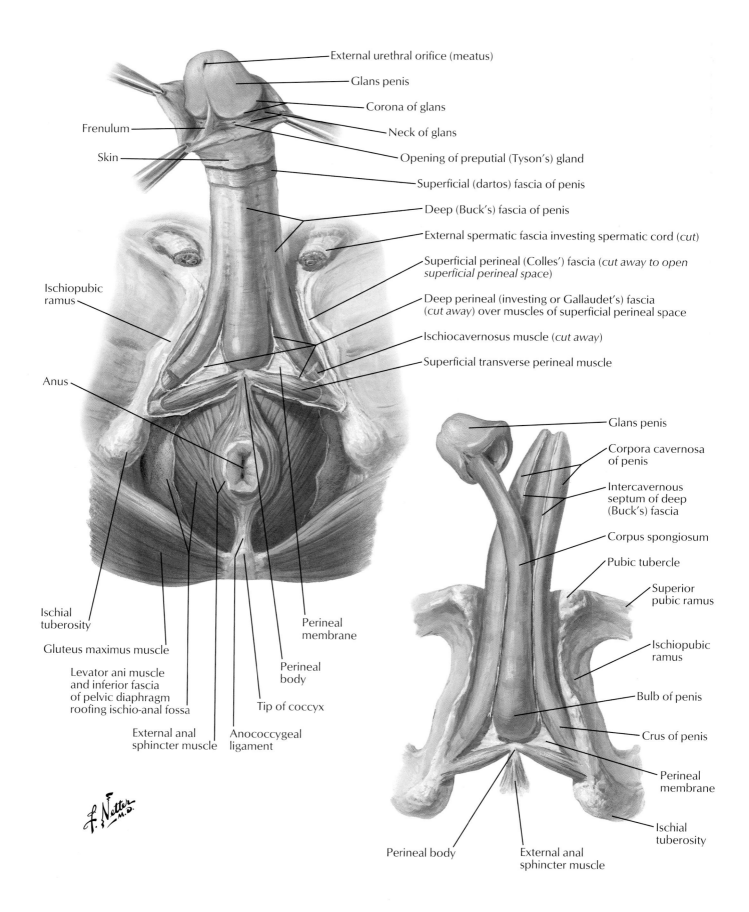

External urethral orifice (meatus)

Glans penis

Corona of glans

Frenulum

Neck of glans

Skin

Opening of preputial (Tyson's) gland

Superficial (dartos) fascia of penis

Deep (Buck's) fascia of penis

External spermatic fascia investing spermatic cord (*cut*)

Superficial perineal (Colles') fascia (*cut away to open superficial perineal space*)

Ischiopubic ramus

Deep perineal (investing or Gallaudet's) fascia (*cut away*) over muscles of superficial perineal space

Ischiocavernosus muscle (*cut away*)

Superficial transverse perineal muscle

Anus

Glans penis

Corpora cavernosa of penis

Intercavernous septum of deep (Buck's) fascia

Corpus spongiosum

Pubic tubercle

Superior pubic ramus

Ischiopubic ramus

Bulb of penis

Crus of penis

Perineal membrane

Ischial tuberosity

Ischial tuberosity

Gluteus maximus muscle

Levator ani muscle and inferior fascia of pelvic diaphragm roofing ischio-anal fossa

External anal sphincter muscle

Anococcygeal ligament

Tip of coccyx

Perineal body

Perineal membrane

Perineal body

External anal sphincter muscle

**Plate 360**

**Perineum and External Genitalia: Male**

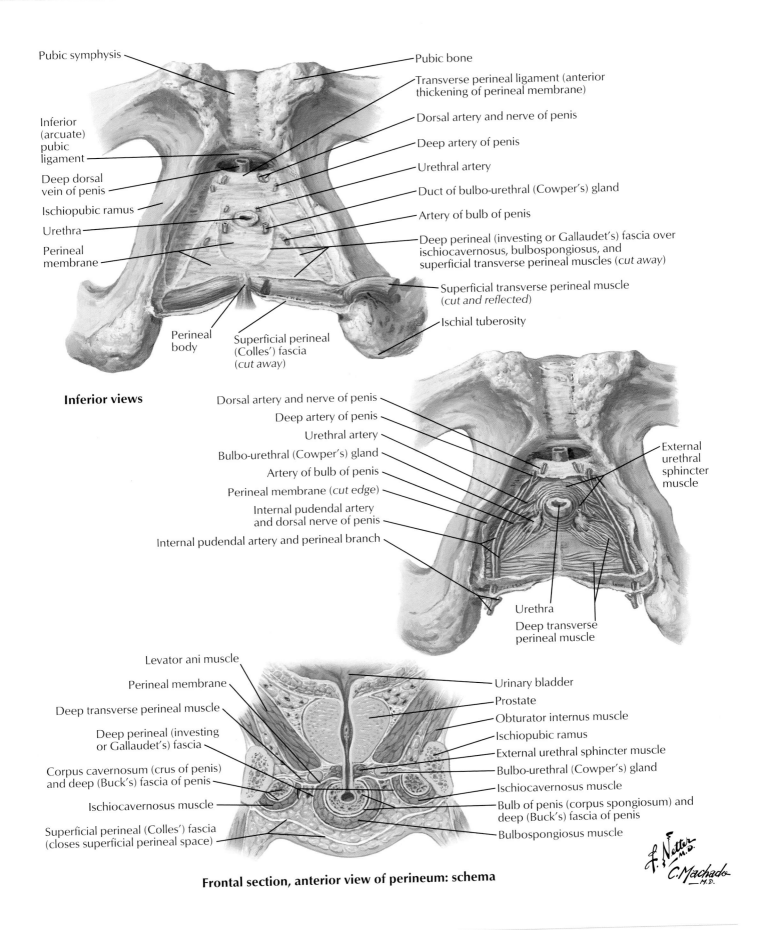

Pubic symphysis

Inferior (arcuate) pubic ligament

Deep dorsal vein of penis

Ischiopubic ramus

Urethra

Perineal membrane

Perineal body

Superficial perineal (Colles') fascia (*cut away*)

**Inferior views**

Pubic bone

Transverse perineal ligament (anterior thickening of perineal membrane)

Dorsal artery and nerve of penis

Deep artery of penis

Urethral artery

Duct of bulbo-urethral (Cowper's) gland

Artery of bulb of penis

Deep perineal (investing or Gallaudet's) fascia over ischiocavernosus, bulbospongiosus, and superficial transverse perineal muscles (*cut away*)

Superficial transverse perineal muscle (*cut and reflected*)

Ischial tuberosity

Dorsal artery and nerve of penis

Deep artery of penis

Urethral artery

Bulbo-urethral (Cowper's) gland

Artery of bulb of penis

Perineal membrane (*cut edge*)

Internal pudendal artery and dorsal nerve of penis

Internal pudendal artery and perineal branch

External urethral sphincter muscle

Urethra

Deep transverse perineal muscle

Levator ani muscle

Perineal membrane

Deep transverse perineal muscle

Deep perineal (investing or Gallaudet's) fascia

Corpus cavernosum (crus of penis) and deep (Buck's) fascia of penis

Ischiocavernosus muscle

Superficial perineal (Colles') fascia (closes superficial perineal space)

Urinary bladder

Prostate

Obturator internus muscle

Ischiopubic ramus

External urethral sphincter muscle

Bulbo-urethral (Cowper's) gland

Ischiocavernosus muscle

Bulb of penis (corpus spongiosum) and deep (Buck's) fascia of penis

Bulbospongiosus muscle

**Frontal section, anterior view of perineum: schema**

**Perineum and External Genitalia: Male**

**Plate 361**

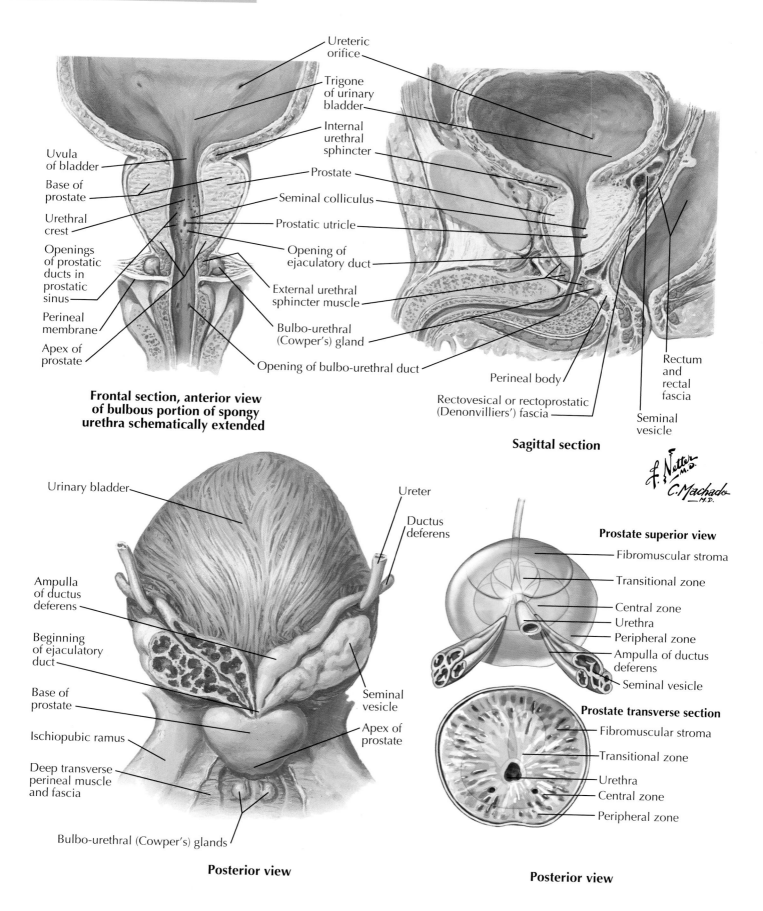

Ureteric orifice

Trigone of urinary bladder

Internal urethral sphincter

Uvula of bladder

Base of prostate

Prostate

Seminal colliculus

Urethral crest

Prostatic utricle

Openings of prostatic ducts in prostatic sinus

Opening of ejaculatory duct

External urethral sphincter muscle

Perineal membrane

Bulbo-urethral (Cowper's) gland

Apex of prostate

Opening of bulbo-urethral duct

**Frontal section, anterior view of bulbous portion of spongy urethra schematically extended**

Perineal body

Rectovesical or rectoprostatic (Denonvilliers') fascia

Rectum and rectal fascia

Seminal vesicle

**Sagittal section**

Urinary bladder

Ureter

Ductus deferens

Ampulla of ductus deferens

Beginning of ejaculatory duct

Base of prostate

Ischiopubic ramus

Deep transverse perineal muscle and fascia

Seminal vesicle

Apex of prostate

Bulbo-urethral (Cowper's) glands

**Posterior view**

**Prostate superior view**

Fibromuscular stroma

Transitional zone

Central zone

Urethra

Peripheral zone

Ampulla of ductus deferens

Seminal vesicle

**Prostate transverse section**

Fibromuscular stroma

Transitional zone

Urethra

Central zone

Peripheral zone

**Posterior view**

**Plate 362**

**Perineum and External Genitalia: Male**

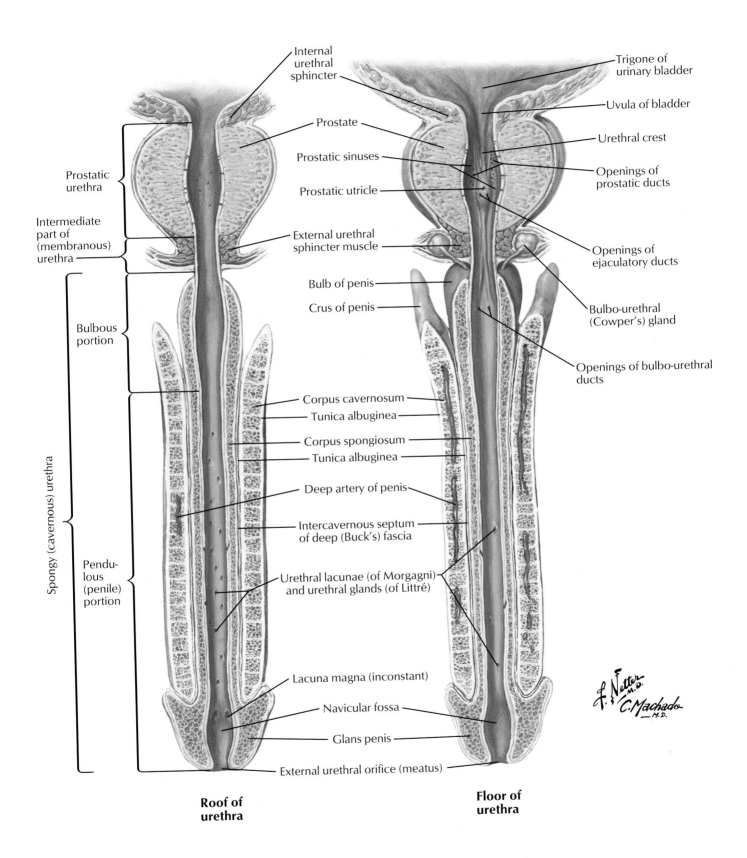

Internal urethral sphincter

Prostate

Prostatic sinuses

Prostatic utricle

External urethral sphincter muscle

Bulb of penis

Crus of penis

Corpus cavernosum

Tunica albuginea

Corpus spongiosum

Tunica albuginea

Deep artery of penis

Intercavernous septum of deep (Buck's) fascia

Urethral lacunae (of Morgagni) and urethral glands (of Littré)

Lacuna magna (inconstant)

Navicular fossa

Glans penis

External urethral orifice (meatus)

Trigone of urinary bladder

Uvula of bladder

Urethral crest

Openings of prostatic ducts

Openings of ejaculatory ducts

Bulbo-urethral (Cowper's) gland

Openings of bulbo-urethral ducts

Prostatic urethra

Intermediate part of (membranous) urethra

Bulbous portion

Spongy (cavernous) urethra

Pendulous (penile) portion

**Roof of urethra**

**Floor of urethra**

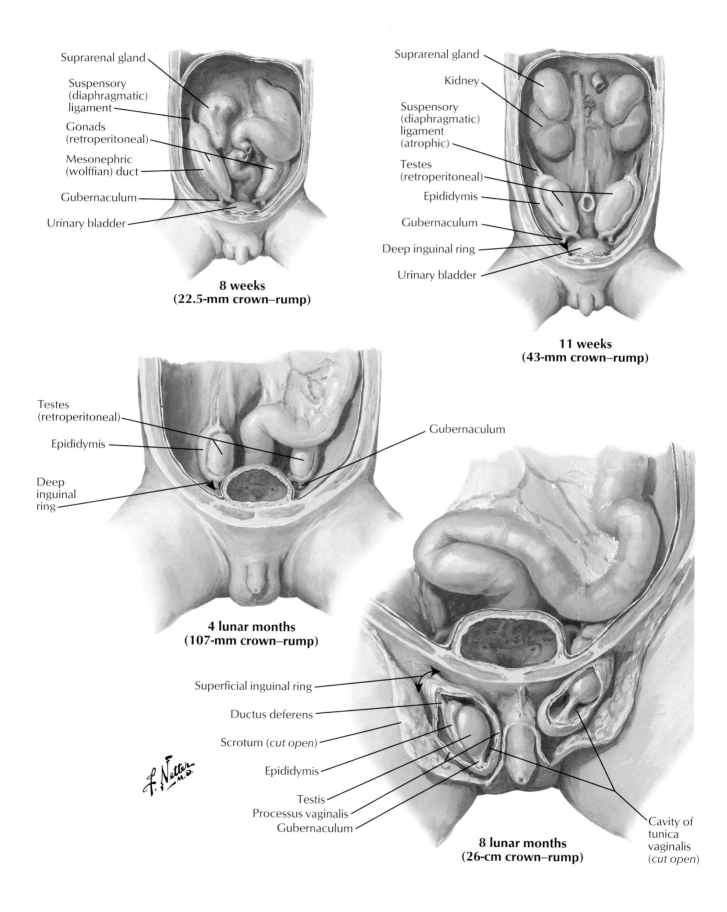

Suprarenal gland

Suspensory (diaphragmatic) ligament

Gonads (retroperitoneal)

Mesonephric (wolffian) duct

Gubernaculum

Urinary bladder

**8 weeks
(22.5-mm crown–rump)**

Suprarenal gland

Kidney

Suspensory (diaphragmatic) ligament (atrophic)

Testes (retroperitoneal)

Epididymis

Gubernaculum

Deep inguinal ring

Urinary bladder

**11 weeks
(43-mm crown–rump)**

Testes (retroperitoneal)

Epididymis

Deep inguinal ring

Gubernaculum

**4 lunar months
(107-mm crown–rump)**

Superficial inguinal ring

Ductus deferens

Scrotum (cut open)

Epididymis

Testis

Processus vaginalis

Gubernaculum

Cavity of tunica vaginalis (cut open)

**8 lunar months
(26-cm crown–rump)**

**Plate 364**

**Perineum and External Genitalia: Male**

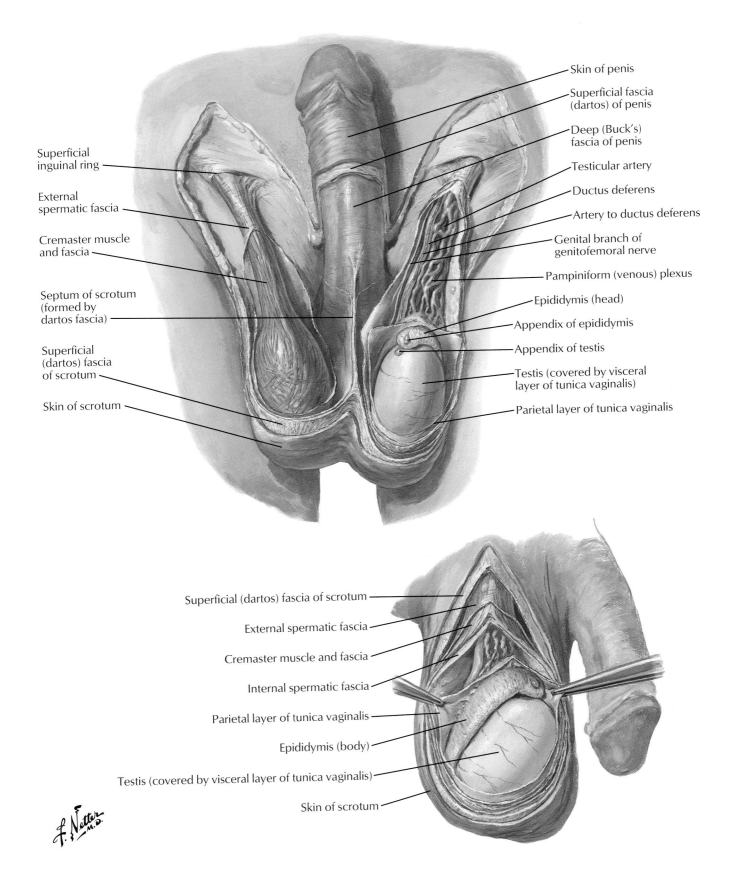

Skin of penis

Superficial fascia (dartos) of penis

Deep (Buck's) fascia of penis

Testicular artery

Ductus deferens

Artery to ductus deferens

Genital branch of genitofemoral nerve

Pampiniform (venous) plexus

Epididymis (head)

Appendix of epididymis

Appendix of testis

Testis (covered by visceral layer of tunica vaginalis)

Parietal layer of tunica vaginalis

Superficial inguinal ring

External spermatic fascia

Cremaster muscle and fascia

Septum of scrotum (formed by dartos fascia)

Superficial (dartos) fascia of scrotum

Skin of scrotum

Superficial (dartos) fascia of scrotum

External spermatic fascia

Cremaster muscle and fascia

Internal spermatic fascia

Parietal layer of tunica vaginalis

Epididymis (body)

Testis (covered by visceral layer of tunica vaginalis)

Skin of scrotum

**Perineum and External Genitalia: Male**

**Plate 365**

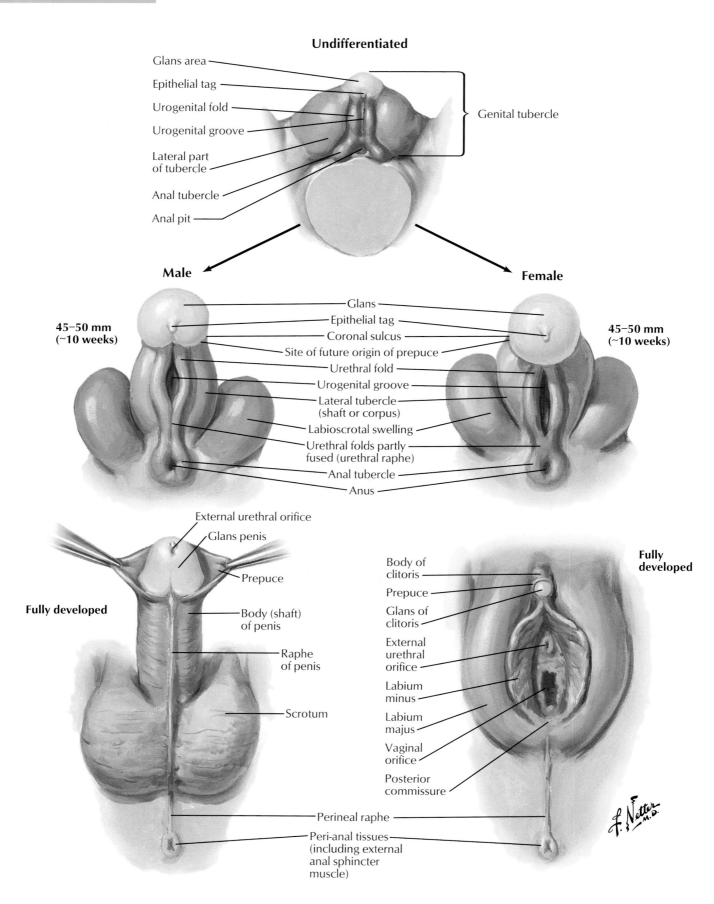

**Undifferentiated**

Glans area
Epithelial tag
Urogenital fold
Urogenital groove
Lateral part of tubercle
Anal tubercle
Anal pit

Genital tubercle

**Male**

45–50 mm (~10 weeks)

**Female**

45–50 mm (~10 weeks)

Glans
Epithelial tag
Coronal sulcus
Site of future origin of prepuce
Urethral fold
Urogenital groove
Lateral tubercle (shaft or corpus)
Labioscrotal swelling
Urethral folds partly fused (urethral raphe)
Anal tubercle
Anus

External urethral orifice
Glans penis
Prepuce
Body (shaft) of penis
Raphe of penis
Scrotum

**Fully developed**

Body of clitoris
Prepuce
Glans of clitoris
External urethral orifice
Labium minus
Labium majus
Vaginal orifice
Posterior commissure

**Fully developed**

Perineal raphe
Peri-anal tissues (including external anal sphincter muscle)

**Plate 366**

**Homologues of Genitalia**

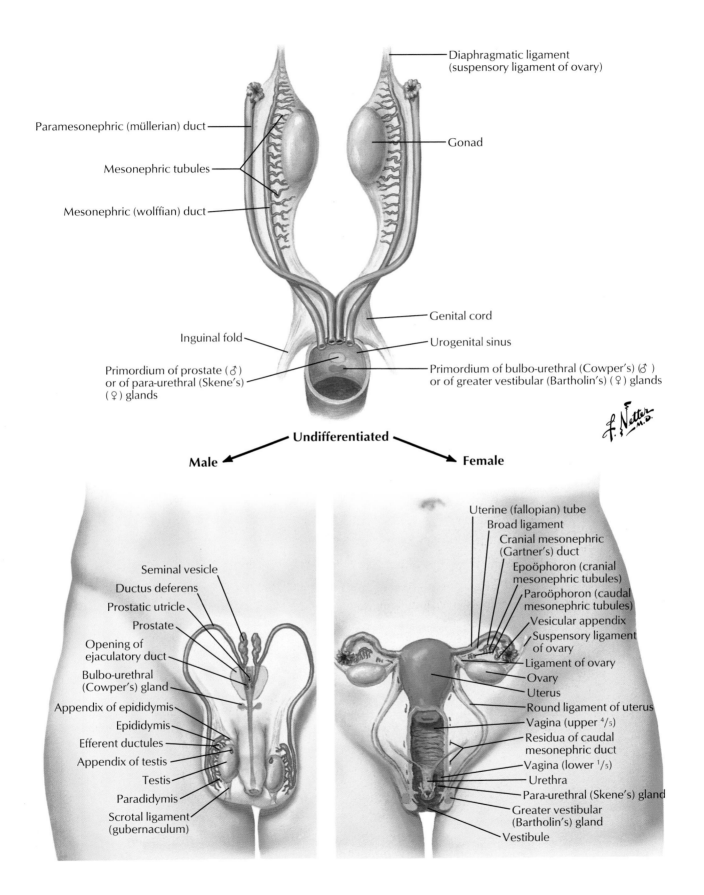

Diaphragmatic ligament (suspensory ligament of ovary)

Paramesonephric (müllerian) duct

Mesonephric tubules

Mesonephric (wolffian) duct

Gonad

Genital cord

Inguinal fold

Urogenital sinus

Primordium of prostate (♂) or of para-urethral (Skene's) (♀) glands

Primordium of bulbo-urethral (Cowper's) (♂) or of greater vestibular (Bartholin's) (♀) glands

**Undifferentiated**

**Male**

**Female**

Seminal vesicle

Ductus deferens

Prostatic utricle

Prostate

Opening of ejaculatory duct

Bulbo-urethral (Cowper's) gland

Appendix of epididymis

Epididymis

Efferent ductules

Appendix of testis

Testis

Paradidymis

Scrotal ligament (gubernaculum)

Uterine (fallopian) tube

Broad ligament

Cranial mesonephric (Gartner's) duct

Epoöphoron (cranial mesonephric tubules)

Paroöphoron (caudal mesonephric tubules)

Vesicular appendix

Suspensory ligament of ovary

Ligament of ovary

Ovary

Uterus

Round ligament of uterus

Vagina (upper ⁴/₅)

Residua of caudal mesonephric duct

Vagina (lower ¹/₅)

Urethra

Para-urethral (Skene's) gland

Greater vestibular (Bartholin's) gland

Vestibule

**Homologues of Genitalia**

**Plate 367**

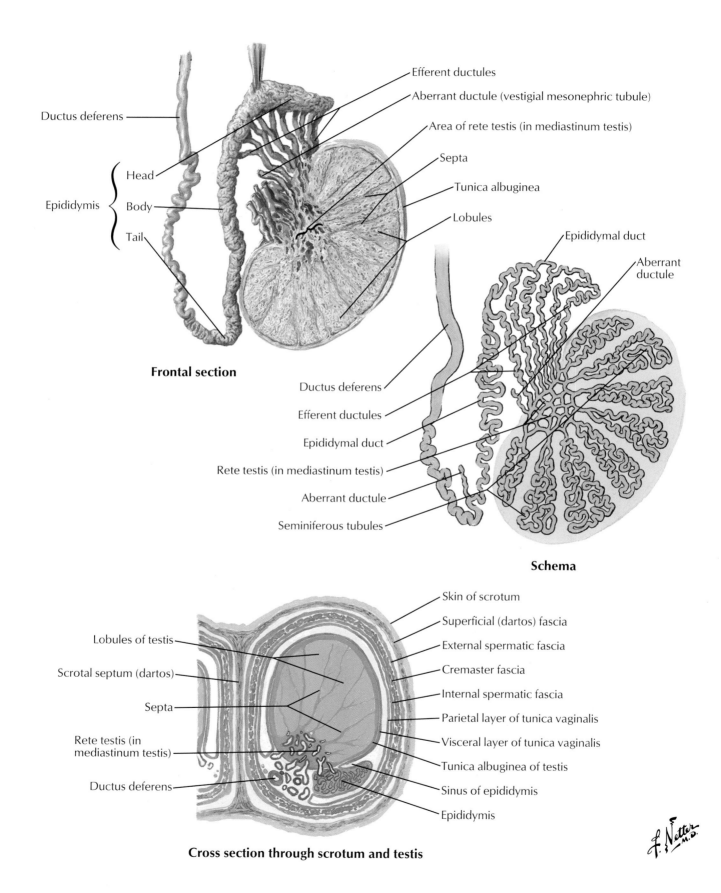

**Frontal section**

Efferent ductules

Aberrant ductule (vestigial mesonephric tubule)

Area of rete testis (in mediastinum testis)

Septa

Tunica albuginea

Lobules

Ductus deferens

Head

Body

Tail

Epididymis

Ductus deferens

Efferent ductules

Epididymal duct

Rete testis (in mediastinum testis)

Aberrant ductule

Seminiferous tubules

Epididymal duct

Aberrant ductule

**Schema**

Lobules of testis

Scrotal septum (dartos)

Septa

Rete testis (in mediastinum testis)

Ductus deferens

Skin of scrotum

Superficial (dartos) fascia

External spermatic fascia

Cremaster fascia

Internal spermatic fascia

Parietal layer of tunica vaginalis

Visceral layer of tunica vaginalis

Tunica albuginea of testis

Sinus of epididymis

Epididymis

**Cross section through scrotum and testis**

**Plate 368**

**Testis, Epididymis, and Ductus Deferens**

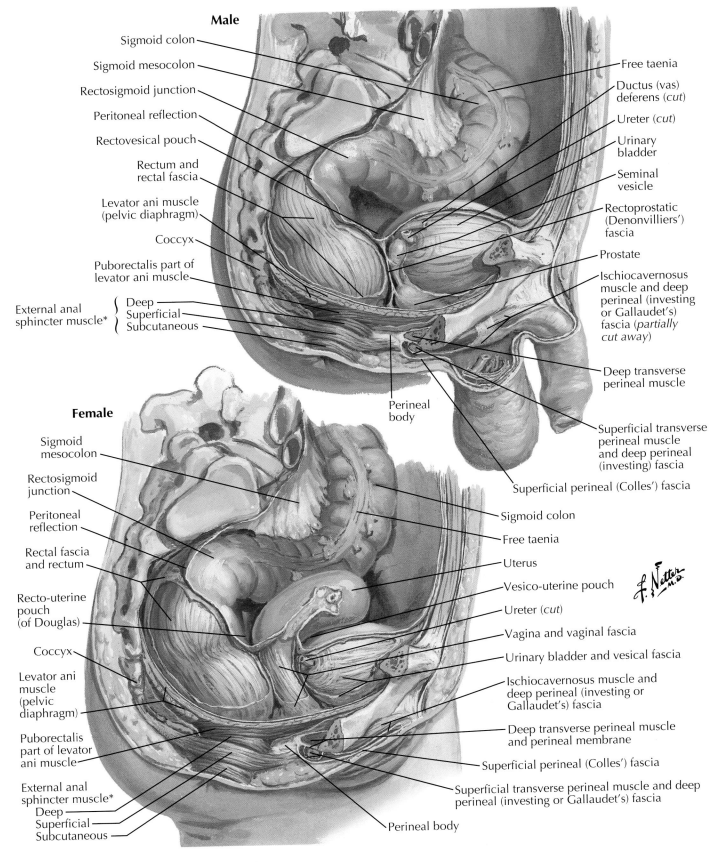

**Male**

Sigmoid colon

Sigmoid mesocolon

Rectosigmoid junction

Peritoneal reflection

Rectovesical pouch

Rectum and rectal fascia

Levator ani muscle (pelvic diaphragm)

Coccyx

Puborectalis part of levator ani muscle

External anal sphincter muscle* { Deep / Superficial / Subcutaneous

Free taenia

Ductus (vas) deferens (cut)

Ureter (cut)

Urinary bladder

Seminal vesicle

Rectoprostatic (Denonvilliers') fascia

Prostate

Ischiocavernosus muscle and deep perineal (investing or Gallaudet's) fascia (partially cut away)

Deep transverse perineal muscle

Perineal body

Superficial transverse perineal muscle and deep perineal (investing) fascia

Superficial perineal (Colles') fascia

**Female**

Sigmoid mesocolon

Rectosigmoid junction

Peritoneal reflection

Rectal fascia and rectum

Recto-uterine pouch (of Douglas)

Coccyx

Levator ani muscle (pelvic diaphragm)

Puborectalis part of levator ani muscle

External anal sphincter muscle* Deep / Superficial / Subcutaneous

Sigmoid colon

Free taenia

Uterus

Vesico-uterine pouch

Ureter (cut)

Vagina and vaginal fascia

Urinary bladder and vesical fascia

Ischiocavernosus muscle and deep perineal (investing or Gallaudet's) fascia

Deep transverse perineal muscle and perineal membrane

Superficial perineal (Colles') fascia

Superficial transverse perineal muscle and deep perineal (investing or Gallaudet's) fascia

Perineal body

*Parts variable and often indistinct

**Rectum**

**Plate 369**

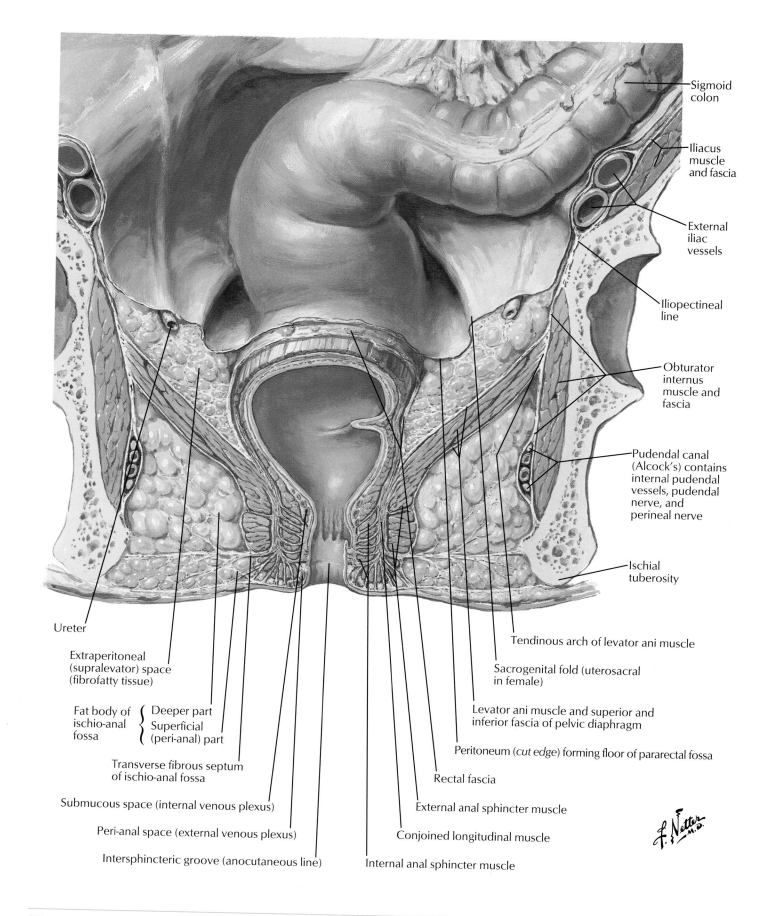

Sigmoid colon

Iliacus muscle and fascia

External iliac vessels

Iliopectineal line

Obturator internus muscle and fascia

Pudendal canal (Alcock's) contains internal pudendal vessels, pudendal nerve, and perineal nerve

Ischial tuberosity

Tendinous arch of levator ani muscle

Sacrogenital fold (uterosacral in female)

Levator ani muscle and superior and inferior fascia of pelvic diaphragm

Peritoneum (*cut edge*) forming floor of pararectal fossa

Rectal fascia

External anal sphincter muscle

Conjoined longitudinal muscle

Internal anal sphincter muscle

Ureter

Extraperitoneal (supralevator) space (fibrofatty tissue)

Fat body of ischio-anal fossa { Deeper part / Superficial (peri-anal) part

Transverse fibrous septum of ischio-anal fossa

Submucous space (internal venous plexus)

Peri-anal space (external venous plexus)

Intersphincteric groove (anocutaneous line)

**Plate 370**

**Rectum**

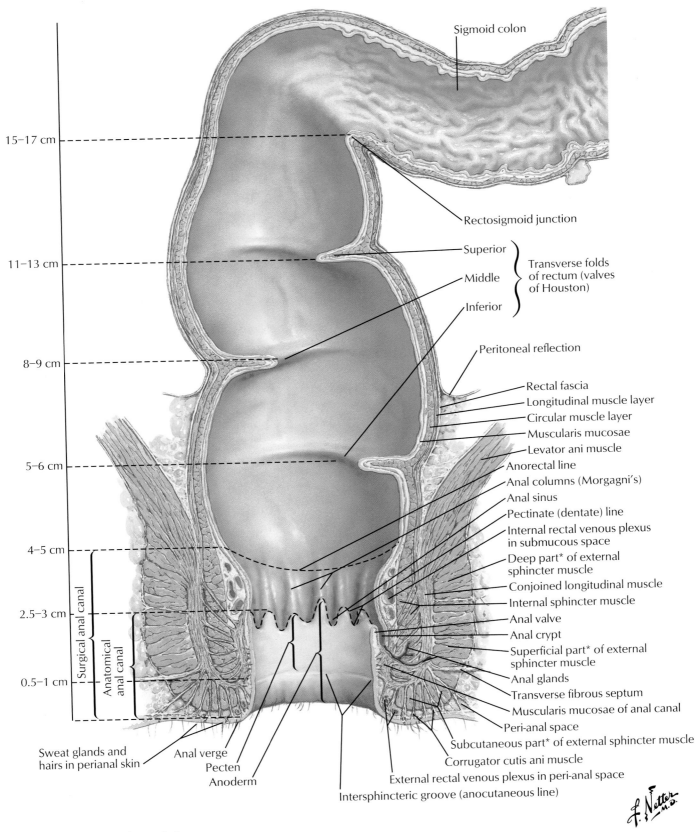

Sigmoid colon

Rectosigmoid junction

15–17 cm

Superior

Transverse folds
of rectum (valves
of Houston)

11–13 cm

Middle

Inferior

Peritoneal reflection

8–9 cm

Rectal fascia

Longitudinal muscle layer

Circular muscle layer

Muscularis mucosae

Levator ani muscle

5–6 cm

Anorectal line

Anal columns (Morgagni's)

Anal sinus

Pectinate (dentate) line

Internal rectal venous plexus
in submucous space

4–5 cm

Deep part* of external
sphincter muscle

Conjoined longitudinal muscle

Internal sphincter muscle

Anal valve

2.5–3 cm

Anal crypt

Superficial part* of external
sphincter muscle

Anal glands

Transverse fibrous septum

0.5–1 cm

Muscularis mucosae of anal canal

Peri-anal space

Subcutaneous part* of external sphincter muscle

Corrugator cutis ani muscle

External rectal venous plexus in peri-anal space

Intersphincteric groove (anocutaneous line)

Sweat glands and
hairs in perianal skin

Anal verge

Pecten

Anoderm

Surgical anal canal

Anatomical
anal canal

*Parts variable and often indistinct

**Plate 371**

**Rectum**

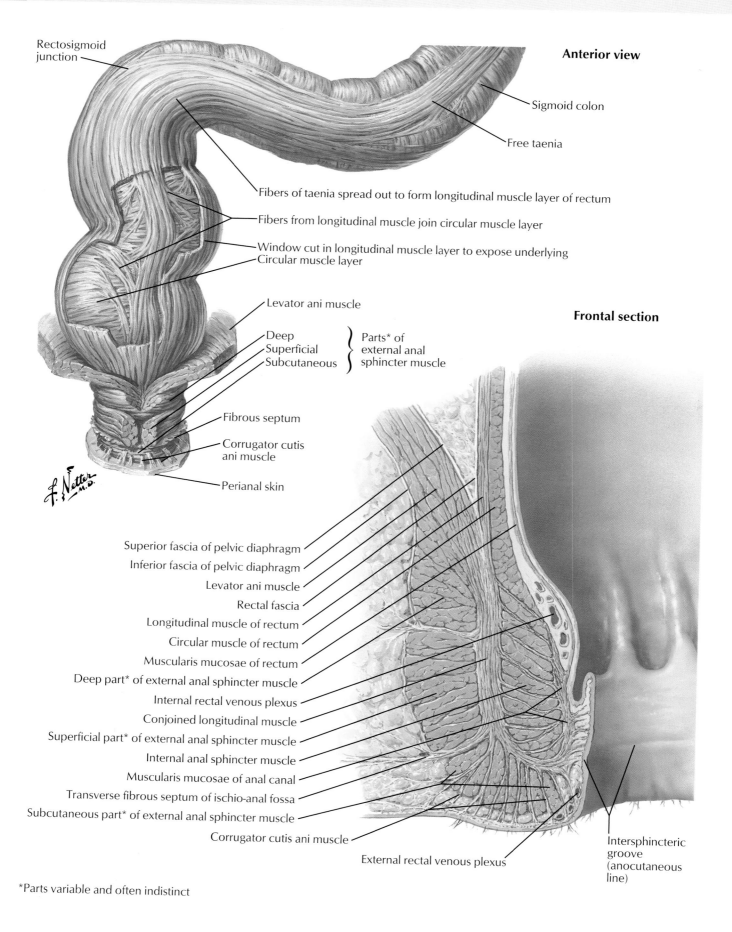

**Anterior view**

Rectosigmoid junction

Sigmoid colon

Free taenia

Fibers of taenia spread out to form longitudinal muscle layer of rectum

Fibers from longitudinal muscle join circular muscle layer

Window cut in longitudinal muscle layer to expose underlying Circular muscle layer

Levator ani muscle

Deep
Superficial    } Parts* of external anal
Subcutaneous    sphincter muscle

Fibrous septum

Corrugator cutis ani muscle

Perianal skin

**Frontal section**

Superior fascia of pelvic diaphragm

Inferior fascia of pelvic diaphragm

Levator ani muscle

Rectal fascia

Longitudinal muscle of rectum

Circular muscle of rectum

Muscularis mucosae of rectum

Deep part* of external anal sphincter muscle

Internal rectal venous plexus

Conjoined longitudinal muscle

Superficial part* of external anal sphincter muscle

Internal anal sphincter muscle

Muscularis mucosae of anal canal

Transverse fibrous septum of ischio-anal fossa

Subcutaneous part* of external anal sphincter muscle

Corrugator cutis ani muscle

External rectal venous plexus

Intersphincteric groove (anocutaneous line)

*Parts variable and often indistinct

**Plate 372**

**Rectum**

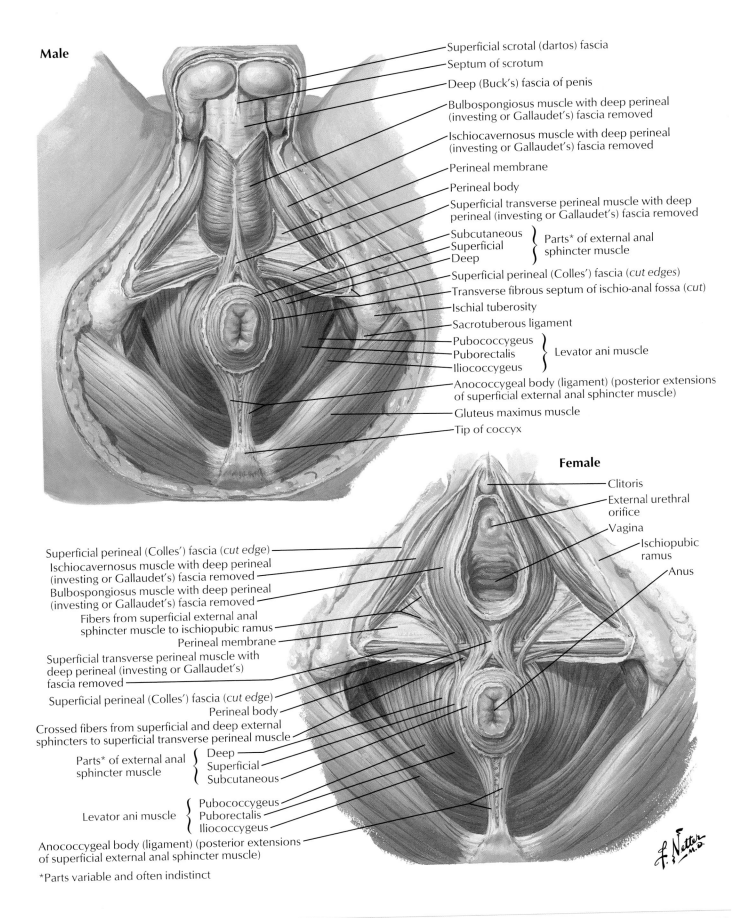

**Male**

Superficial scrotal (dartos) fascia

Septum of scrotum

Deep (Buck's) fascia of penis

Bulbospongiosus muscle with deep perineal (investing or Gallaudet's) fascia removed

Ischiocavernosus muscle with deep perineal (investing or Gallaudet's) fascia removed

Perineal membrane

Perineal body

Superficial transverse perineal muscle with deep perineal (investing or Gallaudet's) fascia removed

Subcutaneous
Superficial    } Parts* of external anal
Deep               sphincter muscle

Superficial perineal (Colles') fascia (*cut edges*)

Transverse fibrous septum of ischio-anal fossa (*cut*)

Ischial tuberosity

Sacrotuberous ligament

Pubococcygeus
Puborectalis    } Levator ani muscle
Iliococcygeus

Anococcygeal body (ligament) (posterior extensions of superficial external anal sphincter muscle)

Gluteus maximus muscle

Tip of coccyx

**Female**

Clitoris

External urethral orifice

Vagina

Ischiopubic ramus

Anus

Superficial perineal (Colles') fascia (*cut edge*)

Ischiocavernosus muscle with deep perineal (investing or Gallaudet's) fascia removed

Bulbospongiosus muscle with deep perineal (investing or Gallaudet's) fascia removed

Fibers from superficial external anal sphincter muscle to ischiopubic ramus

Perineal membrane

Superficial transverse perineal muscle with deep perineal (investing or Gallaudet's) fascia removed

Superficial perineal (Colles') fascia (*cut edge*)

Perineal body

Crossed fibers from superficial and deep external sphincters to superficial transverse perineal muscle

Parts* of external anal sphincter muscle
{ Deep
Superficial
Subcutaneous

Levator ani muscle
{ Pubococcygeus
Puborectalis
Iliococcygeus

Anococcygeal body (ligament) (posterior extensions of superficial external anal sphincter muscle)

*Parts variable and often indistinct

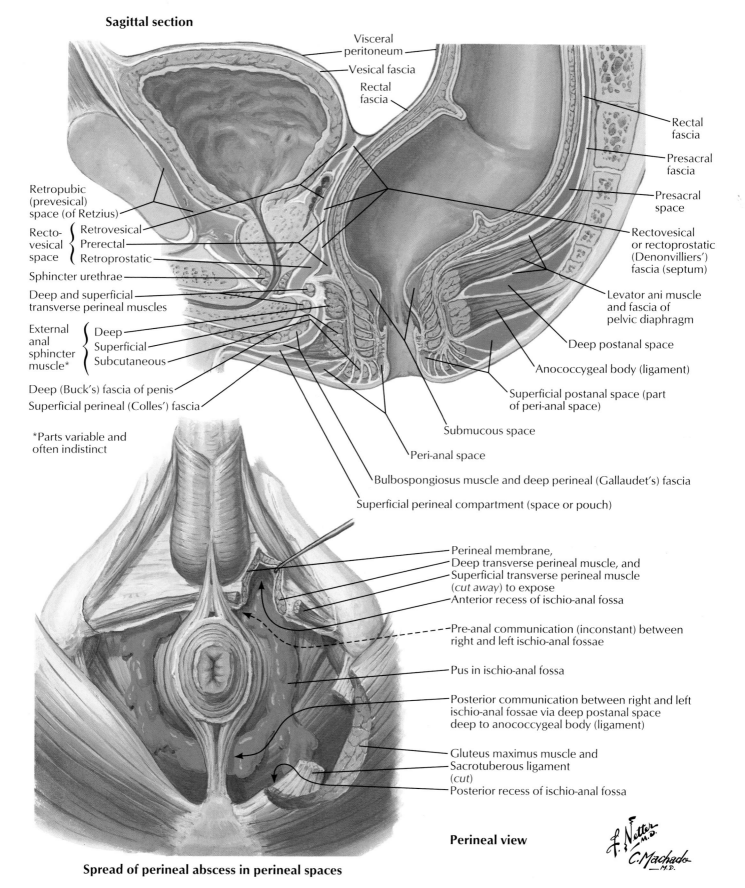

**Sagittal section**

Visceral peritoneum

Vesical fascia

Rectal fascia

Rectal fascia

Presacral fascia

Presacral space

Retropubic (prevesical) space (of Retzius)

Recto-vesical space { Retrovesical / Prerectal / Retroprostatic }

Rectovesical or rectoprostatic (Denonvilliers') fascia (septum)

Sphincter urethrae

Deep and superficial transverse perineal muscles

Levator ani muscle and fascia of pelvic diaphragm

External anal sphincter muscle* { Deep / Superficial / Subcutaneous }

Deep postanal space

Anococcygeal body (ligament)

Deep (Buck's) fascia of penis

Superficial postanal space (part of peri-anal space)

Superficial perineal (Colles') fascia

Submucous space

*Parts variable and often indistinct

Peri-anal space

Bulbospongiosus muscle and deep perineal (Gallaudet's) fascia

Superficial perineal compartment (space or pouch)

Perineal membrane, Deep transverse perineal muscle, and Superficial transverse perineal muscle (*cut away*) to expose Anterior recess of ischio-anal fossa

Pre-anal communication (inconstant) between right and left ischio-anal fossae

Pus in ischio-anal fossa

Posterior communication between right and left ischio-anal fossae via deep postanal space deep to anococcygeal body (ligament)

Gluteus maximus muscle and Sacrotuberous ligament (*cut*)

Posterior recess of ischio-anal fossa

**Perineal view**

**Spread of perineal abscess in perineal spaces**

**Plate 374**

**Rectum**

**Female**

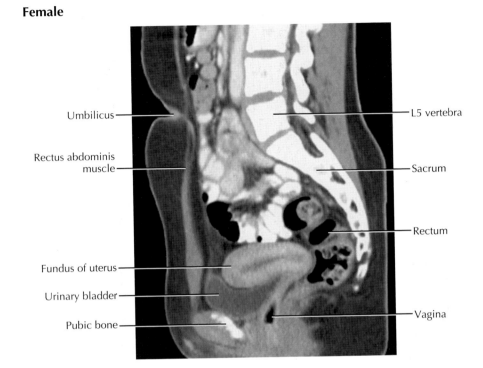

Umbilicus —
Rectus abdominis muscle —
Fundus of uterus —
Urinary bladder —
Pubic bone —

— L5 vertebra
— Sacrum
— Rectum
— Vagina

**Male**

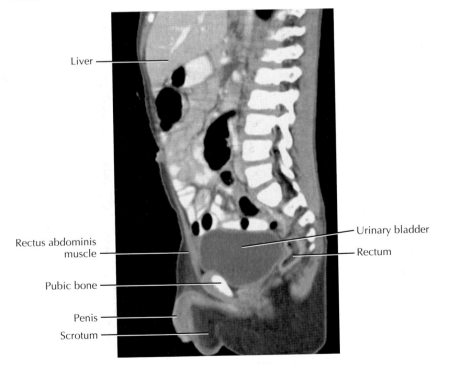

Liver —
Rectus abdominis muscle —
Pubic bone —
Penis —
Scrotum —

— Urinary bladder
— Rectum

**Posterior view**

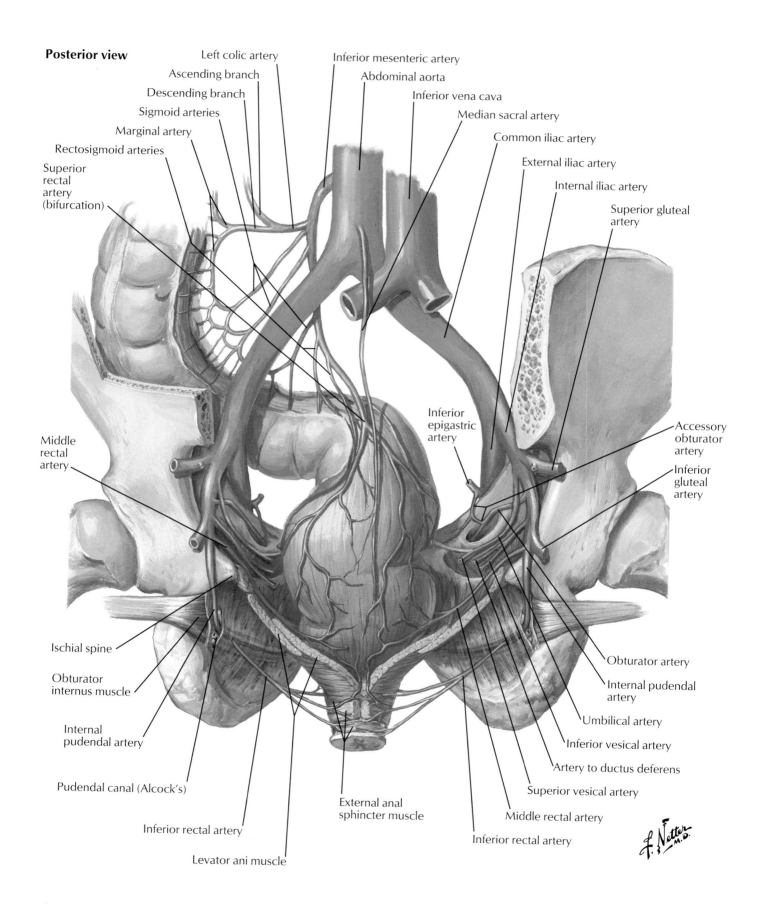

Left colic artery

Ascending branch

Descending branch

Sigmoid arteries

Marginal artery

Rectosigmoid arteries

Superior rectal artery (bifurcation)

Inferior mesenteric artery

Abdominal aorta

Inferior vena cava

Median sacral artery

Common iliac artery

External iliac artery

Internal iliac artery

Superior gluteal artery

Inferior epigastric artery

Accessory obturator artery

Inferior gluteal artery

Middle rectal artery

Ischial spine

Obturator internus muscle

Internal pudendal artery

Pudendal canal (Alcock's)

Inferior rectal artery

Levator ani muscle

External anal sphincter muscle

Obturator artery

Internal pudendal artery

Umbilical artery

Inferior vesical artery

Artery to ductus deferens

Superior vesical artery

Middle rectal artery

Inferior rectal artery

**Plate 376**

**Vasculature**

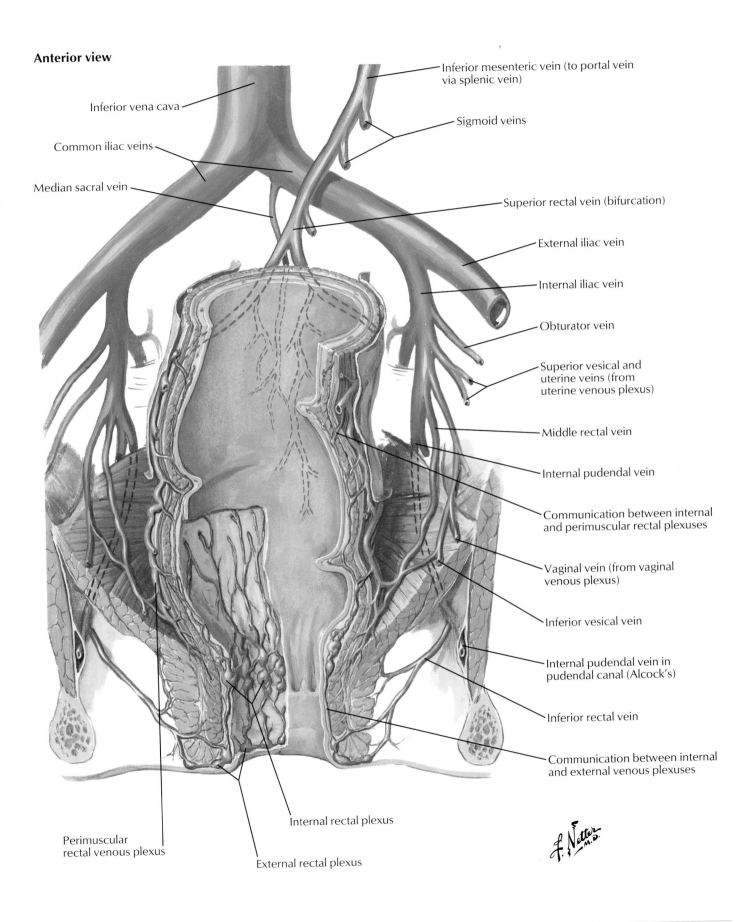

Anterior view

Inferior vena cava

Common iliac veins

Median sacral vein

Inferior mesenteric vein (to portal vein via splenic vein)

Sigmoid veins

Superior rectal vein (bifurcation)

External iliac vein

Internal iliac vein

Obturator vein

Superior vesical and uterine veins (from uterine venous plexus)

Middle rectal vein

Internal pudendal vein

Communication between internal and perimuscular rectal plexuses

Vaginal vein (from vaginal venous plexus)

Inferior vesical vein

Internal pudendal vein in pudendal canal (Alcock's)

Inferior rectal vein

Communication between internal and external venous plexuses

Perimuscular rectal venous plexus

Internal rectal plexus

External rectal plexus

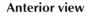

**Anterior view**

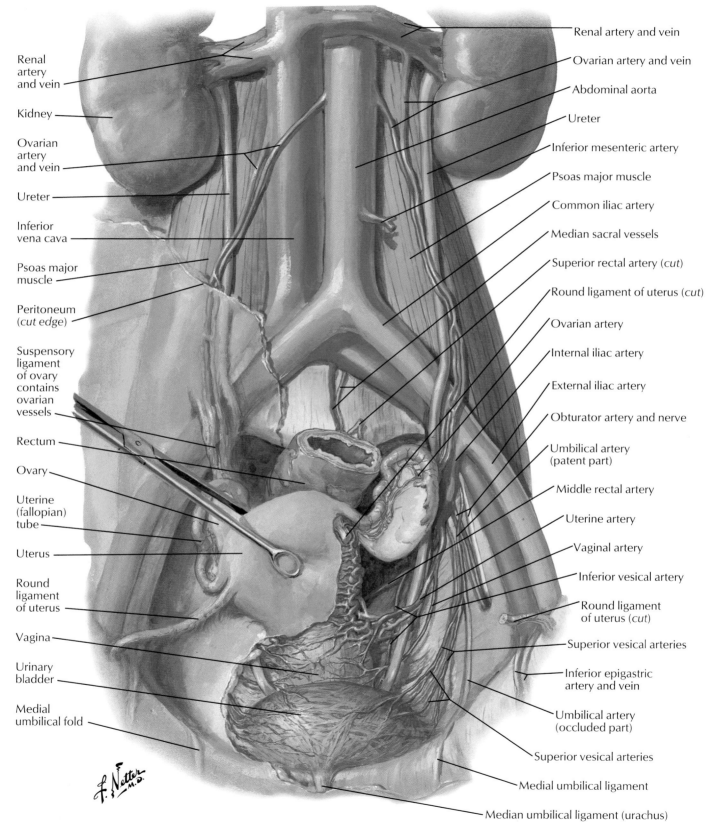

Renal artery and vein

Renal artery and vein

Ovarian artery and vein

Kidney

Abdominal aorta

Ovarian artery and vein

Ureter

Ureter

Inferior mesenteric artery

Inferior vena cava

Psoas major muscle

Psoas major muscle

Common iliac artery

Peritoneum (*cut edge*)

Median sacral vessels

Superior rectal artery (*cut*)

Suspensory ligament of ovary contains ovarian vessels

Round ligament of uterus (*cut*)

Ovarian artery

Rectum

Internal iliac artery

Ovary

External iliac artery

Uterine (fallopian) tube

Obturator artery and nerve

Uterus

Umbilical artery (patent part)

Round ligament of uterus

Middle rectal artery

Uterine artery

Vagina

Vaginal artery

Urinary bladder

Inferior vesical artery

Medial umbilical fold

Round ligament of uterus (*cut*)

Superior vesical arteries

Inferior epigastric artery and vein

Umbilical artery (occluded part)

Superior vesical arteries

Medial umbilical ligament

Median umbilical ligament (urachus)

**Plate 378**

**Vasculature**

**Anterior view**

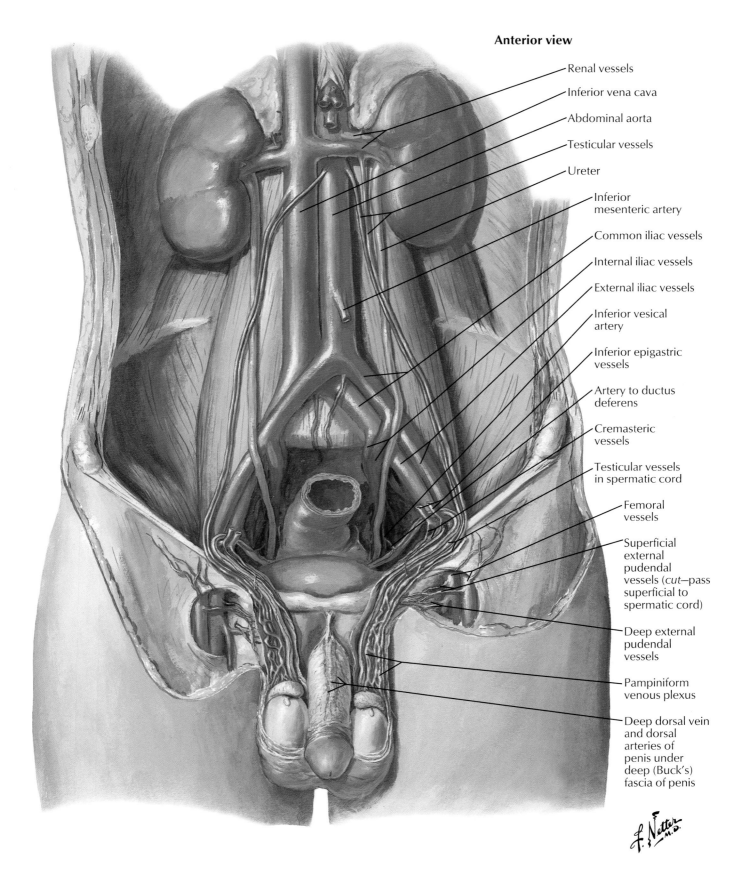

Renal vessels

Inferior vena cava

Abdominal aorta

Testicular vessels

Ureter

Inferior mesenteric artery

Common iliac vessels

Internal iliac vessels

External iliac vessels

Inferior vesical artery

Inferior epigastric vessels

Artery to ductus deferens

Cremasteric vessels

Testicular vessels in spermatic cord

Femoral vessels

Superficial external pudendal vessels (*cut*–pass superficial to spermatic cord)

Deep external pudendal vessels

Pampiniform venous plexus

Deep dorsal vein and dorsal arteries of penis under deep (Buck's) fascia of penis

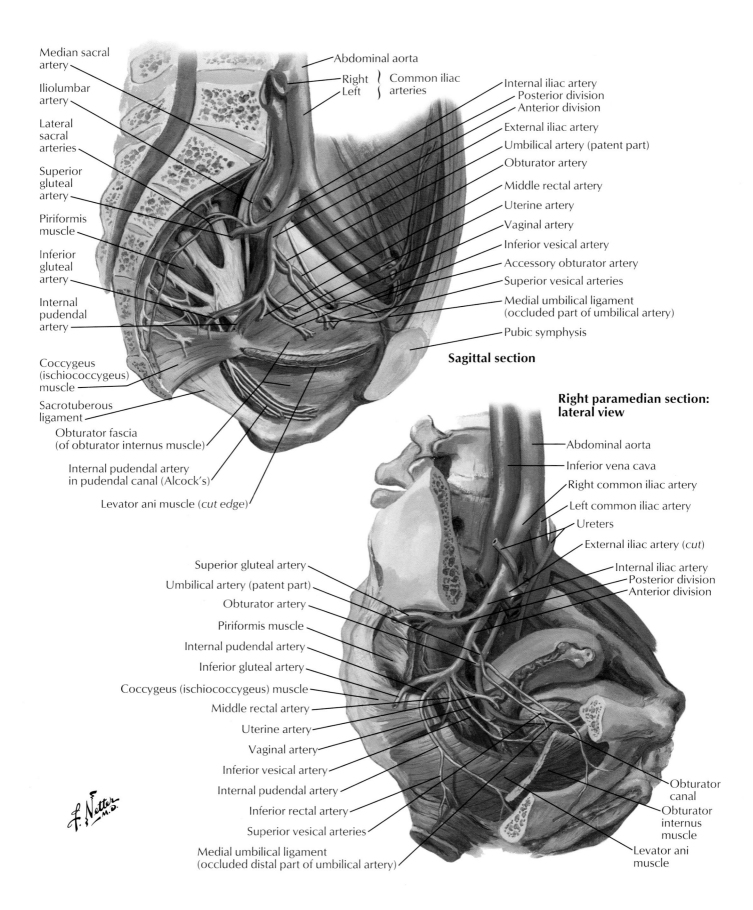

Median sacral artery

Iliolumbar artery

Lateral sacral arteries

Superior gluteal artery

Piriformis muscle

Inferior gluteal artery

Internal pudendal artery

Coccygeus (ischiococcygeus) muscle

Sacrotuberous ligament

Obturator fascia (of obturator internus muscle)

Internal pudendal artery in pudendal canal (Alcock's)

Levator ani muscle (*cut edge*)

Abdominal aorta

Right } Common iliac
Left } arteries

Internal iliac artery
Posterior division
Anterior division

External iliac artery

Umbilical artery (patent part)

Obturator artery

Middle rectal artery

Uterine artery

Vaginal artery

Inferior vesical artery

Accessory obturator artery

Superior vesical arteries

Medial umbilical ligament (occluded part of umbilical artery)

Pubic symphysis

**Sagittal section**

**Right paramedian section: lateral view**

Abdominal aorta

Inferior vena cava

Right common iliac artery

Left common iliac artery

Ureters

External iliac artery (*cut*)

Internal iliac artery
Posterior division
Anterior division

Superior gluteal artery

Umbilical artery (patent part)

Obturator artery

Piriformis muscle

Internal pudendal artery

Inferior gluteal artery

Coccygeus (ischiococcygeus) muscle

Middle rectal artery

Uterine artery

Vaginal artery

Inferior vesical artery

Internal pudendal artery

Inferior rectal artery

Superior vesical arteries

Medial umbilical ligament (occluded distal part of umbilical artery)

Obturator canal

Obturator internus muscle

Levator ani muscle

**Plate 380**

**Vasculature**

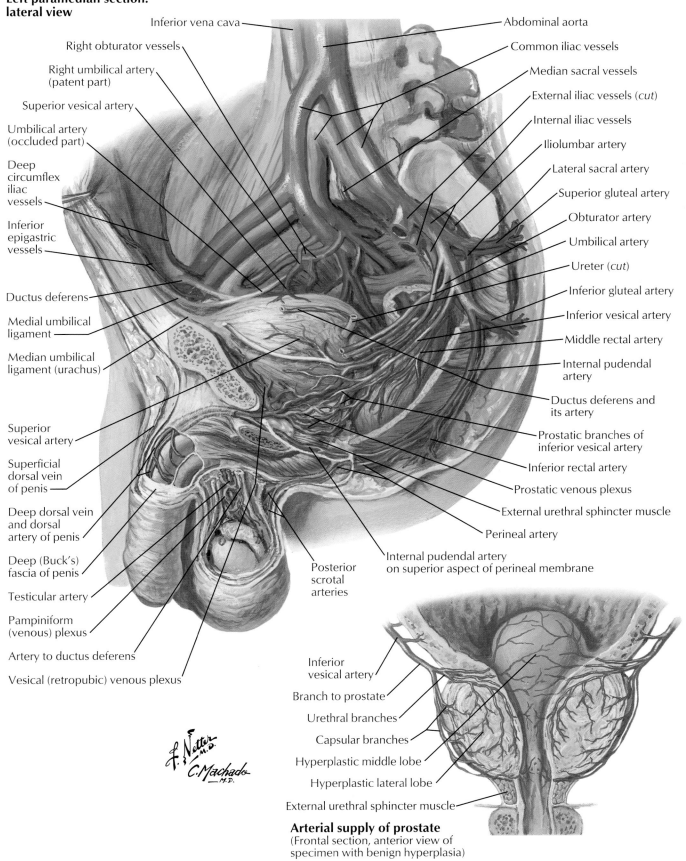

**Left paramedian section: lateral view**

Inferior vena cava

Right obturator vessels

Right umbilical artery (patent part)

Superior vesical artery

Umbilical artery (occluded part)

Deep circumflex iliac vessels

Inferior epigastric vessels

Ductus deferens

Medial umbilical ligament

Median umbilical ligament (urachus)

Superior vesical artery

Superficial dorsal vein of penis

Deep dorsal vein and dorsal artery of penis

Deep (Buck's) fascia of penis

Testicular artery

Pampiniform (venous) plexus

Artery to ductus deferens

Vesical (retropubic) venous plexus

Abdominal aorta

Common iliac vessels

Median sacral vessels

External iliac vessels (cut)

Internal iliac vessels

Iliolumbar artery

Lateral sacral artery

Superior gluteal artery

Obturator artery

Umbilical artery

Ureter (cut)

Inferior gluteal artery

Inferior vesical artery

Middle rectal artery

Internal pudendal artery

Ductus deferens and its artery

Prostatic branches of inferior vesical artery

Inferior rectal artery

Prostatic venous plexus

External urethral sphincter muscle

Perineal artery

Internal pudendal artery on superior aspect of perineal membrane

Posterior scrotal arteries

Inferior vesical artery

Branch to prostate

Urethral branches

Capsular branches

Hyperplastic middle lobe

Hyperplastic lateral lobe

External urethral sphincter muscle

**Arterial supply of prostate**
(Frontal section, anterior view of specimen with benign hyperplasia)

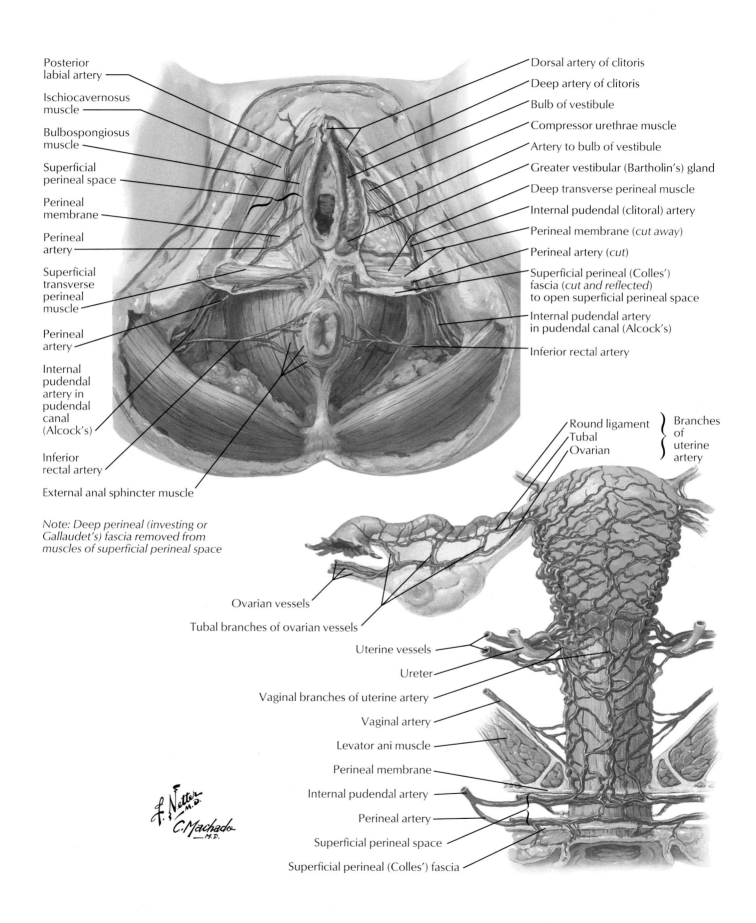

Posterior labial artery

Ischiocavernosus muscle

Bulbospongiosus muscle

Superficial perineal space

Perineal membrane

Perineal artery

Superficial transverse perineal muscle

Perineal artery

Internal pudendal artery in pudendal canal (Alcock's)

Inferior rectal artery

External anal sphincter muscle

Dorsal artery of clitoris

Deep artery of clitoris

Bulb of vestibule

Compressor urethrae muscle

Artery to bulb of vestibule

Greater vestibular (Bartholin's) gland

Deep transverse perineal muscle

Internal pudendal (clitoral) artery

Perineal membrane (cut away)

Perineal artery (cut)

Superficial perineal (Colles') fascia (cut and reflected) to open superficial perineal space

Internal pudendal artery in pudendal canal (Alcock's)

Inferior rectal artery

Note: Deep perineal (investing or Gallaudet's) fascia removed from muscles of superficial perineal space

Round ligament
Tubal
Ovarian
⎫
⎬ Branches of uterine artery
⎭

Ovarian vessels

Tubal branches of ovarian vessels

Uterine vessels

Ureter

Vaginal branches of uterine artery

Vaginal artery

Levator ani muscle

Perineal membrane

Internal pudendal artery

Perineal artery

Superficial perineal space

Superficial perineal (Colles') fascia

**Plate 382**

**Vasculature**

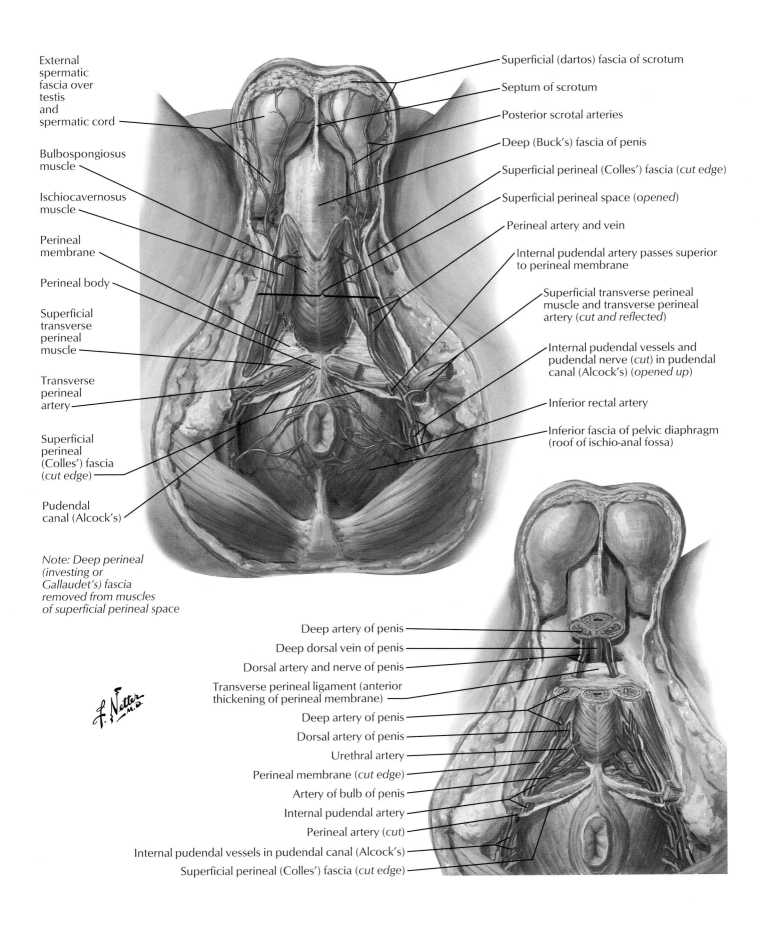

External spermatic fascia over testis and spermatic cord

Bulbospongiosus muscle

Ischiocavernosus muscle

Perineal membrane

Perineal body

Superficial transverse perineal muscle

Transverse perineal artery

Superficial perineal (Colles') fascia (cut edge)

Pudendal canal (Alcock's)

Note: Deep perineal (investing or Gallaudet's) fascia removed from muscles of superficial perineal space

Superficial (dartos) fascia of scrotum

Septum of scrotum

Posterior scrotal arteries

Deep (Buck's) fascia of penis

Superficial perineal (Colles') fascia (cut edge)

Superficial perineal space (opened)

Perineal artery and vein

Internal pudendal artery passes superior to perineal membrane

Superficial transverse perineal muscle and transverse perineal artery (cut and reflected)

Internal pudendal vessels and pudendal nerve (cut) in pudendal canal (Alcock's) (opened up)

Inferior rectal artery

Inferior fascia of pelvic diaphragm (roof of ischio-anal fossa)

Deep artery of penis

Deep dorsal vein of penis

Dorsal artery and nerve of penis

Transverse perineal ligament (anterior thickening of perineal membrane)

Deep artery of penis

Dorsal artery of penis

Urethral artery

Perineal membrane (cut edge)

Artery of bulb of penis

Internal pudendal artery

Perineal artery (cut)

Internal pudendal vessels in pudendal canal (Alcock's)

Superficial perineal (Colles') fascia (cut edge)

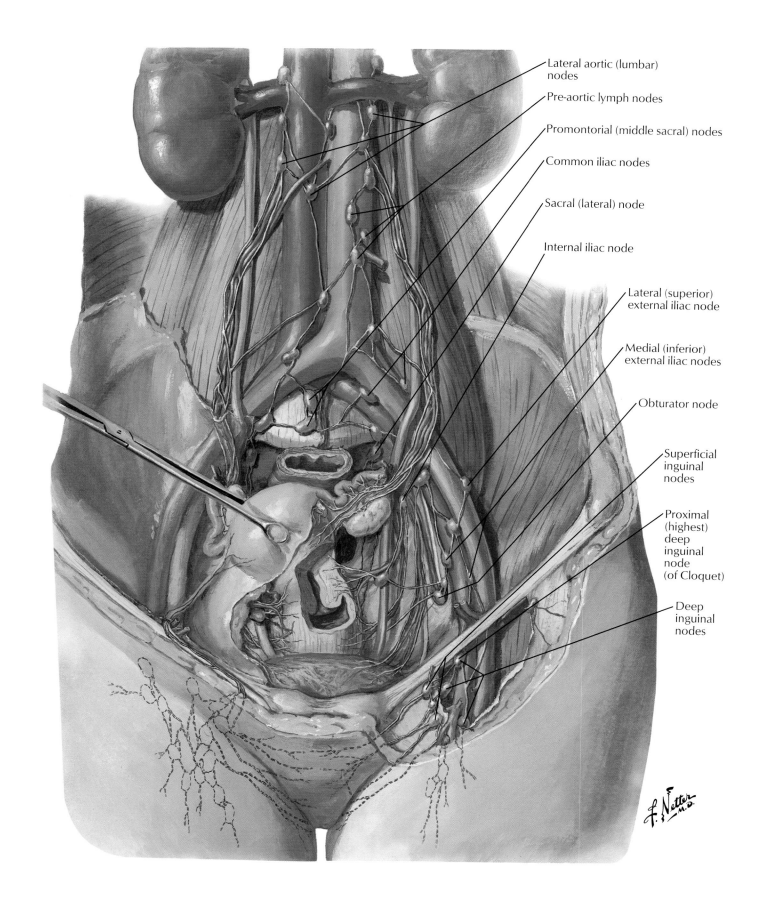

Lateral aortic (lumbar) nodes

Pre-aortic lymph nodes

Promontorial (middle sacral) nodes

Common iliac nodes

Sacral (lateral) node

Internal iliac node

Lateral (superior) external iliac node

Medial (inferior) external iliac nodes

Obturator node

Superficial inguinal nodes

Proximal (highest) deep inguinal node (of Cloquet)

Deep inguinal nodes

**Plate 384**

**Vasculature**

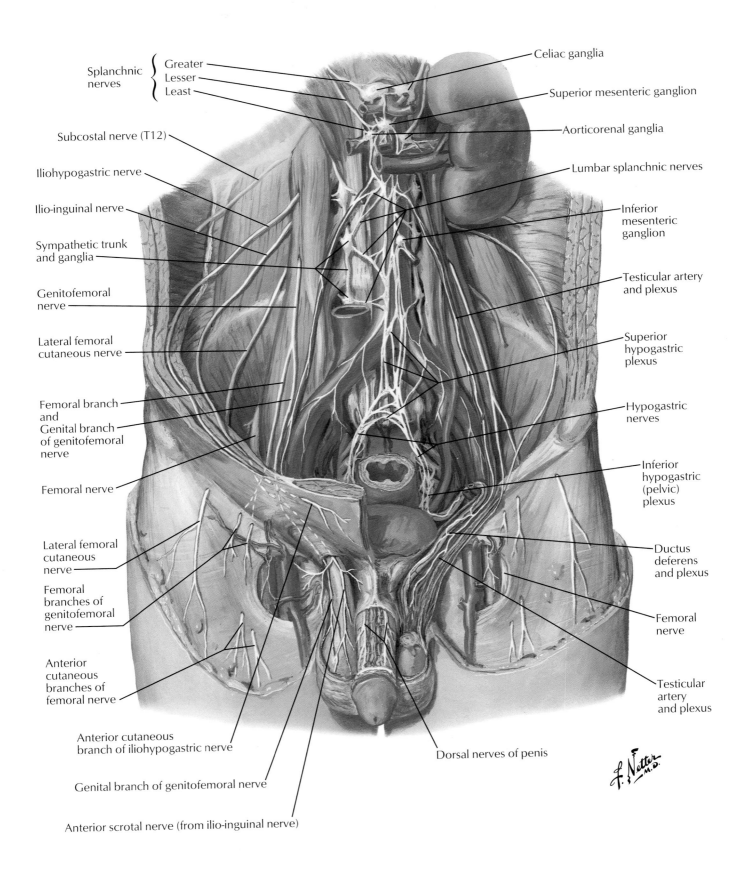

Splanchnic nerves
{ Greater
Lesser
Least

Celiac ganglia

Superior mesenteric ganglion

Subcostal nerve (T12)

Aorticorenal ganglia

Iliohypogastric nerve

Lumbar splanchnic nerves

Ilio-inguinal nerve

Inferior mesenteric ganglion

Sympathetic trunk and ganglia

Testicular artery and plexus

Genitofemoral nerve

Superior hypogastric plexus

Lateral femoral cutaneous nerve

Hypogastric nerves

Femoral branch and Genital branch of genitofemoral nerve

Inferior hypogastric (pelvic) plexus

Femoral nerve

Ductus deferens and plexus

Lateral femoral cutaneous nerve

Femoral nerve

Femoral branches of genitofemoral nerve

Anterior cutaneous branches of femoral nerve

Testicular artery and plexus

Anterior cutaneous branch of iliohypogastric nerve

Dorsal nerves of penis

Genital branch of genitofemoral nerve

Anterior scrotal nerve (from ilio-inguinal nerve)

**Plate 387**

**Innervation**

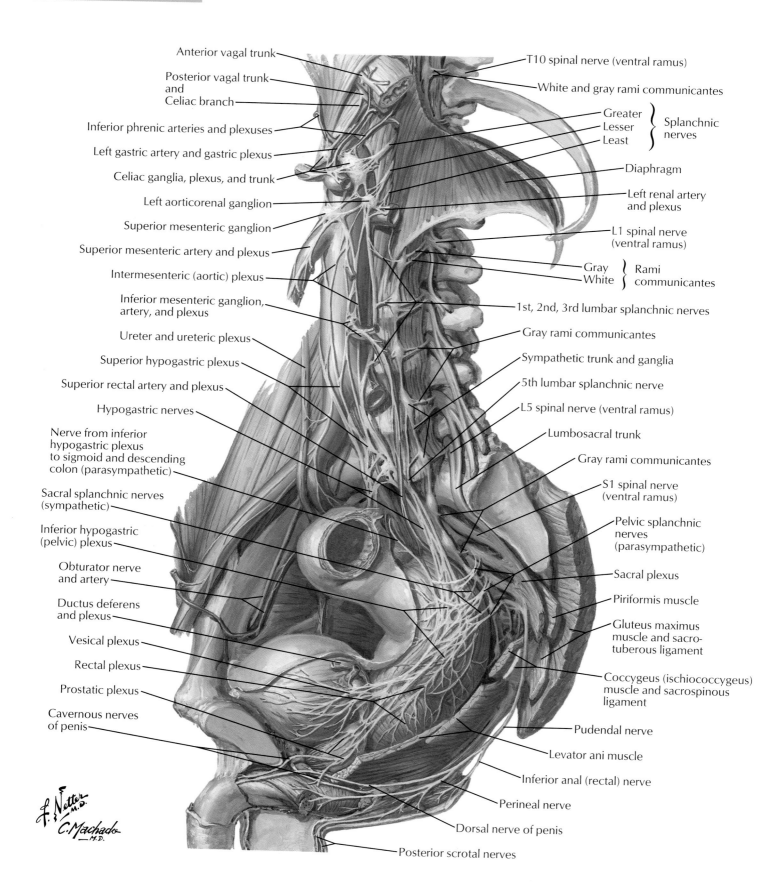

Anterior vagal trunk

Posterior vagal trunk and Celiac branch

Inferior phrenic arteries and plexuses

Left gastric artery and gastric plexus

Celiac ganglia, plexus, and trunk

Left aorticorenal ganglion

Superior mesenteric ganglion

Superior mesenteric artery and plexus

Intermesenteric (aortic) plexus

Inferior mesenteric ganglion, artery, and plexus

Ureter and ureteric plexus

Superior hypogastric plexus

Superior rectal artery and plexus

Hypogastric nerves

Nerve from inferior hypogastric plexus to sigmoid and descending colon (parasympathetic)

Sacral splanchnic nerves (sympathetic)

Inferior hypogastric (pelvic) plexus

Obturator nerve and artery

Ductus deferens and plexus

Vesical plexus

Rectal plexus

Prostatic plexus

Cavernous nerves of penis

T10 spinal nerve (ventral ramus)

White and gray rami communicantes

Greater
Lesser
Least
} Splanchnic nerves

Diaphragm

Left renal artery and plexus

L1 spinal nerve (ventral ramus)

Gray
White
} Rami communicantes

1st, 2nd, 3rd lumbar splanchnic nerves

Gray rami communicantes

Sympathetic trunk and ganglia

5th lumbar splanchnic nerve

L5 spinal nerve (ventral ramus)

Lumbosacral trunk

Gray rami communicantes

S1 spinal nerve (ventral ramus)

Pelvic splanchnic nerves (parasympathetic)

Sacral plexus

Piriformis muscle

Gluteus maximus muscle and sacro-tuberous ligament

Coccygeus (ischiococcygeus) muscle and sacrospinous ligament

Pudendal nerve

Levator ani muscle

Inferior anal (rectal) nerve

Perineal nerve

Dorsal nerve of penis

Posterior scrotal nerves

**Plate 388**

**Innervation**

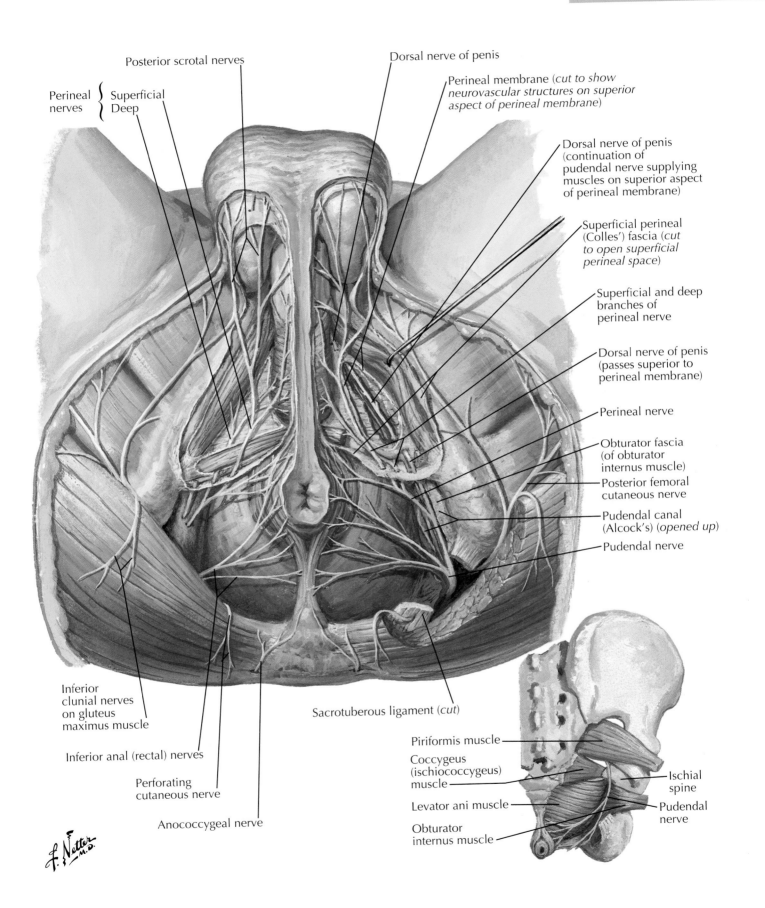

Posterior scrotal nerves

Dorsal nerve of penis

Perineal nerves { Superficial / Deep

Perineal membrane (*cut to show neurovascular structures on superior aspect of perineal membrane*)

Dorsal nerve of penis (continuation of pudendal nerve supplying muscles on superior aspect of perineal membrane)

Superficial perineal (Colles') fascia (*cut to open superficial perineal space*)

Superficial and deep branches of perineal nerve

Dorsal nerve of penis (passes superior to perineal membrane)

Perineal nerve

Obturator fascia (of obturator internus muscle)

Posterior femoral cutaneous nerve

Pudendal canal (Alcock's) (*opened up*)

Pudendal nerve

Inferior clunial nerves on gluteus maximus muscle

Inferior anal (rectal) nerves

Perforating cutaneous nerve

Anococcygeal nerve

Sacrotuberous ligament (*cut*)

Piriformis muscle

Coccygeus (ischiococcygeus) muscle

Levator ani muscle

Obturator internus muscle

Ischial spine

Pudendal nerve

*f. Netter. M.D.*

**Innervation**

**Plate 389**

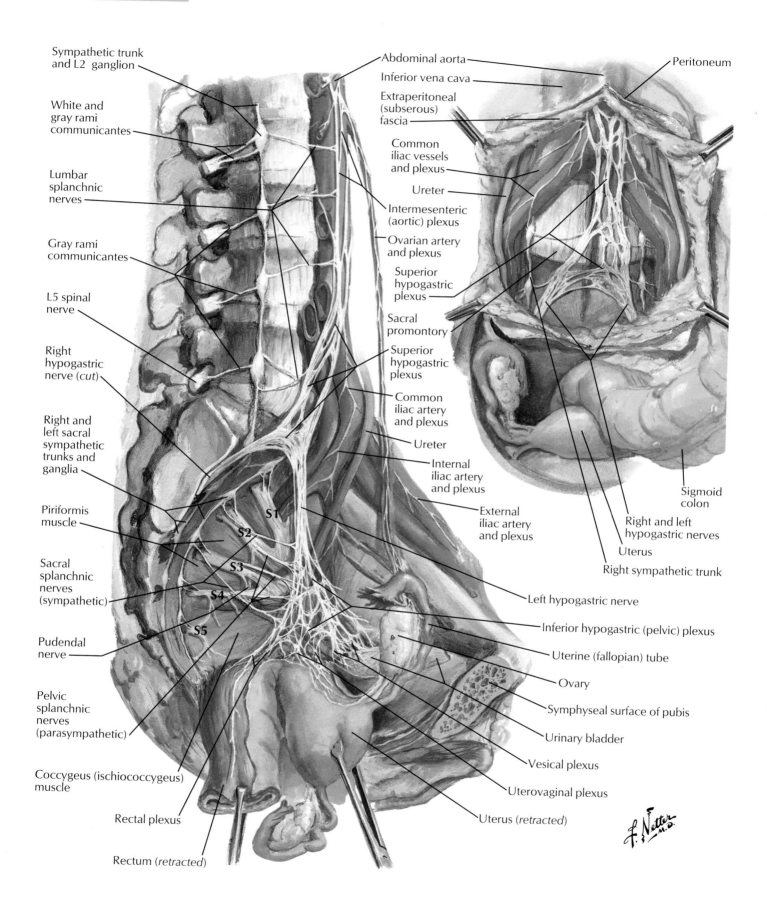

Sympathetic trunk and L2 ganglion

White and gray rami communicantes

Lumbar splanchnic nerves

Gray rami communicantes

L5 spinal nerve

Right hypogastric nerve (*cut*)

Right and left sacral sympathetic trunks and ganglia

Piriformis muscle

Sacral splanchnic nerves (sympathetic)

Pudendal nerve

Pelvic splanchnic nerves (parasympathetic)

Coccygeus (ischiococcygeus) muscle

Rectal plexus

Rectum (*retracted*)

Abdominal aorta

Inferior vena cava

Extraperitoneal (subserous) fascia

Common iliac vessels and plexus

Ureter

Intermesenteric (aortic) plexus

Ovarian artery and plexus

Superior hypogastric plexus

Sacral promontory

Superior hypogastric plexus

Common iliac artery and plexus

Ureter

Internal iliac artery and plexus

External iliac artery and plexus

Left hypogastric nerve

Peritoneum

Sigmoid colon

Right and left hypogastric nerves

Uterus

Right sympathetic trunk

Inferior hypogastric (pelvic) plexus

Uterine (fallopian) tube

Ovary

Symphyseal surface of pubis

Urinary bladder

Vesical plexus

Uterovaginal plexus

Uterus (*retracted*)

S1
S2
S3
S4
S5

**Plate 390**

**Innervation**

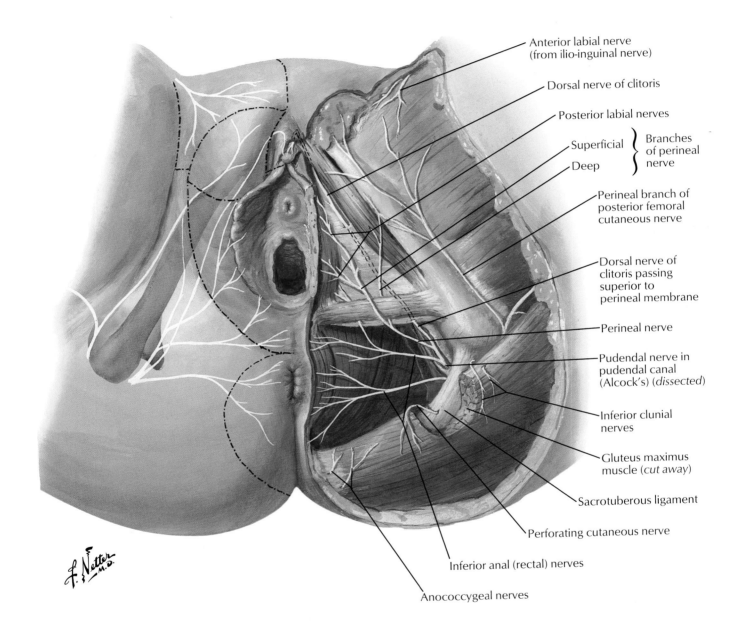

Anterior labial nerve
(from ilio-inguinal nerve)

Dorsal nerve of clitoris

Posterior labial nerves

Superficial ⎱ Branches
⎰ of perineal
Deep    nerve

Perineal branch of
posterior femoral
cutaneous nerve

Dorsal nerve of
clitoris passing
superior to
perineal membrane

Perineal nerve

Pudendal nerve in
pudendal canal
(Alcock's) (dissected)

Inferior clunial
nerves

Gluteus maximus
muscle (cut away)

Sacrotuberous ligament

Perforating cutaneous nerve

Inferior anal (rectal) nerves

Anococcygeal nerves

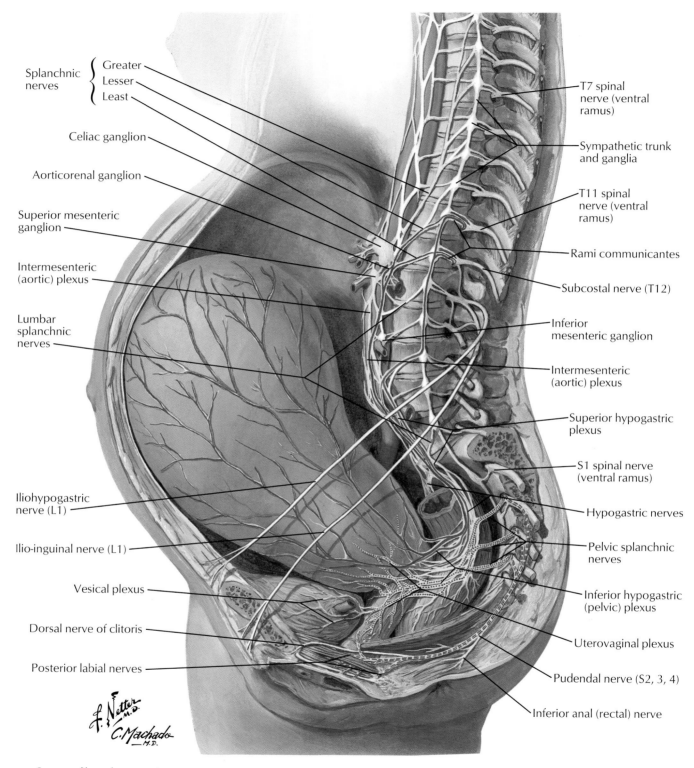

Splanchnic nerves {
Greater
Lesser
Least

Celiac ganglion

Aorticorenal ganglion

Superior mesenteric ganglion

Intermesenteric (aortic) plexus

Lumbar splanchnic nerves

Iliohypogastric nerve (L1)

Ilio-inguinal nerve (L1)

Vesical plexus

Dorsal nerve of clitoris

Posterior labial nerves

T7 spinal nerve (ventral ramus)

Sympathetic trunk and ganglia

T11 spinal nerve (ventral ramus)

Rami communicantes

Subcostal nerve (T12)

Inferior mesenteric ganglion

Intermesenteric (aortic) plexus

Superior hypogastric plexus

S1 spinal nerve (ventral ramus)

Hypogastric nerves

Pelvic splanchnic nerves

Inferior hypogastric (pelvic) plexus

Uterovaginal plexus

Pudendal nerve (S2, 3, 4)

Inferior anal (rectal) nerve

———— Sensory fibers from uterine body and fundus accompany sympathetic fibers via hypogastric plexuses to T11, 12 (L1?)

———— Motor fibers to uterine body and fundus (sympathetic)

·········· Sensory fibers from cervix and upper vagina accompany pelvic splanchnic nerves (parasympathetic) to S2, 3, 4

·········· Motor fibers to lower uterine segment, cervix, and upper vagina (parasympathetic)

– – – – Sensory fibers from lower vagina and perineum accompany somatic fibers via pudendal nerve to S2, 3, 4

– – – – – Motor fibers to lower vagina and perineum via pudendal nerve (somatic)

**Plate 392**

**Innervation**

# Innervation of Female Reproductive Organs: Schema

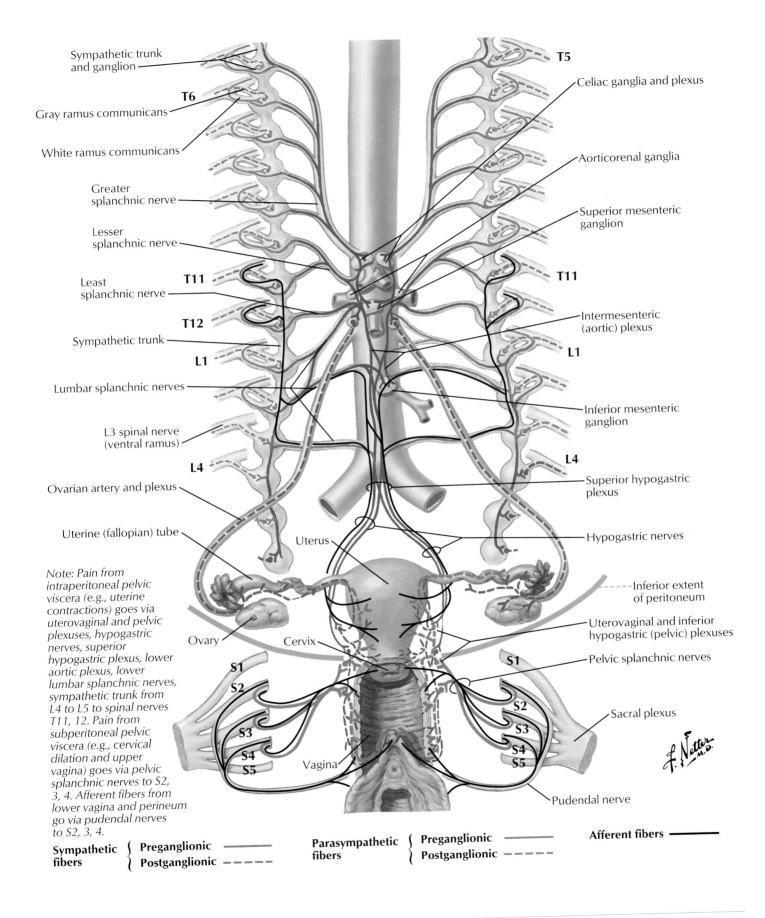

Sympathetic trunk and ganglion

Gray ramus communicans

White ramus communicans

Greater splanchnic nerve

Lesser splanchnic nerve

Least splanchnic nerve

Sympathetic trunk

Lumbar splanchnic nerves

L3 spinal nerve (ventral ramus)

Ovarian artery and plexus

Uterine (fallopian) tube

**T6**

**T11**

**T12**

**L1**

**L4**

*Note: Pain from intraperitoneal pelvic viscera (e.g., uterine contractions) goes via uterovaginal and pelvic plexuses, hypogastric nerves, superior hypogastric plexus, lower aortic plexus, lower lumbar splanchnic nerves, sympathetic trunk from L4 to L5 to spinal nerves T11, 12. Pain from subperitoneal pelvic viscera (e.g., cervical dilation and upper vagina) goes via pelvic splanchnic nerves to S2, 3, 4. Afferent fibers from lower vagina and perineum go via pudendal nerves to S2, 3, 4.*

Uterus

Ovary

Cervix

S1

S2

S3

S4

S5

Vagina

**T5**

Celiac ganglia and plexus

Aorticorenal ganglia

Superior mesenteric ganglion

**T11**

Intermesenteric (aortic) plexus

**L1**

Inferior mesenteric ganglion

**L4**

Superior hypogastric plexus

Hypogastric nerves

Inferior extent of peritoneum

Uterovaginal and inferior hypogastric (pelvic) plexuses

Pelvic splanchnic nerves

S1

S2

S3

S4

S5

Sacral plexus

Pudendal nerve

| Sympathetic fibers | Preganglionic | ———— | Parasympathetic fibers | Preganglionic | ———— | Afferent fibers | ———— |
|---|---|---|---|---|---|---|---|
| | Postganglionic | – – – – | | Postganglionic | – – – – | | |

**Plate 393**

**Innervation**

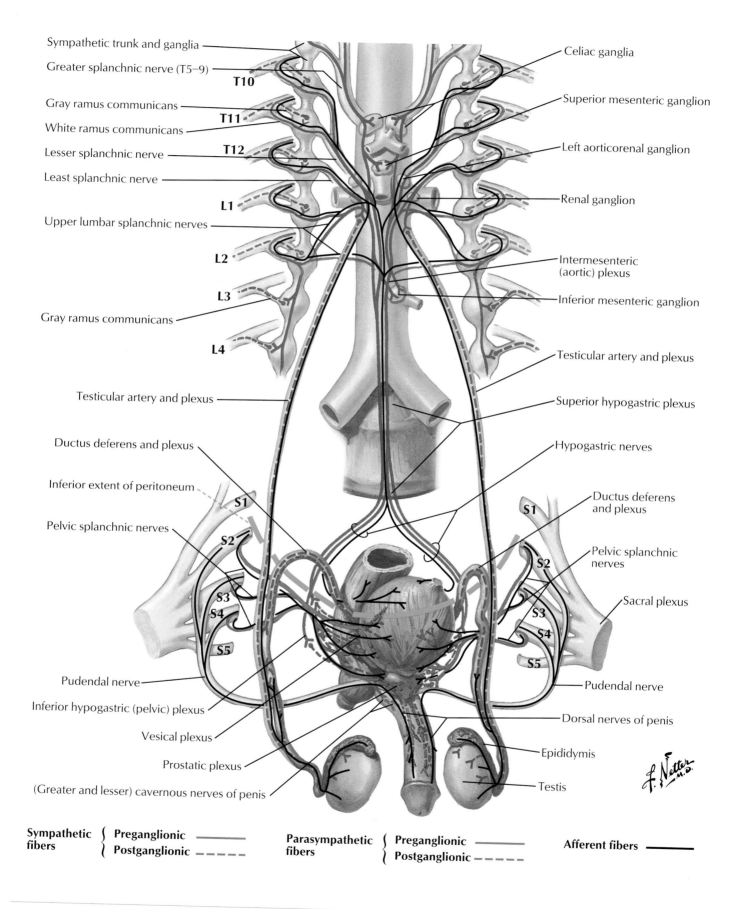

Sympathetic trunk and ganglia

Greater splanchnic nerve (T5–9)

**T10**

Gray ramus communicans

**T11**

White ramus communicans

Lesser splanchnic nerve **T12**

Least splanchnic nerve

**L1**

Upper lumbar splanchnic nerves

**L2**

**L3**

Gray ramus communicans

**L4**

Testicular artery and plexus

Ductus deferens and plexus

Inferior extent of peritoneum

Pelvic splanchnic nerves

Pudendal nerve

Inferior hypogastric (pelvic) plexus

Vesical plexus

Prostatic plexus

(Greater and lesser) cavernous nerves of penis

Celiac ganglia

Superior mesenteric ganglion

Left aorticorenal ganglion

Renal ganglion

Intermesenteric (aortic) plexus

Inferior mesenteric ganglion

Testicular artery and plexus

Superior hypogastric plexus

Hypogastric nerves

Ductus deferens and plexus

Pelvic splanchnic nerves

Sacral plexus

Pudendal nerve

Dorsal nerves of penis

Epididymis

Testis

S1 S2 S3 S4 S5

| Sympathetic fibers | Preganglionic ——— | Parasympathetic fibers | Preganglionic ——— | Afferent fibers ——— |
|---|---|---|---|---|
| | Postganglionic - - - | | Postganglionic - - - | |

**Plate 394**

**Innervation**

# Innervation of Urinary Bladder and Lower Ureter: Schema

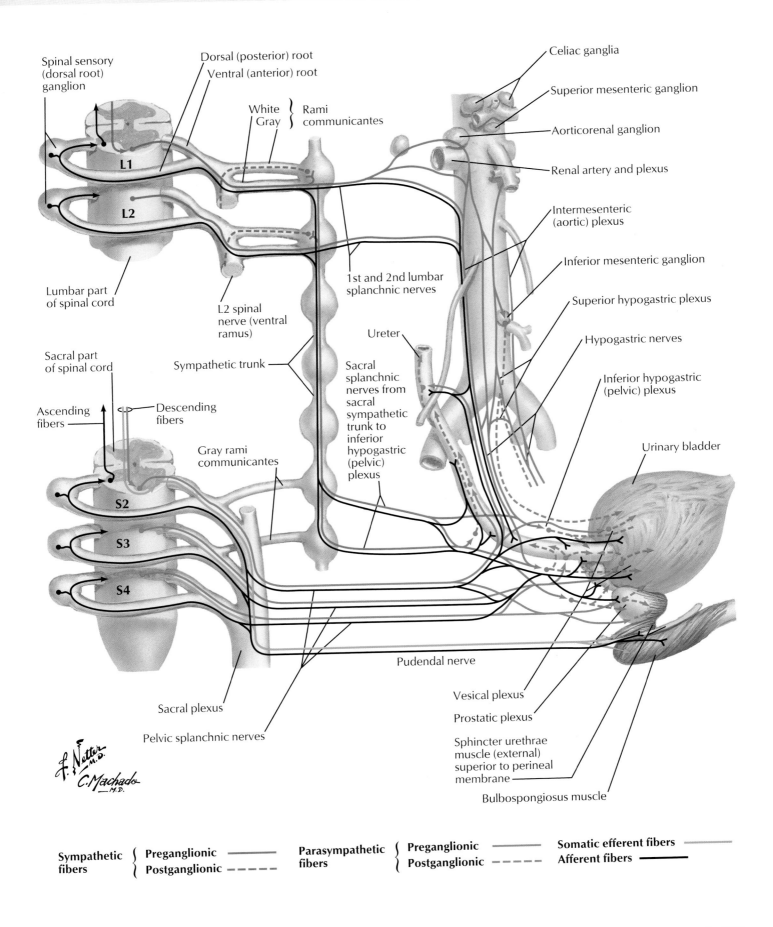

Spinal sensory (dorsal root) ganglion

Dorsal (posterior) root

Ventral (anterior) root

White } Rami
Gray } communicantes

Celiac ganglia

Superior mesenteric ganglion

Aorticorenal ganglion

Renal artery and plexus

Intermesenteric (aortic) plexus

Inferior mesenteric ganglion

Superior hypogastric plexus

Hypogastric nerves

Inferior hypogastric (pelvic) plexus

Urinary bladder

L1

L2

Lumbar part of spinal cord

L2 spinal nerve (ventral ramus)

Sympathetic trunk

1st and 2nd lumbar splanchnic nerves

Ureter

Sacral splanchnic nerves from sacral sympathetic trunk to inferior hypogastric (pelvic) plexus

Sacral part of spinal cord

Ascending fibers

Descending fibers

Gray rami communicantes

S2

S3

S4

Sacral plexus

Pelvic splanchnic nerves

Pudendal nerve

Vesical plexus

Prostatic plexus

Sphincter urethrae muscle (external) superior to perineal membrane

Bulbospongiosus muscle

Sympathetic fibers { Preganglionic ———
Postganglionic - - - - -

Parasympathetic fibers { Preganglionic ———
Postganglionic - - - - -

Somatic efferent fibers ———
Afferent fibers ———

**Plate 395**

**Innervation**

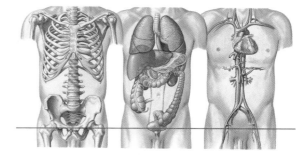

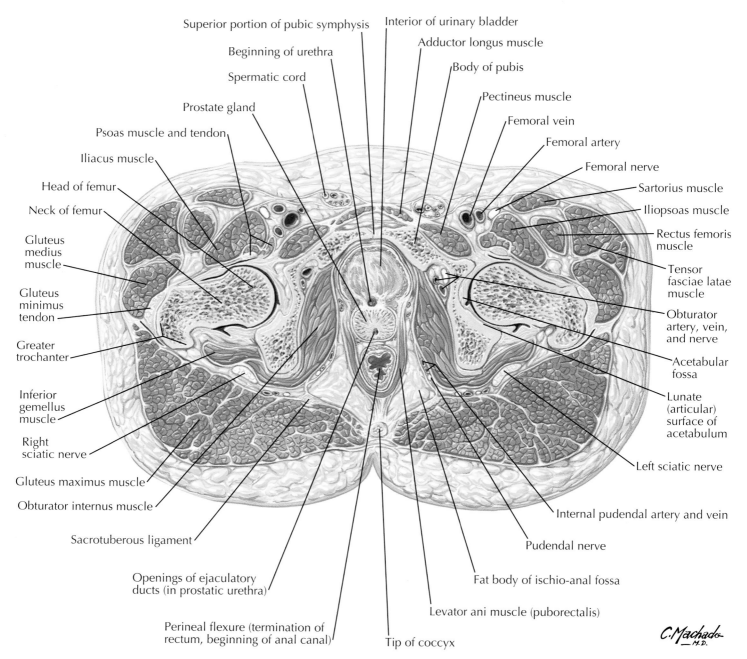

Superior portion of pubic symphysis

Beginning of urethra

Spermatic cord

Prostate gland

Psoas muscle and tendon

Iliacus muscle

Head of femur

Neck of femur

Gluteus medius muscle

Gluteus minimus tendon

Greater trochanter

Inferior gemellus muscle

Right sciatic nerve

Gluteus maximus muscle

Obturator internus muscle

Sacrotuberous ligament

Openings of ejaculatory ducts (in prostatic urethra)

Perineal flexure (termination of rectum, beginning of anal canal)

Interior of urinary bladder

Adductor longus muscle

Body of pubis

Pectineus muscle

Femoral vein

Femoral artery

Femoral nerve

Sartorius muscle

Iliopsoas muscle

Rectus femoris muscle

Tensor fasciae latae muscle

Obturator artery, vein, and nerve

Acetabular fossa

Lunate (articular) surface of acetabulum

Left sciatic nerve

Internal pudendal artery and vein

Pudendal nerve

Fat body of ischio-anal fossa

Levator ani muscle (puborectalis)

Tip of coccyx

**Plate 396**

**Cross-Sectional Anatomy**

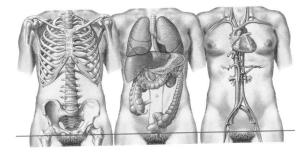

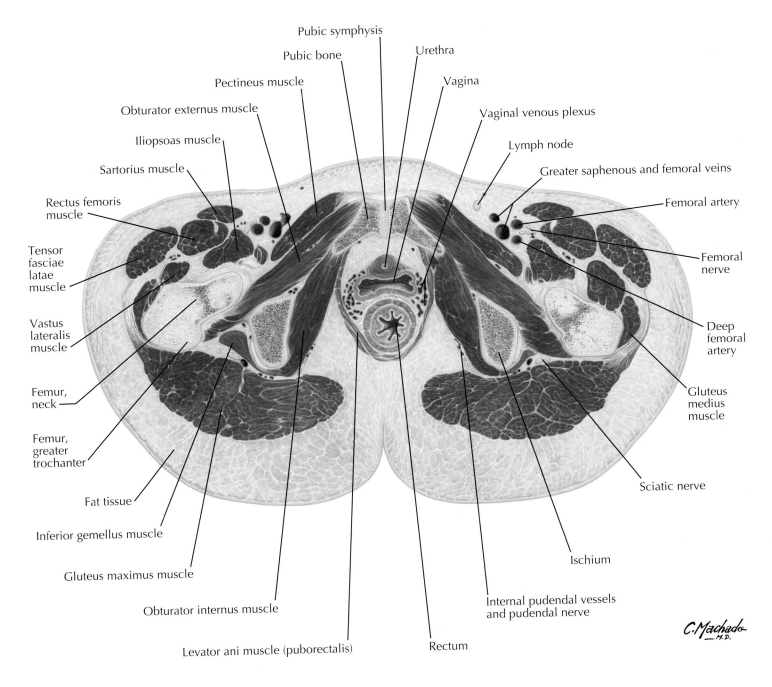

Pubic symphysis

Pubic bone

Urethra

Pectineus muscle

Vagina

Obturator externus muscle

Vaginal venous plexus

Iliopsoas muscle

Lymph node

Sartorius muscle

Greater saphenous and femoral veins

Rectus femoris muscle

Femoral artery

Tensor fasciae latae muscle

Femoral nerve

Vastus lateralis muscle

Deep femoral artery

Femur, neck

Gluteus medius muscle

Femur, greater trochanter

Sciatic nerve

Fat tissue

Inferior gemellus muscle

Ischium

Gluteus maximus muscle

Internal pudendal vessels and pudendal nerve

Obturator internus muscle

Levator ani muscle (puborectalis)

Rectum

| MUSCLE | PROXIMAL ATTACHMENT (ORIGIN) | DISTAL ATTACHMENT (INSERTION) | INNERVATION | MAIN ACTIONS | BLOOD SUPPLY | MUSCLE GROUP |
|---|---|---|---|---|---|---|
| Bulbospongiosus | *Male:* median raphe, bulb of penis, perineal body<br><br>*Female:* perineal body | *Male:* perineal membrane, corpus cavernosum, bulb of penis<br><br>*Female:* dorsum of clitoris, inferior fascia of urogenital diaphragm, bulb of vestibule, pubic arch | Deep branch of perineal nerve from pudendal nerve | *Male:* compresses bulb of penis, forces blood into body of penis during erection, removes urine from urethra and semen during ejaculation<br><br>*Female:* constricts vaginal orifice, assists in expressing secretions of greater vestibular gland, forces blood into body of clitoris | Internal pudendal artery and its branch (perineal artery) | Perineal |
| Coccygeus (ischiococcygeus) | Ischial spine, sacrospinous ligament | Inferior sacrum, coccyx | Ventral rami of lower sacral nerves | Supports pelvic viscera, draws coccyx forward | Inferior gluteal artery | Pelvic floor |
| Compressor urethrae (female only) | Ischiopubic ramus | Anterior aspect of urethra | Perineal branches of pudendal nerve | Sphincter of urethra | Perineal branch of internal pudendal artery | Perineal |
| Cremaster | Lower edge of internal oblique and middle of inguinal ligament | Pubic tubercle, crest of pubis | Genital branch of genitofemoral nerve | Retracts testicle | Cremasteric branch of inferior epigastric artery | Spermatic cord |
| Deep transverse perineal | Inner surface of inferior ischial rami | *Male:* medial tendinous raphe and perineal body<br><br>*Female:* sides of vagina | Perineal branches of pudendal nerve | Stabilizes perineal body, supports prostate/vagina | Perineal branch of internal pudendal artery | Perineal |
| External anal sphincter | Tip of coccyx, anococcygeal ligament | Deeper fibers surround anal canal, attach posteriorly to coccyx and anteriorly to central point of perineum | Perineal and inferior rectal branches of pudendal nerve | Closes anal orifice | Inferior rectal and transverse perineal artery | Perineal |
| Iliacus | Superior 2/3 of iliac fossa, ala of sacrum, anterior sacro-iliac ligaments | Lesser trochanter of femur and shaft inferior to it, to psoas major tendon | Femoral nerve | Flexes thigh at hips and stabilizes hip joint, acts with psoas major | Iliac branches of iliolumbar artery | Anterior thigh |
| Ischiocavernosus | Inferior internal surface of ischiopubic ramus, ischial tuberosity | Crus of penis or clitoris | Deep branch of perineal nerve from pudendal nerve | Forces blood into body of penis and clitoris during erection | Internal pudendal artery and its branch (perineal artery) | Perineal |
| Levator ani (Iliococcygeus, pubococcygeus, and puborectalis) | Body of pubis, tendinous arch of obturator fascia, ischial spine | Perineal body, coccyx, anococcygeal raphe, walls of prostate or vagina, rectum, anal canal | Ventral rami of lower sacral nerves, perineal nerve | Supports pelvic viscera, raises pelvic floor | Inferior gluteal artery, internal pudendal artery and its branches (inferior rectal and perineal arteries) | Pelvic floor |
| Obturator internus | Pelvic surface of obturator membrane and surrounding bone | Medial surface of greater trochanter of femur | Nerve to obturator internus | Laterally rotates extended thigh, abducts flexed thigh at hip | Internal pudendal and obturator arteries | Gluteal region |

Variations in spinal nerve contributions to the innervation of muscles, their arterial supply, their attachments, and their actions are common themes in human anatomy. Therefore, expect differences between texts and realize that anatomical variation is normal.

| MUSCLE | PROXIMAL ATTACHMENT (ORIGIN) | DISTAL ATTACHMENT (INSERTION) | INNERVATION | MAIN ACTIONS | BLOOD SUPPLY | MUSCLE GROUP |
|---|---|---|---|---|---|---|
| Piriformis | Anterior surface of sacral segments 2–4, sacrotuberous ligament | Superior border of greater trochanter of femur | Ventral rami of L5, S1, S2 | Laterally rotates extended thigh, abducts flexed thigh at hip | Superior and inferior gluteal arteries, internal pudendal artery | Gluteal region |
| Sphincter urethrae | External fibers from junction of inferior pubic and ischial rami and adjacent fascia; internal fibers pass medially to surround membranous urethra | *Male:* median raphe in front and behind urethra  *Female:* encloses urethra, attaches to sides of vagina | Perineal branches of pudendal nerve | Compresses urethra at end of micturition; in female also compresses the distal vagina | Perineal branch of internal pudendal artery | Perineal |
| Sphincter urethrovaginalis (female only) | Perineal body | Passes forward and anterior around urethra | Perineal branches of pudendal nerve | Sphincter of urethra and vagina | Perineal branch of pudendal artery | Perineal |
| Superficial transverse perineal | Ischial rami and tuberosities | Central tendon (perineal body) | Perineal branches of pudendal nerve | Stabilizes central tendon | Perineal branch of internal pudendal artery | Perineal |

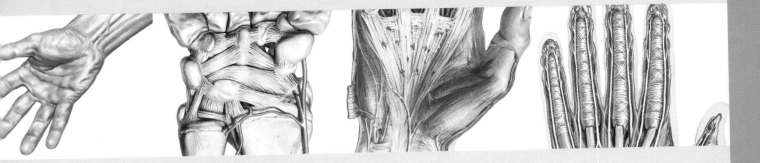

# 6 UPPER LIMB

# UPPER LIMB

## Muscle Tables

**Atlas of Human Anatomy**

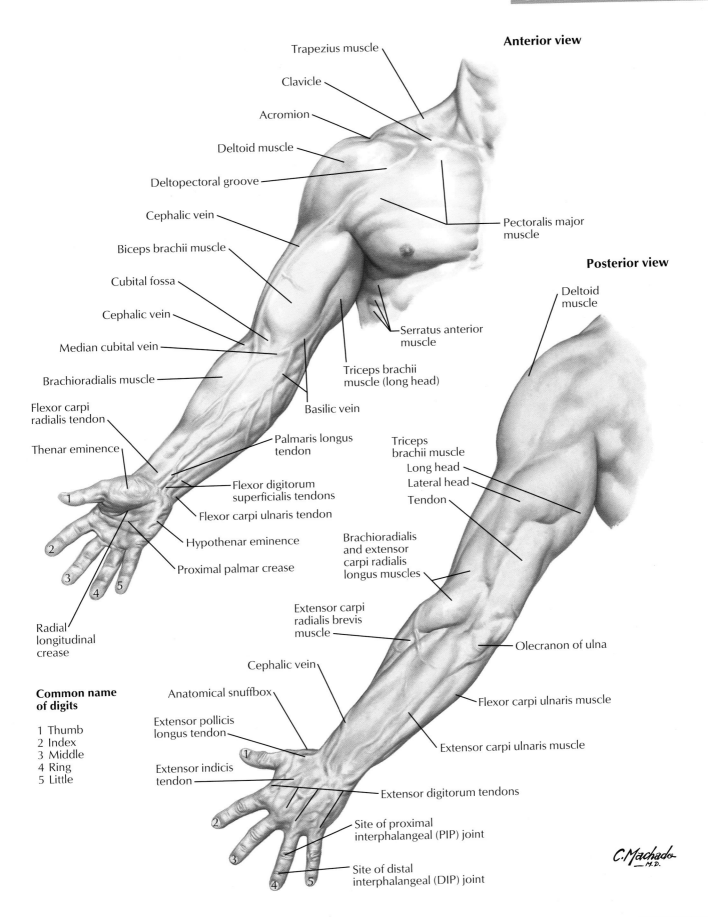

**Anterior view**

Trapezius muscle

Clavicle

Acromion

Deltoid muscle

Deltopectoral groove

Cephalic vein

Biceps brachii muscle

Cubital fossa

Cephalic vein

Median cubital vein

Brachioradialis muscle

Flexor carpi radialis tendon

Thenar eminence

Pectoralis major muscle

**Posterior view**

Deltoid muscle

Serratus anterior muscle

Triceps brachii muscle (long head)

Basilic vein

Palmaris longus tendon

Triceps brachii muscle

Long head

Lateral head

Tendon

Flexor digitorum superficialis tendons

Flexor carpi ulnaris tendon

Hypothenar eminence

Proximal palmar crease

Brachioradialis and extensor carpi radialis longus muscles

Extensor carpi radialis brevis muscle

Olecranon of ulna

Radial longitudinal crease

Cephalic vein

Flexor carpi ulnaris muscle

**Common name of digits**

1 Thumb
2 Index
3 Middle
4 Ring
5 Little

Anatomical snuffbox

Extensor pollicis longus tendon

Extensor indicis tendon

Extensor carpi ulnaris muscle

Extensor digitorum tendons

Site of proximal interphalangeal (PIP) joint

Site of distal interphalangeal (DIP) joint

*C. Machado*
_M.D._

**Topographic Anatomy**

**Plate 398**

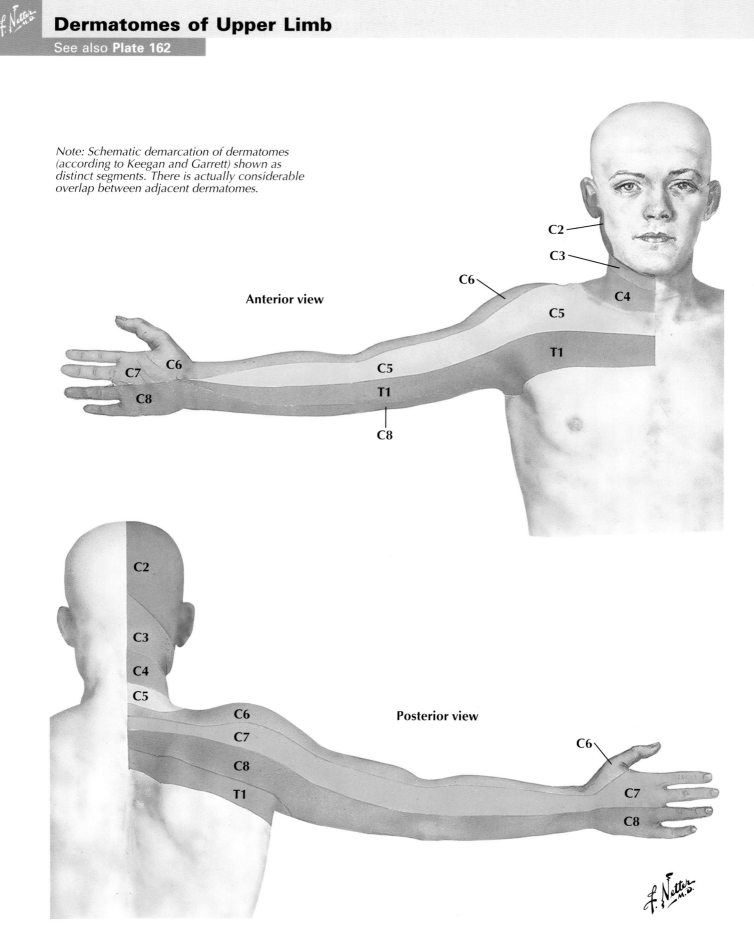

Note: Schematic demarcation of dermatomes (according to Keegan and Garrett) shown as distinct segments. There is actually considerable overlap between adjacent dermatomes.

**Anterior view**

C2
C3
C6
C4
C5
T1
C6
C7
C5
C8
T1
C8

**Posterior view**

C2
C3
C4
C5
C6
C7
C8
T1
C6
C7
C8

**Plate 399**

**Cutaneous Anatomy**

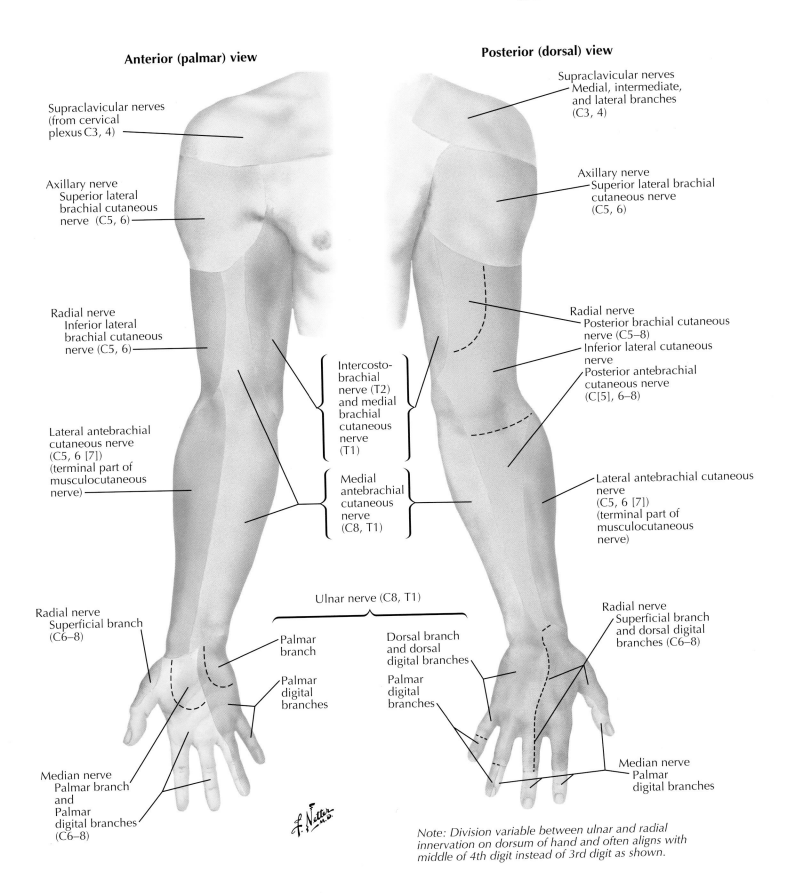

**Anterior (palmar) view**

**Posterior (dorsal) view**

Supraclavicular nerves
(from cervical
plexus C3, 4)

Axillary nerve
Superior lateral
brachial cutaneous
nerve (C5, 6)

Radial nerve
Inferior lateral
brachial cutaneous
nerve (C5, 6)

Lateral antebrachial
cutaneous nerve
(C5, 6 [7])
(terminal part of
musculocutaneous
nerve)

Radial nerve
Superficial branch
(C6–8)

Median nerve
Palmar branch
and
Palmar
digital branches
(C6–8)

Intercosto-
brachial
nerve (T2)
and medial
brachial
cutaneous
nerve
(T1)

Medial
antebrachial
cutaneous
nerve
(C8, T1)

Ulnar nerve (C8, T1)

Palmar
branch

Palmar
digital
branches

Dorsal branch
and dorsal
digital branches

Palmar
digital
branches

Supraclavicular nerves
Medial, intermediate,
and lateral branches
(C3, 4)

Axillary nerve
Superior lateral brachial
cutaneous nerve
(C5, 6)

Radial nerve
Posterior brachial cutaneous
nerve (C5–8)
Inferior lateral cutaneous
nerve
Posterior antebrachial
cutaneous nerve
(C[5], 6–8)

Lateral antebrachial cutaneous
nerve
(C5, 6 [7])
(terminal part of
musculocutaneous
nerve)

Radial nerve
Superficial branch
and dorsal digital
branches (C6–8)

Median nerve
Palmar
digital branches

*Note: Division variable between ulnar and radial
innervation on dorsum of hand and often aligns with
middle of 4th digit instead of 3rd digit as shown.*

**Anterior view**

**Posterior view**

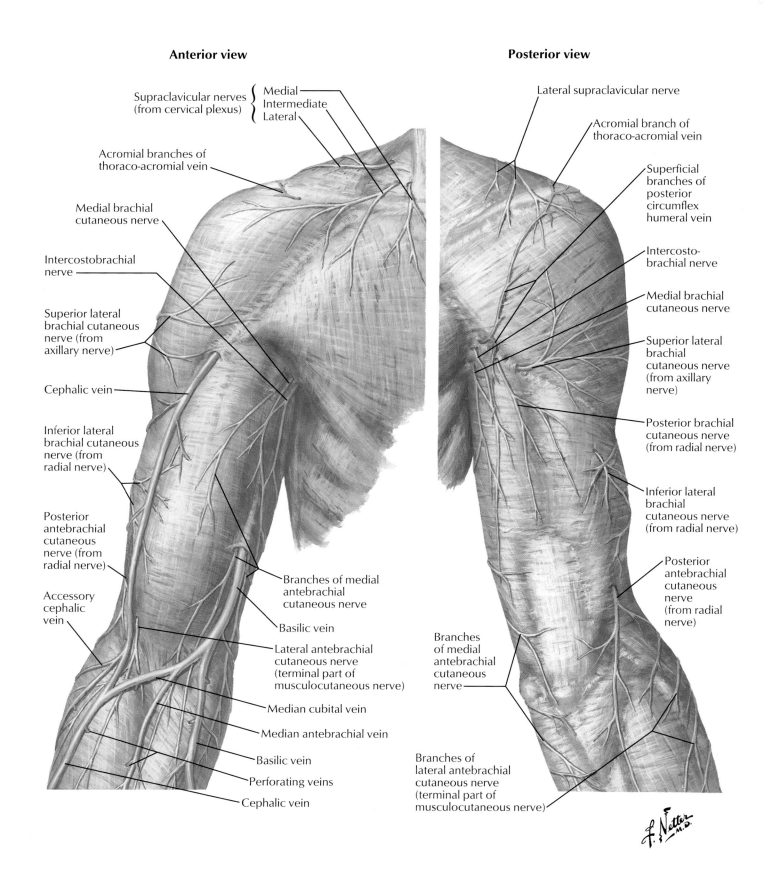

Supraclavicular nerves (from cervical plexus) { Medial / Intermediate / Lateral

Acromial branches of thoraco-acromial vein

Medial brachial cutaneous nerve

Intercostobrachial nerve

Superior lateral brachial cutaneous nerve (from axillary nerve)

Cephalic vein

Inferior lateral brachial cutaneous nerve (from radial nerve)

Posterior antebrachial cutaneous nerve (from radial nerve)

Accessory cephalic vein

Branches of medial antebrachial cutaneous nerve

Basilic vein

Lateral antebrachial cutaneous nerve (terminal part of musculocutaneous nerve)

Median cubital vein

Median antebrachial vein

Basilic vein

Perforating veins

Cephalic vein

Lateral supraclavicular nerve

Acromial branch of thoraco-acromial vein

Superficial branches of posterior circumflex humeral vein

Intercosto-brachial nerve

Medial brachial cutaneous nerve

Superior lateral brachial cutaneous nerve (from axillary nerve)

Posterior brachial cutaneous nerve (from radial nerve)

Inferior lateral brachial cutaneous nerve (from radial nerve)

Posterior antebrachial cutaneous nerve (from radial nerve)

Branches of medial antebrachial cutaneous nerve

Branches of lateral antebrachial cutaneous nerve (terminal part of musculocutaneous nerve)

**Plate 401**

**Cutaneous Anatomy**

**Anterior (palmar) view**

**Posterior (dorsal) view**

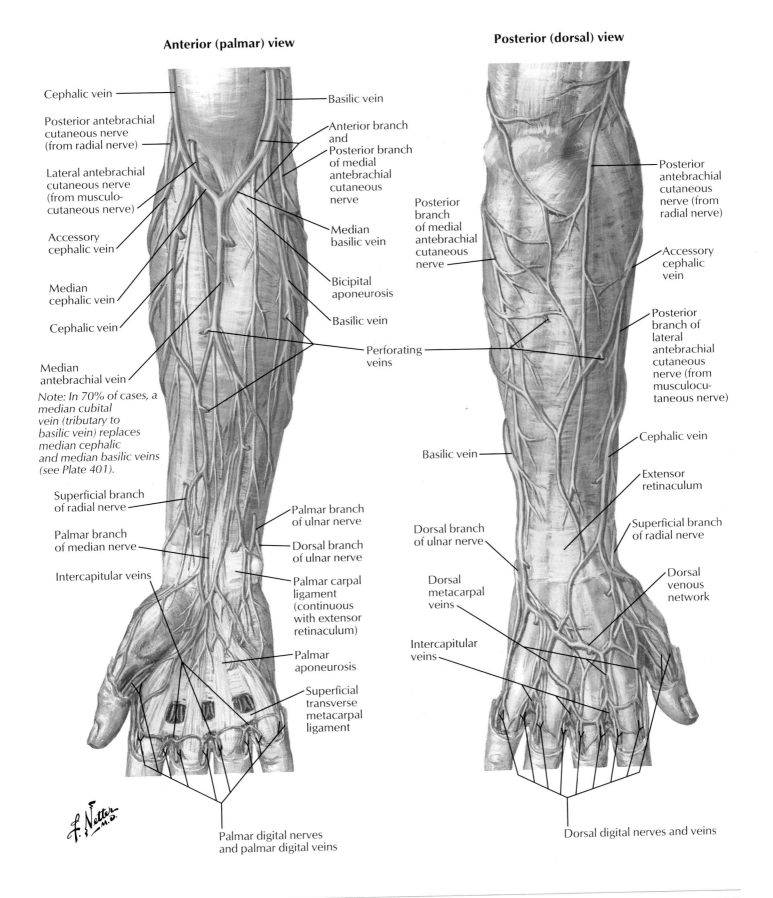

Cephalic vein

Posterior antebrachial cutaneous nerve (from radial nerve)

Lateral antebrachial cutaneous nerve (from musculo-cutaneous nerve)

Accessory cephalic vein

Median cephalic vein

Cephalic vein

Median antebrachial vein

*Note: In 70% of cases, a median cubital vein (tributary to basilic vein) replaces median cephalic and median basilic veins (see Plate 401).*

Superficial branch of radial nerve

Palmar branch of median nerve

Intercapitular veins

Basilic vein

Anterior branch and Posterior branch of medial antebrachial cutaneous nerve

Median basilic vein

Bicipital aponeurosis

Basilic vein

Perforating veins

Palmar branch of ulnar nerve

Dorsal branch of ulnar nerve

Palmar carpal ligament (continuous with extensor retinaculum)

Palmar aponeurosis

Superficial transverse metacarpal ligament

Palmar digital nerves and palmar digital veins

Posterior branch of medial antebrachial cutaneous nerve

Basilic vein

Dorsal branch of ulnar nerve

Dorsal metacarpal veins

Intercapitular veins

Posterior antebrachial cutaneous nerve (from radial nerve)

Accessory cephalic vein

Posterior branch of lateral antebrachial cutaneous nerve (from musculocu-taneous nerve)

Cephalic vein

Extensor retinaculum

Superficial branch of radial nerve

Dorsal venous network

Dorsal digital nerves and veins

**Cutaneous Anatomy**

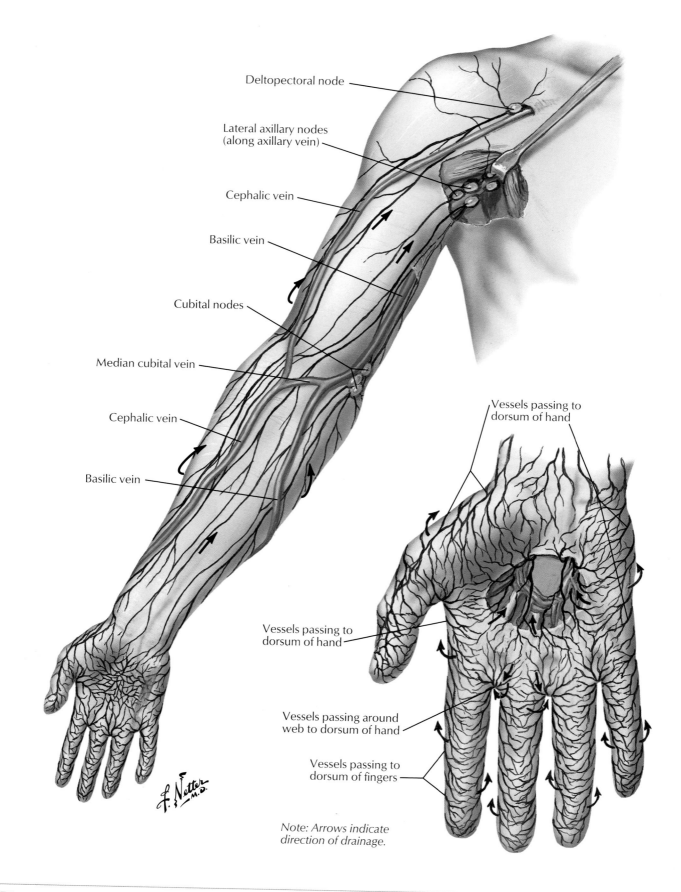

Deltopectoral node

Lateral axillary nodes
(along axillary vein)

Cephalic vein

Basilic vein

Cubital nodes

Median cubital vein

Cephalic vein

Basilic vein

Vessels passing to
dorsum of hand

Vessels passing to
dorsum of hand

Vessels passing around
web to dorsum of hand

Vessels passing to
dorsum of fingers

*Note: Arrows indicate
direction of drainage.*

**Plate 403**

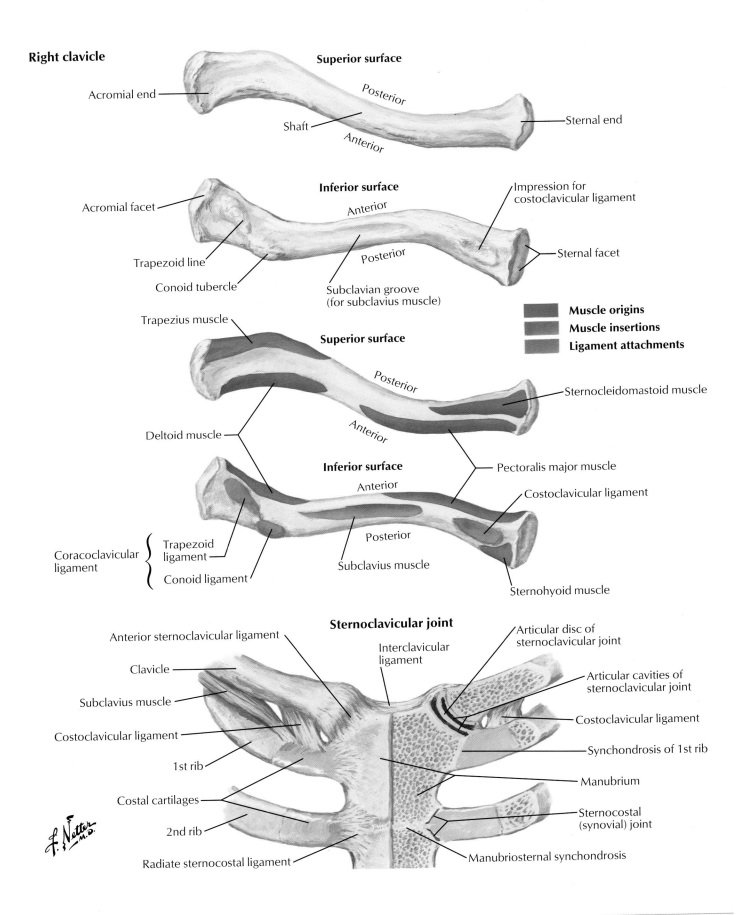

**Right clavicle**

**Superior surface**

Acromial end

Posterior

Shaft

Anterior

Sternal end

**Inferior surface**

Impression for costoclavicular ligament

Acromial facet

Anterior

Trapezoid line

Posterior

Sternal facet

Conoid tubercle

Subclavian groove (for subclavius muscle)

Muscle origins
Muscle insertions
Ligament attachments

Trapezius muscle

**Superior surface**

Posterior

Sternocleidomastoid muscle

Anterior

Deltoid muscle

**Inferior surface**

Anterior

Pectoralis major muscle

Costoclavicular ligament

Coracoclavicular ligament

Trapezoid ligament

Posterior

Conoid ligament

Subclavius muscle

Sternohyoid muscle

**Sternoclavicular joint**

Anterior sternoclavicular ligament

Interclavicular ligament

Articular disc of sternoclavicular joint

Clavicle

Articular cavities of sternoclavicular joint

Subclavius muscle

Costoclavicular ligament

Costoclavicular ligament

Synchondrosis of 1st rib

1st rib

Manubrium

Costal cartilages

Sternocostal (synovial) joint

2nd rib

Radiate sternocostal ligament

Manubriosternal synchondrosis

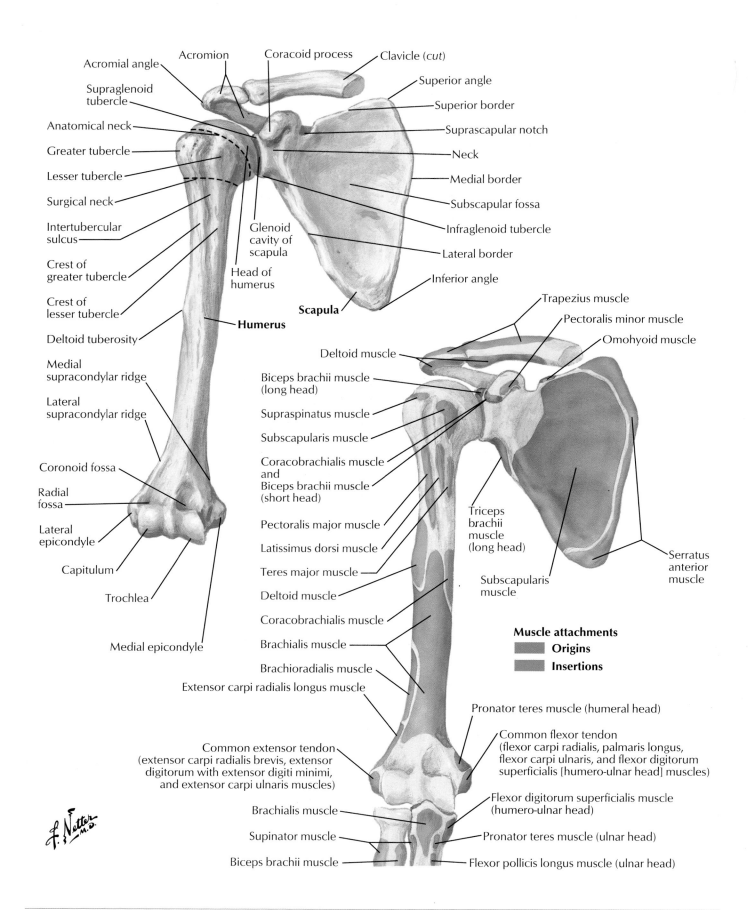

Acromial angle
Acromion
Coracoid process
Clavicle (*cut*)
Superior angle
Supraglenoid tubercle
Superior border
Suprascapular notch
Anatomical neck
Neck
Greater tubercle
Medial border
Lesser tubercle
Subscapular fossa
Surgical neck
Infraglenoid tubercle
Intertubercular sulcus
Lateral border
Glenoid cavity of scapula
Crest of greater tubercle
Head of humerus
Crest of lesser tubercle
**Scapula**
Inferior angle
Deltoid tuberosity
**Humerus**
Medial supracondylar ridge
Lateral supracondylar ridge

Coronoid fossa
Radial fossa
Lateral epicondyle
Capitulum
Trochlea
Medial epicondyle

Trapezius muscle
Pectoralis minor muscle
Omohyoid muscle
Deltoid muscle
Biceps brachii muscle (long head)
Supraspinatus muscle
Subscapularis muscle
Coracobrachialis muscle and Biceps brachii muscle (short head)
Triceps brachii muscle (long head)
Pectoralis major muscle
Latissimus dorsi muscle
Subscapularis muscle
Teres major muscle
Deltoid muscle
Serratus anterior muscle
Coracobrachialis muscle
Brachialis muscle

**Muscle attachments**
Origins
Insertions

Brachioradialis muscle
Extensor carpi radialis longus muscle
Pronator teres muscle (humeral head)
Common flexor tendon (flexor carpi radialis, palmaris longus, flexor carpi ulnaris, and flexor digitorum superficialis [humero-ulnar head] muscles)
Common extensor tendon (extensor carpi radialis brevis, extensor digitorum with extensor digiti minimi, and extensor carpi ulnaris muscles)
Flexor digitorum superficialis muscle (humero-ulnar head)
Brachialis muscle
Pronator teres muscle (ulnar head)
Supinator muscle
Biceps brachii muscle
Flexor pollicis longus muscle (ulnar head)

**Plate 405**

**Shoulder and Axilla**

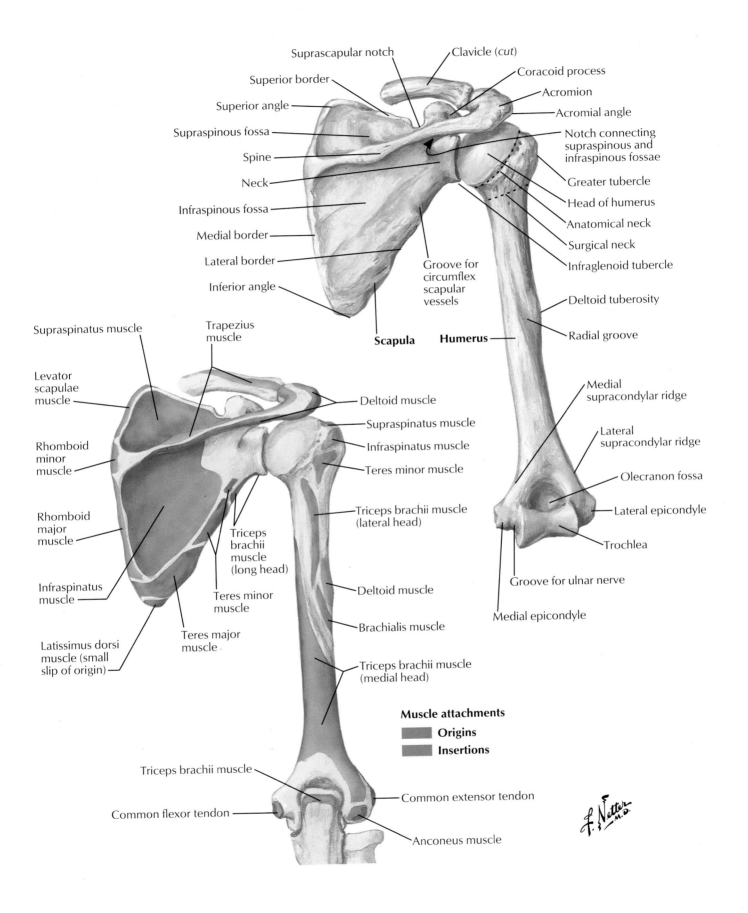

Suprascapular notch

Clavicle (cut)

Coracoid process

Superior border

Acromion

Superior angle

Acromial angle

Supraspinous fossa

Notch connecting
supraspinous and
infraspinous fossae

Spine

Greater tubercle

Neck

Head of humerus

Infraspinous fossa

Anatomical neck

Medial border

Surgical neck

Lateral border

Infraglenoid tubercle

Inferior angle

Groove for
circumflex
scapular
vessels

Deltoid tuberosity

**Scapula**

**Humerus**

Radial groove

Supraspinatus muscle

Trapezius
muscle

Levator
scapulae
muscle

Deltoid muscle

Medial
supracondylar ridge

Supraspinatus muscle

Rhomboid
minor
muscle

Infraspinatus muscle

Lateral
supracondylar ridge

Teres minor muscle

Olecranon fossa

Triceps brachii muscle
(lateral head)

Rhomboid
major
muscle

Lateral epicondyle

Triceps
brachii
muscle
(long head)

Trochlea

Infraspinatus
muscle

Groove for ulnar nerve

Teres minor
muscle

Deltoid muscle

Latissimus dorsi
muscle (small
slip of origin)

Teres major
muscle

Medial epicondyle

Brachialis muscle

Triceps brachii muscle
(medial head)

**Muscle attachments**

**Origins**

**Insertions**

Triceps brachii muscle

Common extensor tendon

Common flexor tendon

Anconeus muscle

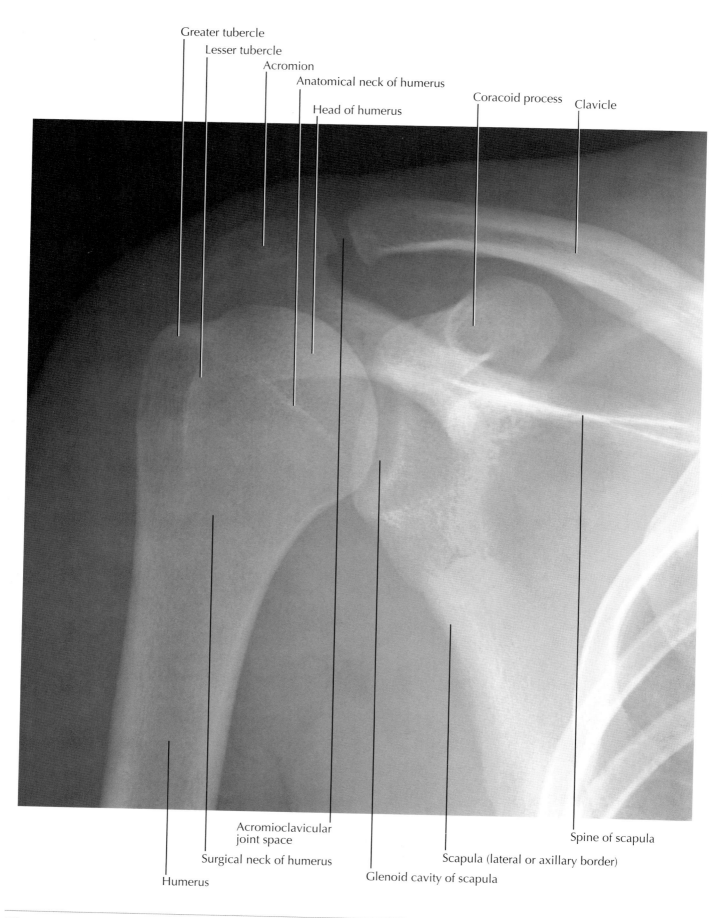

Greater tubercle

Lesser tubercle

Acromion

Anatomical neck of humerus

Head of humerus

Coracoid process  Clavicle

Acromioclavicular joint space

Surgical neck of humerus

Humerus

Glenoid cavity of scapula

Scapula (lateral or axillary border)

Spine of scapula

**Plate 407**

**Shoulder and Axilla**

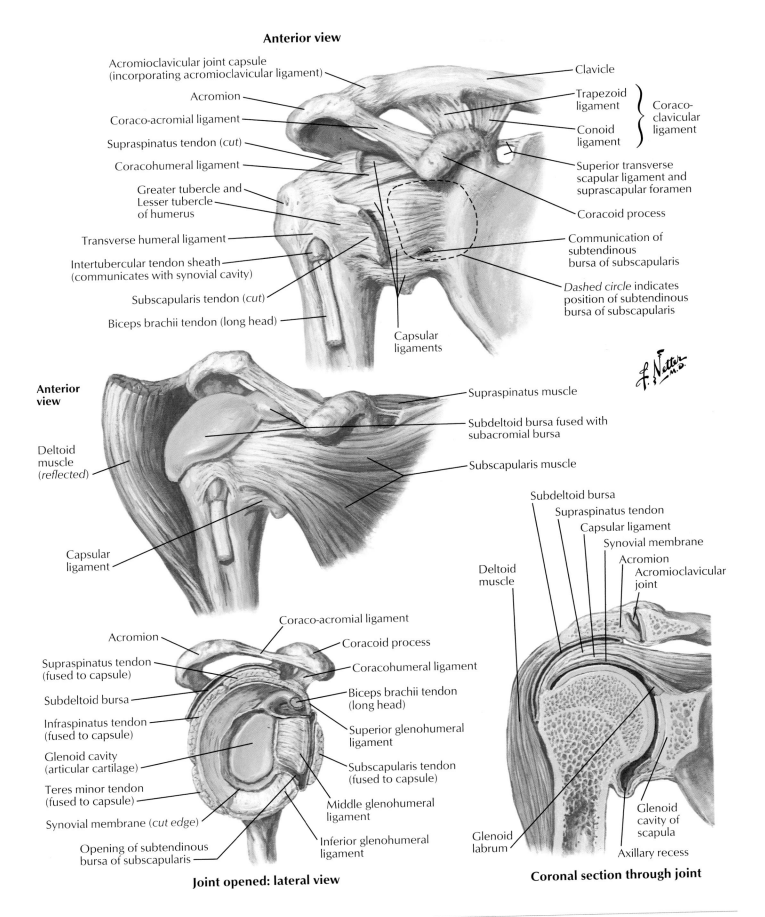

**Anterior view**

Acromioclavicular joint capsule (incorporating acromioclavicular ligament)

Acromion

Coraco-acromial ligament

Supraspinatus tendon (*cut*)

Coracohumeral ligament

Greater tubercle and Lesser tubercle of humerus

Transverse humeral ligament

Intertubercular tendon sheath (communicates with synovial cavity)

Subscapularis tendon (*cut*)

Biceps brachii tendon (long head)

Clavicle

Trapezoid ligament
Conoid ligament } Coraco-clavicular ligament

Superior transverse scapular ligament and suprascapular foramen

Coracoid process

Communication of subtendinous bursa of subscapularis

*Dashed circle* indicates position of subtendinous bursa of subscapularis

Capsular ligaments

**Anterior view**

Deltoid muscle (*reflected*)

Capsular ligament

Supraspinatus muscle

Subdeltoid bursa fused with subacromial bursa

Subscapularis muscle

Acromion

Supraspinatus tendon (fused to capsule)

Subdeltoid bursa

Infraspinatus tendon (fused to capsule)

Glenoid cavity (articular cartilage)

Teres minor tendon (fused to capsule)

Synovial membrane (*cut edge*)

Opening of subtendinous bursa of subscapularis

Coraco-acromial ligament

Coracoid process

Coracohumeral ligament

Biceps brachii tendon (long head)

Superior glenohumeral ligament

Subscapularis tendon (fused to capsule)

Middle glenohumeral ligament

Inferior glenohumeral ligament

**Joint opened: lateral view**

Subdeltoid bursa

Supraspinatus tendon

Capsular ligament

Synovial membrane

Acromion

Acromioclavicular joint

Deltoid muscle

Glenoid labrum

Glenoid cavity of scapula

Axillary recess

**Coronal section through joint**

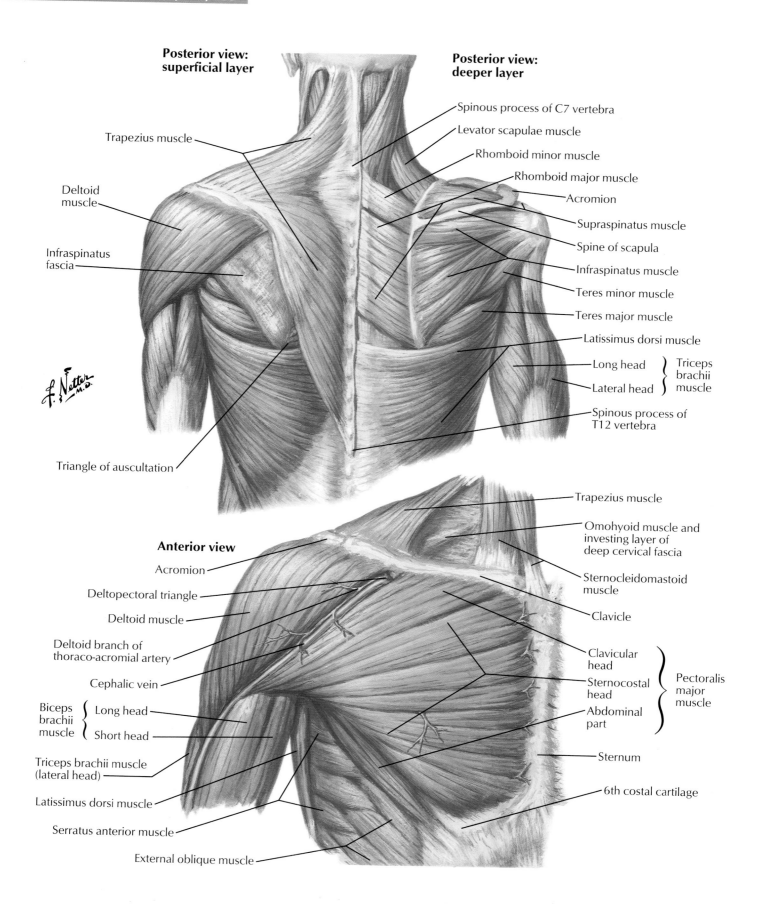

**Posterior view:
superficial layer**

Trapezius muscle

Deltoid
muscle

Infraspinatus
fascia

Triangle of auscultation

**Posterior view:
deeper layer**

Spinous process of C7 vertebra

Levator scapulae muscle

Rhomboid minor muscle

Rhomboid major muscle

Acromion

Supraspinatus muscle

Spine of scapula

Infraspinatus muscle

Teres minor muscle

Teres major muscle

Latissimus dorsi muscle

Long head ⎫ Triceps
          ⎬ brachii
Lateral head ⎭ muscle

Spinous process of
T12 vertebra

**Anterior view**

Acromion

Deltopectoral triangle

Deltoid muscle

Deltoid branch of
thoraco-acromial artery

Cephalic vein

Biceps ⎧ Long head
brachii ⎨
muscle ⎩ Short head

Triceps brachii muscle
(lateral head)

Latissimus dorsi muscle

Serratus anterior muscle

External oblique muscle

Trapezius muscle

Omohyoid muscle and
investing layer of
deep cervical fascia

Sternocleidomastoid
muscle

Clavicle

Clavicular ⎫
head     ⎪
         ⎬ Pectoralis
Sternocostal ⎪ major
head     ⎪ muscle
         ⎪
Abdominal ⎭
part

Sternum

6th costal cartilage

**Plate 409**

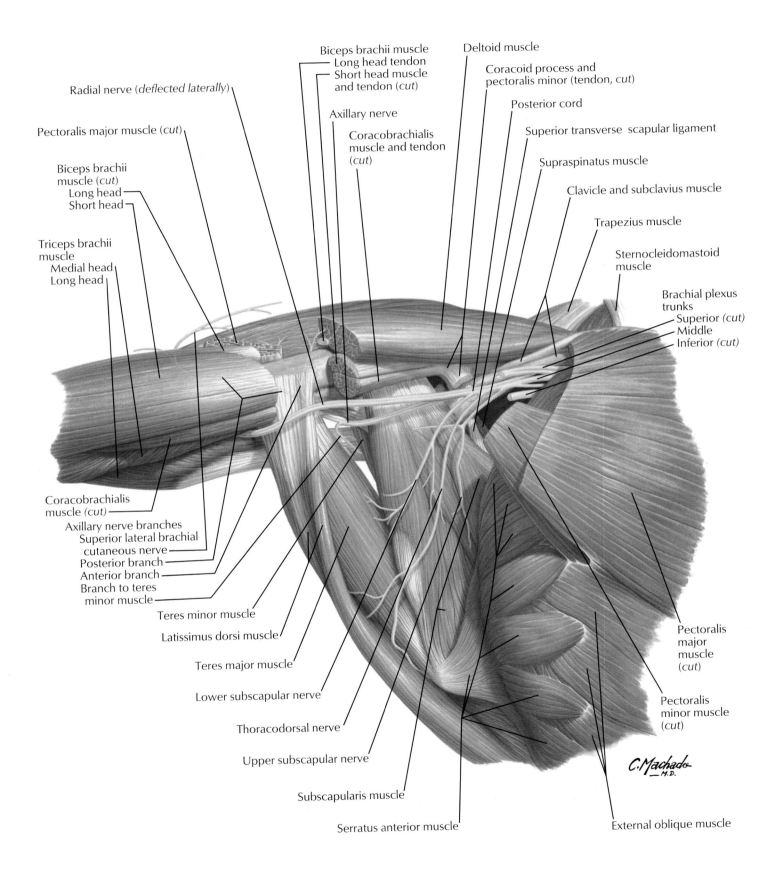

Biceps brachii muscle
— Long head tendon
— Short head muscle and tendon (*cut*)

Deltoid muscle

Coracoid process and pectoralis minor (tendon, *cut*)

Radial nerve (*deflected laterally*)

Posterior cord

Axillary nerve

Superior transverse scapular ligament

Pectoralis major muscle (*cut*)

Coracobrachialis muscle and tendon (*cut*)

Supraspinatus muscle

Biceps brachii muscle (*cut*)
Long head
Short head

Clavicle and subclavius muscle

Trapezius muscle

Triceps brachii muscle
Medial head
Long head

Sternocleidomastoid muscle

Brachial plexus trunks
— Superior (*cut*)
— Middle
— Inferior (*cut*)

Coracobrachialis muscle (*cut*)

Axillary nerve branches
Superior lateral brachial cutaneous nerve
Posterior branch
Anterior branch
Branch to teres minor muscle

Teres minor muscle

Latissimus dorsi muscle

Pectoralis major muscle (*cut*)

Teres major muscle

Pectoralis minor muscle (*cut*)

Lower subscapular nerve

Thoracodorsal nerve

*C. Machado*
_M.D.

Upper subscapular nerve

Subscapularis muscle

Serratus anterior muscle

External oblique muscle

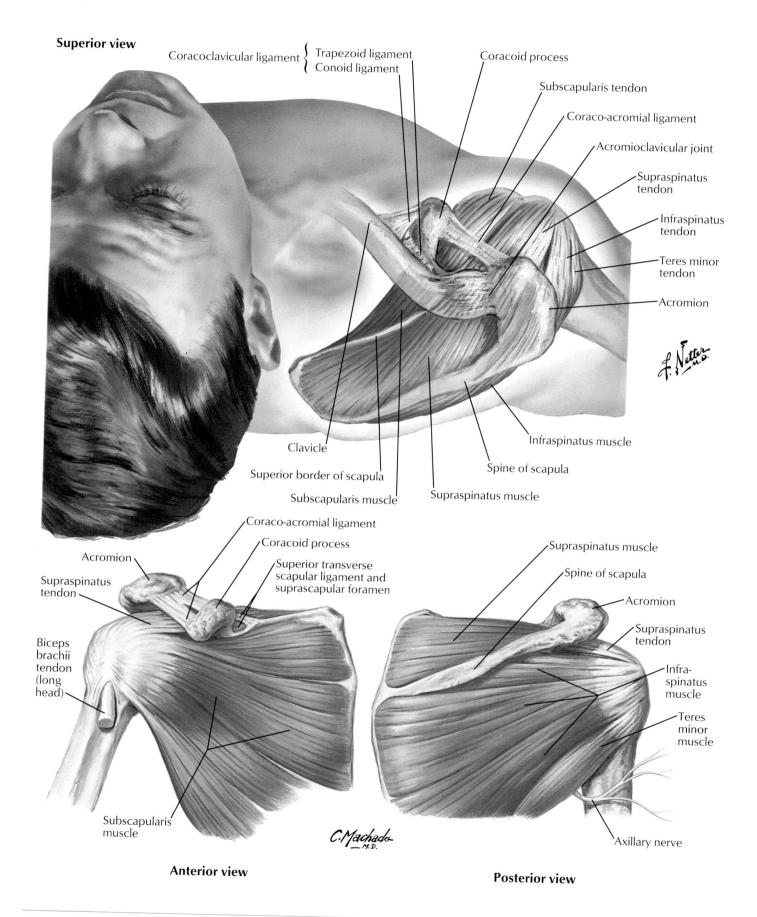

Superior view

Coracoclavicular ligament { Trapezoid ligament / Conoid ligament

Coracoid process

Subscapularis tendon

Coraco-acromial ligament

Acromioclavicular joint

Supraspinatus tendon

Infraspinatus tendon

Teres minor tendon

Acromion

Infraspinatus muscle

Spine of scapula

Supraspinatus muscle

Subscapularis muscle

Superior border of scapula

Clavicle

Coraco-acromial ligament

Coracoid process

Superior transverse scapular ligament and suprascapular foramen

Acromion

Supraspinatus tendon

Biceps brachii tendon (long head)

Subscapularis muscle

Supraspinatus muscle

Spine of scapula

Acromion

Supraspinatus tendon

Infra-spinatus muscle

Teres minor muscle

Axillary nerve

Anterior view

Posterior view

Plate 411

Shoulder and Axilla

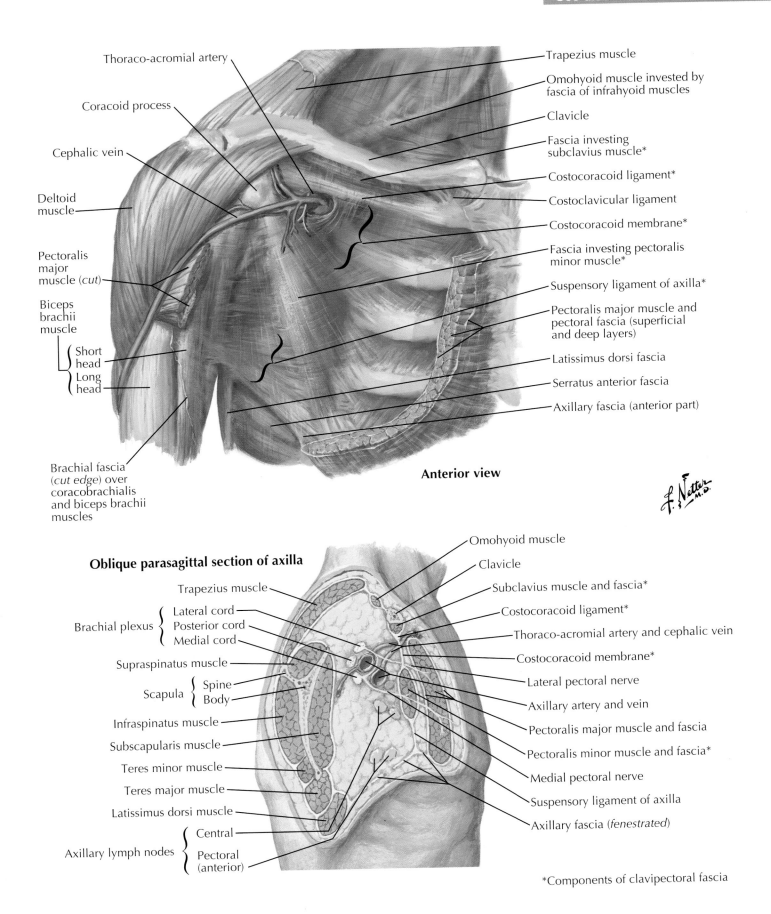

Thoraco-acromial artery

Coracoid process

Cephalic vein

Deltoid muscle

Pectoralis major muscle (*cut*)

Biceps brachii muscle
{ Short head
{ Long head

Brachial fascia (*cut edge*) over coracobrachialis and biceps brachii muscles

Trapezius muscle

Omohyoid muscle invested by fascia of infrahyoid muscles

Clavicle

Fascia investing subclavius muscle*

Costocoracoid ligament*

Costoclavicular ligament

Costocoracoid membrane*

Fascia investing pectoralis minor muscle*

Suspensory ligament of axilla*

Pectoralis major muscle and pectoral fascia (superficial and deep layers)

Latissimus dorsi fascia

Serratus anterior fascia

Axillary fascia (anterior part)

**Anterior view**

**Oblique parasagittal section of axilla**

Brachial plexus {
Lateral cord
Posterior cord
Medial cord

Supraspinatus muscle

Scapula { Spine
{ Body

Infraspinatus muscle

Subscapularis muscle

Teres minor muscle

Teres major muscle

Latissimus dorsi muscle

Axillary lymph nodes {
Central
Pectoral (anterior)

Trapezius muscle

Omohyoid muscle

Clavicle

Subclavius muscle and fascia*

Costocoracoid ligament*

Thoraco-acromial artery and cephalic vein

Costocoracoid membrane*

Lateral pectoral nerve

Axillary artery and vein

Pectoralis major muscle and fascia

Pectoralis minor muscle and fascia*

Medial pectoral nerve

Suspensory ligament of axilla

Axillary fascia (*fenestrated*)

*Components of clavipectoral fascia

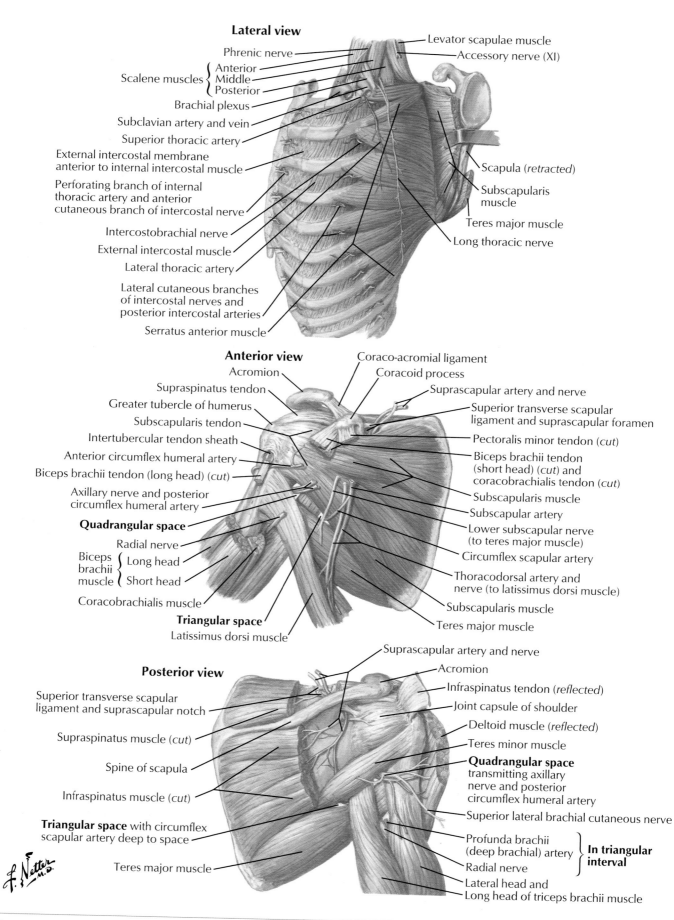

**Lateral view**

Levator scapulae muscle

Phrenic nerve

Accessory nerve (XI)

Scalene muscles { Anterior / Middle / Posterior

Brachial plexus

Subclavian artery and vein

Superior thoracic artery

Scapula (retracted)

Subscapularis muscle

External intercostal membrane anterior to internal intercostal muscle

Perforating branch of internal thoracic artery and anterior cutaneous branch of intercostal nerve

Teres major muscle

Long thoracic nerve

Intercostobrachial nerve

External intercostal muscle

Lateral thoracic artery

Lateral cutaneous branches of intercostal nerves and posterior intercostal arteries

Serratus anterior muscle

**Anterior view**

Coraco-acromial ligament

Acromion

Coracoid process

Supraspinatus tendon

Suprascapular artery and nerve

Greater tubercle of humerus

Superior transverse scapular ligament and suprascapular foramen

Subscapularis tendon

Intertubercular tendon sheath

Pectoralis minor tendon (cut)

Anterior circumflex humeral artery

Biceps brachii tendon (short head) (cut) and coracobrachialis tendon (cut)

Biceps brachii tendon (long head) (cut)

Axillary nerve and posterior circumflex humeral artery

Subscapularis muscle

Subscapular artery

**Quadrangular space**

Lower subscapular nerve (to teres major muscle)

Radial nerve

Biceps brachii muscle { Long head / Short head

Circumflex scapular artery

Thoracodorsal artery and nerve (to latissimus dorsi muscle)

Coracobrachialis muscle

Subscapularis muscle

**Triangular space**

Teres major muscle

Latissimus dorsi muscle

Suprascapular artery and nerve

**Posterior view**

Acromion

Superior transverse scapular ligament and suprascapular notch

Infraspinatus tendon (reflected)

Joint capsule of shoulder

Supraspinatus muscle (cut)

Deltoid muscle (reflected)

Teres minor muscle

Spine of scapula

**Quadrangular space** transmitting axillary nerve and posterior circumflex humeral artery

Infraspinatus muscle (cut)

Superior lateral brachial cutaneous nerve

**Triangular space** with circumflex scapular artery deep to space

Profunda brachii (deep brachial) artery } **In triangular interval**

Radial nerve

Teres major muscle

Lateral head and Long head of triceps brachii muscle

**Plate 413**

**Shoulder and Axilla**

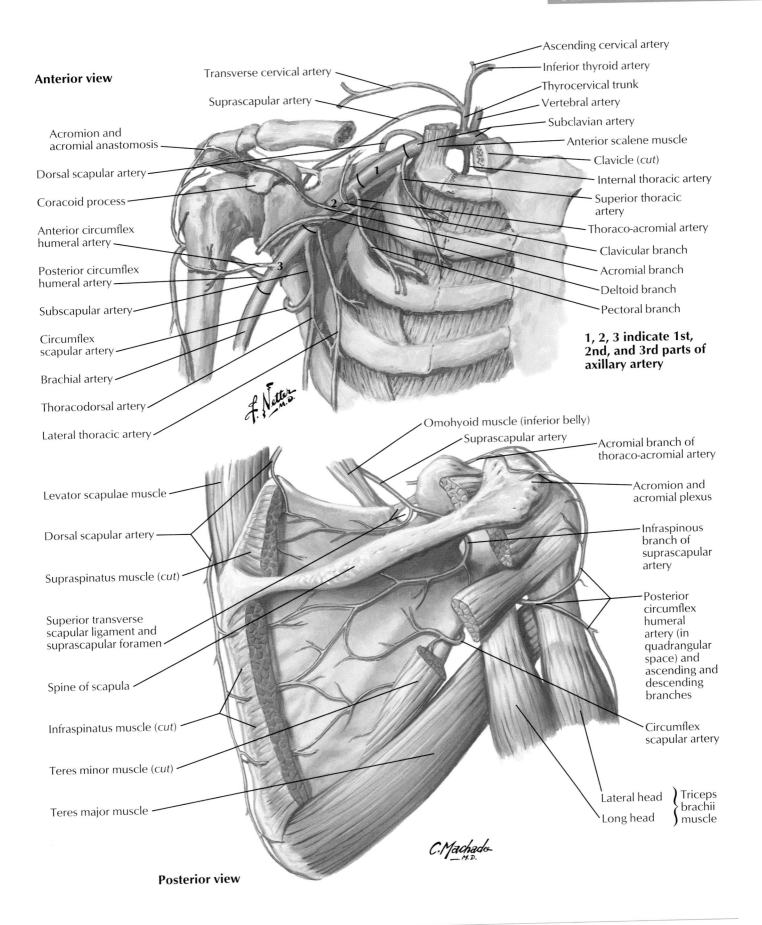

**Anterior view**

Transverse cervical artery
Suprascapular artery

Ascending cervical artery
Inferior thyroid artery
Thyrocervical trunk
Vertebral artery
Subclavian artery
Anterior scalene muscle
Clavicle (*cut*)
Internal thoracic artery
Superior thoracic artery
Thoraco-acromial artery
Clavicular branch
Acromial branch
Deltoid branch
Pectoral branch

Acromion and acromial anastomosis
Dorsal scapular artery
Coracoid process
Anterior circumflex humeral artery
Posterior circumflex humeral artery
Subscapular artery
Circumflex scapular artery
Brachial artery
Thoracodorsal artery
Lateral thoracic artery

**1, 2, 3 indicate 1st, 2nd, and 3rd parts of axillary artery**

*F. Netter M.D.*

Omohyoid muscle (inferior belly)
Suprascapular artery
Acromial branch of thoraco-acromial artery
Acromion and acromial plexus

Levator scapulae muscle

Dorsal scapular artery

Supraspinatus muscle (*cut*)

Superior transverse scapular ligament and suprascapular foramen

Spine of scapula

Infraspinatus muscle (*cut*)

Teres minor muscle (*cut*)

Teres major muscle

Infraspinous branch of suprascapular artery

Posterior circumflex humeral artery (in quadrangular space) and ascending and descending branches

Circumflex scapular artery

Lateral head ⎫ Triceps
Long head ⎬ brachii
⎭ muscle

*C. Machado M.D.*

**Posterior view**

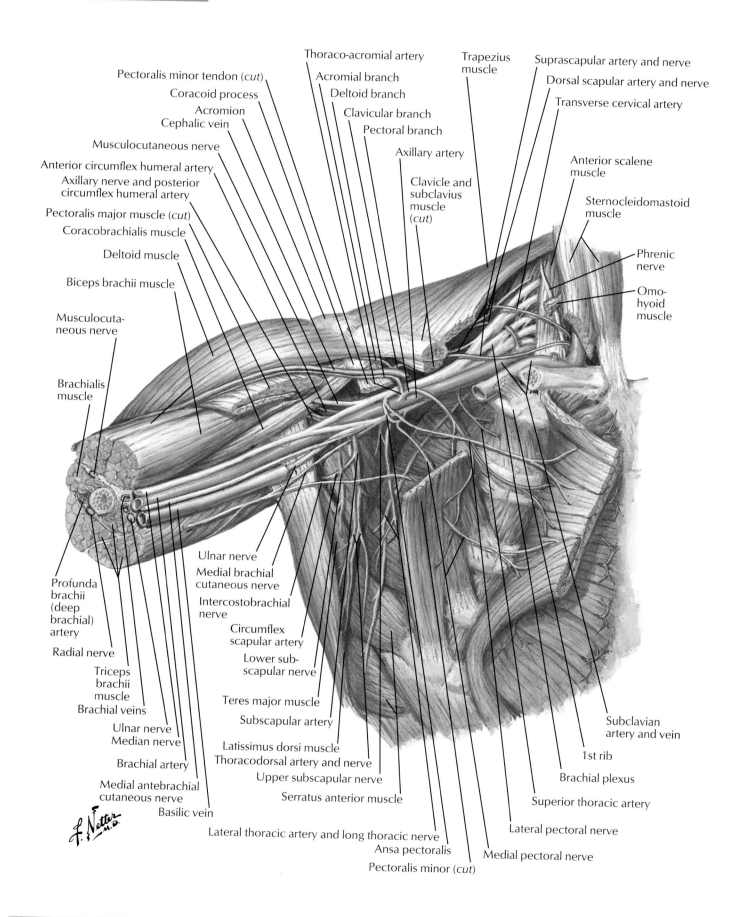

Pectoralis minor tendon (*cut*)
Coracoid process
Acromion
Cephalic vein
Musculocutaneous nerve
Anterior circumflex humeral artery
Axillary nerve and posterior circumflex humeral artery
Pectoralis major muscle (*cut*)
Coracobrachialis muscle
Deltoid muscle
Biceps brachii muscle
Musculocutaneous nerve
Brachialis muscle
Profunda brachii (deep brachial) artery
Radial nerve
Triceps brachii muscle
Brachial veins
Ulnar nerve
Median nerve
Brachial artery
Medial antebrachial cutaneous nerve
Basilic vein

Thoraco-acromial artery
Acromial branch
Deltoid branch
Clavicular branch
Pectoral branch
Axillary artery
Clavicle and subclavius muscle (*cut*)

Trapezius muscle
Suprascapular artery and nerve
Dorsal scapular artery and nerve
Transverse cervical artery
Anterior scalene muscle
Sternocleidomastoid muscle
Phrenic nerve
Omo-hyoid muscle

Ulnar nerve
Medial brachial cutaneous nerve
Intercostobrachial nerve
Circumflex scapular artery
Lower sub-scapular nerve
Teres major muscle
Subscapular artery
Latissimus dorsi muscle
Thoracodorsal artery and nerve
Upper subscapular nerve
Serratus anterior muscle
Lateral thoracic artery and long thoracic nerve
Ansa pectoralis
Pectoralis minor (*cut*)

Subclavian artery and vein
1st rib
Brachial plexus
Superior thoracic artery
Lateral pectoral nerve
Medial pectoral nerve

**Plate 415**

**Shoulder and Axilla**

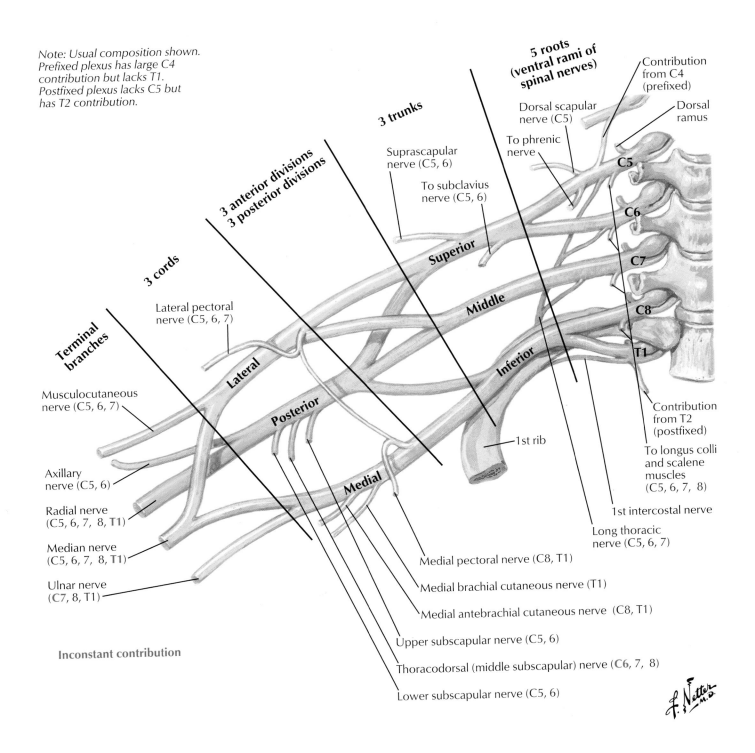

Note: Usual composition shown. *Prefixed plexus has large C4 contribution but lacks T1. Postfixed plexus lacks C5 but has T2 contribution.*

**5 roots (ventral rami of spinal nerves)**

Contribution from C4 (prefixed)

Dorsal ramus

Dorsal scapular nerve (C5)

To phrenic nerve

**3 trunks**

Suprascapular nerve (C5, 6)

To subclavius nerve (C5, 6)

C5

C6

C7

C8

T1

**3 anterior divisions**
**3 posterior divisions**

**Superior**

**Middle**

**Inferior**

**3 cords**

Lateral pectoral nerve (C5, 6, 7)

**Lateral**

**Posterior**

**Terminal branches**

Musculocutaneous nerve (C5, 6, 7)

Axillary nerve (C5, 6)

Radial nerve (C5, 6, 7, 8, **T1**)

Median nerve (C5, 6, 7, 8, **T1**)

Ulnar nerve (**C7**, 8, T1)

**Medial**

1st rib

Contribution from T2 (postfixed)

To longus colli and scalene muscles (C5, 6, 7, 8)

1st intercostal nerve

Long thoracic nerve (C5, 6, 7)

Medial pectoral nerve (C8, T1)

Medial brachial cutaneous nerve (T1)

Medial antebrachial cutaneous nerve (C8, T1)

Upper subscapular nerve (C5, 6)

Inconstant contribution

Thoracodorsal (middle subscapular) nerve (**C6**, 7, 8)

Lower subscapular nerve (C5, 6)

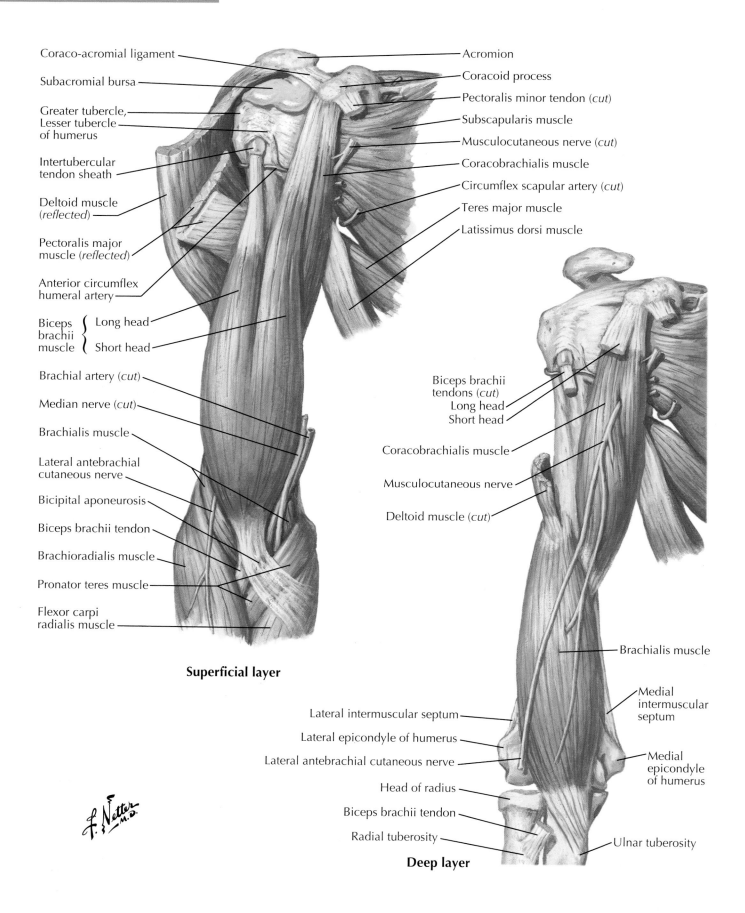

Coraco-acromial ligament

Subacromial bursa

Greater tubercle,
Lesser tubercle
of humerus

Intertubercular
tendon sheath

Deltoid muscle
(reflected)

Pectoralis major
muscle (reflected)

Anterior circumflex
humeral artery

Biceps brachii muscle { Long head / Short head }

Brachial artery (cut)

Median nerve (cut)

Brachialis muscle

Lateral antebrachial
cutaneous nerve

Bicipital aponeurosis

Biceps brachii tendon

Brachioradialis muscle

Pronator teres muscle

Flexor carpi
radialis muscle

Acromion

Coracoid process

Pectoralis minor tendon (cut)

Subscapularis muscle

Musculocutaneous nerve (cut)

Coracobrachialis muscle

Circumflex scapular artery (cut)

Teres major muscle

Latissimus dorsi muscle

**Superficial layer**

Biceps brachii
tendons (cut)
Long head
Short head

Coracobrachialis muscle

Musculocutaneous nerve

Deltoid muscle (cut)

Brachialis muscle

Medial
intermuscular
septum

Lateral intermuscular septum

Lateral epicondyle of humerus

Lateral antebrachial cutaneous nerve

Head of radius

Biceps brachii tendon

Radial tuberosity

Medial
epicondyle
of humerus

Ulnar tuberosity

**Deep layer**

**Plate 417**

**Arm**

**Superficial layer**

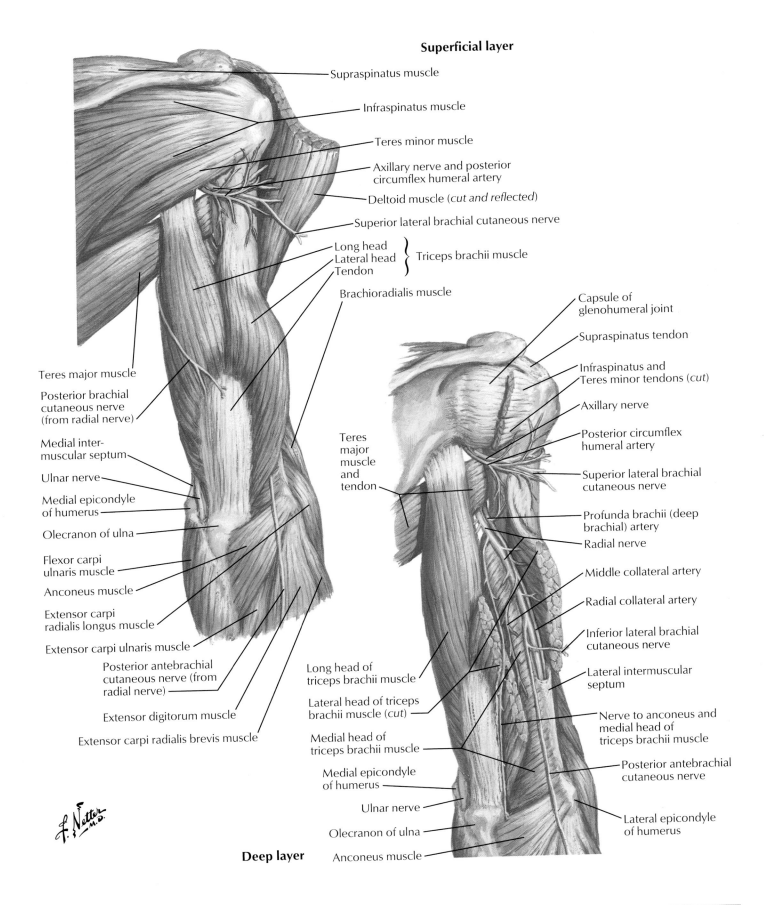

Supraspinatus muscle

Infraspinatus muscle

Teres minor muscle

Axillary nerve and posterior
circumflex humeral artery

Deltoid muscle (*cut and reflected*)

Superior lateral brachial cutaneous nerve

Long head
Lateral head  } Triceps brachii muscle
Tendon

Brachioradialis muscle

Capsule of
glenohumeral joint

Supraspinatus tendon

Infraspinatus and
Teres minor tendons (*cut*)

Axillary nerve

Posterior circumflex
humeral artery

Superior lateral brachial
cutaneous nerve

Profunda brachii (deep
brachial) artery

Radial nerve

Middle collateral artery

Radial collateral artery

Inferior lateral brachial
cutaneous nerve

Lateral intermuscular
septum

Nerve to anconeus and
medial head of
triceps brachii muscle

Posterior antebrachial
cutaneous nerve

Lateral epicondyle
of humerus

Teres major muscle

Posterior brachial
cutaneous nerve
(from radial nerve)

Medial inter-
muscular septum

Ulnar nerve

Medial epicondyle
of humerus

Olecranon of ulna

Flexor carpi
ulnaris muscle

Anconeus muscle

Extensor carpi
radialis longus muscle

Extensor carpi ulnaris muscle

Posterior antebrachial
cutaneous nerve (from
radial nerve)

Extensor digitorum muscle

Extensor carpi radialis brevis muscle

Teres
major
muscle
and
tendon

Long head of
triceps brachii muscle

Lateral head of triceps
brachii muscle (*cut*)

Medial head of
triceps brachii muscle

Medial epicondyle
of humerus

Ulnar nerve

Olecranon of ulna

**Deep layer**   Anconeus muscle

**Plate 418**

**Arm**

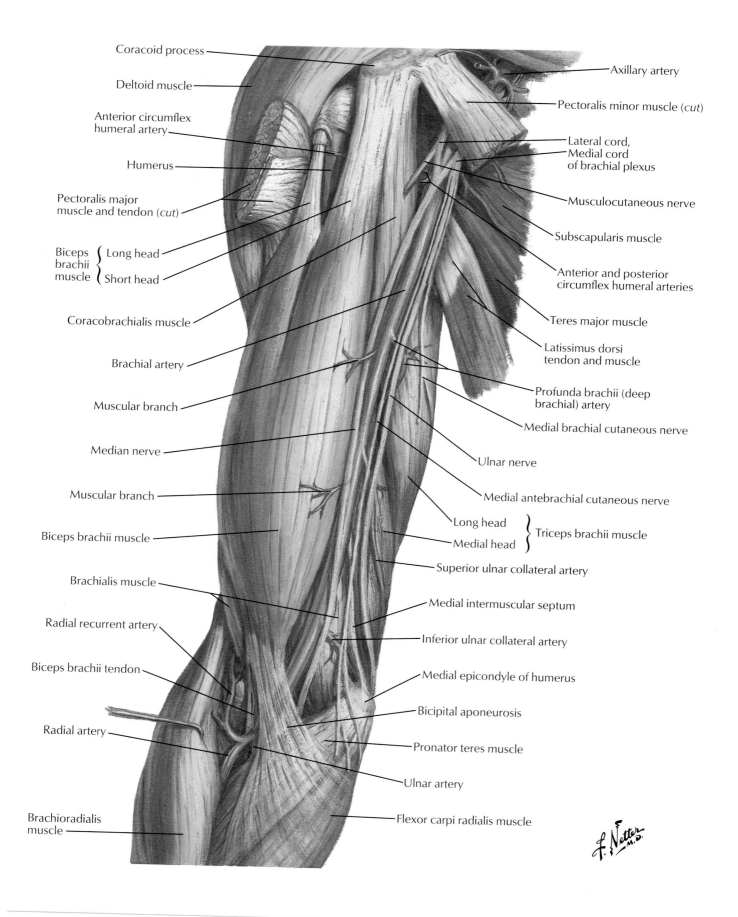

Coracoid process

Deltoid muscle

Anterior circumflex
humeral artery

Humerus

Pectoralis major
muscle and tendon (cut)

Biceps
brachii
muscle { Long head

{ Short head

Coracobrachialis muscle

Brachial artery

Muscular branch

Median nerve

Muscular branch

Biceps brachii muscle

Brachialis muscle

Radial recurrent artery

Biceps brachii tendon

Radial artery

Brachioradialis
muscle

Axillary artery

Pectoralis minor muscle (cut)

Lateral cord,
Medial cord
of brachial plexus

Musculocutaneous nerve

Subscapularis muscle

Anterior and posterior
circumflex humeral arteries

Teres major muscle

Latissimus dorsi
tendon and muscle

Profunda brachii (deep
brachial) artery

Medial brachial cutaneous nerve

Ulnar nerve

Medial antebrachial cutaneous nerve

Long head
Medial head } Triceps brachii muscle

Superior ulnar collateral artery

Medial intermuscular septum

Inferior ulnar collateral artery

Medial epicondyle of humerus

Bicipital aponeurosis

Pronator teres muscle

Ulnar artery

Flexor carpi radialis muscle

**Plate 419**

**Arm**

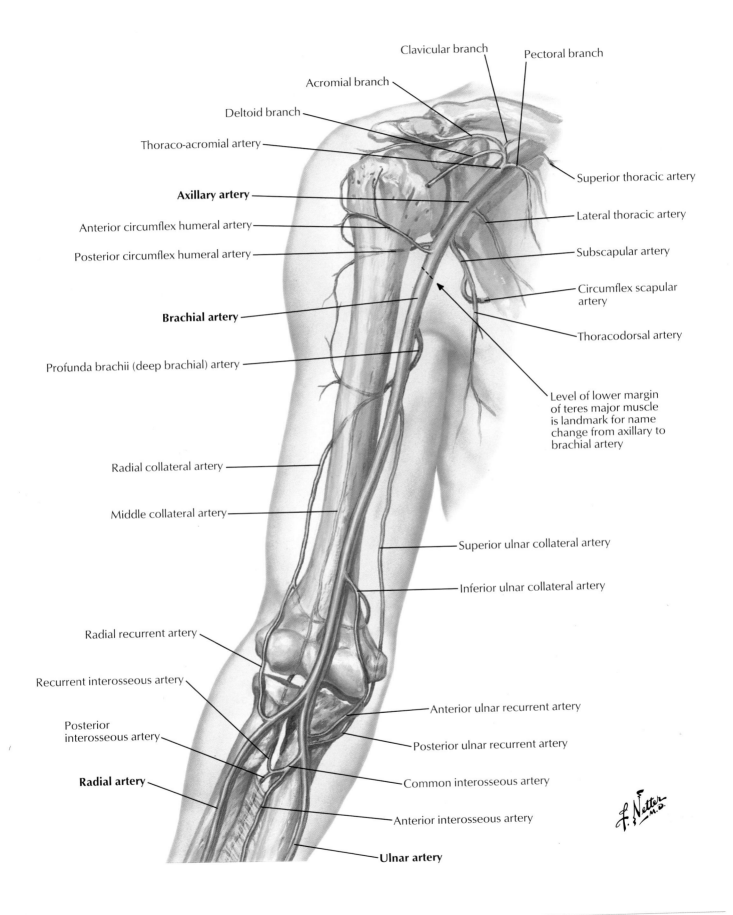

Clavicular branch

Pectoral branch

Acromial branch

Deltoid branch

Thoraco-acromial artery

**Axillary artery**

Anterior circumflex humeral artery

Posterior circumflex humeral artery

**Brachial artery**

Profunda brachii (deep brachial) artery

Radial collateral artery

Middle collateral artery

Radial recurrent artery

Recurrent interosseous artery

Posterior interosseous artery

**Radial artery**

Superior thoracic artery

Lateral thoracic artery

Subscapular artery

Circumflex scapular artery

Thoracodorsal artery

Level of lower margin of teres major muscle is landmark for name change from axillary to brachial artery

Superior ulnar collateral artery

Inferior ulnar collateral artery

Anterior ulnar recurrent artery

Posterior ulnar recurrent artery

Common interosseous artery

Anterior interosseous artery

**Ulnar artery**

*f. Netter*

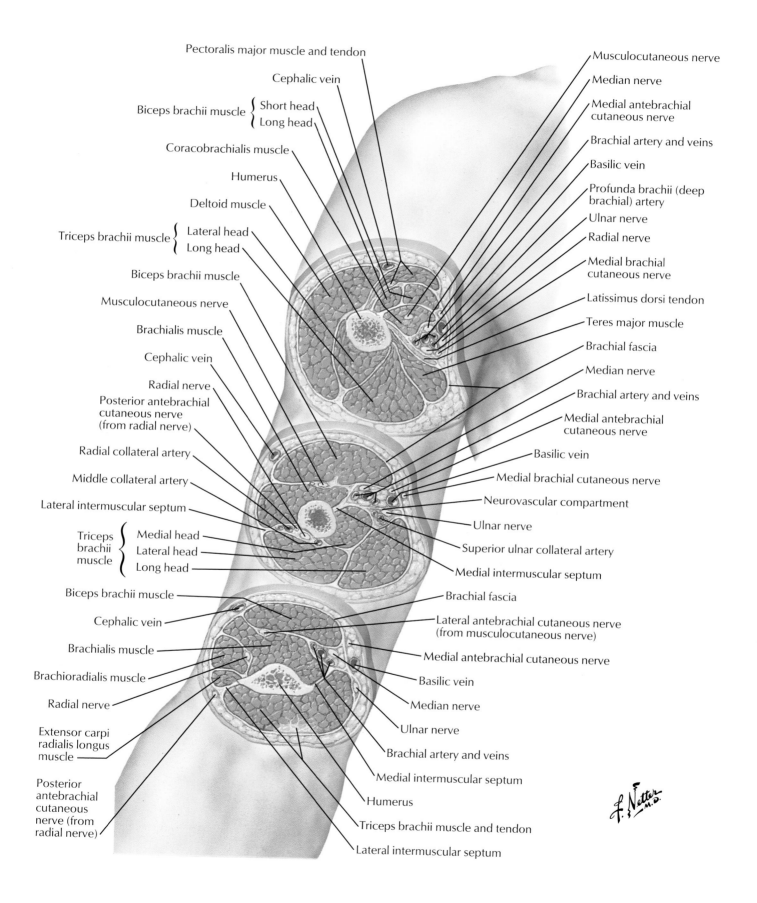

Pectoralis major muscle and tendon

Cephalic vein

Biceps brachii muscle { Short head
Long head

Coracobrachialis muscle

Humerus

Deltoid muscle

Triceps brachii muscle { Lateral head
Long head

Biceps brachii muscle

Musculocutaneous nerve

Brachialis muscle

Cephalic vein

Radial nerve

Posterior antebrachial cutaneous nerve (from radial nerve)

Radial collateral artery

Middle collateral artery

Lateral intermuscular septum

Triceps brachii muscle { Medial head
Lateral head
Long head

Biceps brachii muscle

Cephalic vein

Brachialis muscle

Brachioradialis muscle

Radial nerve

Extensor carpi radialis longus muscle

Posterior antebrachial cutaneous nerve (from radial nerve)

Musculocutaneous nerve

Median nerve

Medial antebrachial cutaneous nerve

Brachial artery and veins

Basilic vein

Profunda brachii (deep brachial) artery

Ulnar nerve

Radial nerve

Medial brachial cutaneous nerve

Latissimus dorsi tendon

Teres major muscle

Brachial fascia

Median nerve

Brachial artery and veins

Medial antebrachial cutaneous nerve

Basilic vein

Medial brachial cutaneous nerve

Neurovascular compartment

Ulnar nerve

Superior ulnar collateral artery

Medial intermuscular septum

Brachial fascia

Lateral antebrachial cutaneous nerve (from musculocutaneous nerve)

Medial antebrachial cutaneous nerve

Basilic vein

Median nerve

Ulnar nerve

Brachial artery and veins

Medial intermuscular septum

Humerus

Triceps brachii muscle and tendon

Lateral intermuscular septum

**Plate 421**

**Arm**

**Right elbow**

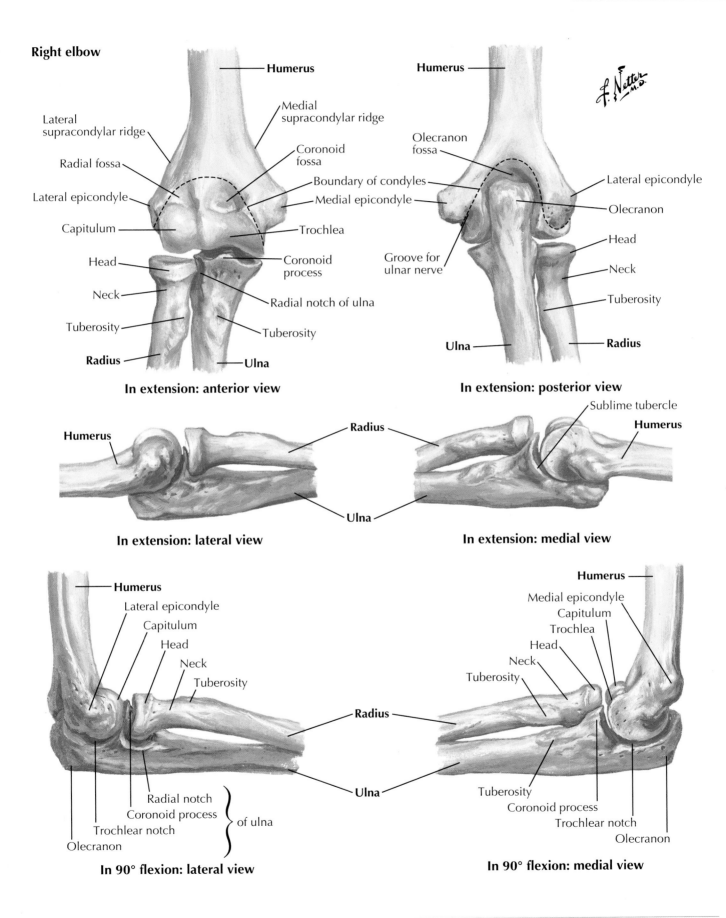

Humerus

Lateral
supracondylar ridge

Medial
supracondylar ridge

Radial fossa

Coronoid
fossa

Lateral epicondyle

Boundary of condyles

Medial epicondyle

Capitulum

Trochlea

Head

Coronoid
process

Neck

Radial notch of ulna

Tuberosity

Tuberosity

**Radius**

**Ulna**

**In extension: anterior view**

Humerus

Olecranon
fossa

Lateral epicondyle

Olecranon

Groove for
ulnar nerve

Head

Neck

Tuberosity

**Ulna**

**Radius**

**In extension: posterior view**

**Humerus**

**Radius**

Sublime tubercle

**Humerus**

**Ulna**

**In extension: lateral view**

**Ulna**

**In extension: medial view**

Humerus

Lateral epicondyle

Capitulum

Head

Neck

Tuberosity

**Radius**

Radial notch
Coronoid process } of ulna
Trochlear notch

Olecranon

**In 90° flexion: lateral view**

Humerus

Medial epicondyle

Capitulum

Trochlea

Head

Neck

Tuberosity

**Radius**

**Ulna**

Tuberosity

Coronoid process

Trochlear notch

Olecranon

**In 90° flexion: medial view**

### Anteroposterior radiograph

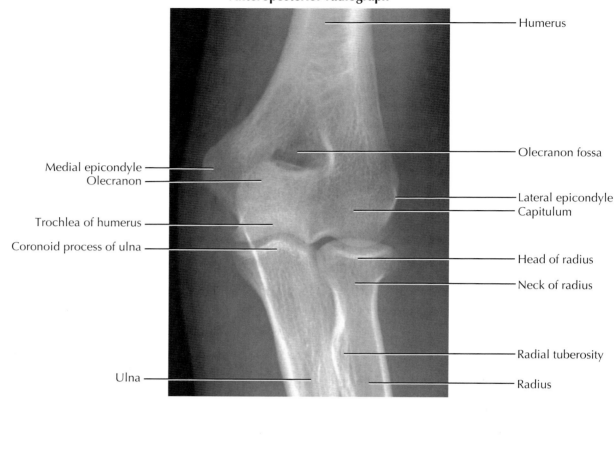

Humerus

Olecranon fossa

Medial epicondyle

Olecranon

Lateral epicondyle

Capitulum

Trochlea of humerus

Coronoid process of ulna

Head of radius

Neck of radius

Radial tuberosity

Ulna

Radius

### Lateral radiograph

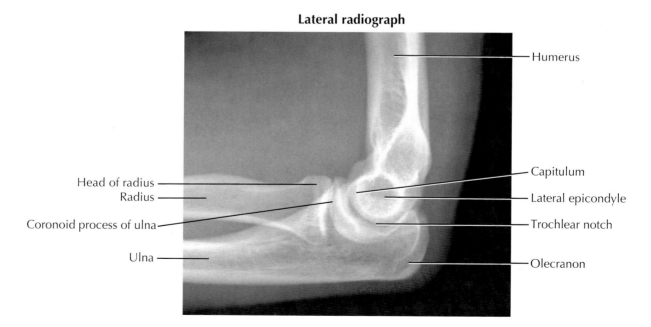

Humerus

Head of radius

Radius

Capitulum

Lateral epicondyle

Coronoid process of ulna

Trochlear notch

Ulna

Olecranon

**Plate 423**

**Elbow and Forearm**

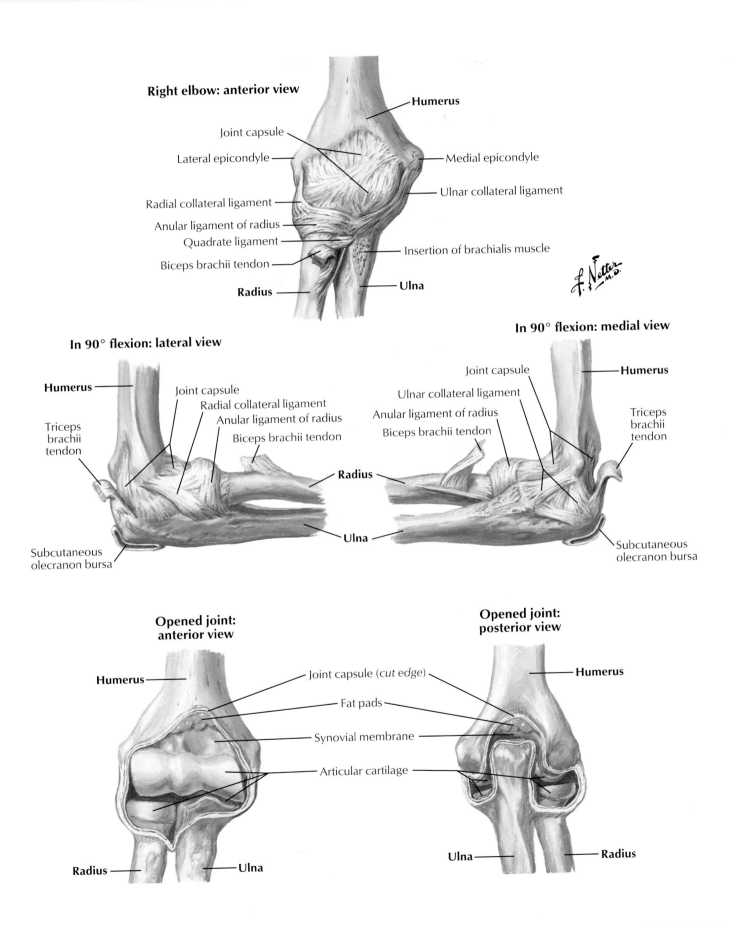

**Right elbow: anterior view**

Joint capsule

Lateral epicondyle

Radial collateral ligament

Anular ligament of radius

Quadrate ligament

Biceps brachii tendon

**Radius**

Humerus

Medial epicondyle

Ulnar collateral ligament

Insertion of brachialis muscle

**Ulna**

**In 90° flexion: lateral view**

**Humerus**

Triceps
brachii
tendon

Joint capsule

Radial collateral ligament

Anular ligament of radius

Biceps brachii tendon

**Radius**

Subcutaneous
olecranon bursa

**Ulna**

**In 90° flexion: medial view**

Joint capsule

Ulnar collateral ligament

Anular ligament of radius

Biceps brachii tendon

**Humerus**

Triceps
brachii
tendon

Subcutaneous
olecranon bursa

**Opened joint:
anterior view**

**Humerus**

Joint capsule (*cut edge*)

Fat pads

Synovial membrane

Articular cartilage

**Radius**

**Ulna**

**Opened joint:
posterior view**

**Humerus**

**Ulna**

**Radius**

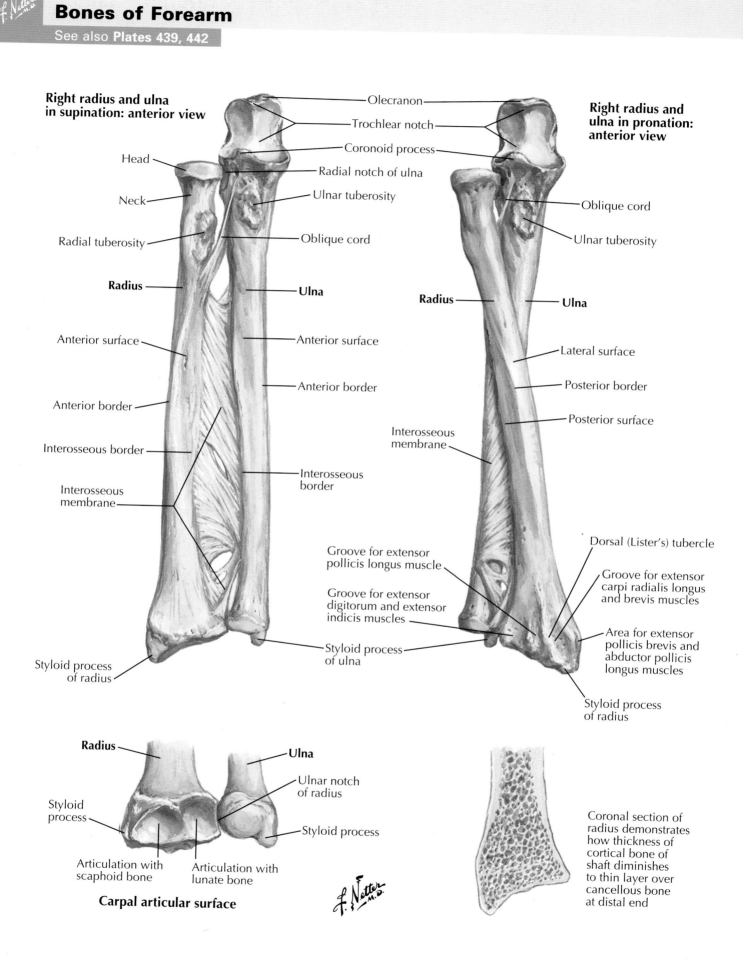

**Right radius and ulna in supination: anterior view**

Olecranon

Trochlear notch

Coronoid process

Head

Radial notch of ulna

Neck

Ulnar tuberosity

Radial tuberosity

Oblique cord

**Radius**

**Ulna**

Anterior surface

Anterior surface

Anterior border

Anterior border

Interosseous border

Interosseous border

Interosseous membrane

Interosseous border

**Right radius and ulna in pronation: anterior view**

Oblique cord

Ulnar tuberosity

**Radius**

**Ulna**

Lateral surface

Posterior border

Posterior surface

Interosseous membrane

Dorsal (Lister's) tubercle

Groove for extensor pollicis longus muscle

Groove for extensor carpi radialis longus and brevis muscles

Groove for extensor digitorum and extensor indicis muscles

Area for extensor pollicis brevis and abductor pollicis longus muscles

Styloid process of ulna

Styloid process of radius

Styloid process of radius

**Radius**

**Ulna**

Styloid process

Ulnar notch of radius

Styloid process

Articulation with scaphoid bone

Articulation with lunate bone

**Carpal articular surface**

Coronal section of radius demonstrates how thickness of cortical bone of shaft diminishes to thin layer over cancellous bone at distal end

**Plate 425**

**Elbow and Forearm**

**Right forearm: anterior view**

Supinated position

Pronated position

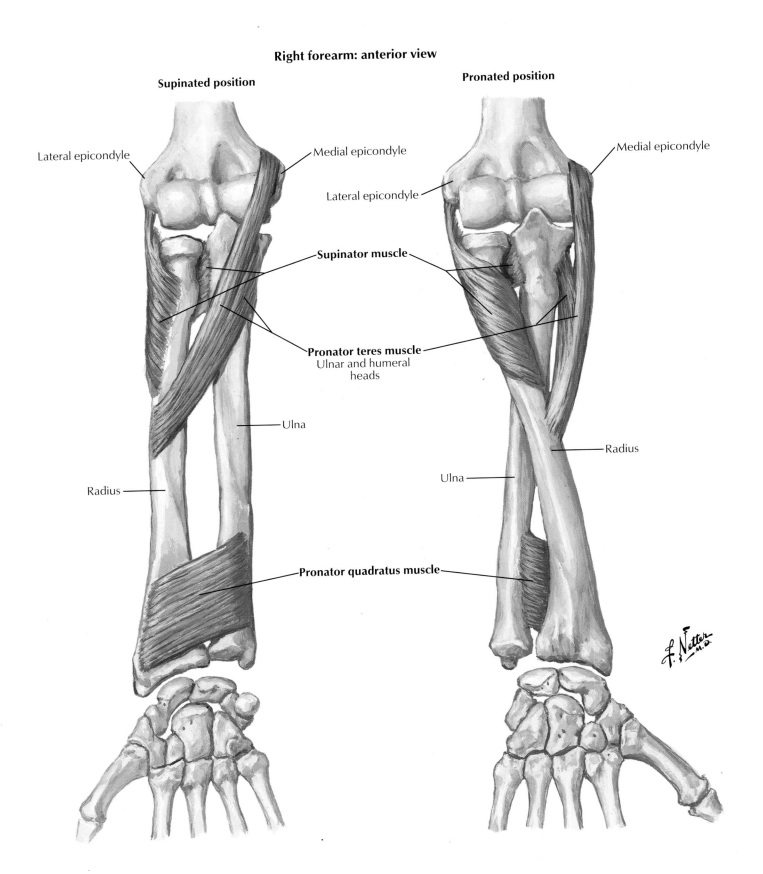

Lateral epicondyle

Medial epicondyle

Medial epicondyle

Lateral epicondyle

**Supinator muscle**

**Pronator teres muscle**
Ulnar and humeral
heads

Ulna

Radius

Ulna

Radius

**Pronator quadratus muscle**

# Individual Muscles of Forearm: Extensors of Wrist and Digits

See also **Plate 438**

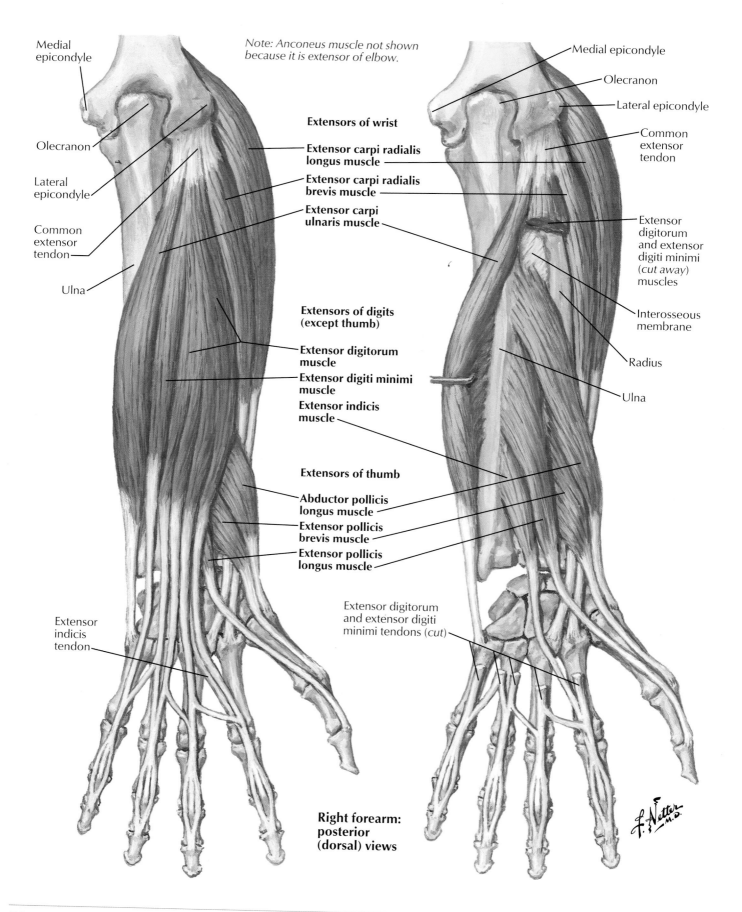

Medial epicondyle

Olecranon

Lateral epicondyle

Common extensor tendon

Ulna

*Note: Anconeus muscle not shown because it is extensor of elbow.*

Extensor indicis tendon

**Extensors of wrist**

**Extensor carpi radialis longus muscle**

**Extensor carpi radialis brevis muscle**

**Extensor carpi ulnaris muscle**

**Extensors of digits (except thumb)**

**Extensor digitorum muscle**

**Extensor digiti minimi muscle**

**Extensor indicis muscle**

**Extensors of thumb**

**Abductor pollicis longus muscle**

**Extensor pollicis brevis muscle**

**Extensor pollicis longus muscle**

Medial epicondyle

Olecranon

Lateral epicondyle

Common extensor tendon

Extensor digitorum and extensor digiti minimi (*cut away*) muscles

Interosseous membrane

Radius

Ulna

Extensor digitorum and extensor digiti minimi tendons (*cut*)

**Right forearm: posterior (dorsal) views**

**Plate 427**

**Elbow and Forearm**

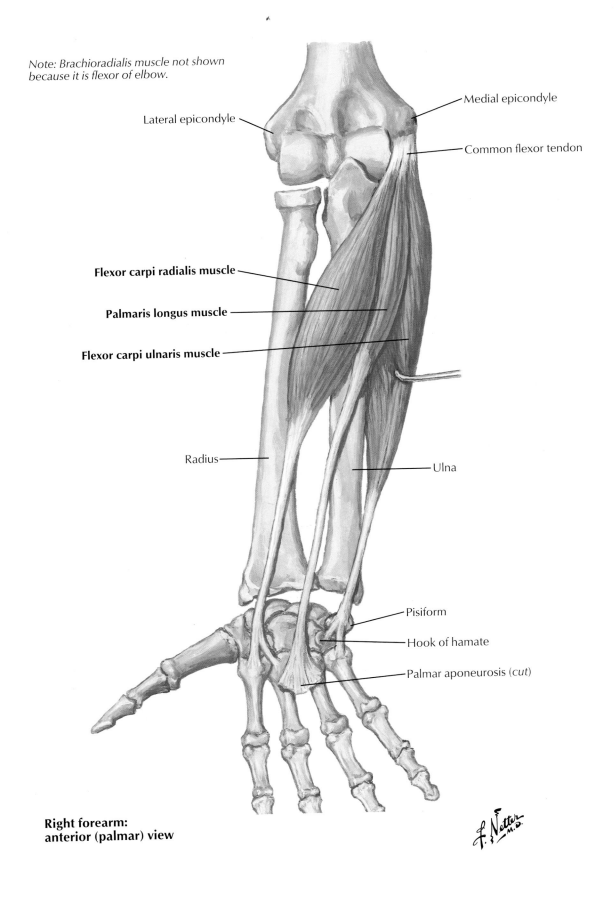

Note: Brachioradialis muscle not shown because it is flexor of elbow.

Lateral epicondyle

Medial epicondyle

Common flexor tendon

**Flexor carpi radialis muscle**

**Palmaris longus muscle**

**Flexor carpi ulnaris muscle**

Radius

Ulna

Pisiform

Hook of hamate

Palmar aponeurosis (cut)

**Right forearm:
anterior (palmar) view**

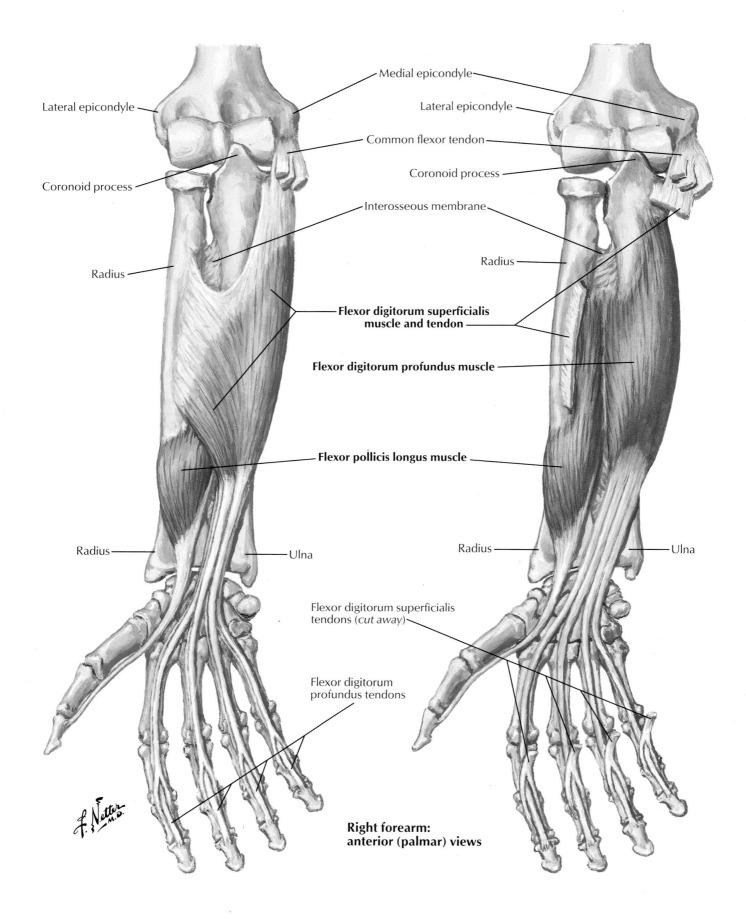

Lateral epicondyle

Coronoid process

Radius

Radius

Medial epicondyle

Lateral epicondyle

Common flexor tendon

Coronoid process

Interosseous membrane

Radius

**Flexor digitorum superficialis muscle and tendon**

**Flexor digitorum profundus muscle**

**Flexor pollicis longus muscle**

Radius

Ulna

Flexor digitorum superficialis tendons (*cut away*)

Flexor digitorum profundus tendons

Ulna

**Right forearm: anterior (palmar) views**

**Plate 429**

**Elbow and Forearm**

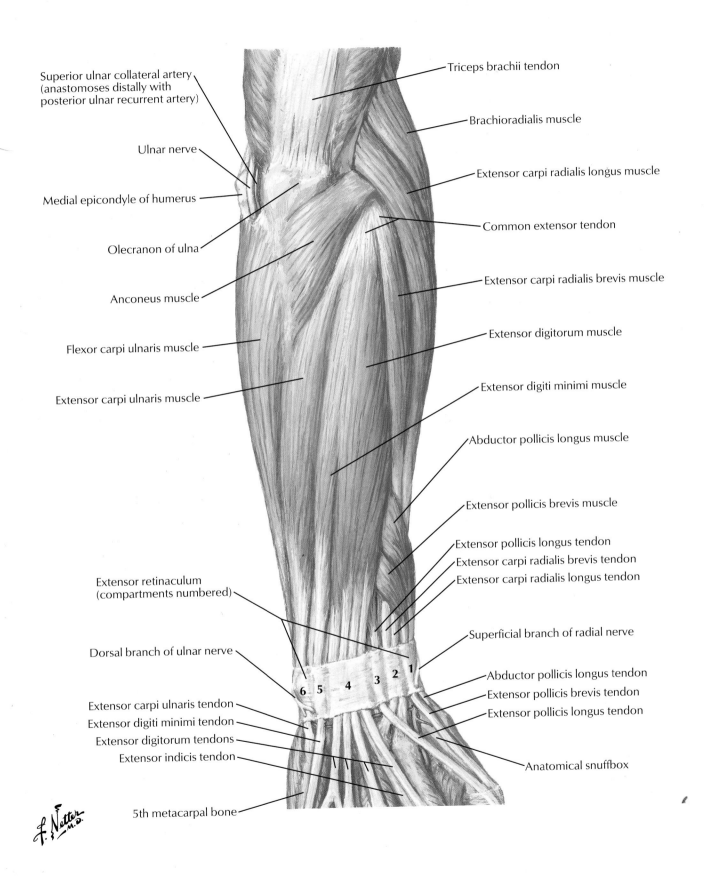

Superior ulnar collateral artery (anastomoses distally with posterior ulnar recurrent artery)

Ulnar nerve

Medial epicondyle of humerus

Olecranon of ulna

Anconeus muscle

Flexor carpi ulnaris muscle

Extensor carpi ulnaris muscle

Extensor retinaculum (compartments numbered)

Dorsal branch of ulnar nerve

Extensor carpi ulnaris tendon
Extensor digiti minimi tendon
Extensor digitorum tendons
Extensor indicis tendon

5th metacarpal bone

Triceps brachii tendon

Brachioradialis muscle

Extensor carpi radialis longus muscle

Common extensor tendon

Extensor carpi radialis brevis muscle

Extensor digitorum muscle

Extensor digiti minimi muscle

Abductor pollicis longus muscle

Extensor pollicis brevis muscle

Extensor pollicis longus tendon
Extensor carpi radialis brevis tendon
Extensor carpi radialis longus tendon

Superficial branch of radial nerve

Abductor pollicis longus tendon
Extensor pollicis brevis tendon
Extensor pollicis longus tendon

Anatomical snuffbox

6 5 4 3 2 1

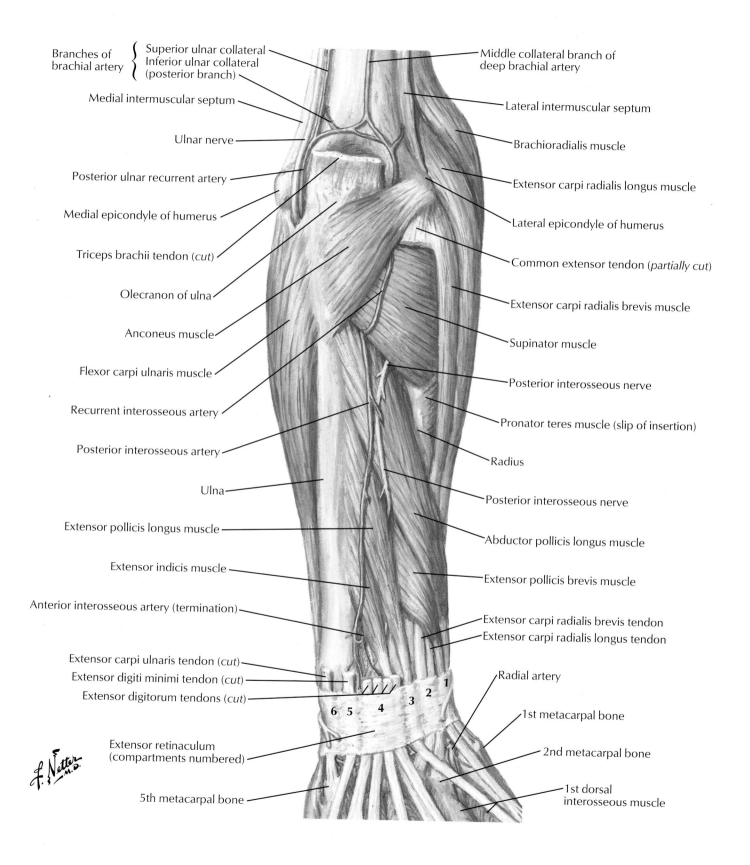

Branches of brachial artery
- Superior ulnar collateral
- Inferior ulnar collateral (posterior branch)

Middle collateral branch of deep brachial artery

Medial intermuscular septum

Lateral intermuscular septum

Ulnar nerve

Brachioradialis muscle

Posterior ulnar recurrent artery

Extensor carpi radialis longus muscle

Medial epicondyle of humerus

Lateral epicondyle of humerus

Triceps brachii tendon (cut)

Common extensor tendon (partially cut)

Olecranon of ulna

Extensor carpi radialis brevis muscle

Anconeus muscle

Supinator muscle

Flexor carpi ulnaris muscle

Posterior interosseous nerve

Recurrent interosseous artery

Pronator teres muscle (slip of insertion)

Posterior interosseous artery

Radius

Ulna

Posterior interosseous nerve

Extensor pollicis longus muscle

Abductor pollicis longus muscle

Extensor indicis muscle

Extensor pollicis brevis muscle

Anterior interosseous artery (termination)

Extensor carpi radialis brevis tendon
Extensor carpi radialis longus tendon

Extensor carpi ulnaris tendon (cut)
Extensor digiti minimi tendon (cut)
Extensor digitorum tendons (cut)

Radial artery

1st metacarpal bone

Extensor retinaculum (compartments numbered)

2nd metacarpal bone

5th metacarpal bone

1st dorsal interosseous muscle

**Plate 431**

**Elbow and Forearm**

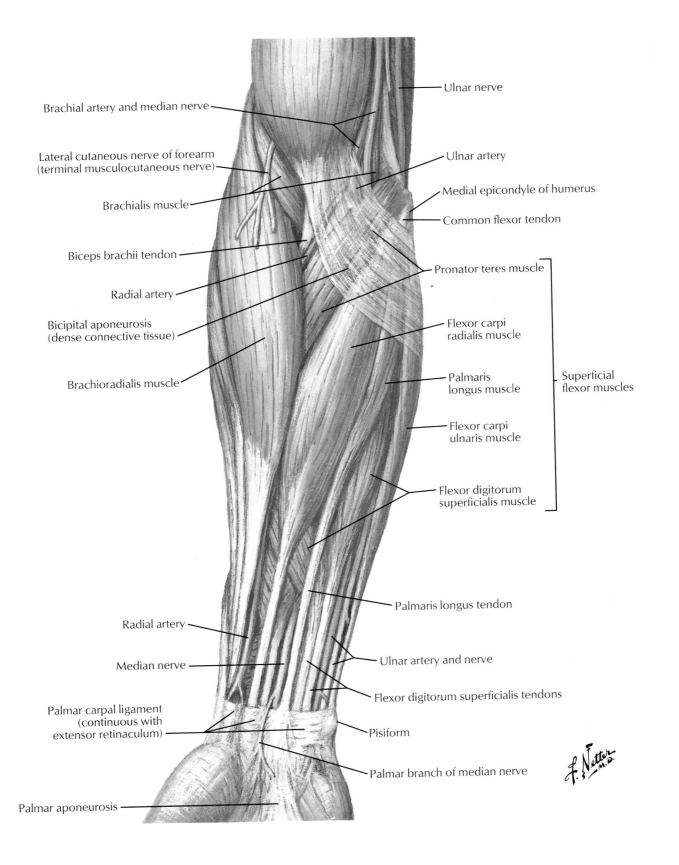

Ulnar nerve

Brachial artery and median nerve

Lateral cutaneous nerve of forearm
(terminal musculocutaneous nerve)

Ulnar artery

Medial epicondyle of humerus

Brachialis muscle

Common flexor tendon

Biceps brachii tendon

Pronator teres muscle

Radial artery

Flexor carpi
radialis muscle

Bicipital aponeurosis
(dense connective tissue)

Palmaris
longus muscle

Superficial
flexor muscles

Brachioradialis muscle

Flexor carpi
ulnaris muscle

Flexor digitorum
superficialis muscle

Palmaris longus tendon

Radial artery

Ulnar artery and nerve

Median nerve

Flexor digitorum superficialis tendons

Palmar carpal ligament
(continuous with
extensor retinaculum)

Pisiform

Palmar branch of median nerve

Palmar aponeurosis

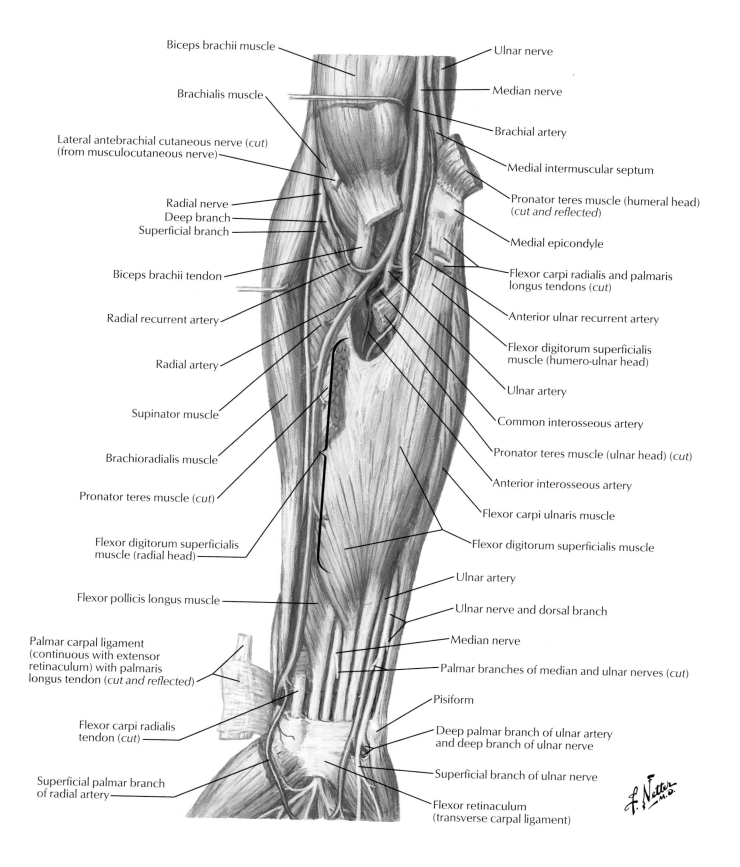

Biceps brachii muscle

Brachialis muscle

Lateral antebrachial cutaneous nerve (cut)
(from musculocutaneous nerve)

Radial nerve
Deep branch
Superficial branch

Biceps brachii tendon

Radial recurrent artery

Radial artery

Supinator muscle

Brachioradialis muscle

Pronator teres muscle (cut)

Flexor digitorum superficialis
muscle (radial head)

Flexor pollicis longus muscle

Palmar carpal ligament
(continuous with extensor
retinaculum) with palmaris
longus tendon (cut and reflected)

Flexor carpi radialis
tendon (cut)

Superficial palmar branch
of radial artery

Ulnar nerve

Median nerve

Brachial artery

Medial intermuscular septum

Pronator teres muscle (humeral head)
(cut and reflected)

Medial epicondyle

Flexor carpi radialis and palmaris
longus tendons (cut)

Anterior ulnar recurrent artery

Flexor digitorum superficialis
muscle (humero-ulnar head)

Ulnar artery

Common interosseous artery

Pronator teres muscle (ulnar head) (cut)

Anterior interosseous artery

Flexor carpi ulnaris muscle

Flexor digitorum superficialis muscle

Ulnar artery

Ulnar nerve and dorsal branch

Median nerve

Palmar branches of median and ulnar nerves (cut)

Pisiform

Deep palmar branch of ulnar artery
and deep branch of ulnar nerve

Superficial branch of ulnar nerve

Flexor retinaculum
(transverse carpal ligament)

**Plate 433**

**Elbow and Forearm**

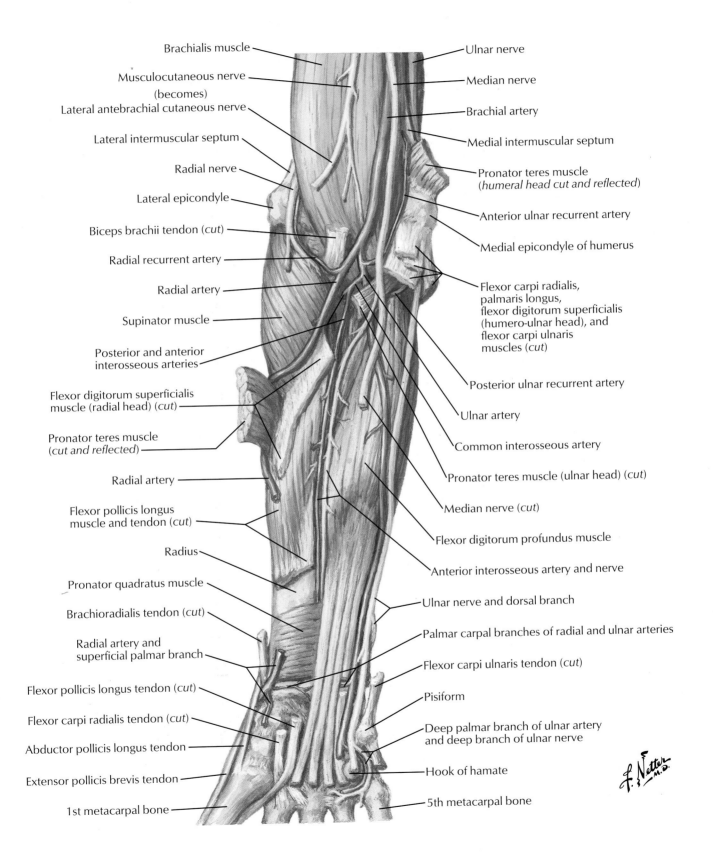

Brachialis muscle

Musculocutaneous nerve (becomes)

Lateral antebrachial cutaneous nerve

Lateral intermuscular septum

Radial nerve

Lateral epicondyle

Biceps brachii tendon (*cut*)

Radial recurrent artery

Radial artery

Supinator muscle

Posterior and anterior interosseous arteries

Flexor digitorum superficialis muscle (radial head) (*cut*)

Pronator teres muscle (*cut and reflected*)

Radial artery

Flexor pollicis longus muscle and tendon (*cut*)

Radius

Pronator quadratus muscle

Brachioradialis tendon (*cut*)

Radial artery and superficial palmar branch

Flexor pollicis longus tendon (*cut*)

Flexor carpi radialis tendon (*cut*)

Abductor pollicis longus tendon

Extensor pollicis brevis tendon

1st metacarpal bone

Ulnar nerve

Median nerve

Brachial artery

Medial intermuscular septum

Pronator teres muscle (*humeral head cut and reflected*)

Anterior ulnar recurrent artery

Medial epicondyle of humerus

Flexor carpi radialis, palmaris longus, flexor digitorum superficialis (humero-ulnar head), and flexor carpi ulnaris muscles (*cut*)

Posterior ulnar recurrent artery

Ulnar artery

Common interosseous artery

Pronator teres muscle (ulnar head) (*cut*)

Median nerve (*cut*)

Flexor digitorum profundus muscle

Anterior interosseous artery and nerve

Ulnar nerve and dorsal branch

Palmar carpal branches of radial and ulnar arteries

Flexor carpi ulnaris tendon (*cut*)

Pisiform

Deep palmar branch of ulnar artery and deep branch of ulnar nerve

Hook of hamate

5th metacarpal bone

*F. Netter M.D.*

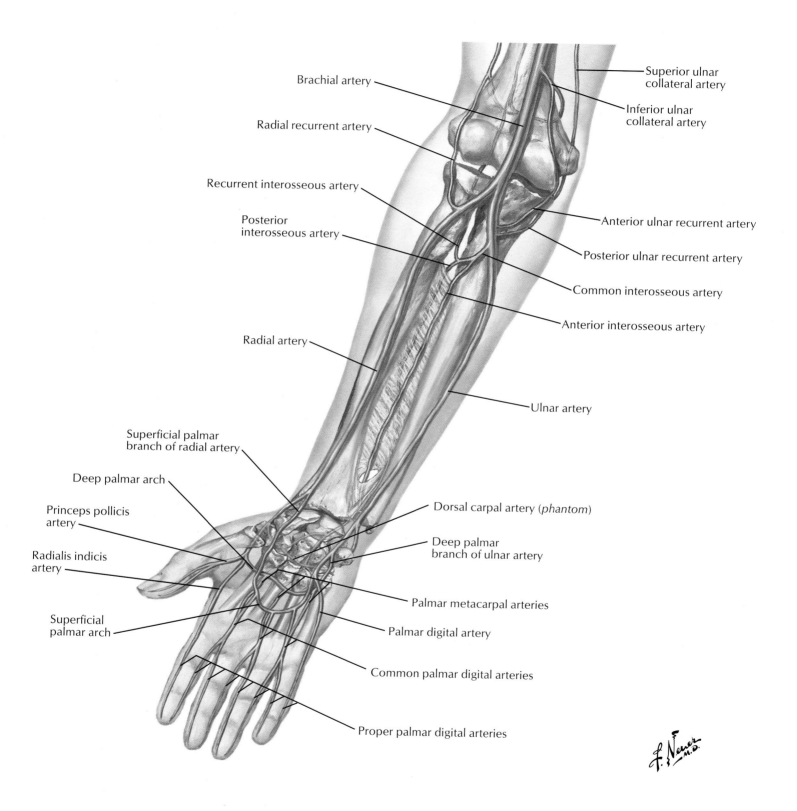

Brachial artery

Radial recurrent artery

Recurrent interosseous artery

Posterior interosseous artery

Radial artery

Superficial palmar branch of radial artery

Deep palmar arch

Princeps pollicis artery

Radialis indicis artery

Superficial palmar arch

Superior ulnar collateral artery

Inferior ulnar collateral artery

Anterior ulnar recurrent artery

Posterior ulnar recurrent artery

Common interosseous artery

Anterior interosseous artery

Ulnar artery

Dorsal carpal artery (*phantom*)

Deep palmar branch of ulnar artery

Palmar metacarpal arteries

Palmar digital artery

Common palmar digital arteries

Proper palmar digital arteries

**Plate 435**

**Elbow and Forearm**

Median antebrachial vein

Pronator teres muscle

Radial artery and superficial branch of radial nerve

Radius

Brachioradialis muscle

Cephalic vein and lateral antebrachial cutaneous nerve (from musculocutaneous nerve)

Supinator muscle

Deep branch of radial nerve

Extensor carpi radialis longus muscle

Extensor carpi radialis brevis muscle

Extensor digitorum muscle

Extensor digiti minimi muscle

Extensor carpi ulnaris muscle

Flexor carpi radialis muscle

Brachioradialis muscle

Radial artery and superficial branch of radial nerve

Flexor pollicis longus muscle

Extensor carpi radialis longus muscle and tendon

Extensor carpi radialis brevis muscle and tendon

Abductor pollicis longus muscle

Extensor digitorum muscle

Extensor digiti minimi muscle

Extensor carpi ulnaris muscle

Flexor carpi radialis tendon

Radial artery

Brachioradialis tendon

Abductor pollicis longus tendon

Superficial branch of radial nerve

Extensor pollicis brevis tendon

Extensor carpi radialis longus tendon

Extensor carpi radialis brevis tendon

Flexor pollicis longus muscle

Extensor pollicis longus tendon

Radius

Flexor digitorum superficialis muscle (radial head)

Anterior branch of medial antebrachial cutaneous nerve

Flexor pollicis longus muscle

Interosseous membrane

Flexor carpi radialis muscle

Ulnar artery and median nerve

Palmaris longus muscle

Flexor digitorum superficialis muscle (humero-ulnar head)

Common interosseous artery

Ulnar nerve

Flexor carpi ulnaris muscle

Basilic vein

Flexor digitorum profundus muscle

Ulna and antebrachial fascia

Anconeus muscle

Posterior antebrachial cutaneous nerve (from radial nerve)

Palmaris longus muscle

Flexor digitorum superficialis muscle

Median nerve

Ulnar artery and nerve

Flexor carpi ulnaris muscle

Anterior interosseous artery and nerve (from median nerve)

Flexor digitorum profundus muscle

Interosseous membrane and extensor pollicis longus muscle

Posterior interosseous artery and nerve (continuation of deep branch of radial nerve)

Palmaris longus tendon

Median nerve

Flexor digitorum superficialis muscle and tendons

Flexor carpi ulnaris muscle and tendon

Ulnar artery and nerve

Dorsal branch of ulnar nerve

Flexor digitorum profundus muscle and tendons

Ulna

Extensor carpi ulnaris tendon

Pronator quadratus muscle and interosseous membrane

Extensor indicis muscle and tendon

Extensor digiti minimi tendon

Extensor digitorum tendons (common tendon to digits 4 and 5 at this level)

*F. Netter, M.D.*

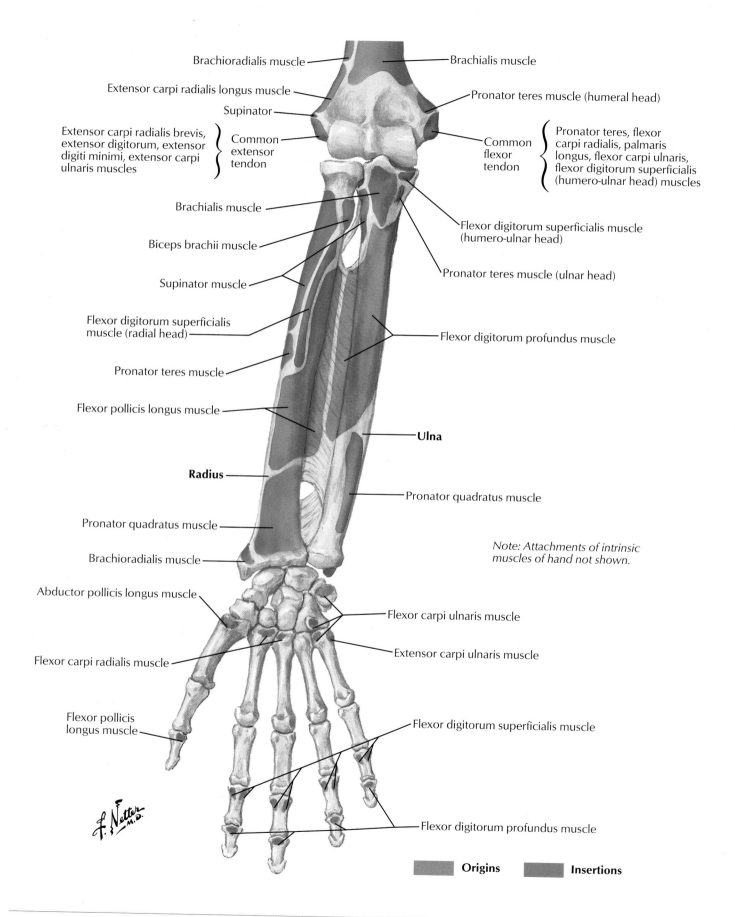

Brachioradialis muscle — Brachialis muscle

Extensor carpi radialis longus muscle — Pronator teres muscle (humeral head)

Supinator

Extensor carpi radialis brevis, extensor digitorum, extensor digiti minimi, extensor carpi ulnaris muscles

Common extensor tendon

Common flexor tendon

Pronator teres, flexor carpi radialis, palmaris longus, flexor carpi ulnaris, flexor digitorum superficialis (humero-ulnar head) muscles

Brachialis muscle

Flexor digitorum superficialis muscle (humero-ulnar head)

Biceps brachii muscle

Supinator muscle

Pronator teres muscle (ulnar head)

Flexor digitorum superficialis muscle (radial head)

Flexor digitorum profundus muscle

Pronator teres muscle

Flexor pollicis longus muscle

**Ulna**

**Radius**

Pronator quadratus muscle

Pronator quadratus muscle

Note: Attachments of intrinsic muscles of hand not shown.

Brachioradialis muscle

Abductor pollicis longus muscle

Flexor carpi ulnaris muscle

Flexor carpi radialis muscle

Extensor carpi ulnaris muscle

Flexor pollicis longus muscle

Flexor digitorum superficialis muscle

Flexor digitorum profundus muscle

Origins          Insertions

**Plate 437**

**Elbow and Forearm**

*Note: Attachments of intrinsic muscles of hand not shown.*

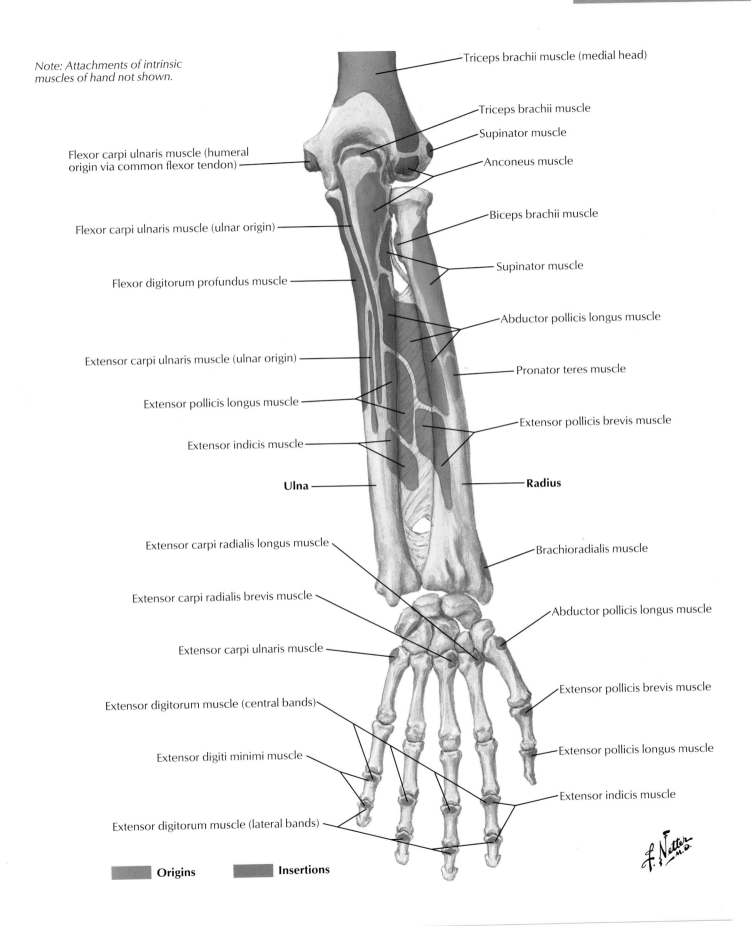

Triceps brachii muscle (medial head)

Triceps brachii muscle

Supinator muscle

Anconeus muscle

Flexor carpi ulnaris muscle (humeral origin via common flexor tendon)

Biceps brachii muscle

Flexor carpi ulnaris muscle (ulnar origin)

Supinator muscle

Flexor digitorum profundus muscle

Abductor pollicis longus muscle

Extensor carpi ulnaris muscle (ulnar origin)

Pronator teres muscle

Extensor pollicis longus muscle

Extensor pollicis brevis muscle

Extensor indicis muscle

**Ulna**

**Radius**

Extensor carpi radialis longus muscle

Brachioradialis muscle

Extensor carpi radialis brevis muscle

Abductor pollicis longus muscle

Extensor carpi ulnaris muscle

Extensor pollicis brevis muscle

Extensor digitorum muscle (central bands)

Extensor pollicis longus muscle

Extensor digiti minimi muscle

Extensor indicis muscle

Extensor digitorum muscle (lateral bands)

**Origins**       **Insertions**

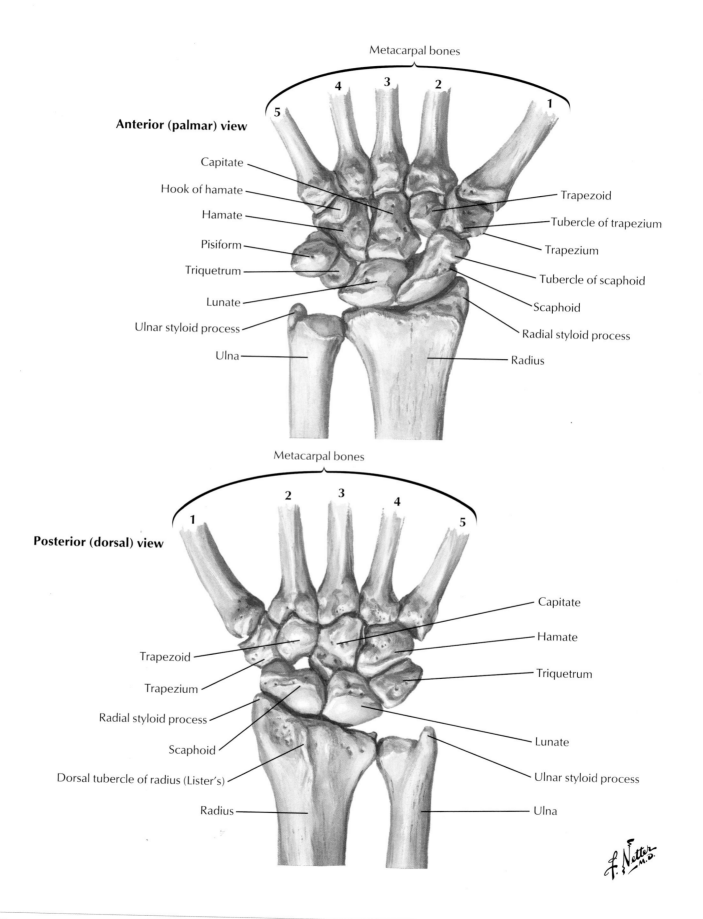

Metacarpal bones

4 3 2

5 1

**Anterior (palmar) view**

Capitate

Hook of hamate

Hamate

Pisiform

Triquetrum

Lunate

Ulnar styloid process

Ulna

Trapezoid

Tubercle of trapezium

Trapezium

Tubercle of scaphoid

Scaphoid

Radial styloid process

Radius

Metacarpal bones

2 3 4

1 5

**Posterior (dorsal) view**

Trapezoid

Trapezium

Radial styloid process

Scaphoid

Dorsal tubercle of radius (Lister's)

Radius

Capitate

Hamate

Triquetrum

Lunate

Ulnar styloid process

Ulna

**Plate 439**

**Wrist and Hand**

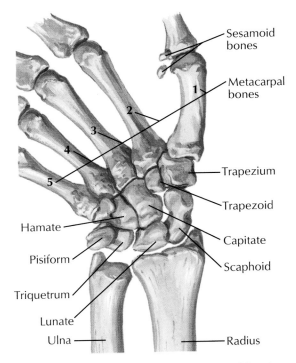

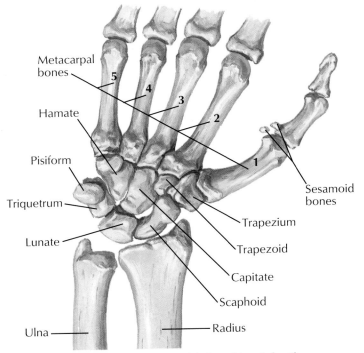

**Position of carpal bones with hand in abduction: anterior (palmar) view**

Metacarpal bones
Hamate
Pisiform
Triquetrum
Lunate
Ulna
5
4
3
2
1
Sesamoid bones
Trapezium
Trapezoid
Capitate
Scaphoid
Radius

**Position of carpal bones with hand in adduction: anterior (palmar) view**

Sesamoid bones
Metacarpal bones
1
2
3
4
5
Trapezium
Trapezoid
Capitate
Scaphoid
Hamate
Pisiform
Triquetrum
Lunate
Ulna
Radius

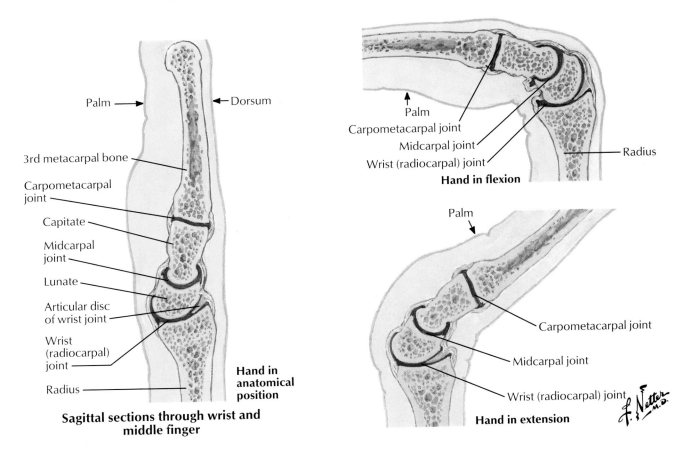

**Sagittal sections through wrist and middle finger**

Palm
Dorsum
3rd metacarpal bone
Carpometacarpal joint
Capitate
Midcarpal joint
Lunate
Articular disc of wrist joint
Wrist (radiocarpal) joint
Radius
**Hand in anatomical position**

Palm
Carpometacarpal joint
Midcarpal joint
Wrist (radiocarpal) joint
Radius
**Hand in flexion**

Palm
Carpometacarpal joint
Midcarpal joint
Wrist (radiocarpal) joint
**Hand in extension**

**Wrist and Hand**

**Plate 440**

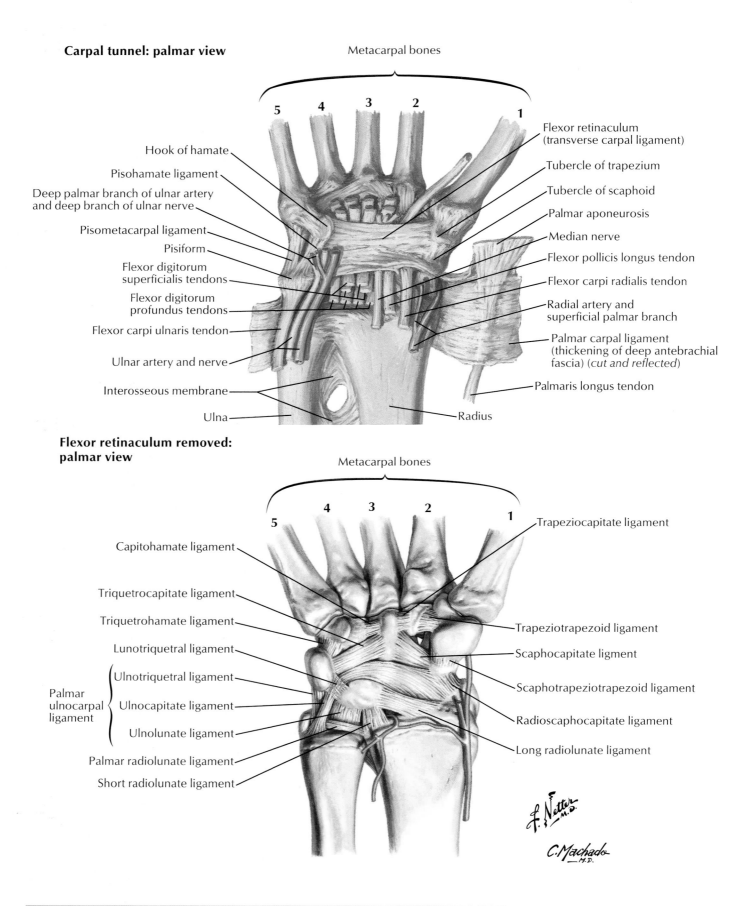

**Carpal tunnel: palmar view**

Metacarpal bones

5 4 3 2 1

Hook of hamate

Pisohamate ligament

Deep palmar branch of ulnar artery and deep branch of ulnar nerve

Pisometacarpal ligament

Pisiform

Flexor digitorum superficialis tendons

Flexor digitorum profundus tendons

Flexor carpi ulnaris tendon

Ulnar artery and nerve

Interosseous membrane

Ulna

Flexor retinaculum (transverse carpal ligament)

Tubercle of trapezium

Tubercle of scaphoid

Palmar aponeurosis

Median nerve

Flexor pollicis longus tendon

Flexor carpi radialis tendon

Radial artery and superficial palmar branch

Palmar carpal ligament (thickening of deep antebrachial fascia) (cut and reflected)

Palmaris longus tendon

Radius

**Flexor retinaculum removed: palmar view**

Metacarpal bones

5 4 3 2 1

Capitohamate ligament

Triquetrocapitate ligament

Triquetrohamate ligament

Lunotriquetral ligament

Ulnotriquetral ligament

Palmar ulnocarpal ligament

Ulnocapitate ligament

Ulnolunate ligament

Palmar radiolunate ligament

Short radiolunate ligament

Trapeziocapitate ligament

Trapeziotrapezoid ligament

Scaphocapitate ligment

Scaphotrapeziotrapezoid ligament

Radioscaphocapitate ligament

Long radiolunate ligament

**Plate 441**

**Wrist and Hand**

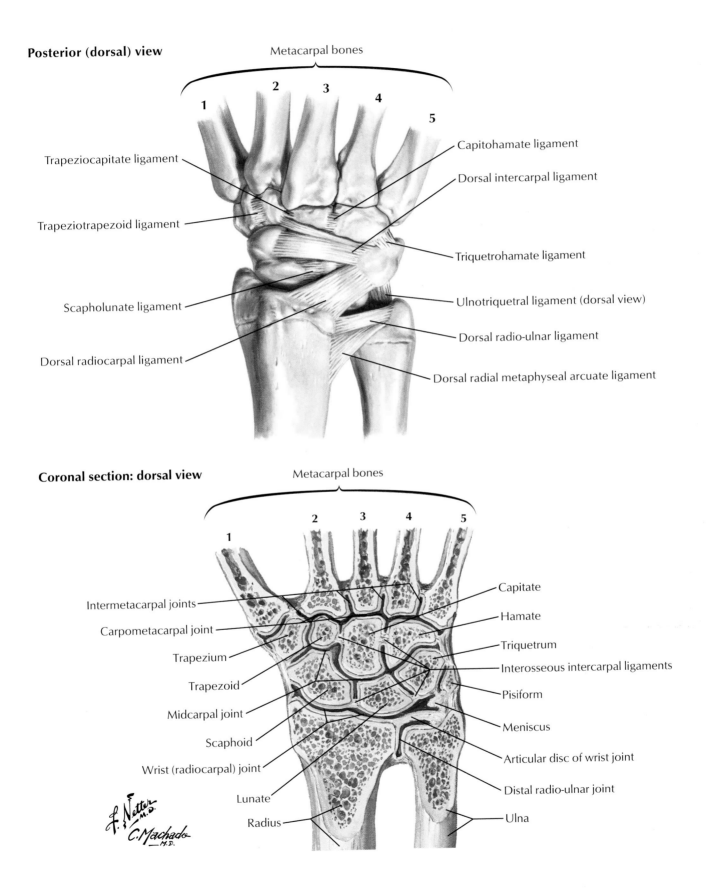

**Posterior (dorsal) view**

Metacarpal bones

1  2  3  4  5

Trapeziocapitate ligament

Trapeziotrapezoid ligament

Scapholunate ligament

Dorsal radiocarpal ligament

Capitohamate ligament

Dorsal intercarpal ligament

Triquetrohamate ligament

Ulnotriquetral ligament (dorsal view)

Dorsal radio-ulnar ligament

Dorsal radial metaphyseal arcuate ligament

**Coronal section: dorsal view**

Metacarpal bones

1  2  3  4  5

Intermetacarpal joints

Carpometacarpal joint

Trapezium

Trapezoid

Midcarpal joint

Scaphoid

Wrist (radiocarpal) joint

Lunate

Radius

Capitate

Hamate

Triquetrum

Interosseous intercarpal ligaments

Pisiform

Meniscus

Articular disc of wrist joint

Distal radio-ulnar joint

Ulna

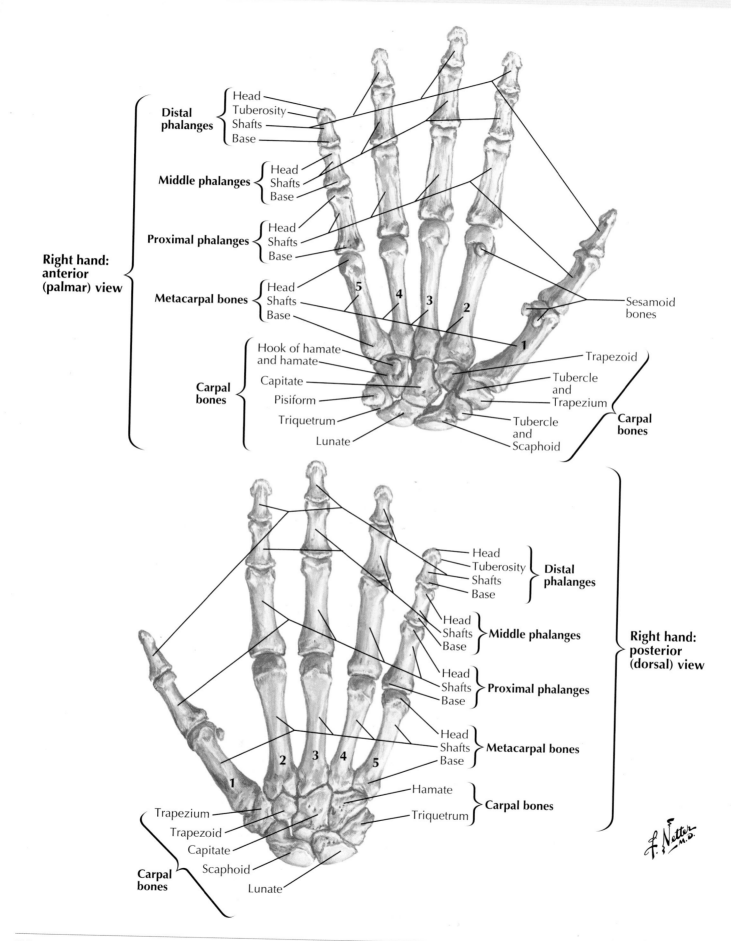

Distal phalanges
Head
Tuberosity
Shafts
Base

Middle phalanges
Head
Shafts
Base

Proximal phalanges
Head
Shafts
Base

Metacarpal bones
Head
Shafts
Base

Right hand: anterior (palmar) view

Carpal bones
Hook of hamate and hamate
Capitate
Pisiform
Triquetrum
Lunate

5 4 3 2 1

Sesamoid bones

Trapezoid
Tubercle and Trapezium
Tubercle and Scaphoid

Carpal bones

Head
Tuberosity
Shafts
Base
Distal phalanges

Head
Shafts
Base
Middle phalanges

Head
Shafts
Base
Proximal phalanges

Head
Shafts
Base
Metacarpal bones

Right hand: posterior (dorsal) view

2 3 4 5
1

Carpal bones
Trapezium
Trapezoid
Capitate
Scaphoid
Lunate

Hamate
Triquetrum
Carpal bones

**Plate 443**

**Wrist and Hand**

**Anteroposterior view**

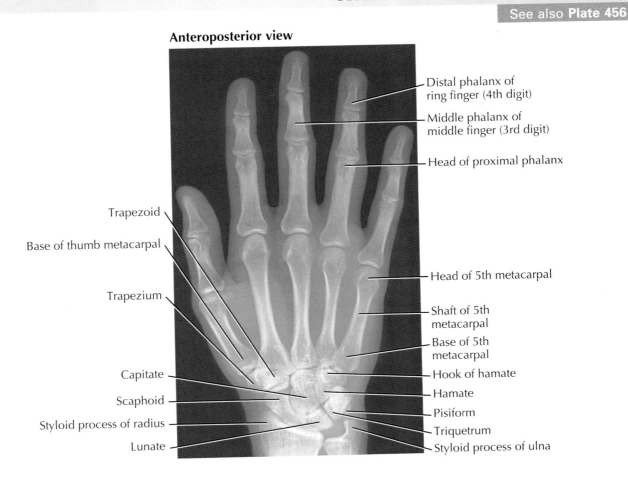

- Distal phalanx of ring finger (4th digit)
- Middle phalanx of middle finger (3rd digit)
- Head of proximal phalanx
- Head of 5th metacarpal
- Shaft of 5th metacarpal
- Base of 5th metacarpal
- Hook of hamate
- Hamate
- Pisiform
- Triquetrum
- Styloid process of ulna

- Trapezoid
- Base of thumb metacarpal
- Trapezium
- Capitate
- Scaphoid
- Styloid process of radius
- Lunate

**Lateral view**

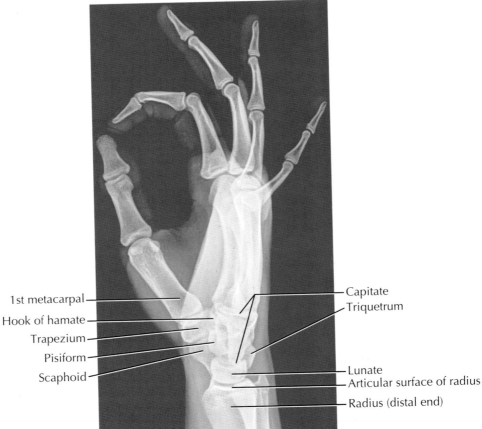

- 1st metacarpal
- Hook of hamate
- Trapezium
- Pisiform
- Scaphoid

- Capitate
- Triquetrum
- Lunate
- Articular surface of radius
- Radius (distal end)

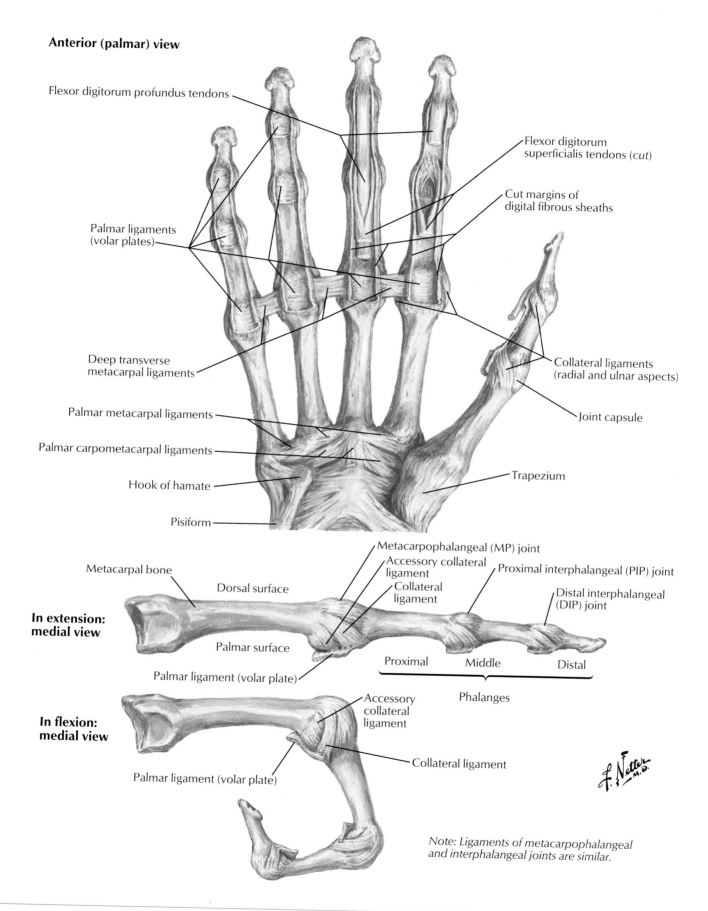

**Anterior (palmar) view**

Flexor digitorum profundus tendons

Flexor digitorum superficialis tendons (*cut*)

Cut margins of digital fibrous sheaths

Palmar ligaments (volar plates)

Deep transverse metacarpal ligaments

Collateral ligaments (radial and ulnar aspects)

Palmar metacarpal ligaments

Palmar carpometacarpal ligaments

Joint capsule

Hook of hamate

Trapezium

Pisiform

Metacarpophalangeal (MP) joint

Accessory collateral ligament

Collateral ligament

Proximal interphalangeal (PIP) joint

Distal interphalangeal (DIP) joint

Metacarpal bone

Dorsal surface

**In extension: medial view**

Palmar surface

Palmar ligament (volar plate)

Proximal    Middle    Distal

Phalanges

**In flexion: medial view**

Accessory collateral ligament

Collateral ligament

Palmar ligament (volar plate)

*Note: Ligaments of metacarpophalangeal and interphalangeal joints are similar.*

**Plate 445**

**Wrist and Hand**

**Anterior (palmar) views**

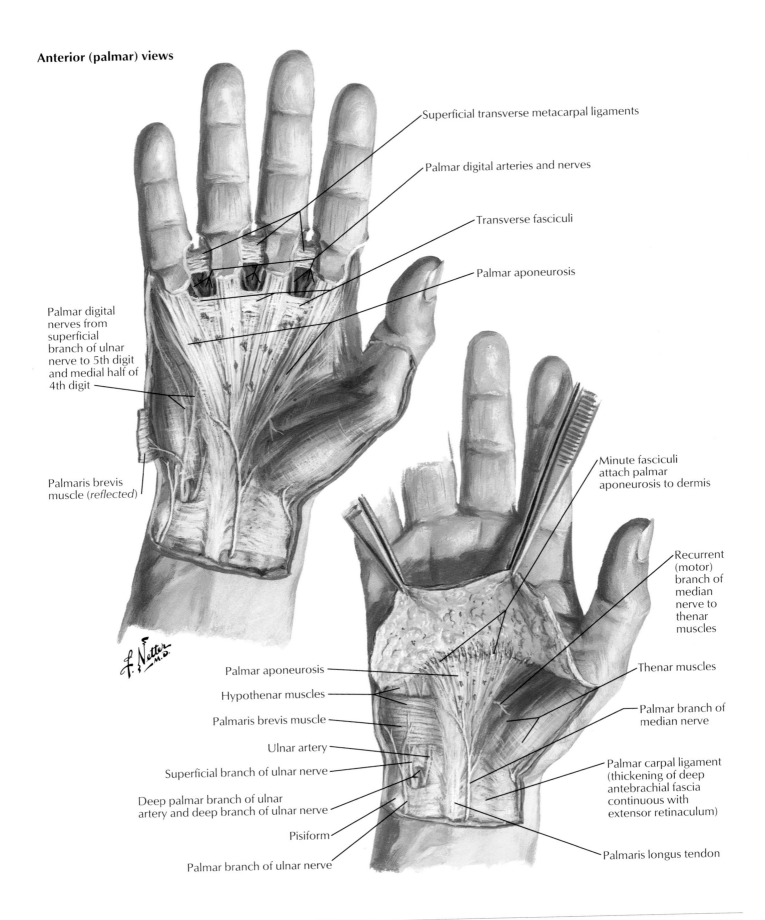

Superficial transverse metacarpal ligaments

Palmar digital arteries and nerves

Transverse fasciculi

Palmar aponeurosis

Palmar digital nerves from superficial branch of ulnar nerve to 5th digit and medial half of 4th digit

Palmaris brevis muscle (*reflected*)

Minute fasciculi attach palmar aponeurosis to dermis

Recurrent (motor) branch of median nerve to thenar muscles

Thenar muscles

Palmar branch of median nerve

Palmar carpal ligament (thickening of deep antebrachial fascia continuous with extensor retinaculum)

Palmaris longus tendon

Palmar aponeurosis

Hypothenar muscles

Palmaris brevis muscle

Ulnar artery

Superficial branch of ulnar nerve

Deep palmar branch of ulnar artery and deep branch of ulnar nerve

Pisiform

Palmar branch of ulnar nerve

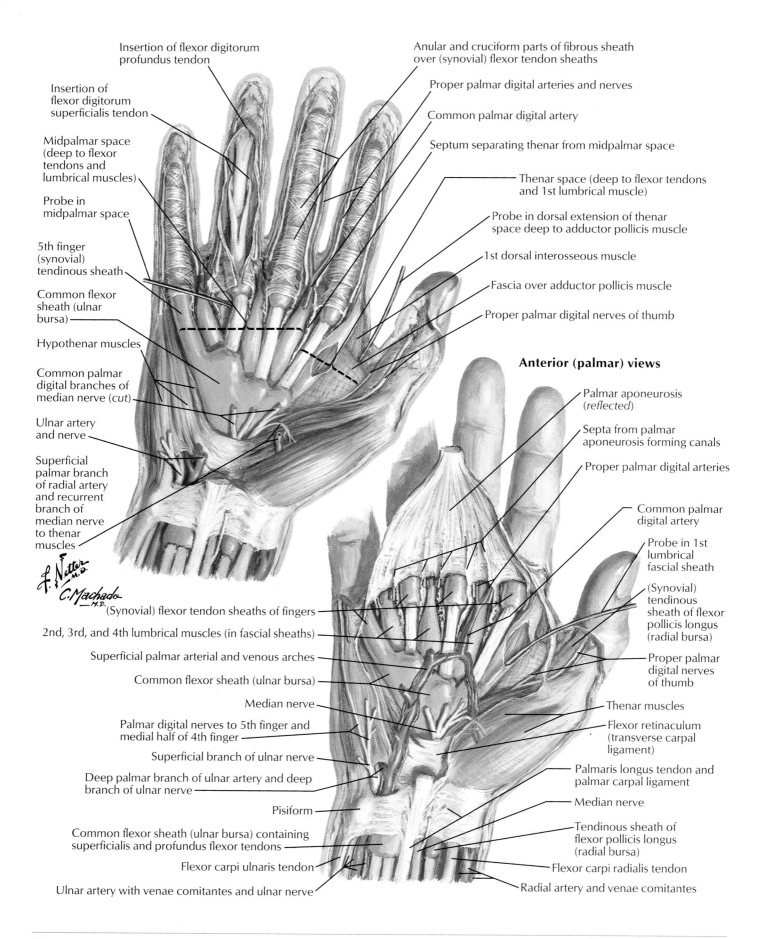

Insertion of flexor digitorum profundus tendon

Insertion of flexor digitorum superficialis tendon

Midpalmar space (deep to flexor tendons and lumbrical muscles)

Probe in midpalmar space

5th finger (synovial) tendinous sheath

Common flexor sheath (ulnar bursa)

Hypothenar muscles

Common palmar digital branches of median nerve (cut)

Ulnar artery and nerve

Superficial palmar branch of radial artery and recurrent branch of median nerve to thenar muscles

Anular and cruciform parts of fibrous sheath over (synovial) flexor tendon sheaths

Proper palmar digital arteries and nerves

Common palmar digital artery

Septum separating thenar from midpalmar space

Thenar space (deep to flexor tendons and 1st lumbrical muscle)

Probe in dorsal extension of thenar space deep to adductor pollicis muscle

1st dorsal interosseous muscle

Fascia over adductor pollicis muscle

Proper palmar digital nerves of thumb

**Anterior (palmar) views**

Palmar aponeurosis (reflected)

Septa from palmar aponeurosis forming canals

Proper palmar digital arteries

Common palmar digital artery

Probe in 1st lumbrical fascial sheath

(Synovial) tendinous sheath of flexor pollicis longus (radial bursa)

Proper palmar digital nerves of thumb

Thenar muscles

Flexor retinaculum (transverse carpal ligament)

Palmaris longus tendon and palmar carpal ligament

Median nerve

Tendinous sheath of flexor pollicis longus (radial bursa)

Flexor carpi radialis tendon

Radial artery and venae comitantes

(Synovial) flexor tendon sheaths of fingers

2nd, 3rd, and 4th lumbrical muscles (in fascial sheaths)

Superficial palmar arterial and venous arches

Common flexor sheath (ulnar bursa)

Median nerve

Palmar digital nerves to 5th finger and medial half of 4th finger

Superficial branch of ulnar nerve

Deep palmar branch of ulnar artery and deep branch of ulnar nerve

Pisiform

Common flexor sheath (ulnar bursa) containing superficialis and profundus flexor tendons

Flexor carpi ulnaris tendon

Ulnar artery with venae comitantes and ulnar nerve

**Plate 447**

**Wrist and Hand**

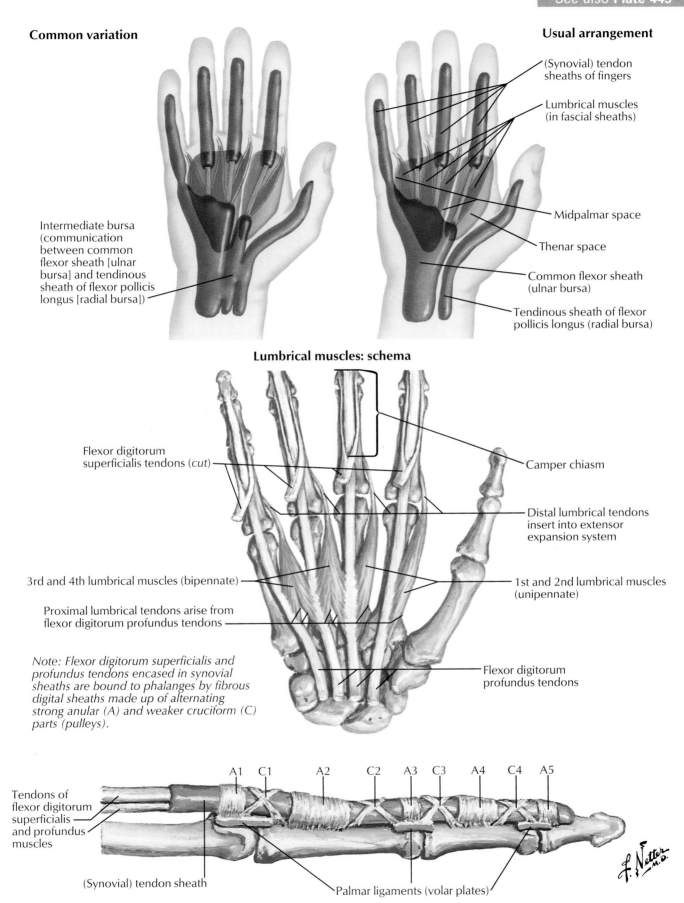

**Common variation**

**Usual arrangement**

(Synovial) tendon sheaths of fingers

Lumbrical muscles (in fascial sheaths)

Intermediate bursa (communication between common flexor sheath [ulnar bursa] and tendinous sheath of flexor pollicis longus [radial bursa])

Midpalmar space

Thenar space

Common flexor sheath (ulnar bursa)

Tendinous sheath of flexor pollicis longus (radial bursa)

**Lumbrical muscles: schema**

Flexor digitorum superficialis tendons (cut)

Camper chiasm

Distal lumbrical tendons insert into extensor expansion system

3rd and 4th lumbrical muscles (bipennate)

Proximal lumbrical tendons arise from flexor digitorum profundus tendons

1st and 2nd lumbrical muscles (unipennate)

Note: Flexor digitorum superficialis and profundus tendons encased in synovial sheaths are bound to phalanges by fibrous digital sheaths made up of alternating strong anular (A) and weaker cruciform (C) parts (pulleys).

Flexor digitorum profundus tendons

A1  C1  A2  C2  A3  C3  A4  C4  A5

Tendons of flexor digitorum superficialis and profundus muscles

(Synovial) tendon sheath

Palmar ligaments (volar plates)

*F. Netter M.D.*

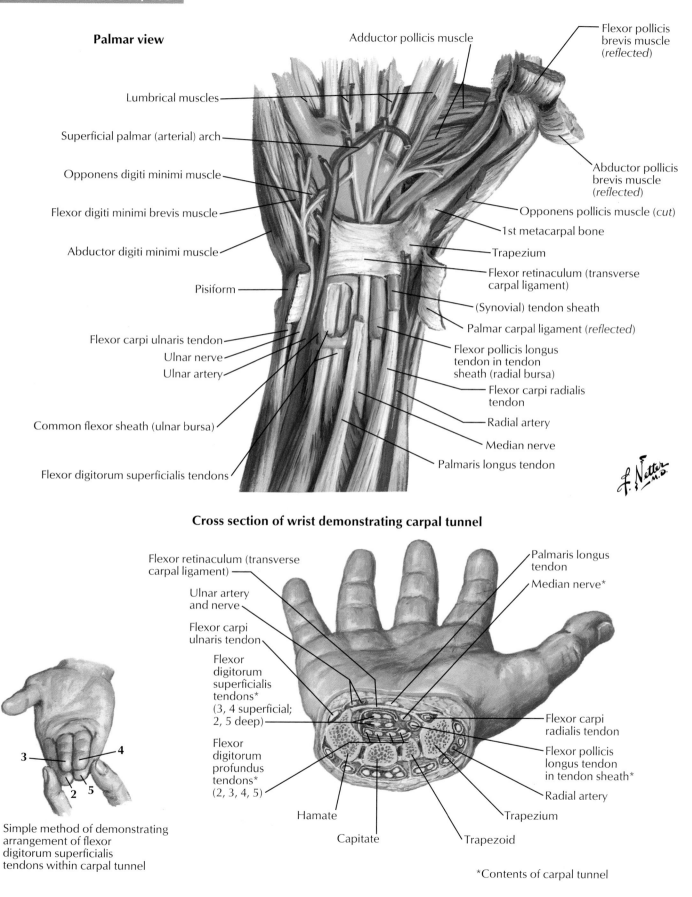

**Palmar view**

Adductor pollicis muscle

Flexor pollicis brevis muscle (*reflected*)

Lumbrical muscles

Superficial palmar (arterial) arch

Opponens digiti minimi muscle

Flexor digiti minimi brevis muscle

Abductor digiti minimi muscle

Abductor pollicis brevis muscle (*reflected*)

Opponens pollicis muscle (*cut*)

1st metacarpal bone

Trapezium

Flexor retinaculum (transverse carpal ligament)

(Synovial) tendon sheath

Palmar carpal ligament (*reflected*)

Pisiform

Flexor carpi ulnaris tendon

Ulnar nerve

Ulnar artery

Flexor pollicis longus tendon in tendon sheath (radial bursa)

Flexor carpi radialis tendon

Radial artery

Common flexor sheath (ulnar bursa)

Median nerve

Palmaris longus tendon

Flexor digitorum superficialis tendons

**Cross section of wrist demonstrating carpal tunnel**

Flexor retinaculum (transverse carpal ligament)

Palmaris longus tendon

Median nerve*

Ulnar artery and nerve

Flexor carpi ulnaris tendon

Flexor digitorum superficialis tendons* (3, 4 superficial; 2, 5 deep)

Flexor carpi radialis tendon

Flexor pollicis longus tendon in tendon sheath*

Flexor digitorum profundus tendons* (2, 3, 4, 5)

Radial artery

Hamate

Trapezium

Capitate

Trapezoid

3    4

2   5

Simple method of demonstrating arrangement of flexor digitorum superficialis tendons within carpal tunnel

*Contents of carpal tunnel

**Plate 449**

**Wrist and Hand**

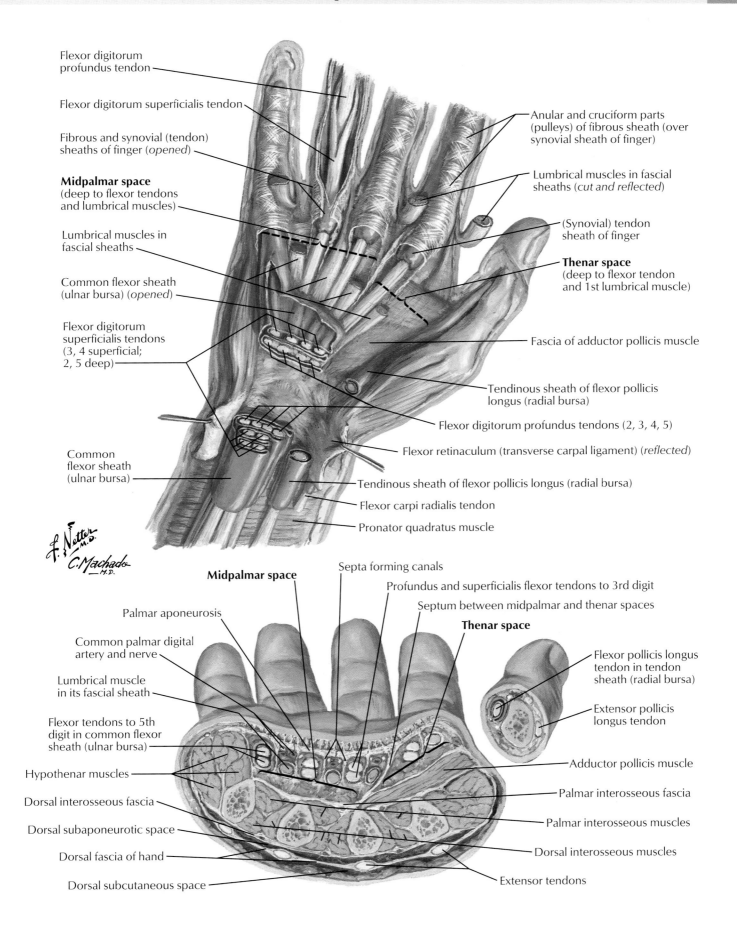

Flexor digitorum profundus tendon

Flexor digitorum superficialis tendon

Fibrous and synovial (tendon) sheaths of finger (*opened*)

**Midpalmar space** (deep to flexor tendons and lumbrical muscles)

Lumbrical muscles in fascial sheaths

Common flexor sheath (ulnar bursa) (*opened*)

Flexor digitorum superficialis tendons (3, 4 superficial; 2, 5 deep)

Common flexor sheath (ulnar bursa)

Anular and cruciform parts (pulleys) of fibrous sheath (over synovial sheath of finger)

Lumbrical muscles in fascial sheaths (*cut and reflected*)

(Synovial) tendon sheath of finger

**Thenar space** (deep to flexor tendon and 1st lumbrical muscle)

Fascia of adductor pollicis muscle

Tendinous sheath of flexor pollicis longus (radial bursa)

Flexor digitorum profundus tendons (2, 3, 4, 5)

Flexor retinaculum (transverse carpal ligament) (*reflected*)

Tendinous sheath of flexor pollicis longus (radial bursa)

Flexor carpi radialis tendon

Pronator quadratus muscle

Septa forming canals

**Midpalmar space**

Profundus and superficialis flexor tendons to 3rd digit

Septum between midpalmar and thenar spaces

**Thenar space**

Palmar aponeurosis

Common palmar digital artery and nerve

Lumbrical muscle in its fascial sheath

Flexor tendons to 5th digit in common flexor sheath (ulnar bursa)

Hypothenar muscles

Dorsal interosseous fascia

Dorsal subaponeurotic space

Dorsal fascia of hand

Dorsal subcutaneous space

Flexor pollicis longus tendon in tendon sheath (radial bursa)

Extensor pollicis longus tendon

Adductor pollicis muscle

Palmar interosseous fascia

Palmar interosseous muscles

Dorsal interosseous muscles

Extensor tendons

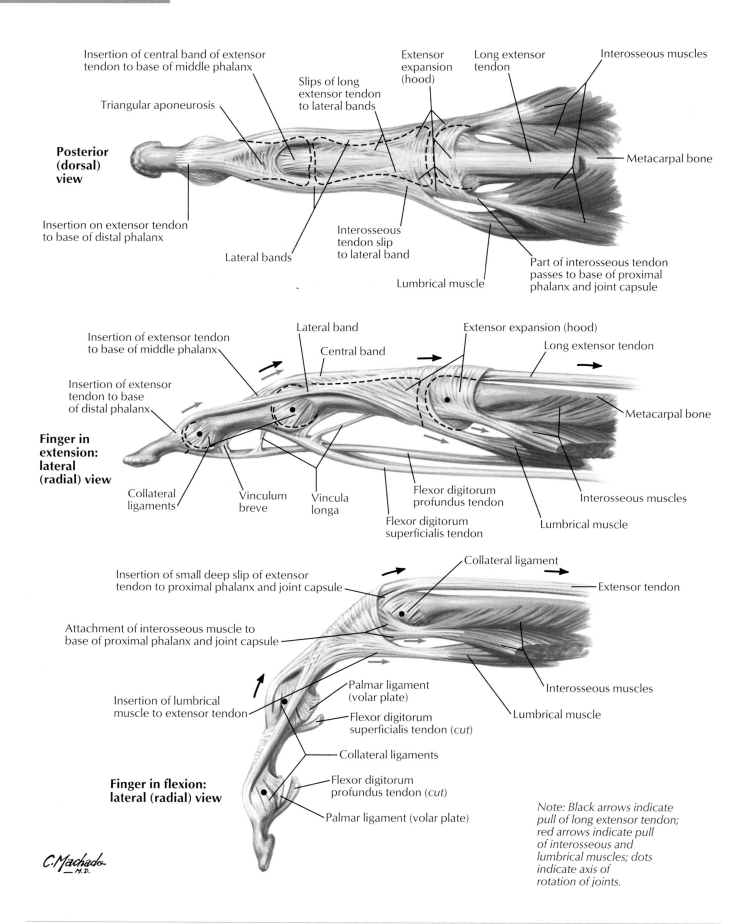

**Posterior (dorsal) view**

Insertion of central band of extensor tendon to base of middle phalanx

Triangular aponeurosis

Slips of long extensor tendon to lateral bands

Extensor expansion (hood)

Long extensor tendon

Interosseous muscles

Metacarpal bone

Insertion on extensor tendon to base of distal phalanx

Lateral bands

Interosseous tendon slip to lateral band

Lumbrical muscle

Part of interosseous tendon passes to base of proximal phalanx and joint capsule

**Finger in extension: lateral (radial) view**

Insertion of extensor tendon to base of middle phalanx

Lateral band

Central band

Extensor expansion (hood)

Long extensor tendon

Insertion of extensor tendon to base of distal phalanx

Metacarpal bone

Collateral ligaments

Vinculum breve

Vincula longa

Flexor digitorum profundus tendon

Flexor digitorum superficialis tendon

Interosseous muscles

Lumbrical muscle

Insertion of small deep slip of extensor tendon to proximal phalanx and joint capsule

Collateral ligament

Extensor tendon

Attachment of interosseous muscle to base of proximal phalanx and joint capsule

Insertion of lumbrical muscle to extensor tendon

Palmar ligament (volar plate)

Flexor digitorum superficialis tendon (cut)

Collateral ligaments

Interosseous muscles

Lumbrical muscle

**Finger in flexion: lateral (radial) view**

Flexor digitorum profundus tendon (cut)

Palmar ligament (volar plate)

*Note: Black arrows indicate pull of long extensor tendon; red arrows indicate pull of interosseous and lumbrical muscles; dots indicate axis of rotation of joints.*

C. Machado M.D.

**Plate 451**

**Wrist and Hand**

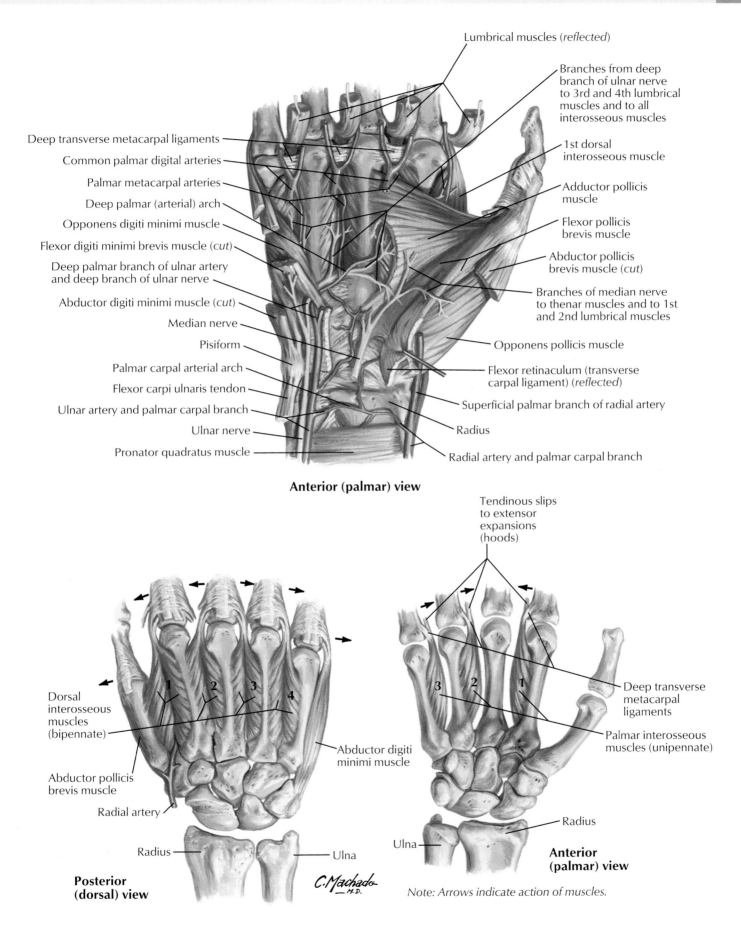

Lumbrical muscles (reflected)

Branches from deep branch of ulnar nerve to 3rd and 4th lumbrical muscles and to all interosseous muscles

Deep transverse metacarpal ligaments

Common palmar digital arteries

Palmar metacarpal arteries

Deep palmar (arterial) arch

Opponens digiti minimi muscle

Flexor digiti minimi brevis muscle (cut)

Deep palmar branch of ulnar artery and deep branch of ulnar nerve

Abductor digiti minimi muscle (cut)

Median nerve

Pisiform

Palmar carpal arterial arch

Flexor carpi ulnaris tendon

Ulnar artery and palmar carpal branch

Ulnar nerve

Pronator quadratus muscle

1st dorsal interosseous muscle

Adductor pollicis muscle

Flexor pollicis brevis muscle

Abductor pollicis brevis muscle (cut)

Branches of median nerve to thenar muscles and to 1st and 2nd lumbrical muscles

Opponens pollicis muscle

Flexor retinaculum (transverse carpal ligament) (reflected)

Superficial palmar branch of radial artery

Radius

Radial artery and palmar carpal branch

**Anterior (palmar) view**

Tendinous slips to extensor expansions (hoods)

Dorsal interosseous muscles (bipennate)

Abductor pollicis brevis muscle

Radial artery

Radius

Ulna

1  2  3  4

Abductor digiti minimi muscle

**Posterior (dorsal) view**

C. Machado —M.D.

Deep transverse metacarpal ligaments

Palmar interosseous muscles (unipennate)

Radius

Ulna

3  2  1

**Anterior (palmar) view**

Note: Arrows indicate action of muscles.

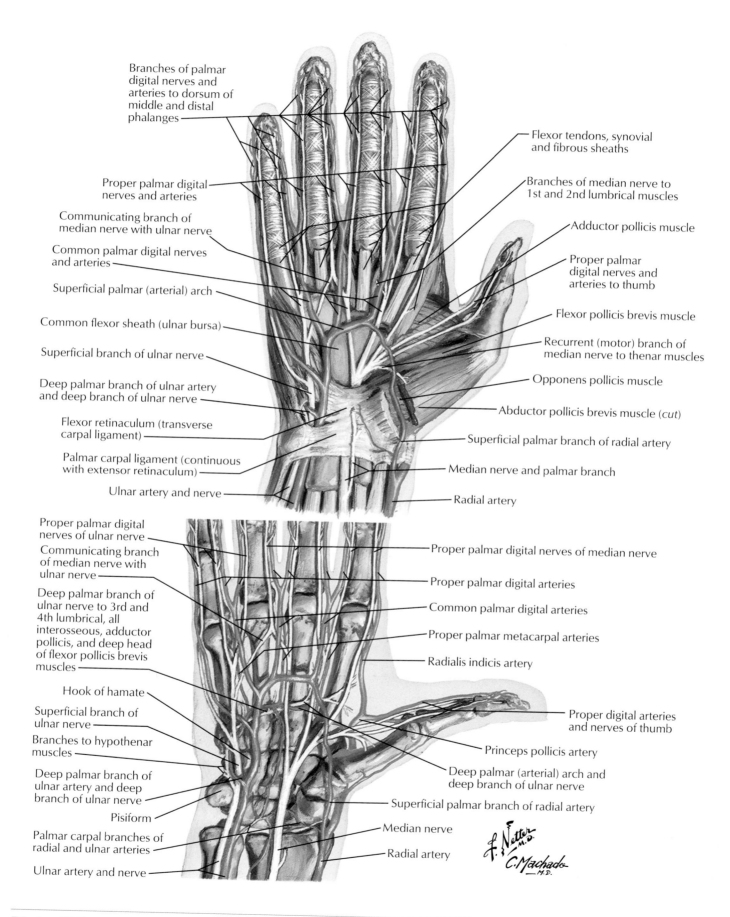

Branches of palmar digital nerves and arteries to dorsum of middle and distal phalanges

Proper palmar digital nerves and arteries

Communicating branch of median nerve with ulnar nerve

Common palmar digital nerves and arteries

Superficial palmar (arterial) arch

Common flexor sheath (ulnar bursa)

Superficial branch of ulnar nerve

Deep palmar branch of ulnar artery and deep branch of ulnar nerve

Flexor retinaculum (transverse carpal ligament)

Palmar carpal ligament (continuous with extensor retinaculum)

Ulnar artery and nerve

Flexor tendons, synovial and fibrous sheaths

Branches of median nerve to 1st and 2nd lumbrical muscles

Adductor pollicis muscle

Proper palmar digital nerves and arteries to thumb

Flexor pollicis brevis muscle

Recurrent (motor) branch of median nerve to thenar muscles

Opponens pollicis muscle

Abductor pollicis brevis muscle (cut)

Superficial palmar branch of radial artery

Median nerve and palmar branch

Radial artery

Proper palmar digital nerves of ulnar nerve

Communicating branch of median nerve with ulnar nerve

Deep palmar branch of ulnar nerve to 3rd and 4th lumbrical, all interosseous, adductor pollicis, and deep head of flexor pollicis brevis muscles

Hook of hamate

Superficial branch of ulnar nerve

Branches to hypothenar muscles

Deep palmar branch of ulnar artery and deep branch of ulnar nerve

Pisiform

Palmar carpal branches of radial and ulnar arteries

Ulnar artery and nerve

Proper palmar digital nerves of median nerve

Proper palmar digital arteries

Common palmar digital arteries

Proper palmar metacarpal arteries

Radialis indicis artery

Proper digital arteries and nerves of thumb

Princeps pollicis artery

Deep palmar (arterial) arch and deep branch of ulnar nerve

Superficial palmar branch of radial artery

Median nerve

Radial artery

**Plate 453**

**Wrist and Hand**

**Lateral (radial) view**

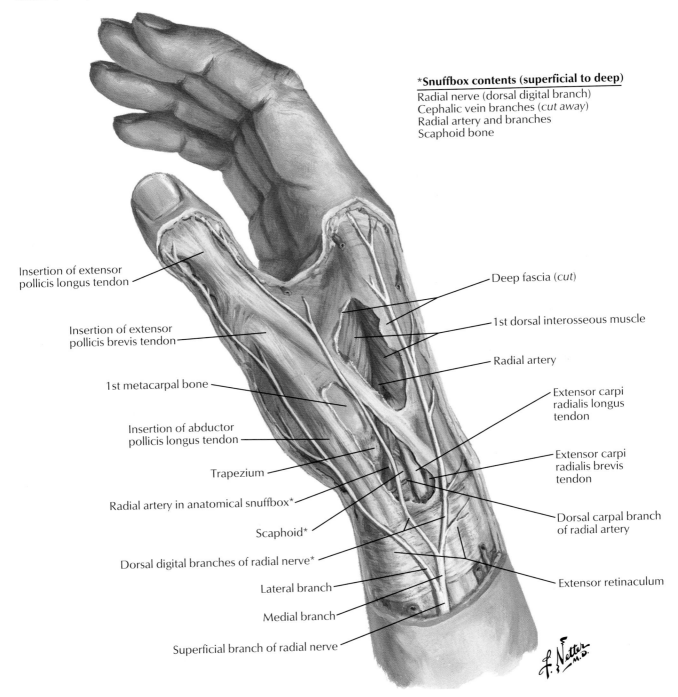

*Snuffbox contents (superficial to deep)
Radial nerve (dorsal digital branch)
Cephalic vein branches (*cut away*)
Radial artery and branches
Scaphoid bone

Insertion of extensor pollicis longus tendon

Insertion of extensor pollicis brevis tendon

1st metacarpal bone

Insertion of abductor pollicis longus tendon

Trapezium

Radial artery in anatomical snuffbox*

Scaphoid*

Dorsal digital branches of radial nerve*

Lateral branch

Medial branch

Superficial branch of radial nerve

Deep fascia (*cut*)

1st dorsal interosseous muscle

Radial artery

Extensor carpi radialis longus tendon

Extensor carpi radialis brevis tendon

Dorsal carpal branch of radial artery

Extensor retinaculum

**Posterior (dorsal) view**

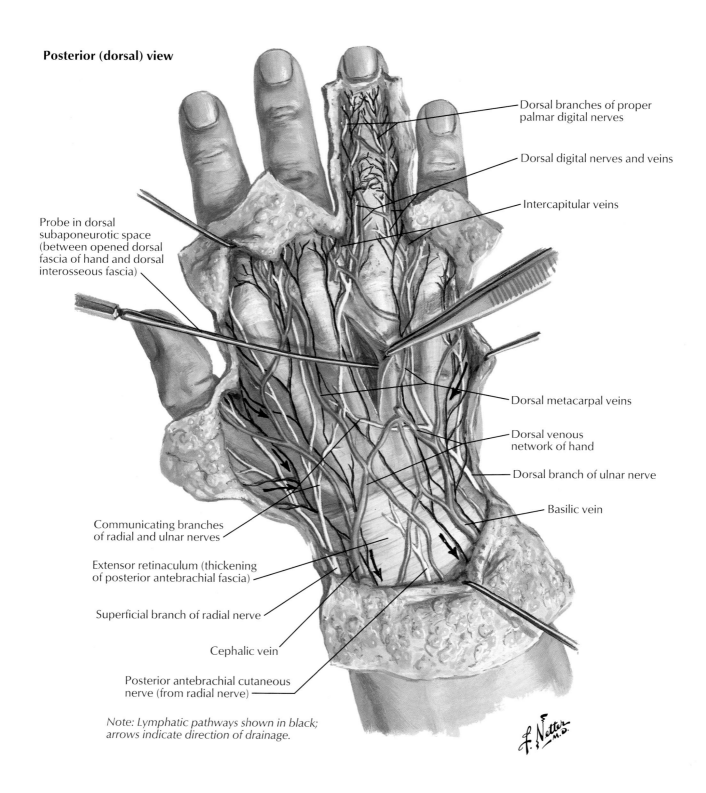

Probe in dorsal subaponeurotic space (between opened dorsal fascia of hand and dorsal interosseous fascia)

Communicating branches of radial and ulnar nerves

Extensor retinaculum (thickening of posterior antebrachial fascia)

Superficial branch of radial nerve

Cephalic vein

Posterior antebrachial cutaneous nerve (from radial nerve)

Dorsal branches of proper palmar digital nerves

Dorsal digital nerves and veins

Intercapitular veins

Dorsal metacarpal veins

Dorsal venous network of hand

Dorsal branch of ulnar nerve

Basilic vein

*Note: Lymphatic pathways shown in black; arrows indicate direction of drainage.*

**Plate 455**

**Wrist and Hand**

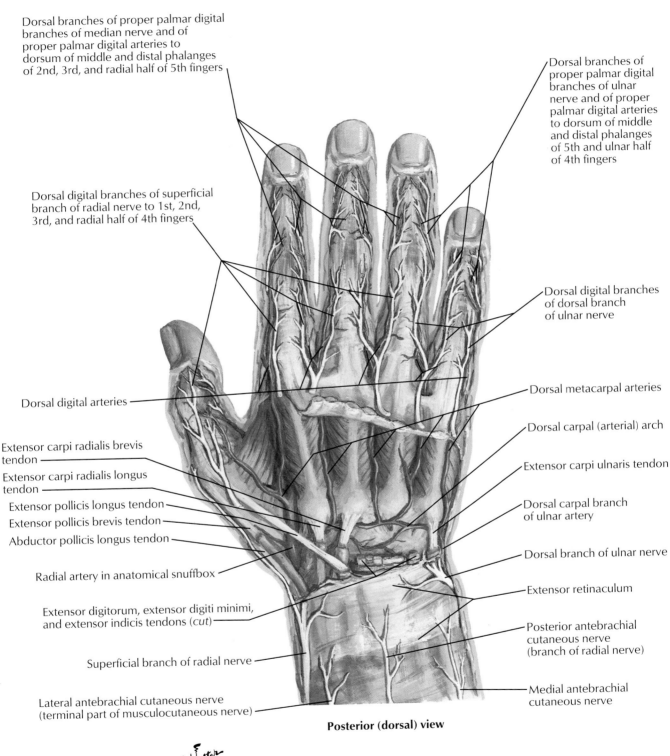

Dorsal branches of proper palmar digital branches of median nerve and of proper palmar digital arteries to dorsum of middle and distal phalanges of 2nd, 3rd, and radial half of 5th fingers

Dorsal branches of proper palmar digital branches of ulnar nerve and of proper palmar digital arteries to dorsum of middle and distal phalanges of 5th and ulnar half of 4th fingers

Dorsal digital branches of superficial branch of radial nerve to 1st, 2nd, 3rd, and radial half of 4th fingers

Dorsal digital branches of dorsal branch of ulnar nerve

Dorsal digital arteries

Dorsal metacarpal arteries

Dorsal carpal (arterial) arch

Extensor carpi radialis brevis tendon

Extensor carpi ulnaris tendon

Extensor carpi radialis longus tendon

Dorsal carpal branch of ulnar artery

Extensor pollicis longus tendon

Extensor pollicis brevis tendon

Abductor pollicis longus tendon

Dorsal branch of ulnar nerve

Radial artery in anatomical snuffbox

Extensor retinaculum

Extensor digitorum, extensor digiti minimi, and extensor indicis tendons (*cut*)

Posterior antebrachial cutaneous nerve (branch of radial nerve)

Superficial branch of radial nerve

Medial antebrachial cutaneous nerve

Lateral antebrachial cutaneous nerve (terminal part of musculocutaneous nerve)

**Posterior (dorsal) view**

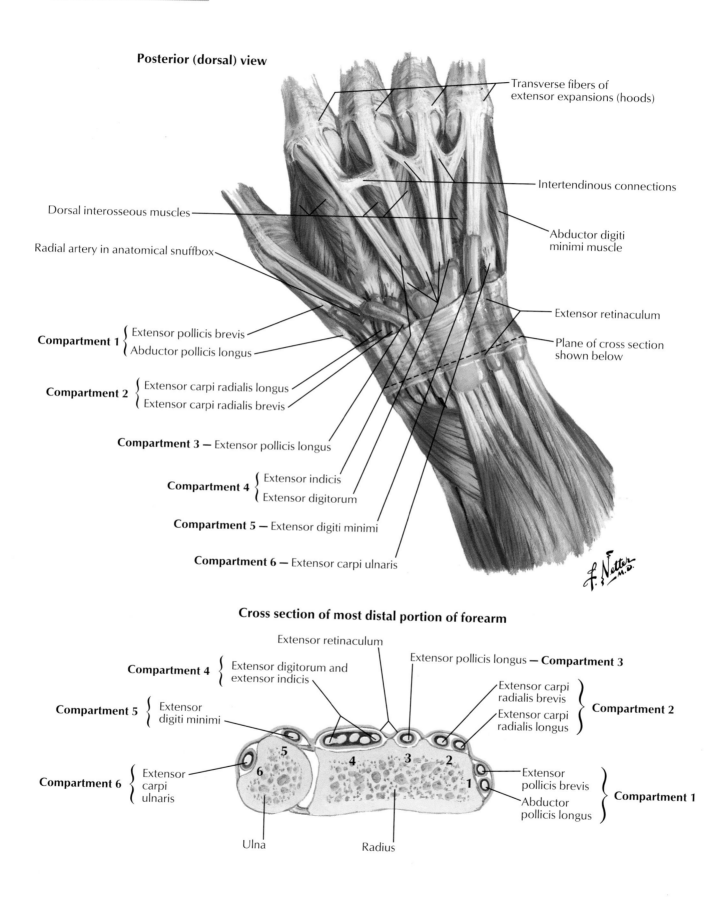

**Posterior (dorsal) view**

Transverse fibers of extensor expansions (hoods)

Intertendinous connections

Abductor digiti minimi muscle

Dorsal interosseous muscles

Radial artery in anatomical snuffbox

Extensor retinaculum

Plane of cross section shown below

**Compartment 1** { Extensor pollicis brevis / Abductor pollicis longus

**Compartment 2** { Extensor carpi radialis longus / Extensor carpi radialis brevis

**Compartment 3** — Extensor pollicis longus

**Compartment 4** { Extensor indicis / Extensor digitorum

**Compartment 5** — Extensor digiti minimi

**Compartment 6** — Extensor carpi ulnaris

**Cross section of most distal portion of forearm**

Extensor retinaculum

Extensor pollicis longus — **Compartment 3**

**Compartment 4** { Extensor digitorum and extensor indicis

Extensor carpi radialis brevis

Extensor carpi radialis longus } **Compartment 2**

**Compartment 5** { Extensor digiti minimi

**Compartment 6** { Extensor carpi ulnaris

Extensor pollicis brevis

Abductor pollicis longus } **Compartment 1**

Ulna

Radius

**Plate 457**

**Wrist and Hand**

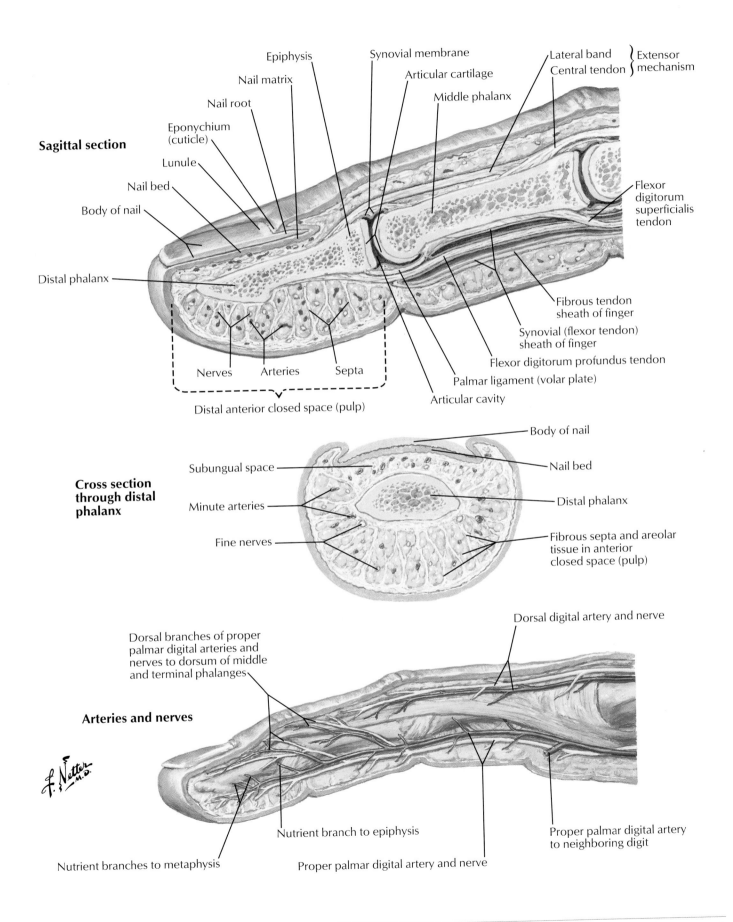

Sagittal section

Epiphysis

Nail matrix

Nail root

Eponychium (cuticle)

Lunule

Nail bed

Body of nail

Distal phalanx

Synovial membrane

Articular cartilage

Middle phalanx

Lateral band ⎫ Extensor
Central tendon ⎬ mechanism

Flexor digitorum superficialis tendon

Fibrous tendon sheath of finger

Synovial (flexor tendon) sheath of finger

Flexor digitorum profundus tendon

Palmar ligament (volar plate)

Articular cavity

Nerves    Arteries    Septa

Distal anterior closed space (pulp)

**Cross section through distal phalanx**

Subungual space

Minute arteries

Fine nerves

Body of nail

Nail bed

Distal phalanx

Fibrous septa and areolar tissue in anterior closed space (pulp)

**Arteries and nerves**

Dorsal branches of proper palmar digital arteries and nerves to dorsum of middle and terminal phalanges

Dorsal digital artery and nerve

Nutrient branch to epiphysis

Nutrient branches to metaphysis

Proper palmar digital artery and nerve

Proper palmar digital artery to neighboring digit

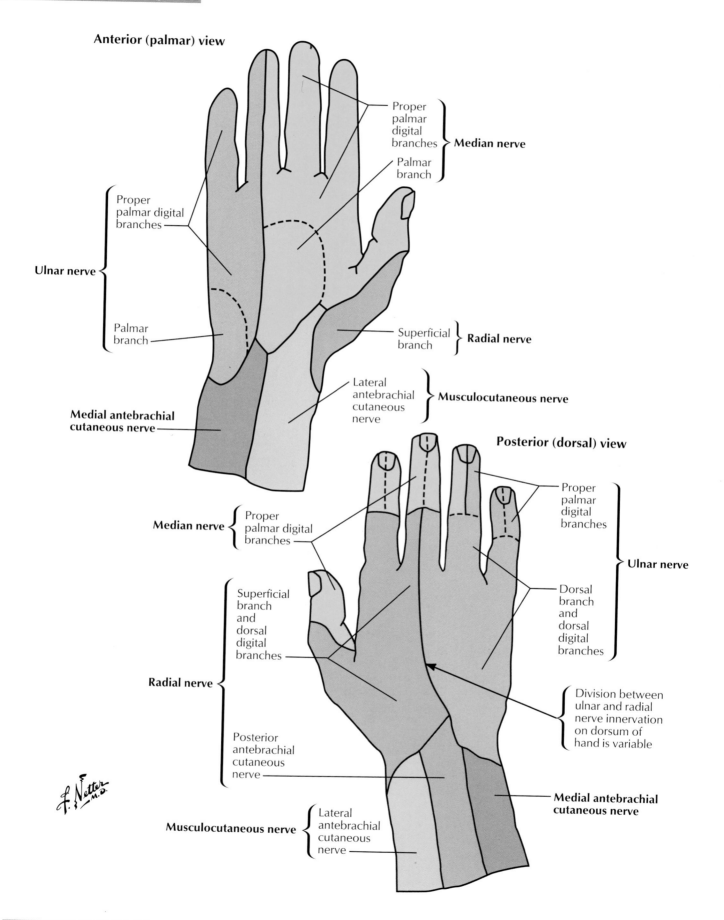

Anterior (palmar) view

Proper palmar digital branches

Palmar branch

} **Median nerve**

Proper palmar digital branches

**Ulnar nerve** {

Palmar branch

Superficial branch } **Radial nerve**

Lateral antebrachial cutaneous nerve } **Musculocutaneous nerve**

**Medial antebrachial cutaneous nerve**

Posterior (dorsal) view

**Median nerve** { Proper palmar digital branches

Proper palmar digital branches

Superficial branch and dorsal digital branches

Dorsal branch and dorsal digital branches

} **Ulnar nerve**

**Radial nerve** {

Division between ulnar and radial nerve innervation on dorsum of hand is variable

Posterior antebrachial cutaneous nerve

Medial antebrachial cutaneous nerve

**Musculocutaneous nerve** { Lateral antebrachial cutaneous nerve

**Plate 459**

**Neurovasculature**

Anterior view

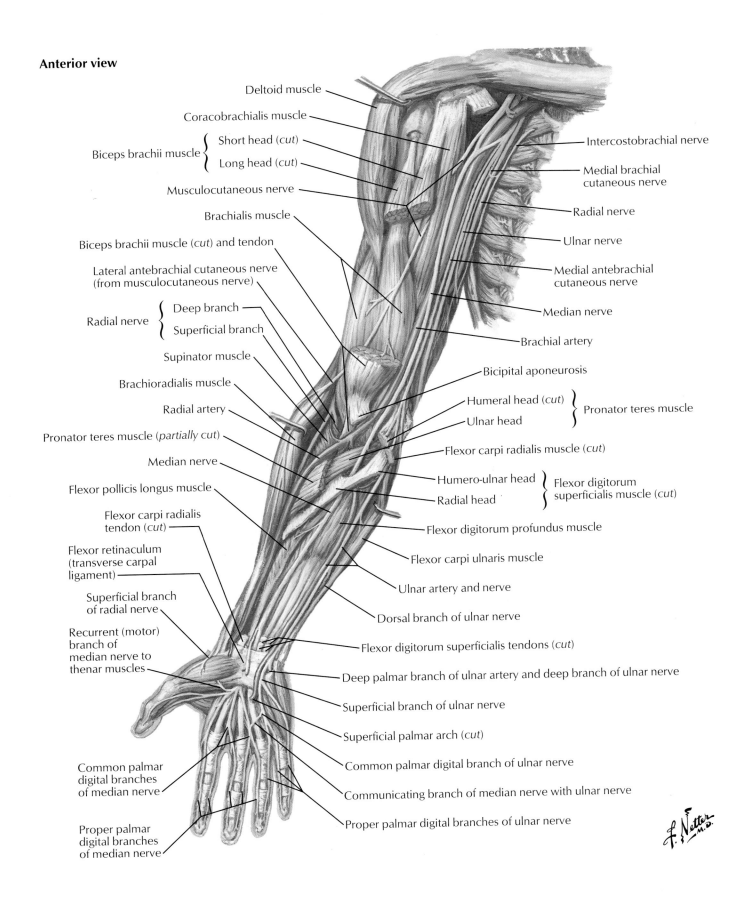

Deltoid muscle

Coracobrachialis muscle

Biceps brachii muscle { Short head (*cut*)

Long head (*cut*)

Musculocutaneous nerve

Brachialis muscle

Biceps brachii muscle (*cut*) and tendon

Lateral antebrachial cutaneous nerve (from musculocutaneous nerve)

Radial nerve { Deep branch

Superficial branch

Supinator muscle

Brachioradialis muscle

Radial artery

Pronator teres muscle (*partially cut*)

Median nerve

Flexor pollicis longus muscle

Flexor carpi radialis tendon (*cut*)

Flexor retinaculum (transverse carpal ligament)

Superficial branch of radial nerve

Recurrent (motor) branch of median nerve to thenar muscles

Common palmar digital branches of median nerve

Proper palmar digital branches of median nerve

Intercostobrachial nerve

Medial brachial cutaneous nerve

Radial nerve

Ulnar nerve

Medial antebrachial cutaneous nerve

Median nerve

Brachial artery

Bicipital aponeurosis

Humeral head (*cut*) } Pronator teres muscle

Ulnar head

Flexor carpi radialis muscle (*cut*)

Humero-ulnar head } Flexor digitorum superficialis muscle (*cut*)

Radial head

Flexor digitorum profundus muscle

Flexor carpi ulnaris muscle

Ulnar artery and nerve

Dorsal branch of ulnar nerve

Flexor digitorum superficialis tendons (*cut*)

Deep palmar branch of ulnar artery and deep branch of ulnar nerve

Superficial branch of ulnar nerve

Superficial palmar arch (*cut*)

Common palmar digital branch of ulnar nerve

Communicating branch of median nerve with ulnar nerve

Proper palmar digital branches of ulnar nerve

**Neurovasculature**

**Plate 460**

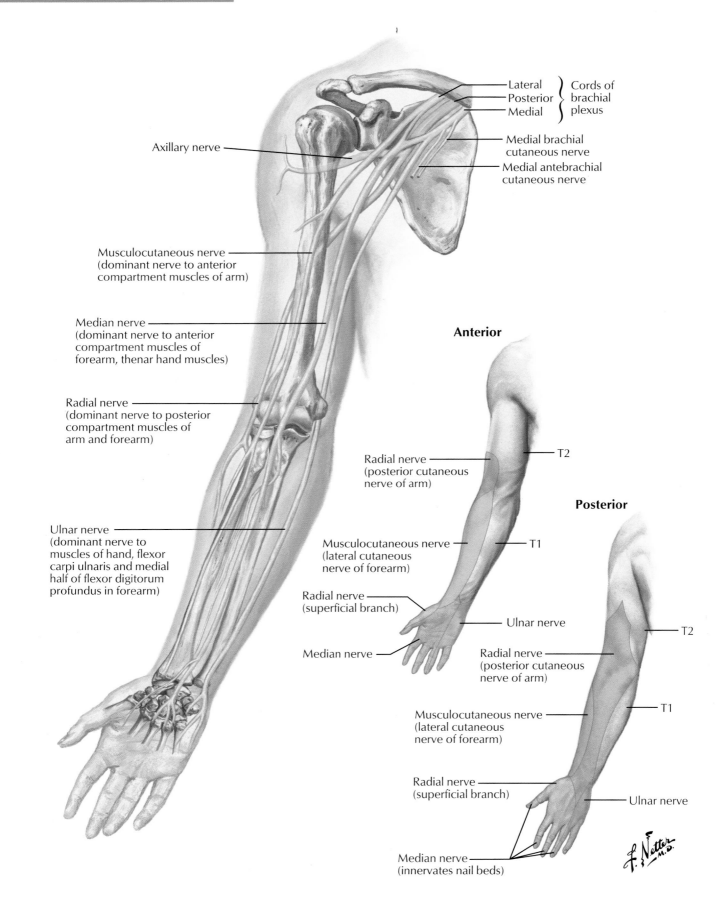

Axillary nerve

Lateral
Posterior
Medial
} Cords of brachial plexus

Medial brachial cutaneous nerve

Medial antebrachial cutaneous nerve

Musculocutaneous nerve (dominant nerve to anterior compartment muscles of arm)

Median nerve (dominant nerve to anterior compartment muscles of forearm, thenar hand muscles)

Radial nerve (dominant nerve to posterior compartment muscles of arm and forearm)

Ulnar nerve (dominant nerve to muscles of hand, flexor carpi ulnaris and medial half of flexor digitorum profundus in forearm)

**Anterior**

Radial nerve (posterior cutaneous nerve of arm)

T2

**Posterior**

Musculocutaneous nerve (lateral cutaneous nerve of forearm)

T1

Radial nerve (superficial branch)

Ulnar nerve

Median nerve

Radial nerve (posterior cutaneous nerve of arm)

T2

Musculocutaneous nerve (lateral cutaneous nerve of forearm)

T1

Radial nerve (superficial branch)

Ulnar nerve

Median nerve (innervates nail beds)

**Plate 461**

**Neurovasculature**

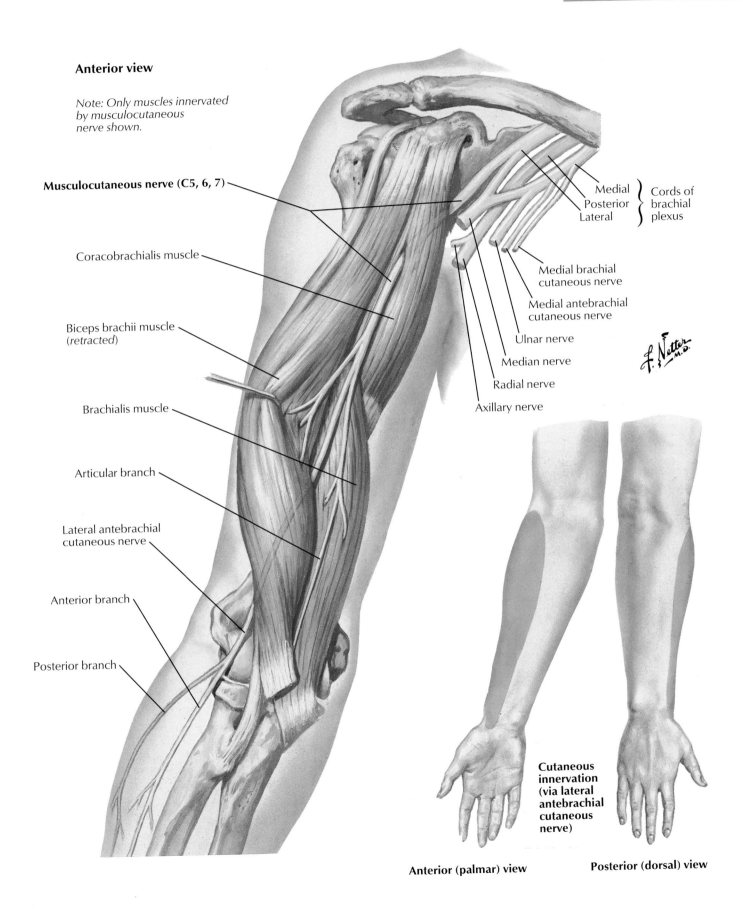

**Anterior view**

*Note: Only muscles innervated by musculocutaneous nerve shown.*

**Musculocutaneous nerve (C5, 6, 7)**

Coracobrachialis muscle

Biceps brachii muscle (*retracted*)

Brachialis muscle

Articular branch

Lateral antebrachial cutaneous nerve

Anterior branch

Posterior branch

Medial } Cords of
Posterior } brachial
Lateral } plexus

Medial brachial cutaneous nerve

Medial antebrachial cutaneous nerve

Ulnar nerve

Median nerve

Radial nerve

Axillary nerve

*f. Netter M.D.*

**Cutaneous innervation (via lateral antebrachial cutaneous nerve)**

**Anterior (palmar) view**

**Posterior (dorsal) view**

**Anterior view**

*Note: Only muscles innervated by median nerve shown.*

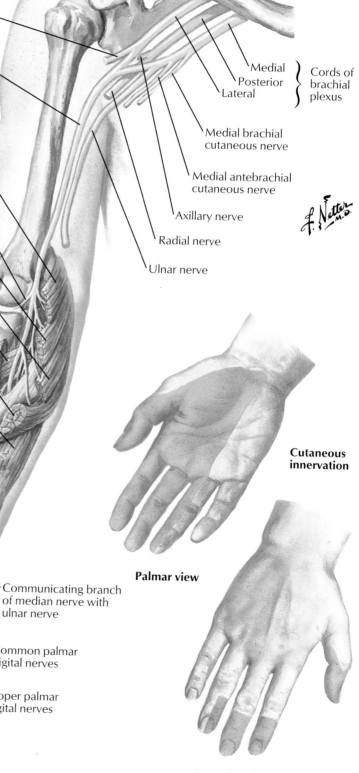

Musculocutaneous nerve

**Median nerve** (C5, 6, 7, **8, T1**)

**Inconstant contribution**

Pronator teres muscle (humeral head)

Articular branch

Flexor carpi radialis muscle

Palmaris longus muscle

Pronator teres muscle (ulnar head)

Flexor digitorum superficialis muscle
(*turned up*)

Flexor digitorum profundus muscle
(lateral part supplied by median
[anterior interosseous] nerve; medial
part supplied by ulnar nerve)

Anterior interosseous nerve

Flexor pollicis longus muscle

Pronator quadratus muscle

Palmar branch of median nerve

Thenar
muscles
{
Abductor pollicis brevis
Opponens pollicis
Superficial head of
flexor pollicis brevis
(deep head
supplied by
ulnar nerve)

1st and 2nd
lumbrical muscles

Dorsal branches to
dorsum of middle and
distal phalanges

Medial
Posterior
Lateral
}
Cords of
brachial
plexus

Medial brachial
cutaneous nerve

Medial antebrachial
cutaneous nerve

Axillary nerve

Radial nerve

Ulnar nerve

Communicating branch
of median nerve with
ulnar nerve

Common palmar
digital nerves

Proper palmar
digital nerves

**Cutaneous
innervation**

**Palmar view**

**Posterior (dorsal) view**

**Plate 463**

**Neurovasculature**

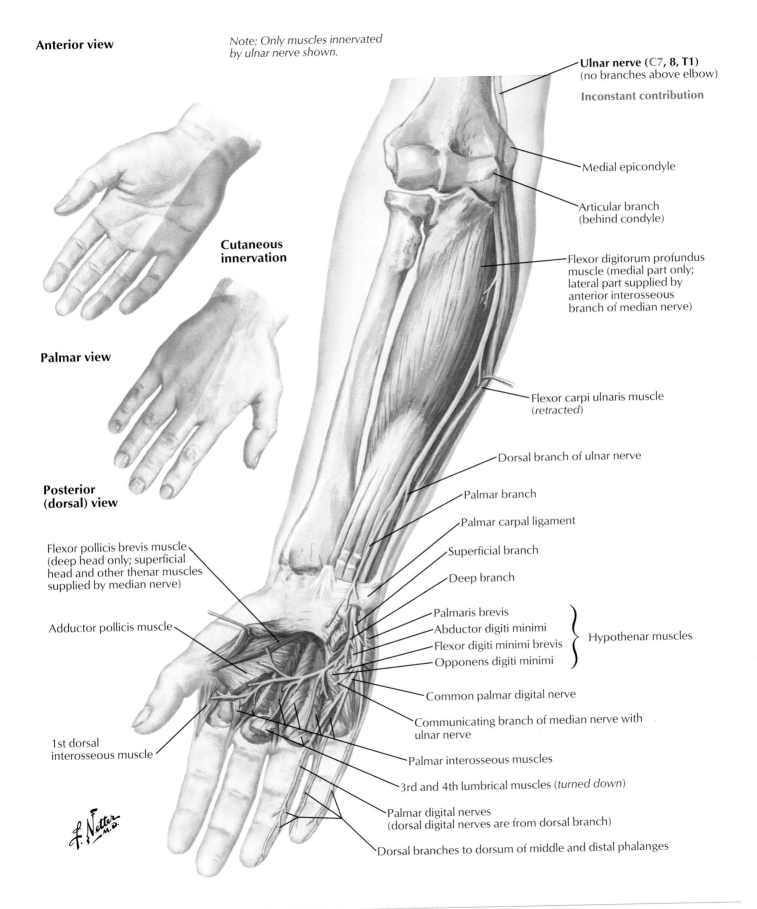

**Anterior view**

*Note: Only muscles innervated by ulnar nerve shown.*

**Ulnar nerve (C7, 8, T1)**
(no branches above elbow)

**Inconstant contribution**

**Cutaneous innervation**

Medial epicondyle

Articular branch
(behind condyle)

Flexor digitorum profundus
muscle (medial part only;
lateral part supplied by
anterior interosseous
branch of median nerve)

**Palmar view**

**Posterior
(dorsal) view**

Flexor carpi ulnaris muscle
(*retracted*)

Dorsal branch of ulnar nerve

Palmar branch

Palmar carpal ligament

Superficial branch

Flexor pollicis brevis muscle
(deep head only; superficial
head and other thenar muscles
supplied by median nerve)

Deep branch

Palmaris brevis

Abductor digiti minimi

Flexor digiti minimi brevis

Opponens digiti minimi

} Hypothenar muscles

Adductor pollicis muscle

Common palmar digital nerve

Communicating branch of median nerve with
ulnar nerve

1st dorsal
interosseous muscle

Palmar interosseous muscles

3rd and 4th lumbrical muscles (*turned down*)

Palmar digital nerves
(dorsal digital nerves are from dorsal branch)

Dorsal branches to dorsum of middle and distal phalanges

*f. Netter*
*m.d.*

**Neurovasculature**

**Plate 464**

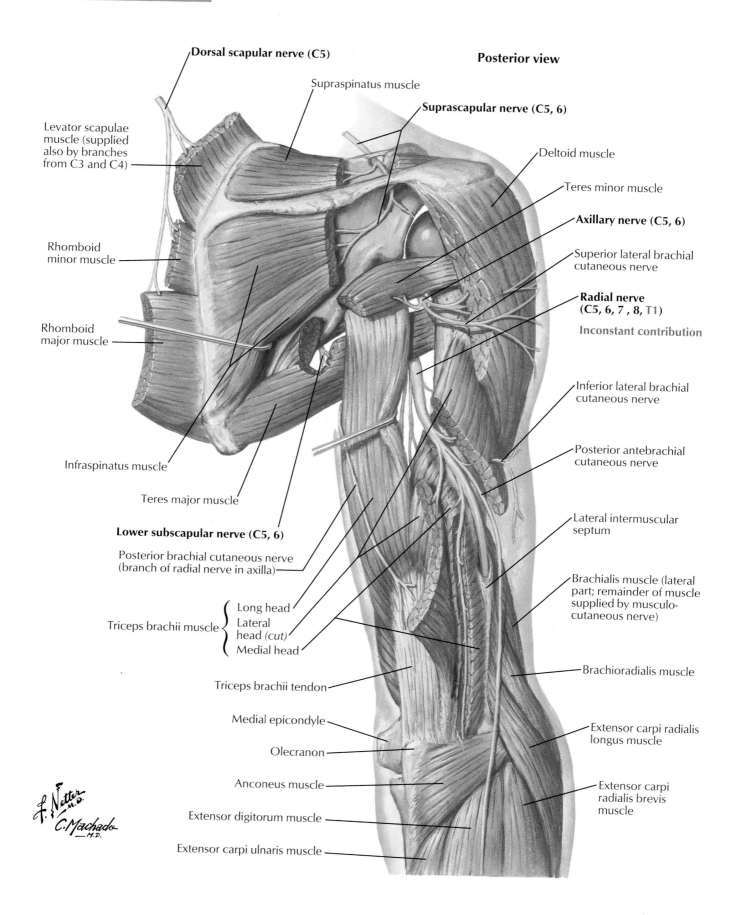

**Dorsal scapular nerve (C5)**

Supraspinatus muscle

**Posterior view**

**Suprascapular nerve (C5, 6)**

Levator scapulae muscle (supplied also by branches from C3 and C4)

Deltoid muscle

Teres minor muscle

**Axillary nerve (C5, 6)**

Superior lateral brachial cutaneous nerve

Rhomboid minor muscle

**Radial nerve (C5, 6, 7, 8, T1)**

Inconstant contribution

Rhomboid major muscle

Inferior lateral brachial cutaneous nerve

Infraspinatus muscle

Posterior antebrachial cutaneous nerve

Teres major muscle

Lateral intermuscular septum

**Lower subscapular nerve (C5, 6)**

Posterior brachial cutaneous nerve (branch of radial nerve in axilla)

Brachialis muscle (lateral part; remainder of muscle supplied by musculo-cutaneous nerve)

Triceps brachii muscle { Long head / Lateral head *(cut)* / Medial head

Brachioradialis muscle

Triceps brachii tendon

Medial epicondyle

Extensor carpi radialis longus muscle

Olecranon

Anconeus muscle

Extensor carpi radialis brevis muscle

Extensor digitorum muscle

Extensor carpi ulnaris muscle

**Plate 465**

**Neurovasculature**

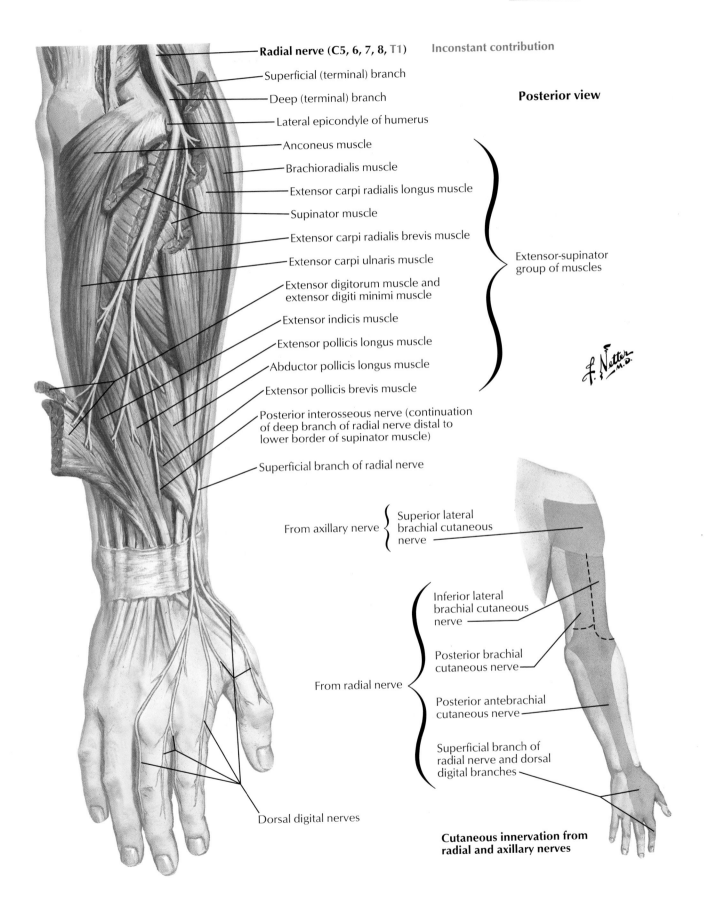

**Radial nerve (C5, 6, 7, 8, T1)**    Inconstant contribution

Superficial (terminal) branch

Deep (terminal) branch

Lateral epicondyle of humerus

**Posterior view**

Anconeus muscle

Brachioradialis muscle

Extensor carpi radialis longus muscle

Supinator muscle

Extensor carpi radialis brevis muscle

Extensor carpi ulnaris muscle

Extensor-supinator group of muscles

Extensor digitorum muscle and extensor digiti minimi muscle

Extensor indicis muscle

Extensor pollicis longus muscle

Abductor pollicis longus muscle

Extensor pollicis brevis muscle

Posterior interosseous nerve (continuation of deep branch of radial nerve distal to lower border of supinator muscle)

Superficial branch of radial nerve

From axillary nerve {
Superior lateral brachial cutaneous nerve

Inferior lateral brachial cutaneous nerve

Posterior brachial cutaneous nerve

From radial nerve {

Posterior antebrachial cutaneous nerve

Superficial branch of radial nerve and dorsal digital branches

Dorsal digital nerves

**Cutaneous innervation from radial and axillary nerves**

**MRI**

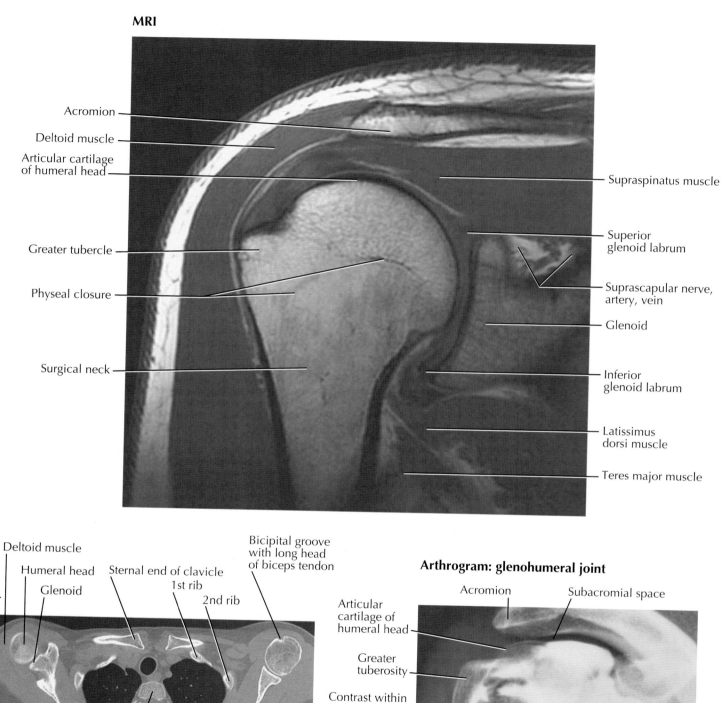

Acromion

Deltoid muscle

Articular cartilage of humeral head

Greater tubercle

Physeal closure

Surgical neck

Supraspinatus muscle

Superior glenoid labrum

Suprascapular nerve, artery, vein

Glenoid

Inferior glenoid labrum

Latissimus dorsi muscle

Teres major muscle

**CT**

Deltoid muscle

Humeral head

Glenoid

Sternal end of clavicle

1st rib

2nd rib

Bicipital groove with long head of biceps tendon

Scapula

Vertebral border of scapula

Body of T2

Subscapularis muscle

Infraspinatus muscle

**Arthrogram: glenohumeral joint**

Acromion

Subacromial space

Articular cartilage of humeral head

Greater tuberosity

Contrast within glenohumeral joint capsule

Bicipital groove

Contrast within sheath of biceps long head

Surgical neck

Axillary recess

Subscapular recess

**Plate 467**

**Regional Scans**

| MUSCLE | PROXIMAL ATTACHMENT (ORIGIN) | DISTAL ATTACHMENT (INSERTION) | INNERVATION | MAIN ACTIONS | BLOOD SUPPLY | MUSCLE GROUP |
|---|---|---|---|---|---|---|
| Abductor digiti minimi | Pisiform bone and tendon of flexor carpi ulnaris | Medial side of base of proximal phalanx of little finger (5th digit) | Ulnar nerve (deep branch) | Abducts little finger | Deep palmar branch of ulnar artery | Hand |
| Abductor pollicis brevis | Flexor retinaculum, tubercles of scaphoid and trapezium | Lateral side of base of proximal phalanx of thumb | Median nerve (recurrent branch) | Abducts thumb | Superficial palmar branch of radial artery | Hand |
| Abductor pollicis longus | Posterior surface of ulna, radius, and interosseous membrane | Base of 1st metacarpal | Radial nerve (posterior interosseous) | Abducts and extends thumb at carpometacarpal joint | Posterior interosseous artery | Posterior forearm |
| Adductor pollicis | *Oblique head*: bases of 2nd and 3rd metacarpals and capitate and adjacent bones<br><br>*Transverse head*: anterior surface of 3rd metacarpal | Medial side of base of proximal phalanx of thumb | Ulnar nerve (deep branch) | Adducts thumb | Deep palmar arch | Hand |
| Anconeus | Posterior surface of lateral epicondyle of humerus | Lateral surface of olecranon and posterior proximal ulna | Radial nerve (C5–T1) | Assists triceps in extending elbow, abducts ulna in pronation | Deep brachial artery | Arm |
| Biceps brachii | *Long head*: supraglenoid tubercle of scapula<br><br>*Short head*: tip of coracoid process of scapula | Radial tuberosity, fascia of forearm via bicipital aponeurosis | Musculocutaneous nerve (C5,C6) | Flexes and supinates forearm at elbow | Muscular branches of brachial artery | Arm |
| Brachialis | Distal half of anterior surface of humerus | Coronoid process and tuberosity of ulna | Musculocutaneous nerve and radial nerve (C7) | Flexes forearm at elbow | Radial recurrent artery, muscular branches of brachial artery | Arm |
| Brachioradialis | Proximal 2/3 of lateral supracondylar ridge of humerus | Lateral side of distal end of radius | Radial nerve | Weak flexion of forearm when forearm is midpronated | Radial recurrent artery | Posterior forearm |
| Coracobrachialis | Tip of coracoid process of scapula | Middle third of medial surface of humerus | Musculocutaneous nerve | Flexes and adducts arm at shoulder | Muscular branches of brachial artery | Arm |
| Deltoid | Lateral third of anterior clavicle, lateral acromion, inferior edge of spine of scapula | Deltoid tuberosity of humerus | Axillary nerve | *Clavicular part*: flexes and medially rotates arm<br><br>*Acromial part*: abducts arm beyond initial 15 degrees done by supraspinatus<br><br>*Spinal part*: extends and laterally rotates arm | Posterior circumflex humeral artery, deltoid branch of thoraco-acromial artery | Shoulder |
| Dorsal interosseous muscles | Adjacent sides of two metacarpal bones | Base of proximal phalanges, extensor expansion of digits 2–4 | Ulnar nerve (deep branch) | Abduct digits from axial line of hand (3rd digit); flex digits at metacarpophalangeal joint and extend interphalangeal joints | Deep palmar arch | Hand |
| Extensor carpi radialis brevis | Lateral epicondyle of humerus | Dorsal base of 3rd metacarpal and slip to 2nd metacarpal | Radial nerve (deep branch) | Extends and abducts hand at wrist | Radial artery, radial recurrent artery | Posterior forearm |
| Extensor carpi radialis longus | Distal third of lateral supracondylar ridge of humerus | Dorsal base of 2nd metacarpal and slip to 3rd metacarpal | Radial nerve | Extends and abducts hand at wrist | Radial artery, radial recurrent artery | Posterior forearm |

Variations in spinal nerve contributions to the innervation of muscles, their arterial supply, their attachments, and their actions are common themes in human anatomy. Therefore, expect differences between texts and realize that anatomical variation is normal.

**Muscle Tables**

**Table 6-1**

# Muscle Tables

| MUSCLE | PROXIMAL ATTACHMENT (ORIGIN) | DISTAL ATTACHMENT (INSERTION) | INNERVATION | MAIN ACTIONS | BLOOD SUPPLY | MUSCLE GROUP |
|---|---|---|---|---|---|---|
| Extensor carpi ulnaris | Lateral epicondyle of humerus and posterior border of ulna | Dorsal base of 5th metacarpal | Radial nerve (posterior interosseous) | Extends and adducts hand at wrist | Posterior interosseous artery | Posterior forearm |
| Extensor digiti minimi | Lateral epicondyle of humerus | Extensor expansion of 5th digit | Radial nerve (posterior interosseous) | Extends 5th digit | Posterior interosseous artery | Posterior forearm |
| Extensor digitorum | Lateral epicondyle of humerus | Extensor expansions of medial four digits | Radial nerve (posterior interosseous) | Extends medial four digits, assists in wrist extension | Posterior interosseous artery | Posterior forearm |
| Extensor indicis | Posterior surface of ulna and interosseous membrane | Extensor expansion of 2nd digit | Radial nerve (posterior interosseous) | Extends 2nd digit and helps extend hand at wrist | Posterior interosseous artery | Posterior forearm |
| Extensor pollicis brevis | Posterior surface of radius and interosseous membrane | Dorsal base of proximal phalanx of thumb | Radial nerve (posterior interosseous) | Extends proximal phalanx of thumb at carpometacarpal joint | Posterior interosseous artery | Posterior forearm |
| Extensor pollicis longus | Posterior surface of middle third of ulna, interosseous membrane | Dorsal base of distal phalanx of thumb | Radial nerve (posterior interosseous) | Extends distal phalanx of thumb at interphalangeal and metacarpophalangeal joints | Posterior interosseous artery | Posterior forearm |
| Flexor carpi radialis | Medial epicondyle of humerus | Base of 2nd metacarpal | Median nerve | Flexes and abducts hand at wrist | Radial artery | Anterior forearm |
| Flexor carpi ulnaris | *Humeral head:* medial epicondyle of humerus  *Ulnar head:* olecranon and posterior border of ulna | Pisiform bone, hook of hamate, base of 5th metacarpal | Ulnar nerve | Flexes and adducts hand at wrist | Posterior ulnar recurrent artery | Anterior forearm |
| Flexor digiti minimi brevis | Flexor retinaculum and hook of hamate bone | Medial side of base of proximal phalanx of little finger | Ulnar nerve (deep branch) | Flexes proximal phalanx of little finger | Deep palmar branch of ulnar artery | Hand |
| Flexor digitorum profundus | Medial and anterior surface of proximal 3/4 of ulna and interosseous membrane | Palmar base of distal phalanges of medial four digits | *Medial part:* ulnar nerve  *Lateral part:* median nerve | Flexes distal phalanges of medial four digits, assists with flexion of hand at wrist | Anterior interosseous artery, muscular branches of ulnar artery | Anterior forearm |
| Flexor digitorum superficialis | *Humero-ulnar head:* medial epicondyle of humerus and coronoid process of ulna  *Radial head:* superior half of anterior radius | Bodies of middle phalanges of medial four digits | Median nerve | Flexes middle and proximal phalanges of medial four digits, flexes hand at wrist | Ulnar and radial arteries | Anterior forearm |
| Flexor pollicis brevis | Flexor retinaculum and tubercle of trapezium | Lateral side of base of proximal phalanx of thumb | Median nerve (recurrent branch) | Flexes proximal phalanx of thumb | Superficial palmar branch of radial artery | Hand |
| Flexor pollicis longus | Anterior surface of radius and interosseous membrane | Palmar base of distal phalanx of thumb | Median nerve (anterior interosseous) | Flexes phalanges of thumb | Anterior interosseous artery | Anterior forearm |
| Infraspinatus | Infraspinous fossa of scapula and deep fascia | Middle facet of greater tubercle of humerus | Suprascapular nerve | Lateral rotation of arm (with teres minor) | Suprascapular artery | Shoulder |

**Table 6-2**                                              **Muscle Tables**

| MUSCLE | PROXIMAL ATTACHMENT (ORIGIN) | DISTAL ATTACHMENT (INSERTION) | INNERVATION | MAIN ACTIONS | BLOOD SUPPLY | MUSCLE GROUP |
|---|---|---|---|---|---|---|
| Latissimus dorsi | Spinous processes of T7–L5 vertebrae, thoracolumbar fascia, iliac crest, last 3 ribs | Intertubercular sulcus of humerus | Thoracodorsal nerve | Extends, adducts, and medially rotates humerus at shoulder | Thoracodorsal artery, dorsal perforating branches of 9th, 10th, and 11th posterior intercostal, subcostal, and first three lumbar arteries | Shoulder |
| Levator scapulae | Posterior tubercles of transverse processes of C1–C4 | Medial border of scapula from superior angle to spine | Ventral rami of C3–C4 and dorsal scapular nerve | Elevates scapula medially, inferiorly rotates glenoid cavity | Dorsal scapular artery, transverse cervical artery, ascending cervical artery | Superficial back |
| Lumbrical, first and second | Lateral two tendons of flexor digitorum profundus | Lateral sides of extensor expansion of digits 2 and 3 | Median nerve (digital branches) | Extend digits at interphalangeal joints, flex metacarpophalangeal joints | Superficial and deep palmar arches | Hand |
| Lumbrical, third and fourth | Medial three tendons of flexor digitorum profundus | Lateral sides of extensor expansion of digits 4 and 5 | Ulnar nerve (deep branch) | Extend digits at interphalangeal joints, flex metacarpophalangeal joints | Superficial and deep palmar arches | Hand |
| Opponens digiti minimi | Flexor retinaculum and hook of hamate bone | Palmar surface of 5th metacarpal | Ulnar nerve (deep branch) | Draws 5th metacarpal anteriorly and rotates it to face thumb | Deep palmar branch of ulnar artery | Hand |
| Opponens pollicis | Flexor retinaculum and tubercle of trapezium | Lateral side of 1st metacarpal | Median nerve (recurrent branch) | Draws 1st metacarpal forward and rotates it medially | Superficial palmar branch of radial artery | Hand |
| Palmar interosseous muscles | Sides of metacarpals 2, 4, and 5 | Bases of proximal phalanx and extensor expansion of digits 2, 4, and 5 | Ulnar nerve (deep branch) | Adducts digits toward axial line of hand (3rd digit); flexes digits at metacarpophalngeal joint and extends interphalangeal joints | Deep palmar arch | Hand |
| Palmaris brevis | Palmar aponeurosis and flexor retinaculum | Skin of medial border of palm | Superficial palmar branch of ulnar nerve | Deepens hollow of hand, assists grip | Superficial palmar arch | Hand |
| Palmaris longus | Medial epicondyle of humerus | Distal half of flexor retinaculum and palmar aponeurosis | Median nerve | Flexes hand at wrist and tenses palmar aponeurosis | Posterior ulnar recurrent artery | Anterior forearm |
| Pectoralis major | Sternal half of clavicle, sternum to 7th rib, cartilages of true ribs, aponeurosis of external oblique muscle | Lateral lip of intertubercular sulcus of humerus | Medial and lateral pectoral nerves | Flexes and adducts arm, rotates arm medially | Pectoral branch of thoraco-acromial artery, perforating branches of internal thoracic artery | Pectoral region/axilla |
| Pectoralis minor | Outer surface of upper margin of ribs 3–5 | Coracoid process of scapula | Medial pectoral nerve | Lowers lateral angle of scapula and protracts scapula | Pectoral branch of thoraco-acromial and intercostal lateral thoracic arteries | Pectoral region/axilla |
| Pronator quadratus | Distal fourth of anterior ulna | Distal fourth of anterior radius | Median nerve (anterior interosseous) | Pronates forearm | Anterior interosseous artery | Anterior forearm |
| Pronator teres | Two heads: medial epicondyle of humerus and coronoid process of ulna | Midway along lateral surface of radius | Median nerve | Pronates forearm and assists with elbow flexion | Anterior ulnar recurrent artery | Anterior forearm |

| MUSCLE | PROXIMAL ATTACHMENT (ORIGIN) | DISTAL ATTACHMENT (INSERTION) | INNERVATION | MAIN ACTIONS | BLOOD SUPPLY | MUSCLE GROUP |
|---|---|---|---|---|---|---|
| Rhomboid major | Spinous processes of T2–T5 vertebrae | Medial border of scapula below base of spine of scapula | Dorsal scapular nerve | Fixes scapula to thoracic wall and retracts and rotates it to depress glenoid cavity | Dorsal scapular OR deep branch of transverse cervical artery, dorsal perforating branches of the upper five or six posterior intercostal arteries artery | Superficial back |
| Rhomboid minor | Ligamentum nuchae, spines of C7 and T1 vertebrae | Medial border of scapula at spine of scapula | Dorsal scapular nerve | Fixes scapula to thoracic wall and retracts and rotates it to depress glenoid cavity | Dorsal scapular artery OR deep branch of transverse cervical artery, dorsal perforating branches of the upper five or six posterior intercostal arteries | Superficial back |
| Serratus anterior | Lateral surfaces of upper 8–9 ribs | Costal surface of medial border of scapula | Long thoracic nerve | Protracts and rotates scapula and holds it against thoracic wall | Lateral thoracic artery | Shoulder |
| Subclavius | Upper border of 1st rib and its cartilage | Inferior surface of middle third of clavicle | Nerve to subclavius | Anchors and depresses clavicle | Clavicular branch of thoraco-acromial artery | Shoulder |
| Subscapularis | Subscapular fossa | Lesser tubercle of humerus | Upper and lower subscapular nerves | Medially rotates arm at shoulder and adducts it, helps hold humeral head in glenoid cavity | Subscapular artery, lateral thoracic artery | Shoulder |
| Supinator | Lateral epicondyle of humerus, supinator crest of ulna | Lateral, posterior, and anterior surfaces of proximal third of radius | Radial nerve (deep branch) | Supinates forearm | Radial recurrent artery, posterior interosseous arteries | Posterior forearm |
| Supraspinatus | Supraspinous fossa of scapula and deep fascia | Superior facet of greater tubercle of humerus | Suprascapular nerve | Initiates arm abduction, acts with rotator cuff muscles | Suprascapular artery | Shoulder |
| Teres major | Posterior surface of inferior angle of scapula | Medial lip of intertubercular sulcus of humerus | Lower subscapular nerve | Adducts and medially rotates arm | Circumflex scapular artery | Shoulder |
| Teres minor | Upper 2/3 of posterior surface of lateral border of scapula | Inferior facet of greater tubercle of humerus | Axillary nerve | Laterally rotates arm | Circumflex scapular artery | Shoulder |
| Trapezius | Superior nuchal line, external occipital protuberance, nuchal ligament, spinous processes of C7–T12 | Lateral third of clavicle, acromion, and spine of scapula | Accessory nerve (cranial nerve XI) | Elevates, retracts, and rotates scapula; lower fibers depress scapula | Transverse cervical artery, dorsal perforating branches of posterior intercostal arteries | Superficial back |
| Triceps brachii | *Long head:* infraglenoid tubercle of scapula<br><br>*Lateral head:* upper half of posterior humerus<br><br>*Medial head:* distal 2/3 of medial and posterior humerus | Posterior surface of olecranon process of ulna | Radial nerve | Extends forearm at elbow; long head stabilizes head of abducted humerus and extends and adducts arm at shoulder | Branch of profunda brachii artery | Arm |

**Table 6-4**

**Muscle Tables**

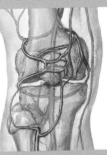

# 7 LOWER LIMB

## Topographic Anatomy
**Plate 468**

## Cutaneous Anatomy
**Plates 469–472**

## Hip and Thigh
**Plates 473–492**

## Muscle Tables

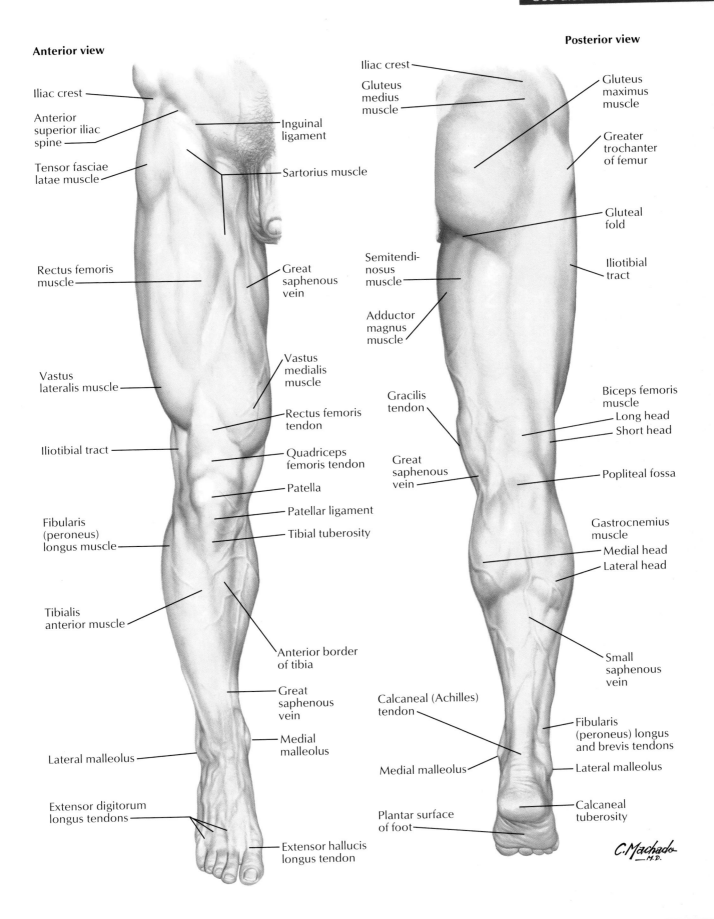

**Anterior view**

Iliac crest

Anterior superior iliac spine

Tensor fasciae latae muscle

Inguinal ligament

Sartorius muscle

Rectus femoris muscle

Great saphenous vein

Vastus lateralis muscle

Vastus medialis muscle

Rectus femoris tendon

Iliotibial tract

Quadriceps femoris tendon

Patella

Patellar ligament

Tibial tuberosity

Fibularis (peroneus) longus muscle

Tibialis anterior muscle

Anterior border of tibia

Great saphenous vein

Medial malleolus

Lateral malleolus

Extensor digitorum longus tendons

Extensor hallucis longus tendon

**Posterior view**

Iliac crest

Gluteus medius muscle

Gluteus maximus muscle

Greater trochanter of femur

Gluteal fold

Iliotibial tract

Semitendinosus muscle

Adductor magnus muscle

Gracilis tendon

Biceps femoris muscle
Long head
Short head

Great saphenous vein

Popliteal fossa

Gastrocnemius muscle
Medial head
Lateral head

Small saphenous vein

Calcaneal (Achilles) tendon

Fibularis (peroneus) longus and brevis tendons

Medial malleolus

Lateral malleolus

Plantar surface of foot

Calcaneal tuberosity

C. Machado M.D.

**Topographic Anatomy**

**Plate 468**

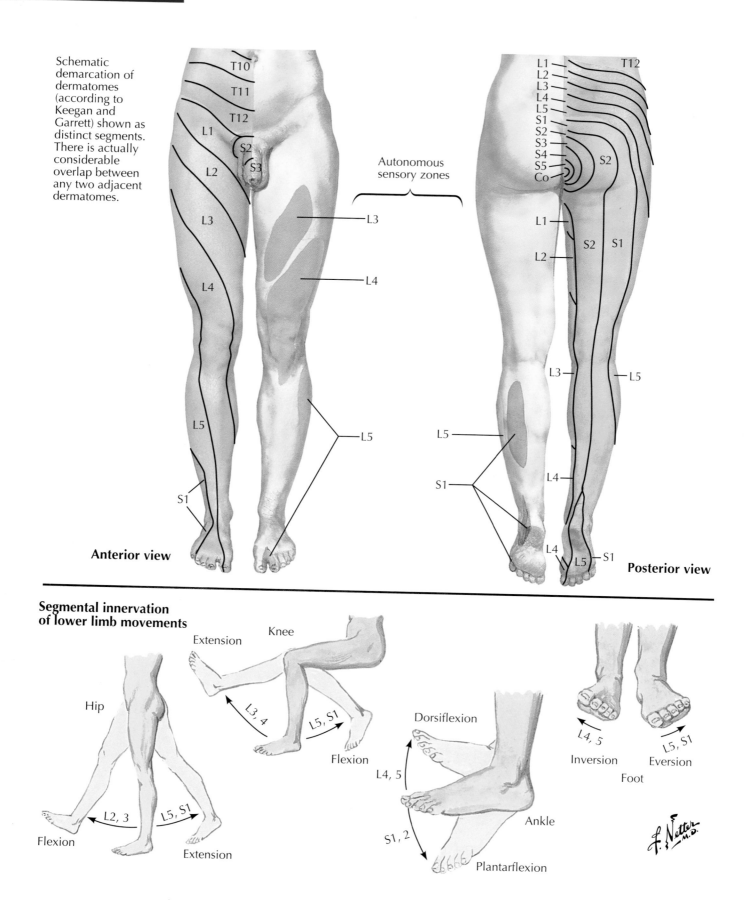

Schematic demarcation of dermatomes (according to Keegan and Garrett) shown as distinct segments. There is actually considerable overlap between any two adjacent dermatomes.

Autonomous sensory zones

**Anterior view**

**Posterior view**

**Segmental innervation of lower limb movements**

Hip

Knee

Extension

L3, 4

L5, S1

Flexion

Dorsiflexion

L4, 5

Inversion

L4, 5

Eversion

L5, S1

Foot

Flexion

L2, 3

L5, S1

Extension

S1, 2

Ankle

Plantarflexion

**Plate 469**

**Cutaneous Anatomy**

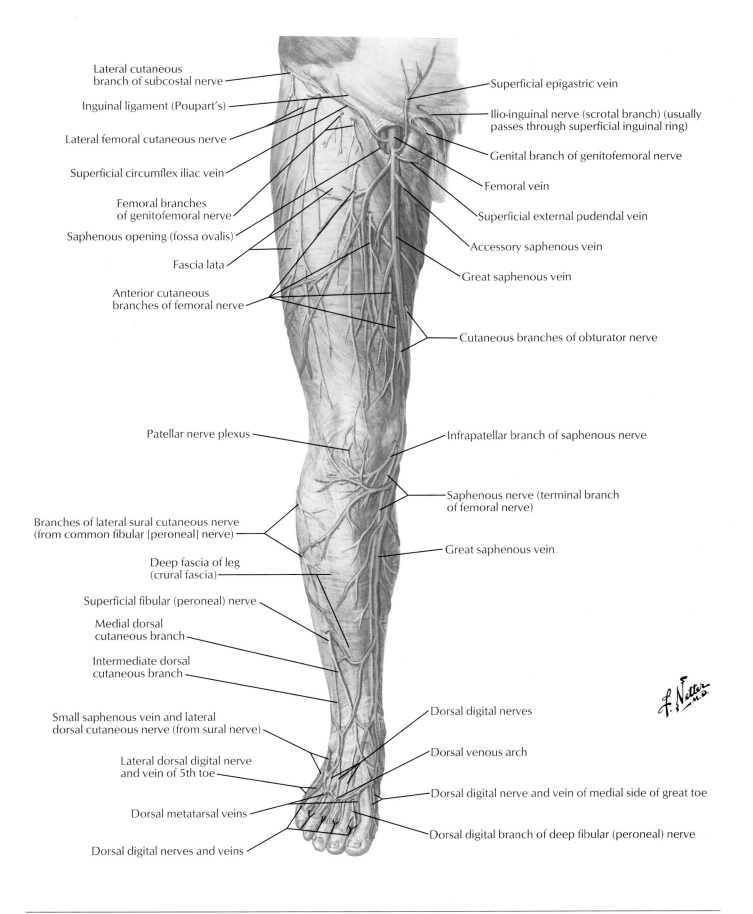

Lateral cutaneous branch of subcostal nerve

Inguinal ligament (Poupart's)

Lateral femoral cutaneous nerve

Superficial circumflex iliac vein

Femoral branches of genitofemoral nerve

Saphenous opening (fossa ovalis)

Fascia lata

Anterior cutaneous branches of femoral nerve

Patellar nerve plexus

Branches of lateral sural cutaneous nerve (from common fibular [peroneal] nerve)

Deep fascia of leg (crural fascia)

Superficial fibular (peroneal) nerve

Medial dorsal cutaneous branch

Intermediate dorsal cutaneous branch

Small saphenous vein and lateral dorsal cutaneous nerve (from sural nerve)

Lateral dorsal digital nerve and vein of 5th toe

Dorsal metatarsal veins

Dorsal digital nerves and veins

Superficial epigastric vein

Ilio-inguinal nerve (scrotal branch) (usually passes through superficial inguinal ring)

Genital branch of genitofemoral nerve

Femoral vein

Superficial external pudendal vein

Accessory saphenous vein

Great saphenous vein

Cutaneous branches of obturator nerve

Infrapatellar branch of saphenous nerve

Saphenous nerve (terminal branch of femoral nerve)

Great saphenous vein

Dorsal digital nerves

Dorsal venous arch

Dorsal digital nerve and vein of medial side of great toe

Dorsal digital branch of deep fibular (peroneal) nerve

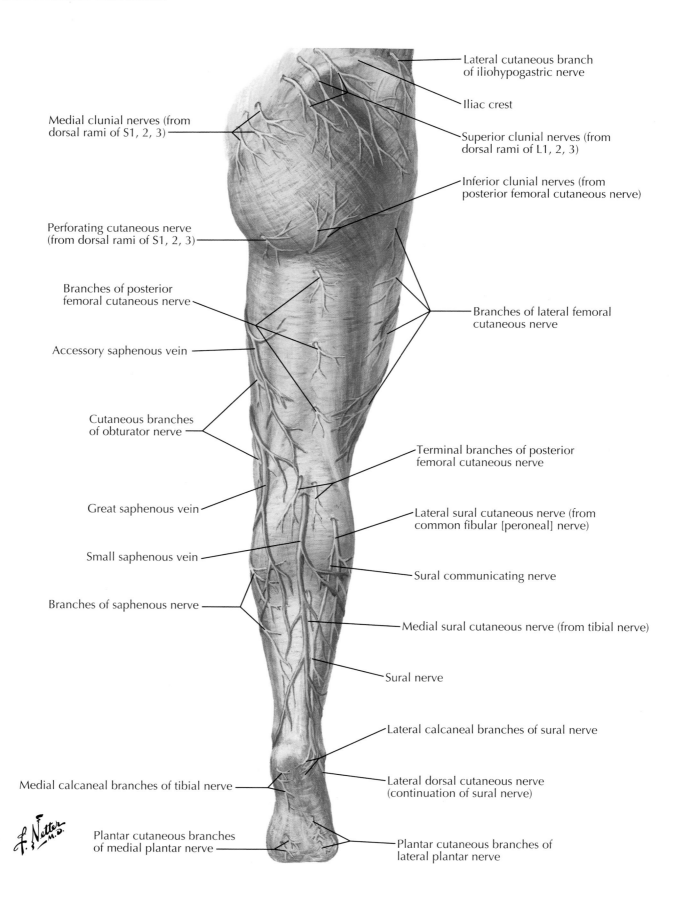

Lateral cutaneous branch
of iliohypogastric nerve

Iliac crest

Medial clunial nerves (from
dorsal rami of S1, 2, 3)

Superior clunial nerves (from
dorsal rami of L1, 2, 3)

Inferior clunial nerves (from
posterior femoral cutaneous nerve)

Perforating cutaneous nerve
(from dorsal rami of S1, 2, 3)

Branches of posterior
femoral cutaneous nerve

Branches of lateral femoral
cutaneous nerve

Accessory saphenous vein

Cutaneous branches
of obturator nerve

Terminal branches of posterior
femoral cutaneous nerve

Great saphenous vein

Lateral sural cutaneous nerve (from
common fibular [peroneal] nerve)

Small saphenous vein

Sural communicating nerve

Branches of saphenous nerve

Medial sural cutaneous nerve (from tibial nerve)

Sural nerve

Lateral calcaneal branches of sural nerve

Medial calcaneal branches of tibial nerve

Lateral dorsal cutaneous nerve
(continuation of sural nerve)

Plantar cutaneous branches
of medial plantar nerve

Plantar cutaneous branches of
lateral plantar nerve

**Plate 471**

**Cutaneous Anatomy**

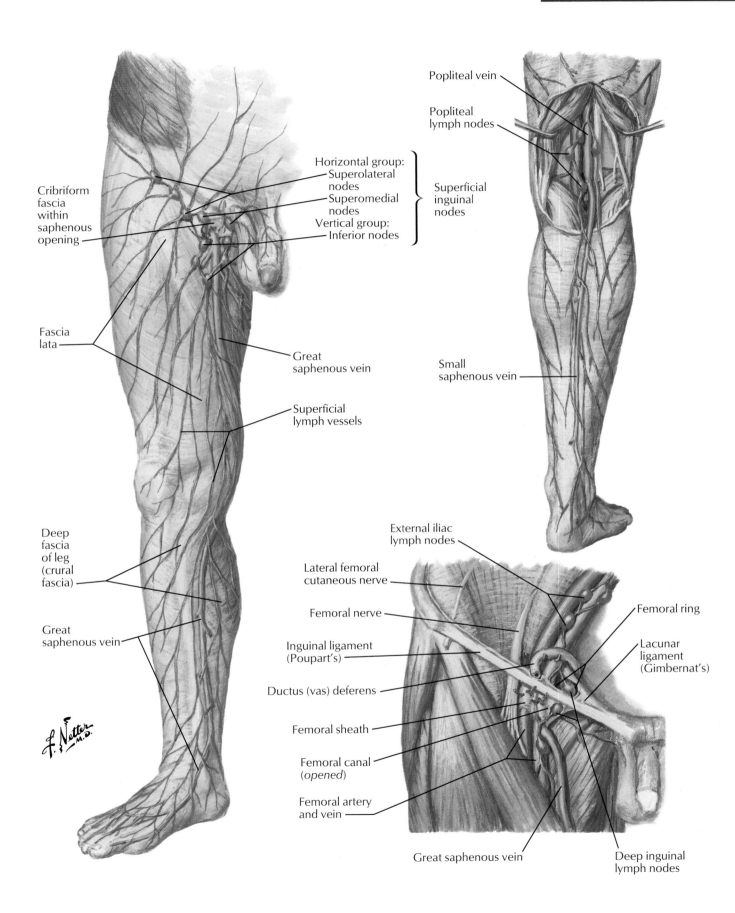

Popliteal vein

Popliteal
lymph nodes

Cribriform
fascia
within
saphenous
opening

Horizontal group:
Superolateral
nodes
Superomedial
nodes
Vertical group:
Inferior nodes

Superficial
inguinal
nodes

Fascia
lata

Great
saphenous vein

Small
saphenous vein

Superficial
lymph vessels

Deep
fascia
of leg
(crural
fascia)

External iliac
lymph nodes

Great
saphenous vein

Lateral femoral
cutaneous nerve

Femoral ring

Femoral nerve

Lacunar
ligament
(Gimbernat's)

Inguinal ligament
(Poupart's)

Ductus (vas) deferens

Femoral sheath

Femoral canal
(*opened*)

Femoral artery
and vein

Great saphenous vein

Deep inguinal
lymph nodes

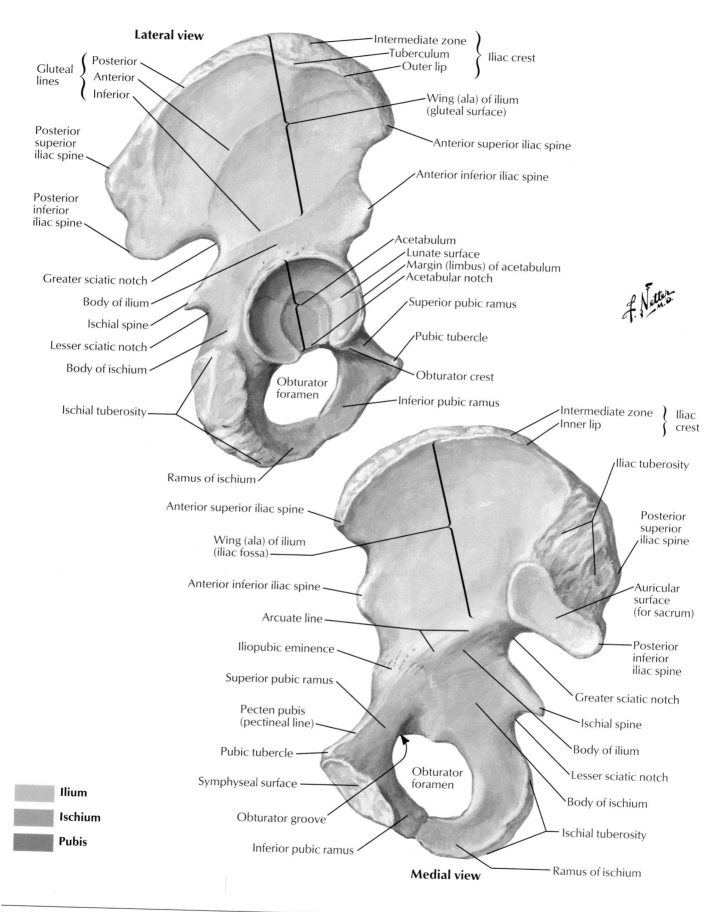

**Lateral view**

Gluteal lines { Posterior / Anterior / Inferior

Intermediate zone
Tuberculum
Outer lip
} Iliac crest

Wing (ala) of ilium (gluteal surface)

Anterior superior iliac spine

Posterior superior iliac spine

Anterior inferior iliac spine

Posterior inferior iliac spine

Acetabulum
Lunate surface
Margin (limbus) of acetabulum
Acetabular notch

Greater sciatic notch

Superior pubic ramus

Body of ilium

Ischial spine

Pubic tubercle

Lesser sciatic notch

Obturator crest

Body of ischium

Inferior pubic ramus

Obturator foramen

Ischial tuberosity

Ramus of ischium

Anterior superior iliac spine

Wing (ala) of ilium (iliac fossa)

Intermediate zone
Inner lip
} Iliac crest

Iliac tuberosity

Posterior superior iliac spine

Anterior inferior iliac spine

Arcuate line

Iliopubic eminence

Auricular surface (for sacrum)

Superior pubic ramus

Posterior inferior iliac spine

Pecten pubis (pectineal line)

Greater sciatic notch

Pubic tubercle

Ischial spine

Symphyseal surface

Body of ilium

Obturator groove

Obturator foramen

Lesser sciatic notch

Body of ischium

Ischial tuberosity

Inferior pubic ramus

Ramus of ischium

**Medial view**

Ilium

Ischium

Pubis

**Plate 473**

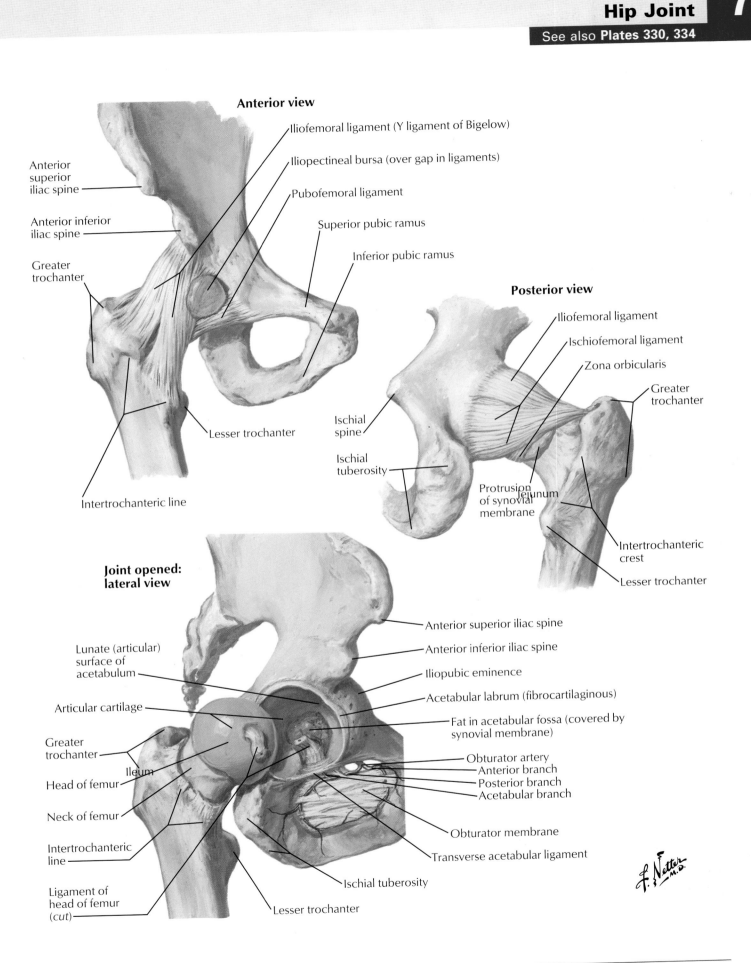

**Anterior view**

Iliofemoral ligament (Y ligament of Bigelow)

Iliopectineal bursa (over gap in ligaments)

Pubofemoral ligament

Superior pubic ramus

Inferior pubic ramus

Anterior superior iliac spine

Anterior inferior iliac spine

Greater trochanter

Lesser trochanter

Intertrochanteric line

**Posterior view**

Iliofemoral ligament

Ischiofemoral ligament

Zona orbicularis

Greater trochanter

Ischial spine

Ischial tuberosity

Protrusion of synovial membrane

Jejunum

Intertrochanteric crest

Lesser trochanter

**Joint opened: lateral view**

Lunate (articular) surface of acetabulum

Articular cartilage

Greater trochanter

Ileum

Head of femur

Neck of femur

Intertrochanteric line

Ligament of head of femur (cut)

Anterior superior iliac spine

Anterior inferior iliac spine

Iliopubic eminence

Acetabular labrum (fibrocartilaginous)

Fat in acetabular fossa (covered by synovial membrane)

Obturator artery

Anterior branch

Posterior branch

Acetabular branch

Obturator membrane

Transverse acetabular ligament

Ischial tuberosity

Lesser trochanter

*F. Netter M.D.*

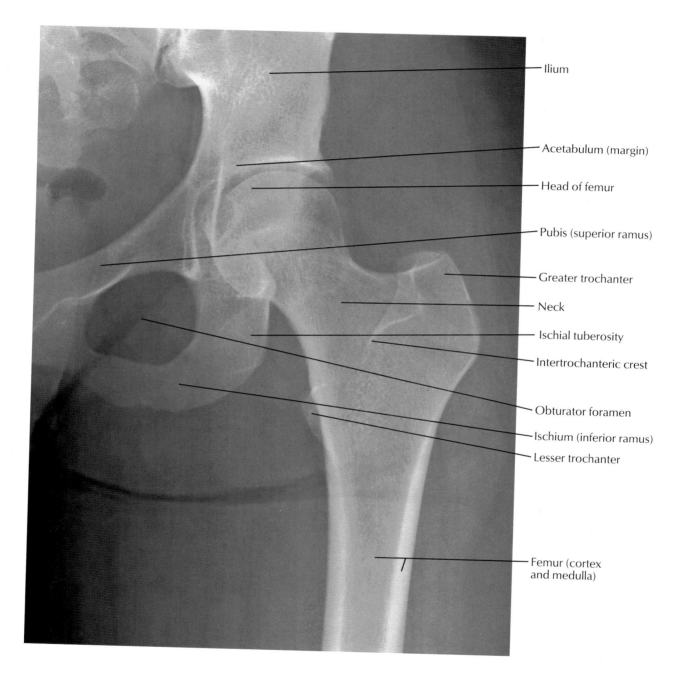

Ilium

Acetabulum (margin)

Head of femur

Pubis (superior ramus)

Greater trochanter

Neck

Ischial tuberosity

Intertrochanteric crest

Obturator foramen

Ischium (inferior ramus)

Lesser trochanter

Femur (cortex and medulla)

**Plate 475**

**Hip and Thigh**

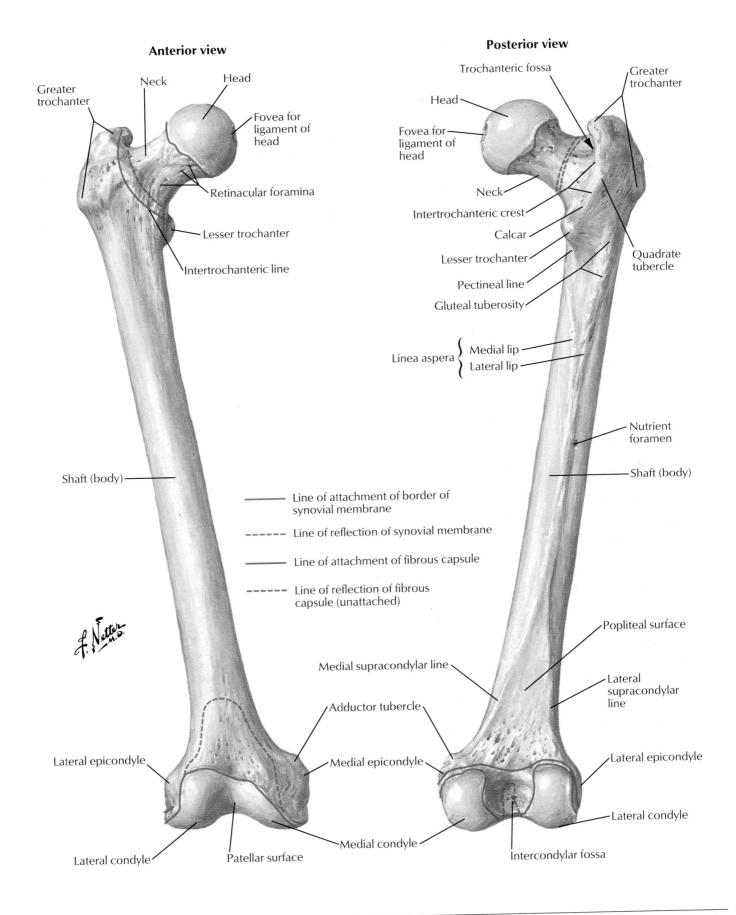

**Anterior view**

Greater trochanter

Neck

Head

Fovea for ligament of head

Retinacular foramina

Lesser trochanter

Intertrochanteric line

Shaft (body)

Line of attachment of border of synovial membrane

Line of reflection of synovial membrane

Line of attachment of fibrous capsule

Line of reflection of fibrous capsule (unattached)

Medial supracondylar line

Adductor tubercle

Lateral epicondyle

Medial epicondyle

Lateral condyle

Patellar surface

Medial condyle

**Posterior view**

Trochanteric fossa

Greater trochanter

Head

Fovea for ligament of head

Neck

Intertrochanteric crest

Calcar

Lesser trochanter

Pectineal line

Gluteal tuberosity

Quadrate tubercle

Linea aspera { Medial lip / Lateral lip }

Nutrient foramen

Shaft (body)

Popliteal surface

Lateral supracondylar line

Lateral epicondyle

Lateral condyle

Intercondylar fossa

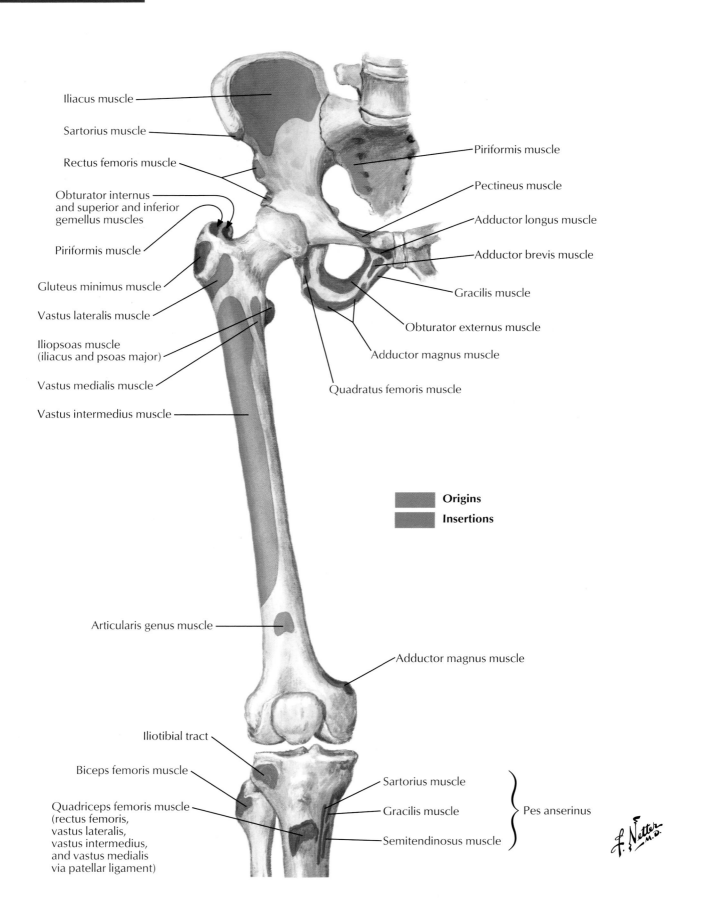

Iliacus muscle

Sartorius muscle

Rectus femoris muscle

Obturator internus
and superior and inferior
gemellus muscles

Piriformis muscle

Gluteus minimus muscle

Vastus lateralis muscle

Iliopsoas muscle
(iliacus and psoas major)

Vastus medialis muscle

Vastus intermedius muscle

Piriformis muscle

Pectineus muscle

Adductor longus muscle

Adductor brevis muscle

Gracilis muscle

Obturator externus muscle

Adductor magnus muscle

Quadratus femoris muscle

Origins
Insertions

Articularis genus muscle

Adductor magnus muscle

Iliotibial tract

Biceps femoris muscle

Quadriceps femoris muscle
(rectus femoris,
vastus lateralis,
vastus intermedius,
and vastus medialis
via patellar ligament)

Sartorius muscle

Gracilis muscle

Semitendinosus muscle

Pes anserinus

**Plate 477**

**Hip and Thigh**

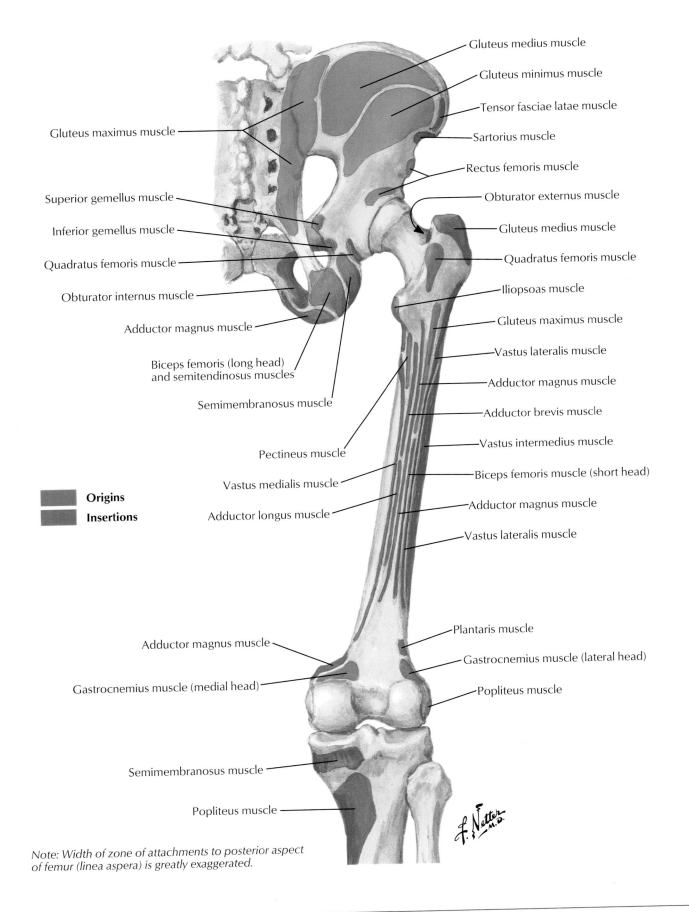

Gluteus medius muscle

Gluteus minimus muscle

Tensor fasciae latae muscle

Sartorius muscle

Rectus femoris muscle

Obturator externus muscle

Gluteus medius muscle

Quadratus femoris muscle

Iliopsoas muscle

Gluteus maximus muscle

Vastus lateralis muscle

Adductor magnus muscle

Adductor brevis muscle

Vastus intermedius muscle

Biceps femoris muscle (short head)

Adductor magnus muscle

Vastus lateralis muscle

Plantaris muscle

Gastrocnemius muscle (lateral head)

Popliteus muscle

Gluteus maximus muscle

Superior gemellus muscle

Inferior gemellus muscle

Quadratus femoris muscle

Obturator internus muscle

Adductor magnus muscle

Biceps femoris (long head) and semitendinosus muscles

Semimembranosus muscle

Pectineus muscle

Vastus medialis muscle

Adductor longus muscle

Origins
Insertions

Adductor magnus muscle

Gastrocnemius muscle (medial head)

Semimembranosus muscle

Popliteus muscle

*Note: Width of zone of attachments to posterior aspect of femur (linea aspera) is greatly exaggerated.*

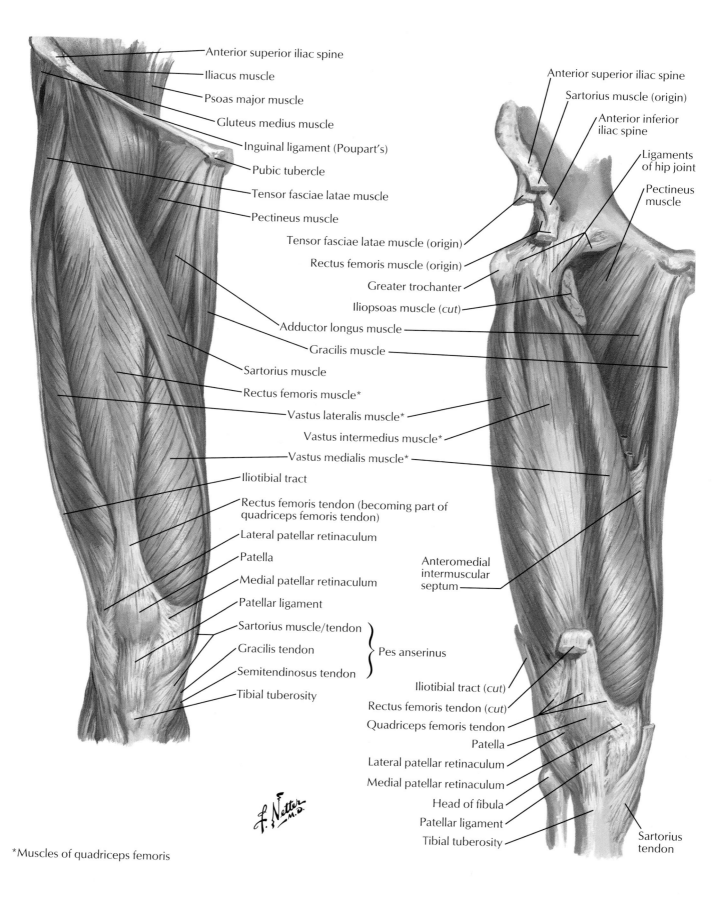

Anterior superior iliac spine

Iliacus muscle

Psoas major muscle

Gluteus medius muscle

Inguinal ligament (Poupart's)

Pubic tubercle

Tensor fasciae latae muscle

Pectineus muscle

Tensor fasciae latae muscle (origin)

Rectus femoris muscle (origin)

Greater trochanter

Iliopsoas muscle (cut)

Adductor longus muscle

Gracilis muscle

Sartorius muscle

Rectus femoris muscle*

Vastus lateralis muscle*

Vastus intermedius muscle*

Vastus medialis muscle*

Iliotibial tract

Rectus femoris tendon (becoming part of quadriceps femoris tendon)

Lateral patellar retinaculum

Patella

Medial patellar retinaculum

Patellar ligament

Sartorius muscle/tendon

Gracilis tendon

Semitendinosus tendon

Tibial tuberosity

Anterior superior iliac spine

Sartorius muscle (origin)

Anterior inferior iliac spine

Ligaments of hip joint

Pectineus muscle

Anteromedial intermuscular septum

} Pes anserinus

Iliotibial tract (cut)

Rectus femoris tendon (cut)

Quadriceps femoris tendon

Patella

Lateral patellar retinaculum

Medial patellar retinaculum

Head of fibula

Patellar ligament

Tibial tuberosity

Sartorius tendon

*Muscles of quadriceps femoris

**Plate 479**

**Hip and Thigh**

**Deep dissection**

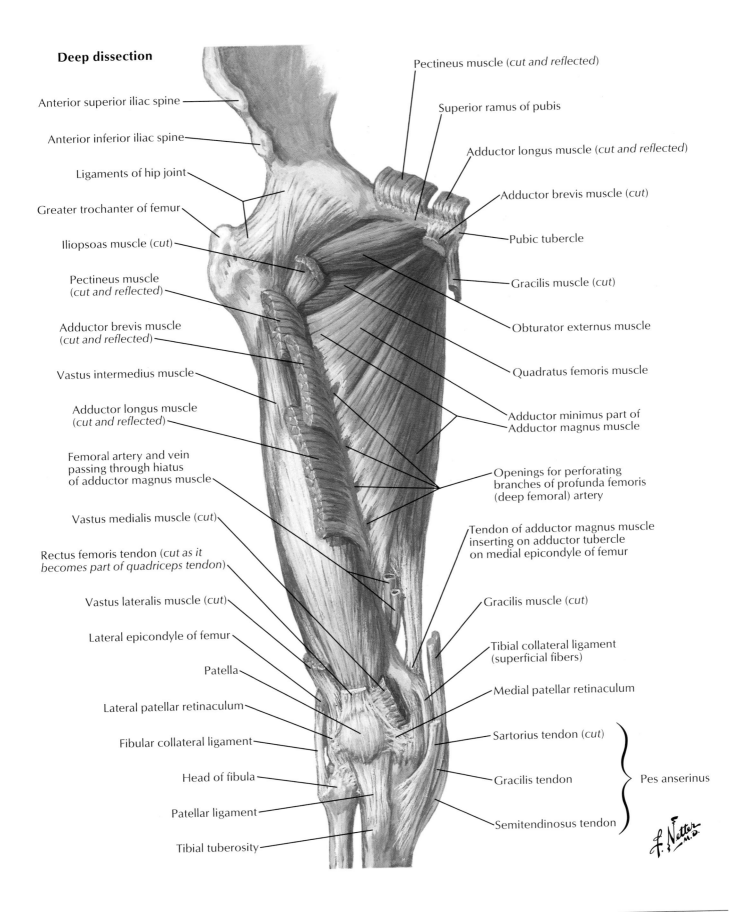

Pectineus muscle (*cut and reflected*)

Superior ramus of pubis

Adductor longus muscle (*cut and reflected*)

Adductor brevis muscle (*cut*)

Pubic tubercle

Gracilis muscle (*cut*)

Obturator externus muscle

Quadratus femoris muscle

Adductor minimus part of Adductor magnus muscle

Openings for perforating branches of profunda femoris (deep femoral) artery

Tendon of adductor magnus muscle inserting on adductor tubercle on medial epicondyle of femur

Gracilis muscle (*cut*)

Tibial collateral ligament (superficial fibers)

Medial patellar retinaculum

Sartorius tendon (*cut*)

Gracilis tendon

Semitendinosus tendon

Pes anserinus

Anterior superior iliac spine

Anterior inferior iliac spine

Ligaments of hip joint

Greater trochanter of femur

Iliopsoas muscle (*cut*)

Pectineus muscle (*cut and reflected*)

Adductor brevis muscle (*cut and reflected*)

Vastus intermedius muscle

Adductor longus muscle (*cut and reflected*)

Femoral artery and vein passing through hiatus of adductor magnus muscle

Vastus medialis muscle (*cut*)

Rectus femoris tendon (*cut as it becomes part of quadriceps tendon*)

Vastus lateralis muscle (*cut*)

Lateral epicondyle of femur

Patella

Lateral patellar retinaculum

Fibular collateral ligament

Head of fibula

Patellar ligament

Tibial tuberosity

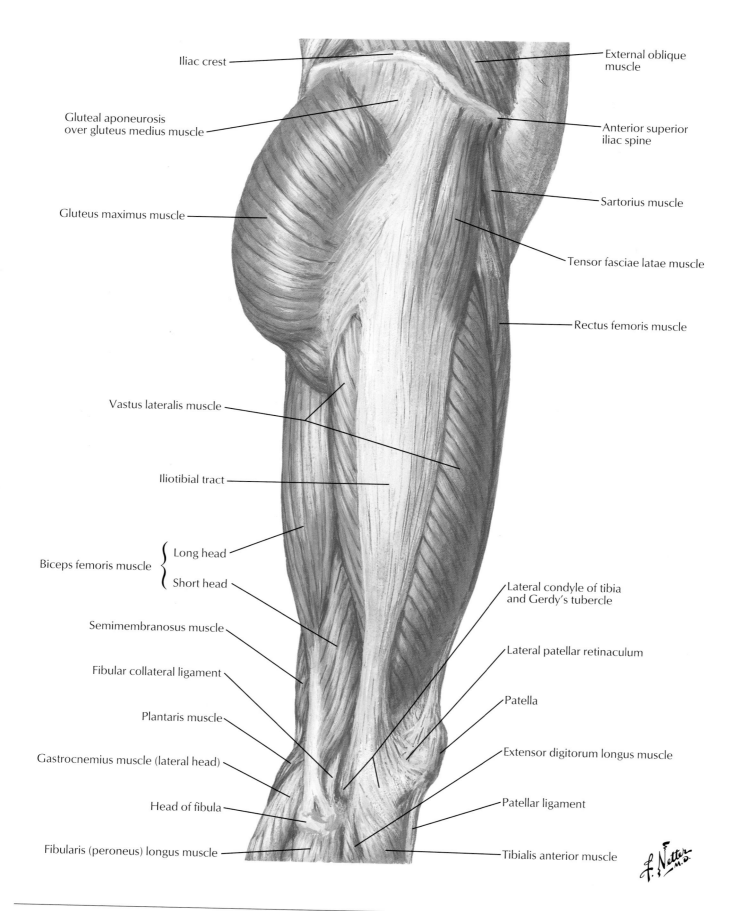

Iliac crest

External oblique muscle

Gluteal aponeurosis over gluteus medius muscle

Anterior superior iliac spine

Gluteus maximus muscle

Sartorius muscle

Tensor fasciae latae muscle

Rectus femoris muscle

Vastus lateralis muscle

Iliotibial tract

Biceps femoris muscle { Long head

Short head

Lateral condyle of tibia and Gerdy's tubercle

Semimembranosus muscle

Lateral patellar retinaculum

Fibular collateral ligament

Plantaris muscle

Patella

Gastrocnemius muscle (lateral head)

Extensor digitorum longus muscle

Head of fibula

Patellar ligament

Fibularis (peroneus) longus muscle

Tibialis anterior muscle

**Plate 481**

**Hip and Thigh**

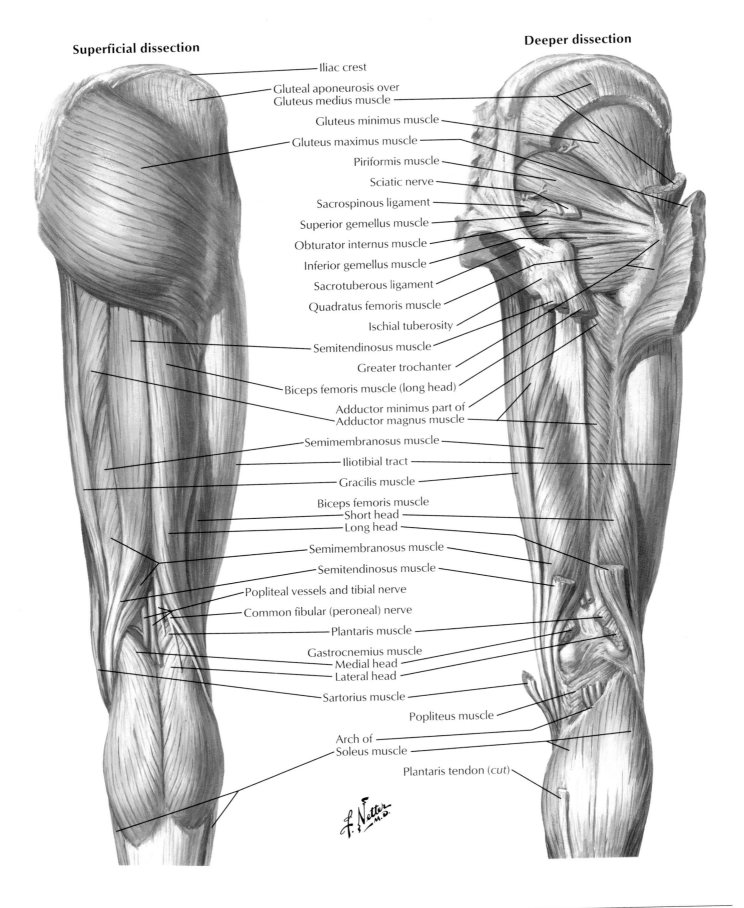

**Superficial dissection**

**Deeper dissection**

Iliac crest

Gluteal aponeurosis over Gluteus medius muscle

Gluteus minimus muscle

Gluteus maximus muscle

Piriformis muscle

Sciatic nerve

Sacrospinous ligament

Superior gemellus muscle

Obturator internus muscle

Inferior gemellus muscle

Sacrotuberous ligament

Quadratus femoris muscle

Ischial tuberosity

Semitendinosus muscle

Greater trochanter

Biceps femoris muscle (long head)

Adductor minimus part of Adductor magnus muscle

Semimembranosus muscle

Iliotibial tract

Gracilis muscle

Biceps femoris muscle
Short head
Long head

Semimembranosus muscle

Semitendinosus muscle

Popliteal vessels and tibial nerve

Common fibular (peroneal) nerve

Plantaris muscle

Gastrocnemius muscle
Medial head
Lateral head

Sartorius muscle

Popliteus muscle

Arch of
Soleus muscle

Plantaris tendon (*cut*)

*f. Netter, m.d.*

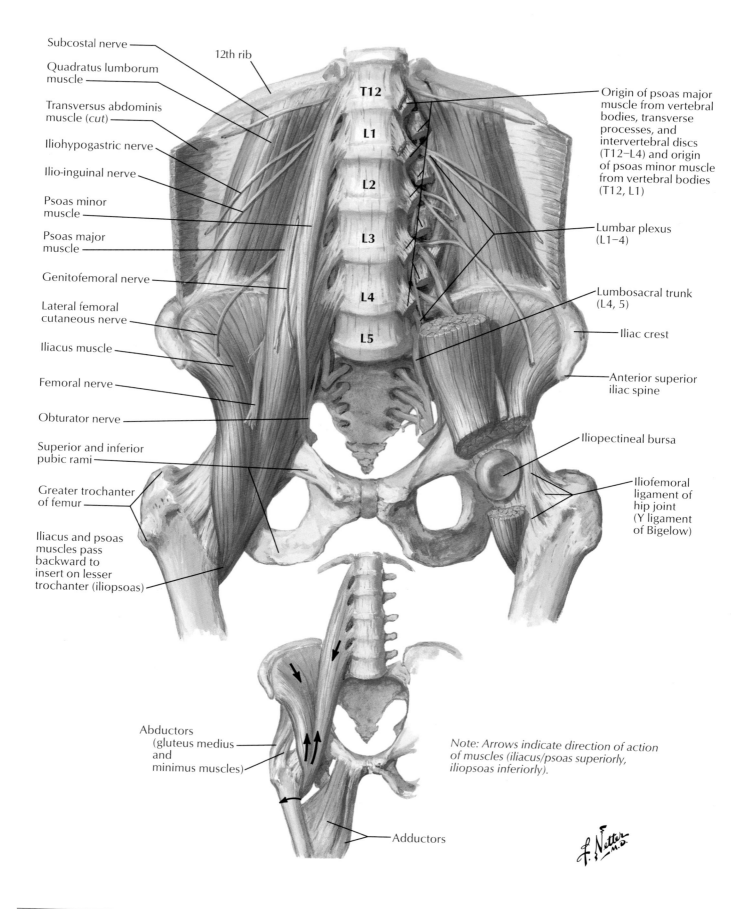

Subcostal nerve

Quadratus lumborum muscle

Transversus abdominis muscle (*cut*)

Iliohypogastric nerve

Ilio-inguinal nerve

Psoas minor muscle

Psoas major muscle

Genitofemoral nerve

Lateral femoral cutaneous nerve

Iliacus muscle

Femoral nerve

Obturator nerve

Superior and inferior pubic rami

Greater trochanter of femur

Iliacus and psoas muscles pass backward to insert on lesser trochanter (iliopsoas)

12th rib

T12

L1

L2

L3

L4

L5

Origin of psoas major muscle from vertebral bodies, transverse processes, and intervertebral discs (T12–L4) and origin of psoas minor muscle from vertebral bodies (T12, L1)

Lumbar plexus (L1–4)

Lumbosacral trunk (L4, 5)

Iliac crest

Anterior superior iliac spine

Iliopectineal bursa

Iliofemoral ligament of hip joint (Y ligament of Bigelow)

Abductors (gluteus medius and minimus muscles)

Adductors

*Note: Arrows indicate direction of action of muscles (iliacus/psoas superiorly, iliopsoas inferiorly).*

**Plate 483**

**Hip and Thigh**

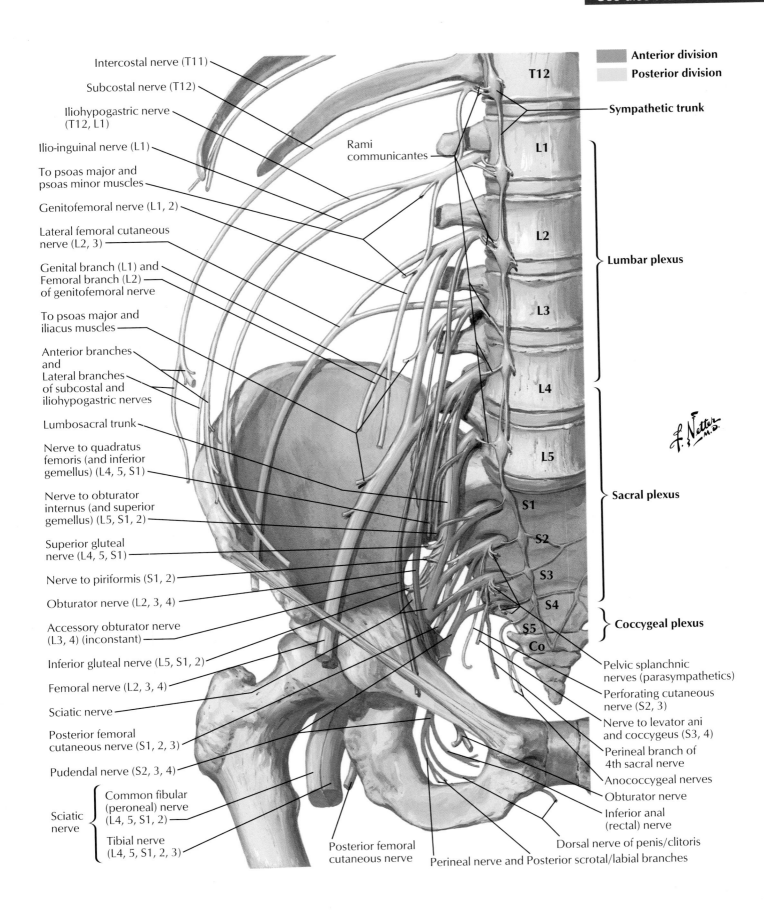

Anterior division
Posterior division

Intercostal nerve (T11)

Subcostal nerve (T12)

Iliohypogastric nerve (T12, L1)

Ilio-inguinal nerve (L1)

To psoas major and psoas minor muscles

Genitofemoral nerve (L1, 2)

Lateral femoral cutaneous nerve (L2, 3)

Genital branch (L1) and Femoral branch (L2) of genitofemoral nerve

To psoas major and iliacus muscles

Anterior branches and Lateral branches of subcostal and iliohypogastric nerves

Lumbosacral trunk

Nerve to quadratus femoris (and inferior gemellus) (L4, 5, S1)

Nerve to obturator internus (and superior gemellus) (L5, S1, 2)

Superior gluteal nerve (L4, 5, S1)

Nerve to piriformis (S1, 2)

Obturator nerve (L2, 3, 4)

Accessory obturator nerve (L3, 4) (inconstant)

Inferior gluteal nerve (L5, S1, 2)

Femoral nerve (L2, 3, 4)

Sciatic nerve

Posterior femoral cutaneous nerve (S1, 2, 3)

Pudendal nerve (S2, 3, 4)

Sciatic nerve {
Common fibular (peroneal) nerve (L4, 5, S1, 2)

Tibial nerve (L4, 5, S1, 2, 3)
}

Rami communicantes

T12

L1

L2

L3

L4

L5

S1

S2

S3

S4

S5

Co

Sympathetic trunk

Lumbar plexus

Sacral plexus

Coccygeal plexus

Pelvic splanchnic nerves (parasympathetics)

Perforating cutaneous nerve (S2, 3)

Nerve to levator ani and coccygeus (S3, 4)

Perineal branch of 4th sacral nerve

Anococcygeal nerves

Obturator nerve

Inferior anal (rectal) nerve

Dorsal nerve of penis/clitoris

Posterior femoral cutaneous nerve

Perineal nerve and Posterior scrotal/labial branches

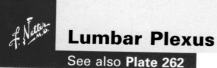
**Schema**

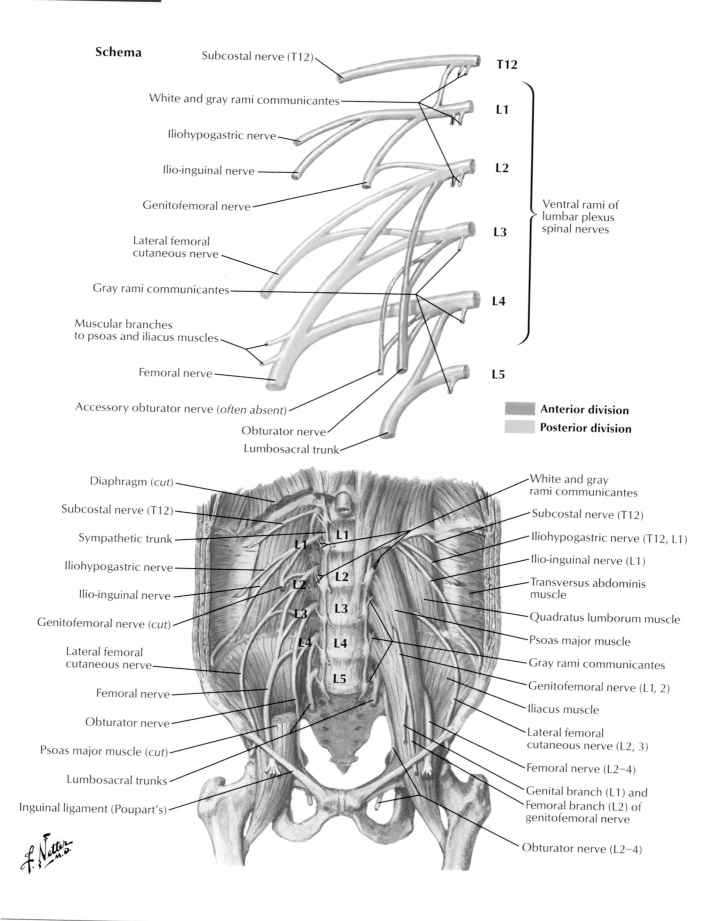

Subcostal nerve (T12)

White and gray rami communicantes

Iliohypogastric nerve

Ilio-inguinal nerve

Genitofemoral nerve

Lateral femoral cutaneous nerve

Gray rami communicantes

Muscular branches to psoas and iliacus muscles

Femoral nerve

Accessory obturator nerve (often absent)

Obturator nerve

Lumbosacral trunk

T12

L1

L2

L3

L4

L5

Ventral rami of lumbar plexus spinal nerves

**Anterior division**
**Posterior division**

Diaphragm (cut)

Subcostal nerve (T12)

Sympathetic trunk

Iliohypogastric nerve

Ilio-inguinal nerve

Genitofemoral nerve (cut)

Lateral femoral cutaneous nerve

Femoral nerve

Obturator nerve

Psoas major muscle (cut)

Lumbosacral trunks

Inguinal ligament (Poupart's)

White and gray rami communicantes

Subcostal nerve (T12)

Iliohypogastric nerve (T12, L1)

Ilio-inguinal nerve (L1)

Transversus abdominis muscle

Quadratus lumborum muscle

Psoas major muscle

Gray rami communicantes

Genitofemoral nerve (L1, 2)

Iliacus muscle

Lateral femoral cutaneous nerve (L2, 3)

Femoral nerve (L2–4)

Genital branch (L1) and Femoral branch (L2) of genitofemoral nerve

Obturator nerve (L2–4)

L1
L1
L2
L2
L3
L3
L4
L4
L5

**Plate 485**

**Hip and Thigh**

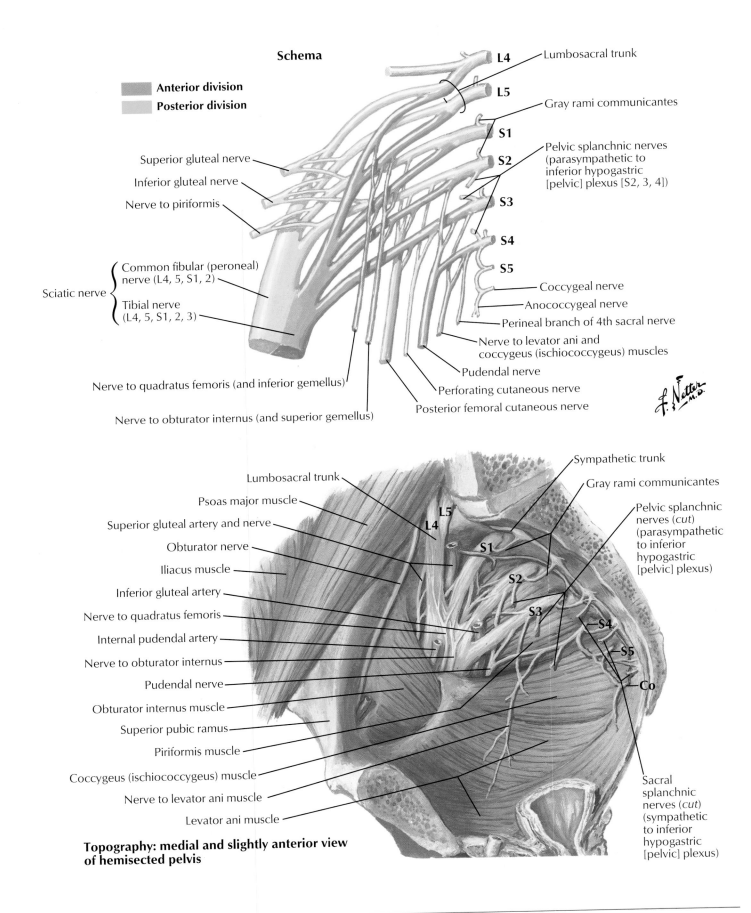

Schema

Anterior division
Posterior division

L4 — Lumbosacral trunk

L5 — Gray rami communicantes

S1

S2 — Pelvic splanchnic nerves (parasympathetic to inferior hypogastric [pelvic] plexus [S2, 3, 4])

S3

S4

S5

Superior gluteal nerve
Inferior gluteal nerve
Nerve to piriformis

Coccygeal nerve
Anococcygeal nerve
Perineal branch of 4th sacral nerve
Nerve to levator ani and coccygeus (ischiococcygeus) muscles
Pudendal nerve
Perforating cutaneous nerve
Posterior femoral cutaneous nerve

Sciatic nerve { Common fibular (peroneal) nerve (L4, 5, S1, 2)
Tibial nerve (L4, 5, S1, 2, 3)

Nerve to quadratus femoris (and inferior gemellus)

Nerve to obturator internus (and superior gemellus)

Lumbosacral trunk
Psoas major muscle
Superior gluteal artery and nerve
Obturator nerve
Iliacus muscle
Inferior gluteal artery
Nerve to quadratus femoris
Internal pudendal artery
Nerve to obturator internus
Pudendal nerve
Obturator internus muscle
Superior pubic ramus
Piriformis muscle
Coccygeus (ischiococcygeus) muscle
Nerve to levator ani muscle
Levator ani muscle

L4
L5
S1
S2
S3
S4
S5
Co

Sympathetic trunk
Gray rami communicantes
Pelvic splanchnic nerves (cut) (parasympathetic to inferior hypogastric [pelvic] plexus)

Sacral splanchnic nerves (cut) (sympathetic to inferior hypogastric [pelvic] plexus)

**Topography: medial and slightly anterior view of hemisected pelvis**

**Superficial dissections**

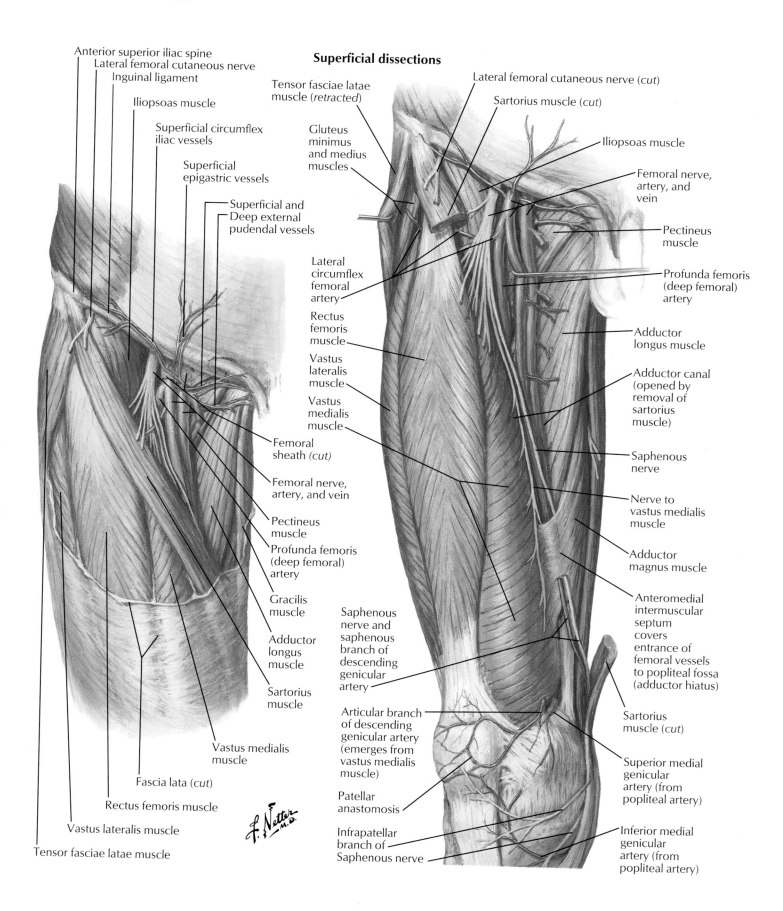

Anterior superior iliac spine

Lateral femoral cutaneous nerve

Inguinal ligament

Iliopsoas muscle

Superficial circumflex iliac vessels

Superficial epigastric vessels

Superficial and Deep external pudendal vessels

Tensor fasciae latae muscle (*retracted*)

Gluteus minimus and medius muscles

Lateral circumflex femoral artery

Rectus femoris muscle

Vastus lateralis muscle

Vastus medialis muscle

Femoral sheath (*cut*)

Femoral nerve, artery, and vein

Pectineus muscle

Profunda femoris (deep femoral) artery

Gracilis muscle

Adductor longus muscle

Sartorius muscle

Vastus medialis muscle

Fascia lata (*cut*)

Rectus femoris muscle

Vastus lateralis muscle

Tensor fasciae latae muscle

Lateral femoral cutaneous nerve (*cut*)

Sartorius muscle (*cut*)

Iliopsoas muscle

Femoral nerve, artery, and vein

Pectineus muscle

Profunda femoris (deep femoral) artery

Adductor longus muscle

Adductor canal (opened by removal of sartorius muscle)

Saphenous nerve

Nerve to vastus medialis muscle

Adductor magnus muscle

Anteromedial intermuscular septum covers entrance of femoral vessels to popliteal fossa (adductor hiatus)

Sartorius muscle (*cut*)

Superior medial genicular artery (from popliteal artery)

Inferior medial genicular artery (from popliteal artery)

Saphenous nerve and saphenous branch of descending genicular artery

Articular branch of descending genicular artery (emerges from vastus medialis muscle)

Patellar anastomosis

Infrapatellar branch of Saphenous nerve

*f. Netter*

**Plate 487**

**Hip and Thigh**

**Deep dissection**

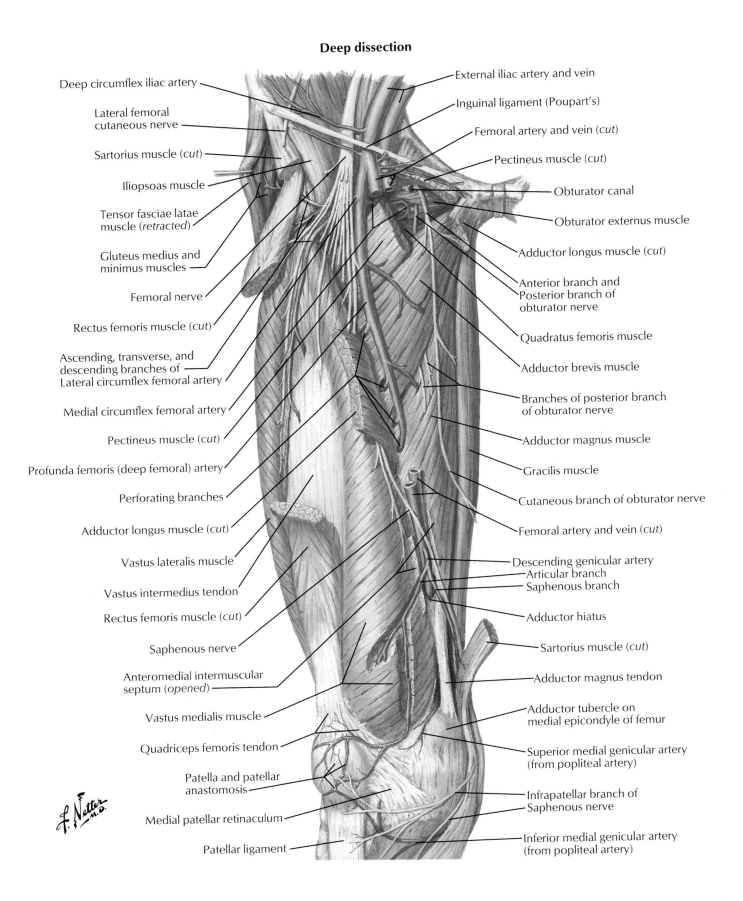

Deep circumflex iliac artery

Lateral femoral cutaneous nerve

Sartorius muscle (*cut*)

Iliopsoas muscle

Tensor fasciae latae muscle (*retracted*)

Gluteus medius and minimus muscles

Femoral nerve

Rectus femoris muscle (*cut*)

Ascending, transverse, and descending branches of Lateral circumflex femoral artery

Medial circumflex femoral artery

Pectineus muscle (*cut*)

Profunda femoris (deep femoral) artery

Perforating branches

Adductor longus muscle (*cut*)

Vastus lateralis muscle

Vastus intermedius tendon

Rectus femoris muscle (*cut*)

Saphenous nerve

Anteromedial intermuscular septum (*opened*)

Vastus medialis muscle

Quadriceps femoris tendon

Patella and patellar anastomosis

Medial patellar retinaculum

Patellar ligament

External iliac artery and vein

Inguinal ligament (Poupart's)

Femoral artery and vein (*cut*)

Pectineus muscle (*cut*)

Obturator canal

Obturator externus muscle

Adductor longus muscle (*cut*)

Anterior branch and Posterior branch of obturator nerve

Quadratus femoris muscle

Adductor brevis muscle

Branches of posterior branch of obturator nerve

Adductor magnus muscle

Gracilis muscle

Cutaneous branch of obturator nerve

Femoral artery and vein (*cut*)

Descending genicular artery
Articular branch
Saphenous branch

Adductor hiatus

Sartorius muscle (*cut*)

Adductor magnus tendon

Adductor tubercle on medial epicondyle of femur

Superior medial genicular artery (from popliteal artery)

Infrapatellar branch of Saphenous nerve

Inferior medial genicular artery (from popliteal artery)

**Deep dissection**

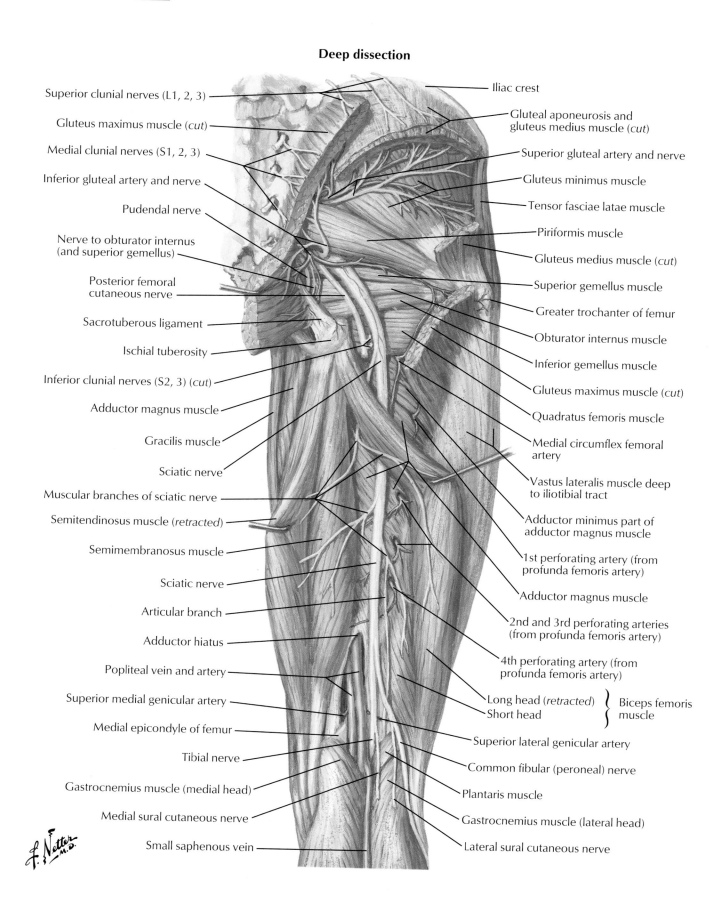

Superior clunial nerves (L1, 2, 3)

Gluteus maximus muscle (*cut*)

Medial clunial nerves (S1, 2, 3)

Inferior gluteal artery and nerve

Pudendal nerve

Nerve to obturator internus
(and superior gemellus)

Posterior femoral
cutaneous nerve

Sacrotuberous ligament

Ischial tuberosity

Inferior clunial nerves (S2, 3) (*cut*)

Adductor magnus muscle

Gracilis muscle

Sciatic nerve

Muscular branches of sciatic nerve

Semitendinosus muscle (*retracted*)

Semimembranosus muscle

Sciatic nerve

Articular branch

Adductor hiatus

Popliteal vein and artery

Superior medial genicular artery

Medial epicondyle of femur

Tibial nerve

Gastrocnemius muscle (medial head)

Medial sural cutaneous nerve

Small saphenous vein

Iliac crest

Gluteal aponeurosis and
gluteus medius muscle (*cut*)

Superior gluteal artery and nerve

Gluteus minimus muscle

Tensor fasciae latae muscle

Piriformis muscle

Gluteus medius muscle (*cut*)

Superior gemellus muscle

Greater trochanter of femur

Obturator internus muscle

Inferior gemellus muscle

Gluteus maximus muscle (*cut*)

Quadratus femoris muscle

Medial circumflex femoral
artery

Vastus lateralis muscle deep
to iliotibial tract

Adductor minimus part of
adductor magnus muscle

1st perforating artery (from
profunda femoris artery)

Adductor magnus muscle

2nd and 3rd perforating arteries
(from profunda femoris artery)

4th perforating artery (from
profunda femoris artery)

Long head (*retracted*) } Biceps femoris
Short head } muscle

Superior lateral genicular artery

Common fibular (peroneal) nerve

Plantaris muscle

Gastrocnemius muscle (lateral head)

Lateral sural cutaneous nerve

**Plate 489**

**Hip and Thigh**

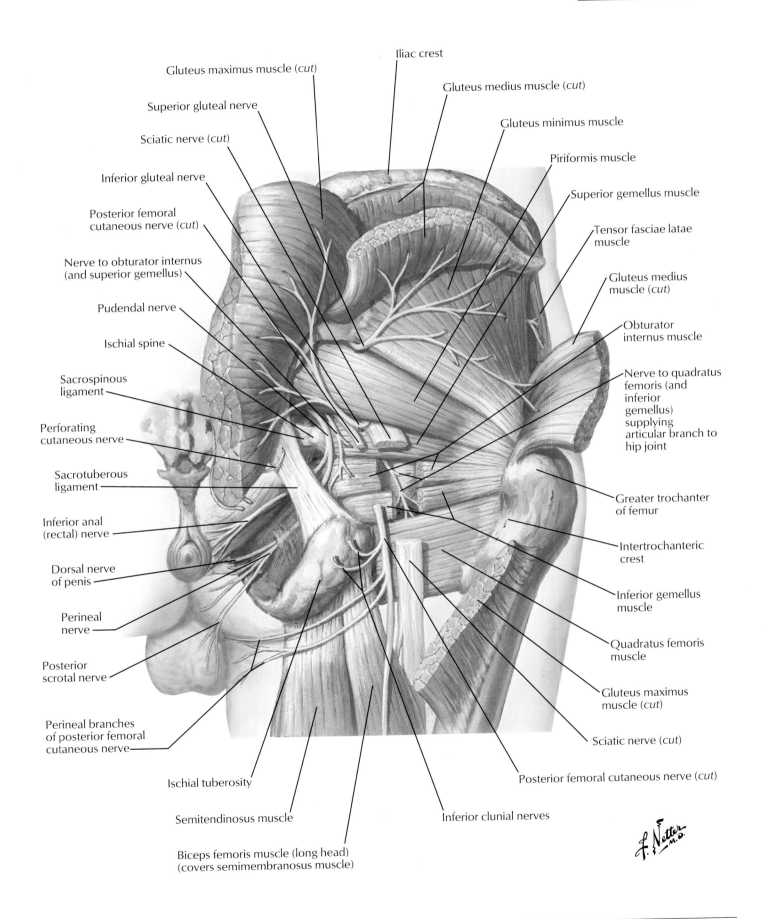

Iliac crest

Gluteus maximus muscle (*cut*)

Gluteus medius muscle (*cut*)

Superior gluteal nerve

Gluteus minimus muscle

Sciatic nerve (*cut*)

Piriformis muscle

Inferior gluteal nerve

Superior gemellus muscle

Posterior femoral cutaneous nerve (*cut*)

Tensor fasciae latae muscle

Nerve to obturator internus (and superior gemellus)

Gluteus medius muscle (*cut*)

Pudendal nerve

Obturator internus muscle

Ischial spine

Nerve to quadratus femoris (and inferior gemellus) supplying articular branch to hip joint

Sacrospinous ligament

Perforating cutaneous nerve

Sacrotuberous ligament

Greater trochanter of femur

Inferior anal (rectal) nerve

Intertrochanteric crest

Dorsal nerve of penis

Inferior gemellus muscle

Perineal nerve

Quadratus femoris muscle

Posterior scrotal nerve

Gluteus maximus muscle (*cut*)

Perineal branches of posterior femoral cutaneous nerve

Sciatic nerve (*cut*)

Posterior femoral cutaneous nerve (*cut*)

Ischial tuberosity

Semitendinosus muscle

Inferior clunial nerves

Biceps femoris muscle (long head) (covers semimembranosus muscle)

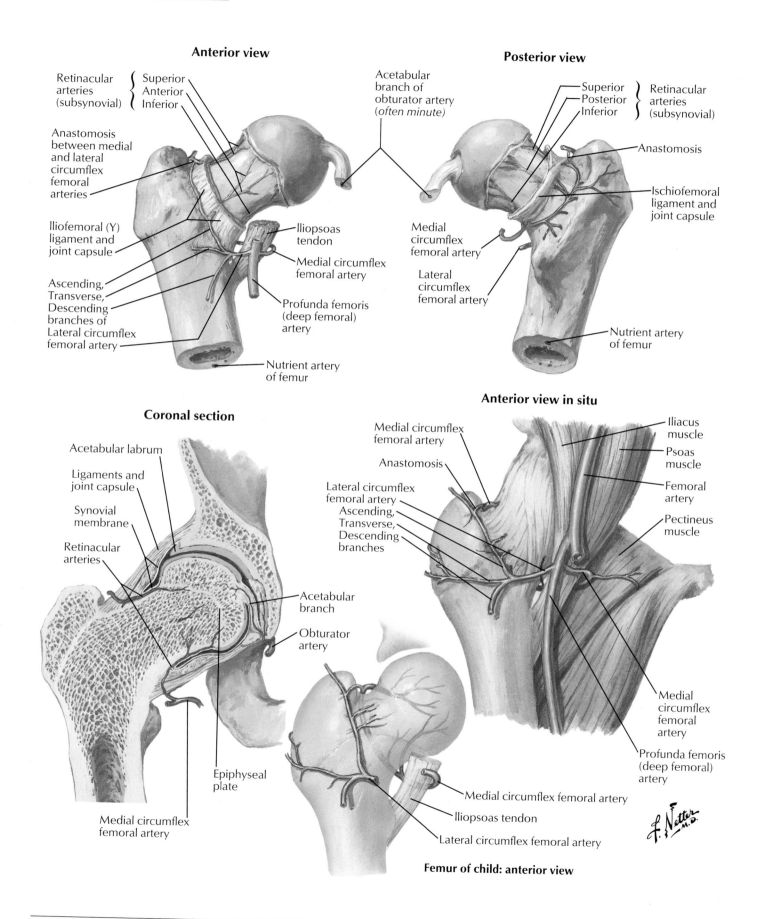

**Anterior view**

Retinacular arteries (subsynovial) { Superior / Anterior / Inferior

Anastomosis between medial and lateral circumflex femoral arteries

Iliofemoral (Y) ligament and joint capsule

Ascending, Transverse, Descending branches of Lateral circumflex femoral artery

Acetabular branch of obturator artery (often minute)

Iliopsoas tendon

Medial circumflex femoral artery

Profunda femoris (deep femoral) artery

Nutrient artery of femur

**Posterior view**

Superior / Posterior / Inferior } Retinacular arteries (subsynovial)

Anastomosis

Ischiofemoral ligament and joint capsule

Medial circumflex femoral artery

Lateral circumflex femoral artery

Nutrient artery of femur

**Coronal section**

Acetabular labrum

Ligaments and joint capsule

Synovial membrane

Retinacular arteries

Medial circumflex femoral artery

Acetabular branch

Obturator artery

Epiphyseal plate

**Anterior view in situ**

Medial circumflex femoral artery

Anastomosis

Lateral circumflex femoral artery / Ascending, Transverse, Descending branches

Iliacus muscle

Psoas muscle

Femoral artery

Pectineus muscle

Medial circumflex femoral artery

Profunda femoris (deep femoral) artery

Medial circumflex femoral artery

Iliopsoas tendon

Lateral circumflex femoral artery

**Femur of child: anterior view**

**Plate 491**

**Hip and Thigh**

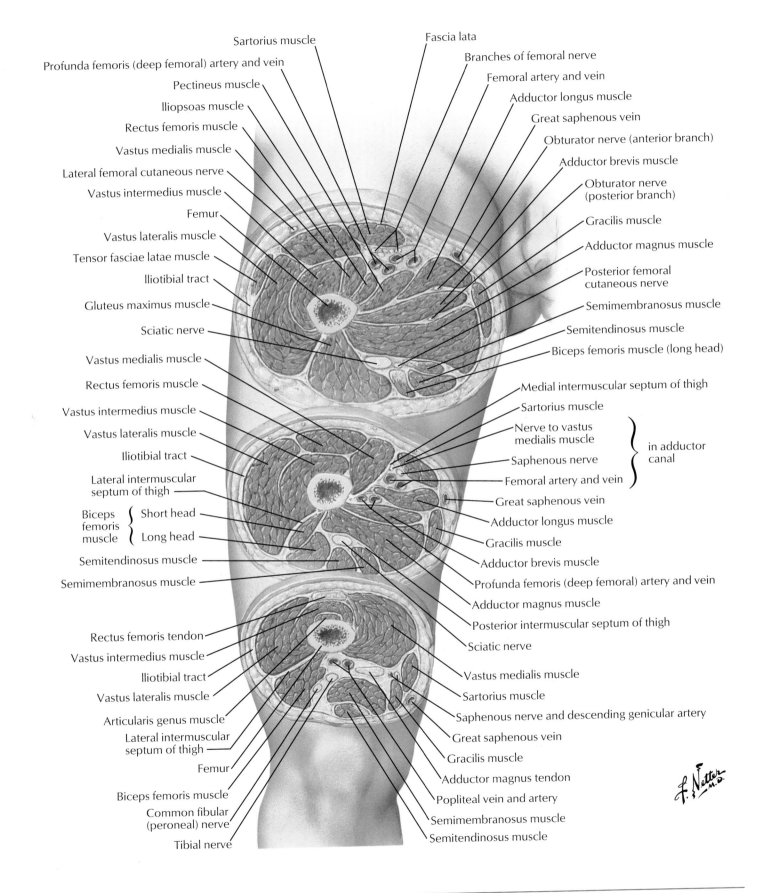

Sartorius muscle

Profunda femoris (deep femoral) artery and vein

Pectineus muscle

Iliopsoas muscle

Rectus femoris muscle

Vastus medialis muscle

Lateral femoral cutaneous nerve

Vastus intermedius muscle

Femur

Vastus lateralis muscle

Tensor fasciae latae muscle

Iliotibial tract

Gluteus maximus muscle

Sciatic nerve

Vastus medialis muscle

Rectus femoris muscle

Vastus intermedius muscle

Vastus lateralis muscle

Iliotibial tract

Lateral intermuscular septum of thigh

Biceps femoris muscle { Short head / Long head }

Semitendinosus muscle

Semimembranosus muscle

Rectus femoris tendon

Vastus intermedius muscle

Iliotibial tract

Vastus lateralis muscle

Articularis genus muscle

Lateral intermuscular septum of thigh

Femur

Biceps femoris muscle

Common fibular (peroneal) nerve

Tibial nerve

Fascia lata

Branches of femoral nerve

Femoral artery and vein

Adductor longus muscle

Great saphenous vein

Obturator nerve (anterior branch)

Adductor brevis muscle

Obturator nerve (posterior branch)

Gracilis muscle

Adductor magnus muscle

Posterior femoral cutaneous nerve

Semimembranosus muscle

Semitendinosus muscle

Biceps femoris muscle (long head)

Medial intermuscular septum of thigh

Sartorius muscle

Nerve to vastus medialis muscle

Saphenous nerve

Femoral artery and vein

} in adductor canal

Great saphenous vein

Adductor longus muscle

Gracilis muscle

Adductor brevis muscle

Profunda femoris (deep femoral) artery and vein

Adductor magnus muscle

Posterior intermuscular septum of thigh

Sciatic nerve

Vastus medialis muscle

Sartorius muscle

Saphenous nerve and descending genicular artery

Great saphenous vein

Gracilis muscle

Adductor magnus tendon

Popliteal vein and artery

Semimembranosus muscle

Semitendinosus muscle

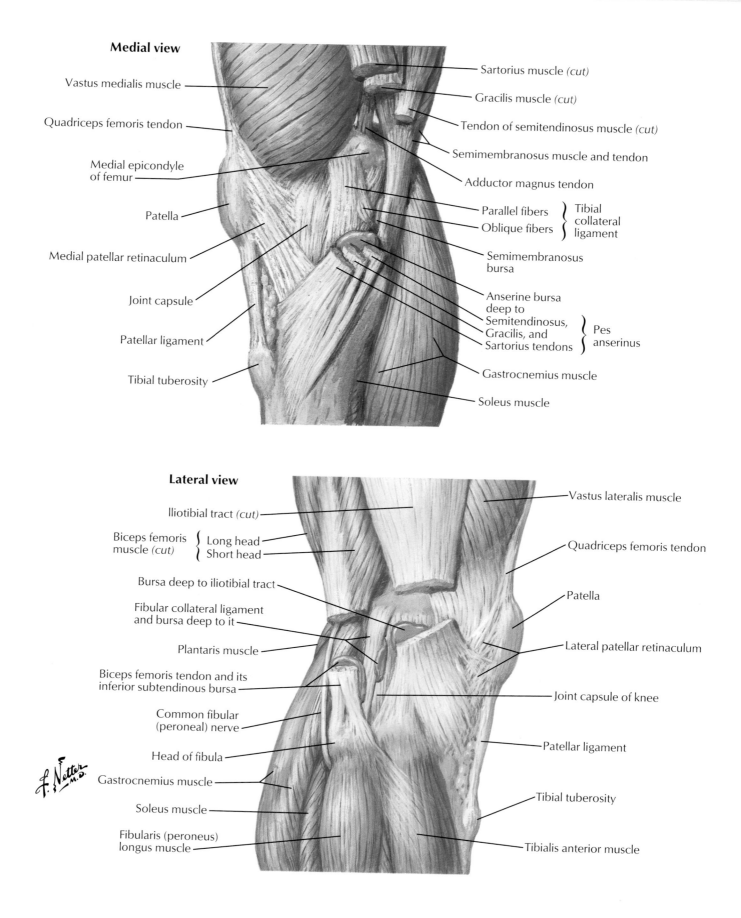

**Medial view**

Vastus medialis muscle

Quadriceps femoris tendon

Medial epicondyle of femur

Patella

Medial patellar retinaculum

Joint capsule

Patellar ligament

Tibial tuberosity

Sartorius muscle (cut)

Gracilis muscle (cut)

Tendon of semitendinosus muscle (cut)

Semimembranosus muscle and tendon

Adductor magnus tendon

Parallel fibers ⎫
Oblique fibers ⎭ Tibial collateral ligament

Semimembranosus bursa

Anserine bursa deep to Semitendinosus, Gracilis, and Sartorius tendons ⎫ Pes anserinus

Gastrocnemius muscle

Soleus muscle

**Lateral view**

Iliotibial tract (cut)

Biceps femoris muscle (cut) ⎧ Long head
⎩ Short head

Bursa deep to iliotibial tract

Fibular collateral ligament and bursa deep to it

Plantaris muscle

Biceps femoris tendon and its inferior subtendinous bursa

Common fibular (peroneal) nerve

Head of fibula

Gastrocnemius muscle

Soleus muscle

Fibularis (peroneus) longus muscle

Vastus lateralis muscle

Quadriceps femoris tendon

Patella

Lateral patellar retinaculum

Joint capsule of knee

Patellar ligament

Tibial tuberosity

Tibialis anterior muscle

**Plate 493**

**Knee**

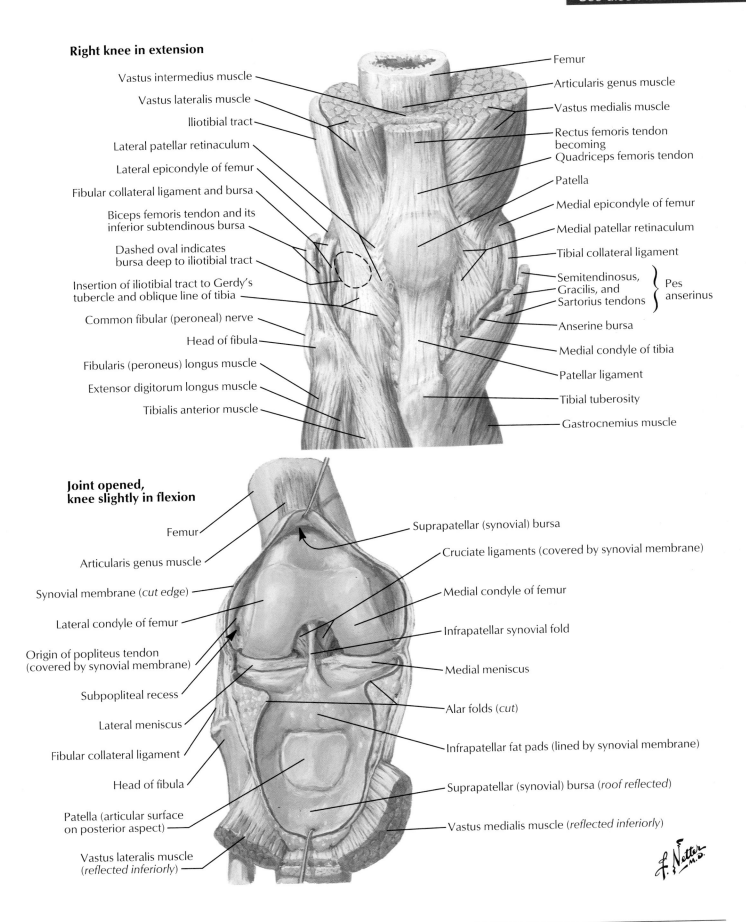

**Right knee in extension**

Vastus intermedius muscle

Vastus lateralis muscle

Iliotibial tract

Lateral patellar retinaculum

Lateral epicondyle of femur

Fibular collateral ligament and bursa

Biceps femoris tendon and its inferior subtendinous bursa

Dashed oval indicates bursa deep to iliotibial tract

Insertion of iliotibial tract to Gerdy's tubercle and oblique line of tibia

Common fibular (peroneal) nerve

Head of fibula

Fibularis (peroneus) longus muscle

Extensor digitorum longus muscle

Tibialis anterior muscle

Femur

Articularis genus muscle

Vastus medialis muscle

Rectus femoris tendon becoming Quadriceps femoris tendon

Patella

Medial epicondyle of femur

Medial patellar retinaculum

Tibial collateral ligament

Semitendinosus, Gracilis, and Sartorius tendons } Pes anserinus

Anserine bursa

Medial condyle of tibia

Patellar ligament

Tibial tuberosity

Gastrocnemius muscle

**Joint opened, knee slightly in flexion**

Femur

Articularis genus muscle

Synovial membrane (*cut edge*)

Lateral condyle of femur

Origin of popliteus tendon (covered by synovial membrane)

Subpopliteal recess

Lateral meniscus

Fibular collateral ligament

Head of fibula

Patella (articular surface on posterior aspect)

Vastus lateralis muscle (*reflected inferiorly*)

Suprapatellar (synovial) bursa

Cruciate ligaments (covered by synovial membrane)

Medial condyle of femur

Infrapatellar synovial fold

Medial meniscus

Alar folds (*cut*)

Infrapatellar fat pads (lined by synovial membrane)

Suprapatellar (synovial) bursa (*roof reflected*)

Vastus medialis muscle (*reflected inferiorly*)

*f. Netter M.D.*

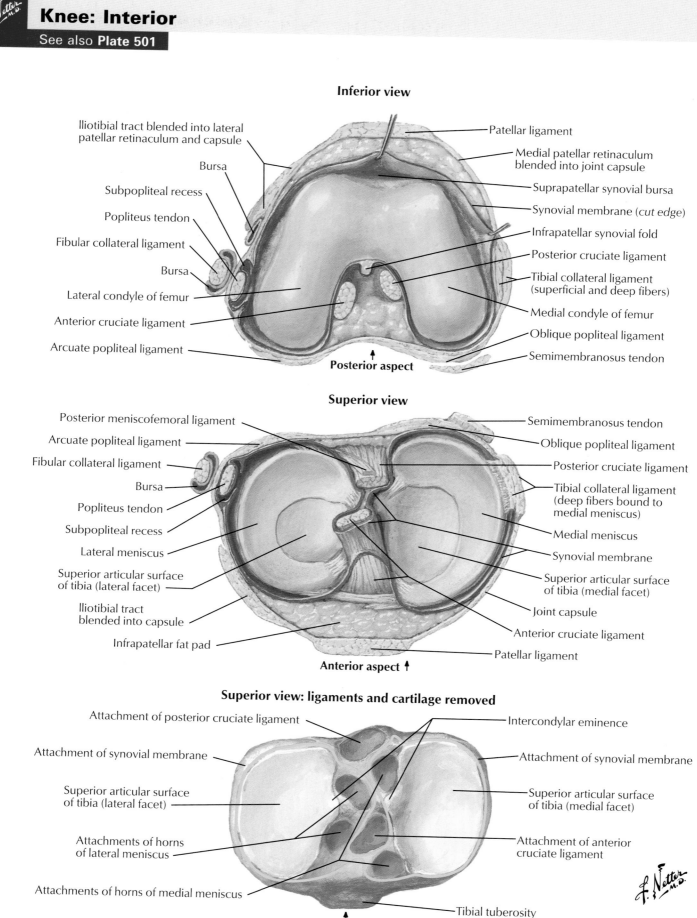

**Inferior view**

Iliotibial tract blended into lateral patellar retinaculum and capsule

Bursa

Subpopliteal recess

Popliteus tendon

Fibular collateral ligament

Bursa

Lateral condyle of femur

Anterior cruciate ligament

Arcuate popliteal ligament

Patellar ligament

Medial patellar retinaculum blended into joint capsule

Suprapatellar synovial bursa

Synovial membrane (*cut edge*)

Infrapatellar synovial fold

Posterior cruciate ligament

Tibial collateral ligament (superficial and deep fibers)

Medial condyle of femur

Oblique popliteal ligament

Semimembranosus tendon

**Posterior aspect**

**Superior view**

Posterior meniscofemoral ligament

Arcuate popliteal ligament

Fibular collateral ligament

Bursa

Popliteus tendon

Subpopliteal recess

Lateral meniscus

Superior articular surface of tibia (lateral facet)

Iliotibial tract blended into capsule

Infrapatellar fat pad

Semimembranosus tendon

Oblique popliteal ligament

Posterior cruciate ligament

Tibial collateral ligament (deep fibers bound to medial meniscus)

Medial meniscus

Synovial membrane

Superior articular surface of tibia (medial facet)

Joint capsule

Anterior cruciate ligament

Patellar ligament

**Anterior aspect**

**Superior view: ligaments and cartilage removed**

Attachment of posterior cruciate ligament

Attachment of synovial membrane

Superior articular surface of tibia (lateral facet)

Attachments of horns of lateral meniscus

Attachments of horns of medial meniscus

Intercondylar eminence

Attachment of synovial membrane

Superior articular surface of tibia (medial facet)

Attachment of anterior cruciate ligament

Tibial tuberosity

**Anterior aspect**

**Plate 495**

**Knee**

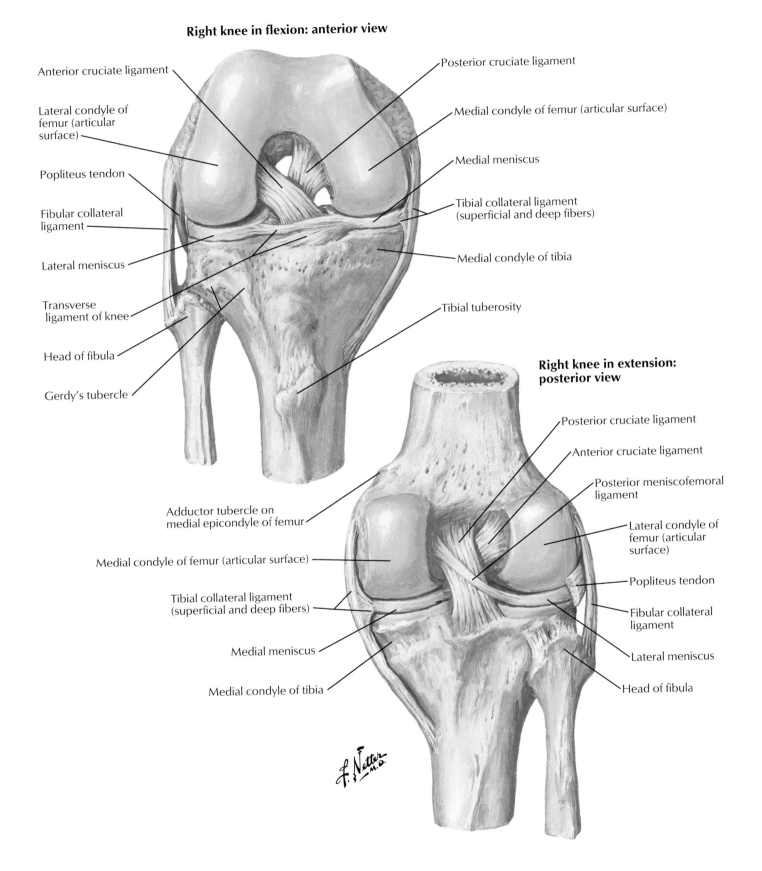

**Right knee in flexion: anterior view**

Anterior cruciate ligament

Lateral condyle of femur (articular surface)

Popliteus tendon

Fibular collateral ligament

Lateral meniscus

Transverse ligament of knee

Head of fibula

Gerdy's tubercle

Posterior cruciate ligament

Medial condyle of femur (articular surface)

Medial meniscus

Tibial collateral ligament (superficial and deep fibers)

Medial condyle of tibia

Tibial tuberosity

**Right knee in extension: posterior view**

Adductor tubercle on medial epicondyle of femur

Medial condyle of femur (articular surface)

Tibial collateral ligament (superficial and deep fibers)

Medial meniscus

Medial condyle of tibia

Posterior cruciate ligament

Anterior cruciate ligament

Posterior meniscofemoral ligament

Lateral condyle of femur (articular surface)

Popliteus tendon

Fibular collateral ligament

Lateral meniscus

Head of fibula

**Knee**

**Plate 496**

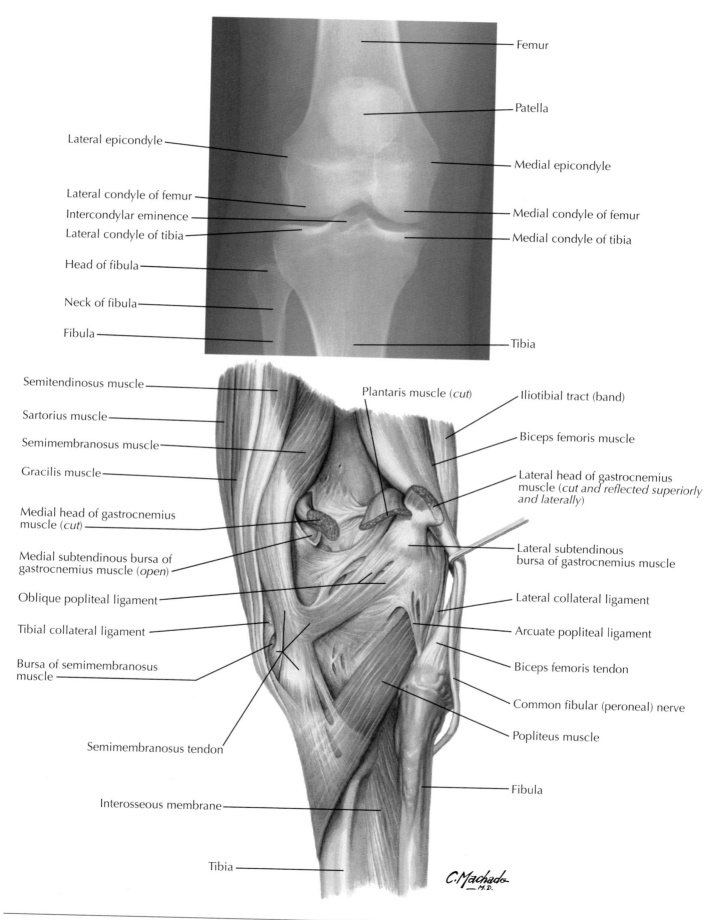

Femur

Patella

Lateral epicondyle

Medial epicondyle

Lateral condyle of femur

Intercondylar eminence

Lateral condyle of tibia

Medial condyle of femur

Medial condyle of tibia

Head of fibula

Neck of fibula

Fibula

Tibia

Semitendinosus muscle

Plantaris muscle (*cut*)

Iliotibial tract (band)

Sartorius muscle

Semimembranosus muscle

Biceps femoris muscle

Gracilis muscle

Lateral head of gastrocnemius muscle (*cut and reflected superiorly and laterally*)

Medial head of gastrocnemius muscle (*cut*)

Medial subtendinous bursa of gastrocnemius muscle (*open*)

Lateral subtendinous bursa of gastrocnemius muscle

Oblique popliteal ligament

Lateral collateral ligament

Tibial collateral ligament

Arcuate popliteal ligament

Bursa of semimembranosus muscle

Biceps femoris tendon

Common fibular (peroneal) nerve

Semimembranosus tendon

Popliteus muscle

Fibula

Interosseous membrane

Tibia

C. Machado
_M.D.

**Plate 497**

**Knee**

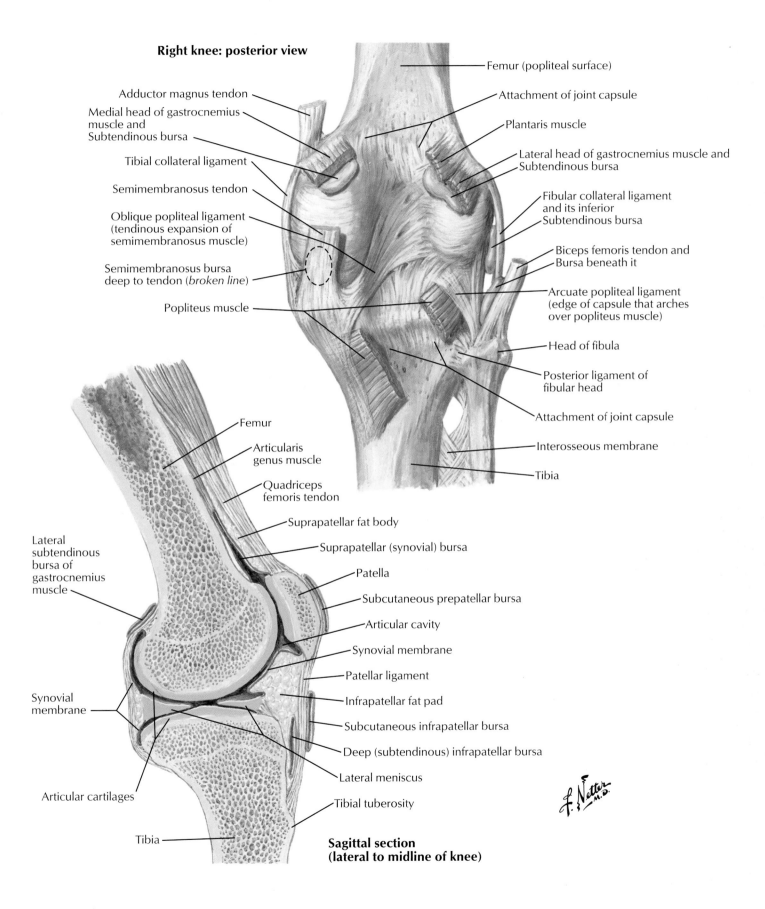

**Right knee: posterior view**

Adductor magnus tendon

Medial head of gastrocnemius muscle and Subtendinous bursa

Tibial collateral ligament

Semimembranosus tendon

Oblique popliteal ligament (tendinous expansion of semimembranosus muscle)

Semimembranosus bursa deep to tendon (*broken line*)

Popliteus muscle

Femur (popliteal surface)

Attachment of joint capsule

Plantaris muscle

Lateral head of gastrocnemius muscle and Subtendinous bursa

Fibular collateral ligament and its inferior Subtendinous bursa

Biceps femoris tendon and Bursa beneath it

Arcuate popliteal ligament (edge of capsule that arches over popliteus muscle)

Head of fibula

Posterior ligament of fibular head

Attachment of joint capsule

Interosseous membrane

Tibia

Femur

Articularis genus muscle

Quadriceps femoris tendon

Suprapatellar fat body

Suprapatellar (synovial) bursa

Patella

Subcutaneous prepatellar bursa

Articular cavity

Synovial membrane

Patellar ligament

Infrapatellar fat pad

Subcutaneous infrapatellar bursa

Deep (subtendinous) infrapatellar bursa

Lateral meniscus

Tibial tuberosity

Lateral subtendinous bursa of gastrocnemius muscle

Synovial membrane

Articular cartilages

Tibia

**Sagittal section (lateral to midline of knee)**

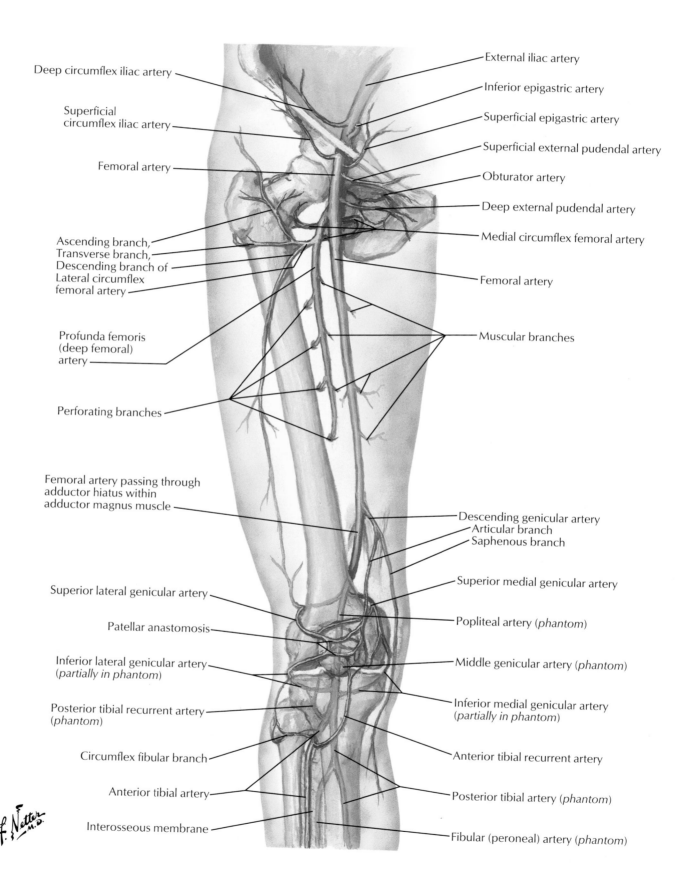

Deep circumflex iliac artery

Superficial circumflex iliac artery

Femoral artery

Ascending branch,
Transverse branch,
Descending branch of
Lateral circumflex
femoral artery

Profunda femoris
(deep femoral)
artery

Perforating branches

Femoral artery passing through
adductor hiatus within
adductor magnus muscle

Superior lateral genicular artery

Patellar anastomosis

Inferior lateral genicular artery
(partially in phantom)

Posterior tibial recurrent artery
(phantom)

Circumflex fibular branch

Anterior tibial artery

Interosseous membrane

External iliac artery

Inferior epigastric artery

Superficial epigastric artery

Superficial external pudendal artery

Obturator artery

Deep external pudendal artery

Medial circumflex femoral artery

Femoral artery

Muscular branches

Descending genicular artery
Articular branch
Saphenous branch

Superior medial genicular artery

Popliteal artery (phantom)

Middle genicular artery (phantom)

Inferior medial genicular artery
(partially in phantom)

Anterior tibial recurrent artery

Posterior tibial artery (phantom)

Fibular (peroneal) artery (phantom)

**Plate 499**

**Knee**

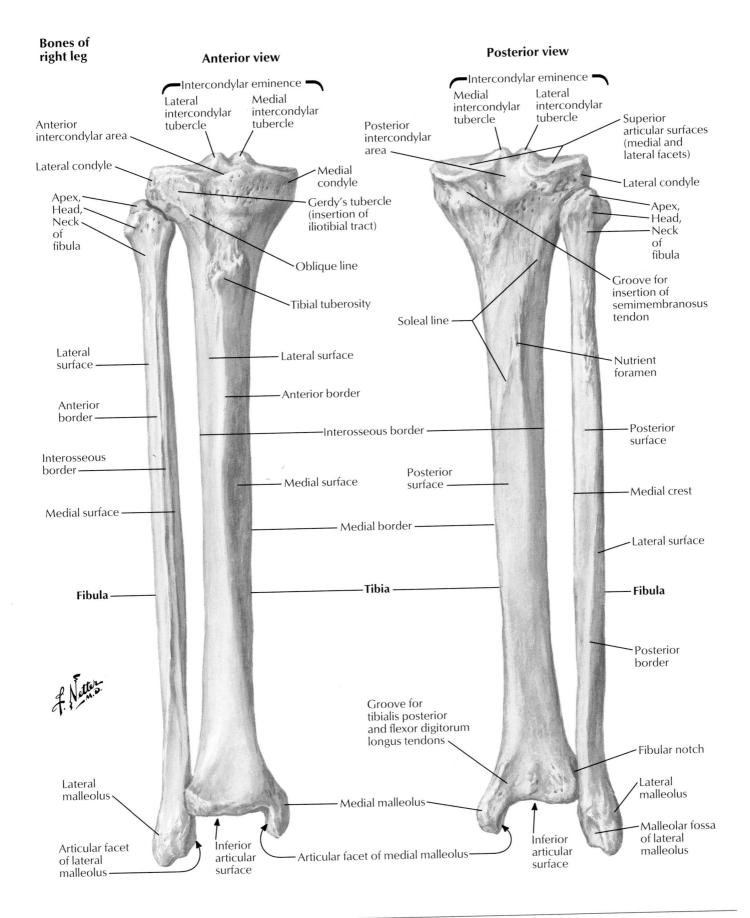

**Bones of right leg**

**Anterior view**

**Posterior view**

Intercondylar eminence

Lateral intercondylar tubercle

Medial intercondylar tubercle

Anterior intercondylar area

Lateral condyle

Apex, Head, Neck of fibula

Medial condyle

Gerdy's tubercle (insertion of iliotibial tract)

Oblique line

Tibial tuberosity

Lateral surface

Anterior border

Lateral surface

Anterior border

Interosseous border

Medial surface

Interosseous border

Medial surface

Medial border

**Fibula**

**Tibia**

Lateral malleolus

Articular facet of lateral malleolus

Inferior articular surface

Medial malleolus

Groove for tibialis posterior and flexor digitorum longus tendons

Articular facet of medial malleolus

Intercondylar eminence

Medial intercondylar tubercle

Lateral intercondylar tubercle

Posterior intercondylar area

Superior articular surfaces (medial and lateral facets)

Lateral condyle

Apex, Head, Neck of fibula

Groove for insertion of semimembranosus tendon

Soleal line

Nutrient foramen

Posterior surface

Posterior surface

Medial crest

Lateral surface

**Fibula**

Posterior border

Fibular notch

Lateral malleolus

Malleolar fossa of lateral malleolus

Inferior articular surface

f. Netter M.D.

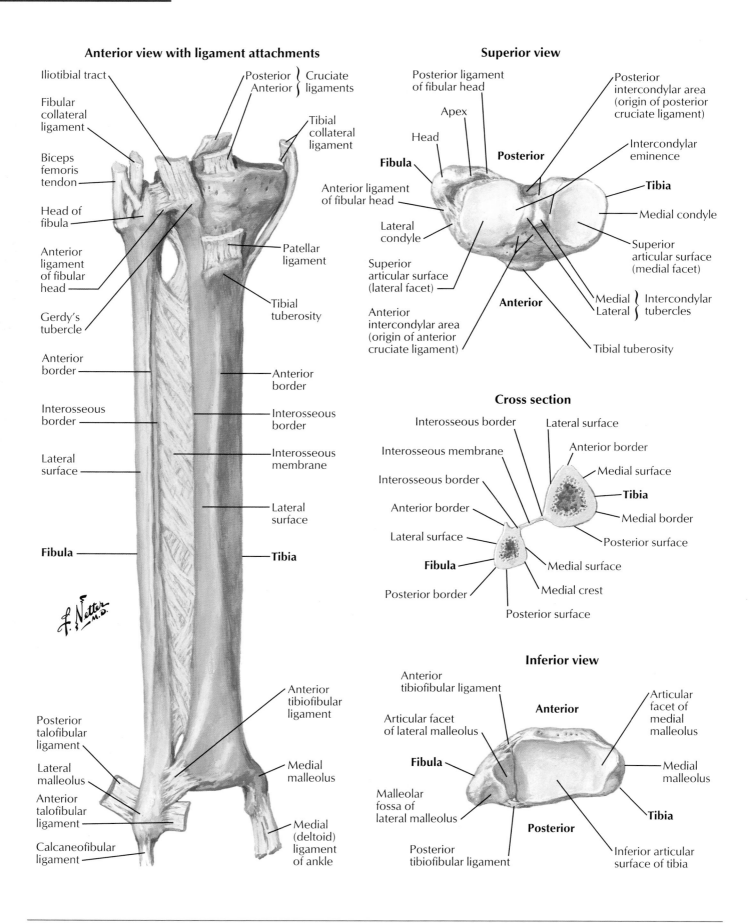

**Anterior view with ligament attachments**

Iliotibial tract

Fibular collateral ligament

Biceps femoris tendon

Head of fibula

Anterior ligament of fibular head

Gerdy's tubercle

Anterior border

Interosseous border

Lateral surface

**Fibula**

Posterior talofibular ligament

Lateral malleolus

Anterior talofibular ligament

Calcaneofibular ligament

Posterior } Cruciate
Anterior } ligaments

Tibial collateral ligament

Patellar ligament

Tibial tuberosity

Anterior border

Interosseous border

Interosseous membrane

Lateral surface

**Tibia**

Anterior tibiofibular ligament

Medial malleolus

Medial (deltoid) ligament of ankle

**Superior view**

Posterior ligament of fibular head

Apex

Head

**Fibula**

Anterior ligament of fibular head

Lateral condyle

Superior articular surface (lateral facet)

Anterior intercondylar area (origin of anterior cruciate ligament)

Posterior intercondylar area (origin of posterior cruciate ligament)

Intercondylar eminence

**Posterior**

**Tibia**

Medial condyle

Superior articular surface (medial facet)

Medial } Intercondylar
Lateral } tubercles

**Anterior**

Tibial tuberosity

**Cross section**

Interosseous border

Interosseous membrane

Interosseous border

Anterior border

Lateral surface

**Fibula**

Posterior border

Lateral surface

Anterior border

Medial surface

**Tibia**

Medial border

Posterior surface

Medial surface

Medial crest

Posterior surface

**Inferior view**

Anterior tibiofibular ligament

Articular facet of lateral malleolus

**Fibula**

Malleolar fossa of lateral malleolus

Posterior tibiofibular ligament

**Anterior**

Articular facet of medial malleolus

Medial malleolus

**Tibia**

**Posterior**

Inferior articular surface of tibia

**Plate 501**

**Leg**

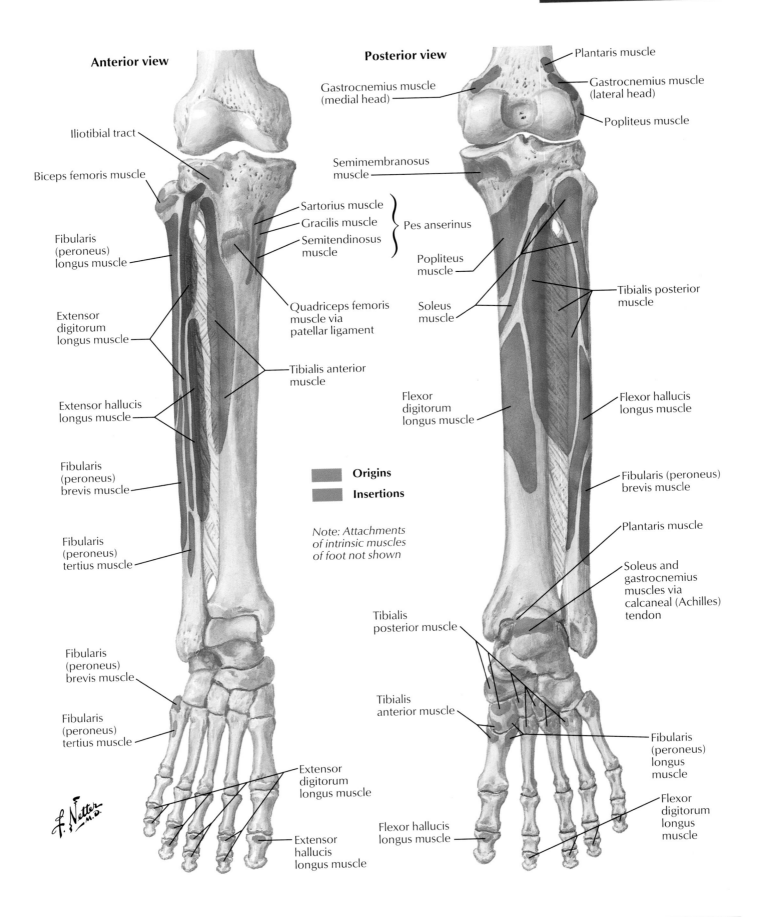

Anterior view

Posterior view

Plantaris muscle

Gastrocnemius muscle (medial head)

Gastrocnemius muscle (lateral head)

Iliotibial tract

Popliteus muscle

Biceps femoris muscle

Semimembranosus muscle

Sartorius muscle

Gracilis muscle

Pes anserinus

Fibularis (peroneus) longus muscle

Semitendinosus muscle

Popliteus muscle

Extensor digitorum longus muscle

Quadriceps femoris muscle via patellar ligament

Soleus muscle

Tibialis posterior muscle

Extensor hallucis longus muscle

Tibialis anterior muscle

Flexor digitorum longus muscle

Flexor hallucis longus muscle

Fibularis (peroneus) brevis muscle

**Origins**

**Insertions**

Fibularis (peroneus) brevis muscle

Fibularis (peroneus) tertius muscle

Note: Attachments of intrinsic muscles of foot not shown

Plantaris muscle

Soleus and gastrocnemius muscles via calcaneal (Achilles) tendon

Fibularis (peroneus) brevis muscle

Tibialis posterior muscle

Fibularis (peroneus) tertius muscle

Tibialis anterior muscle

Fibularis (peroneus) longus muscle

Extensor digitorum longus muscle

Flexor digitorum longus muscle

Extensor hallucis longus muscle

Flexor hallucis longus muscle

F. Netter M.D.

**Right leg**

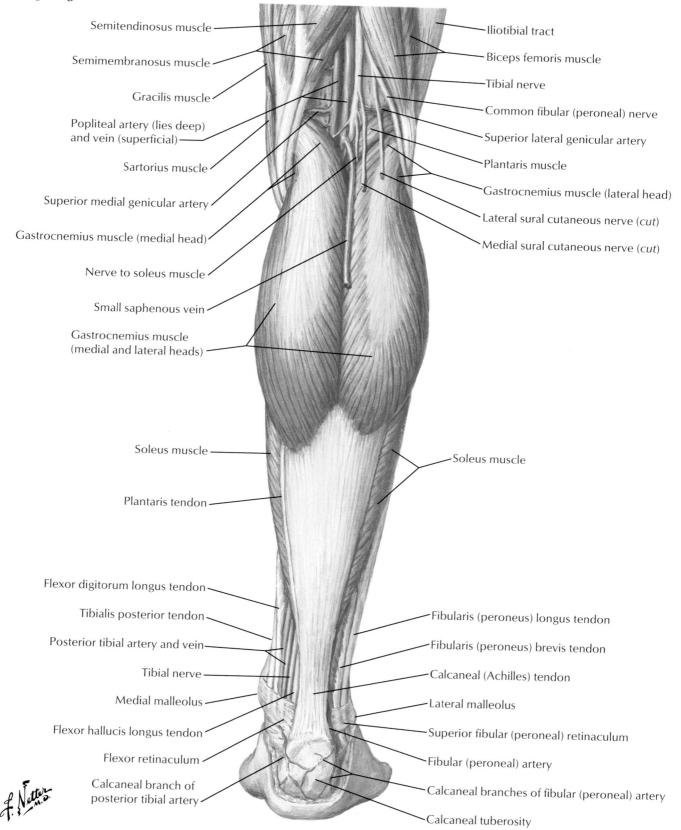

Semitendinosus muscle

Semimembranosus muscle

Gracilis muscle

Popliteal artery (lies deep)
and vein (superficial)

Sartorius muscle

Superior medial genicular artery

Gastrocnemius muscle (medial head)

Nerve to soleus muscle

Small saphenous vein

Gastrocnemius muscle
(medial and lateral heads)

Soleus muscle

Plantaris tendon

Flexor digitorum longus tendon

Tibialis posterior tendon

Posterior tibial artery and vein

Tibial nerve

Medial malleolus

Flexor hallucis longus tendon

Flexor retinaculum

Calcaneal branch of
posterior tibial artery

Iliotibial tract

Biceps femoris muscle

Tibial nerve

Common fibular (peroneal) nerve

Superior lateral genicular artery

Plantaris muscle

Gastrocnemius muscle (lateral head)

Lateral sural cutaneous nerve (*cut*)

Medial sural cutaneous nerve (*cut*)

Soleus muscle

Fibularis (peroneus) longus tendon

Fibularis (peroneus) brevis tendon

Calcaneal (Achilles) tendon

Lateral malleolus

Superior fibular (peroneal) retinaculum

Fibular (peroneal) artery

Calcaneal branches of fibular (peroneal) artery

Calcaneal tuberosity

**Plate 503**

**Leg**

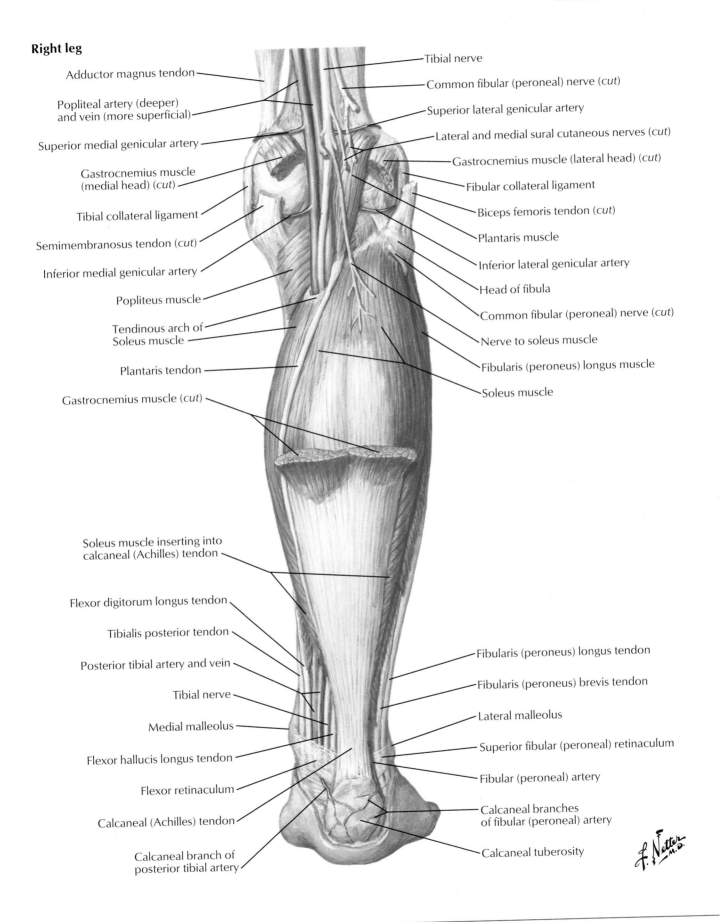

Right leg

Adductor magnus tendon

Popliteal artery (deeper) and vein (more superficial)

Superior medial genicular artery

Gastrocnemius muscle (medial head) (*cut*)

Tibial collateral ligament

Semimembranosus tendon (*cut*)

Inferior medial genicular artery

Popliteus muscle

Tendinous arch of Soleus muscle

Plantaris tendon

Gastrocnemius muscle (*cut*)

Soleus muscle inserting into calcaneal (Achilles) tendon

Flexor digitorum longus tendon

Tibialis posterior tendon

Posterior tibial artery and vein

Tibial nerve

Medial malleolus

Flexor hallucis longus tendon

Flexor retinaculum

Calcaneal (Achilles) tendon

Calcaneal branch of posterior tibial artery

Tibial nerve

Common fibular (peroneal) nerve (*cut*)

Superior lateral genicular artery

Lateral and medial sural cutaneous nerves (*cut*)

Gastrocnemius muscle (lateral head) (*cut*)

Fibular collateral ligament

Biceps femoris tendon (*cut*)

Plantaris muscle

Inferior lateral genicular artery

Head of fibula

Common fibular (peroneal) nerve (*cut*)

Nerve to soleus muscle

Fibularis (peroneus) longus muscle

Soleus muscle

Fibularis (peroneus) longus tendon

Fibularis (peroneus) brevis tendon

Lateral malleolus

Superior fibular (peroneal) retinaculum

Fibular (peroneal) artery

Calcaneal branches of fibular (peroneal) artery

Calcaneal tuberosity

**Plate 504**

**Leg**

**Right leg**

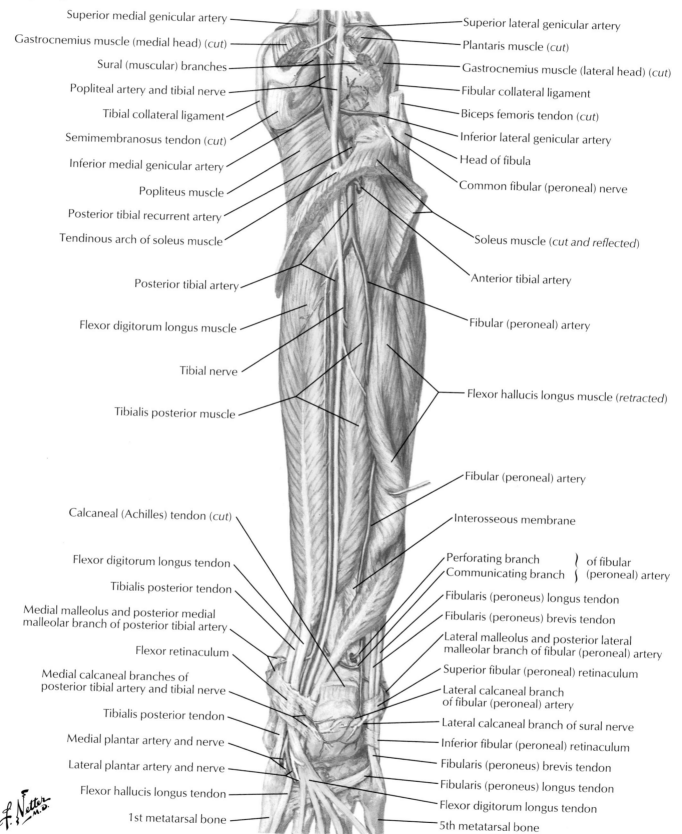

Superior medial genicular artery

Gastrocnemius muscle (medial head) (*cut*)

Sural (muscular) branches

Popliteal artery and tibial nerve

Tibial collateral ligament

Semimembranosus tendon (*cut*)

Inferior medial genicular artery

Popliteus muscle

Posterior tibial recurrent artery

Tendinous arch of soleus muscle

Posterior tibial artery

Flexor digitorum longus muscle

Tibial nerve

Tibialis posterior muscle

Calcaneal (Achilles) tendon (*cut*)

Flexor digitorum longus tendon

Tibialis posterior tendon

Medial malleolus and posterior medial malleolar branch of posterior tibial artery

Flexor retinaculum

Medial calcaneal branches of posterior tibial artery and tibial nerve

Tibialis posterior tendon

Medial plantar artery and nerve

Lateral plantar artery and nerve

Flexor hallucis longus tendon

1st metatarsal bone

Superior lateral genicular artery

Plantaris muscle (*cut*)

Gastrocnemius muscle (lateral head) (*cut*)

Fibular collateral ligament

Biceps femoris tendon (*cut*)

Inferior lateral genicular artery

Head of fibula

Common fibular (peroneal) nerve

Soleus muscle (*cut and reflected*)

Anterior tibial artery

Fibular (peroneal) artery

Flexor hallucis longus muscle (*retracted*)

Fibular (peroneal) artery

Interosseous membrane

Perforating branch ⎫ of fibular
Communicating branch ⎭ (peroneal) artery

Fibularis (peroneus) longus tendon

Fibularis (peroneus) brevis tendon

Lateral malleolus and posterior lateral malleolar branch of fibular (peroneal) artery

Superior fibular (peroneal) retinaculum

Lateral calcaneal branch of fibular (peroneal) artery

Lateral calcaneal branch of sural nerve

Inferior fibular (peroneal) retinaculum

Fibularis (peroneus) brevis tendon

Fibularis (peroneus) longus tendon

Flexor digitorum longus tendon

5th metatarsal bone

**Plate 505**

**Leg**

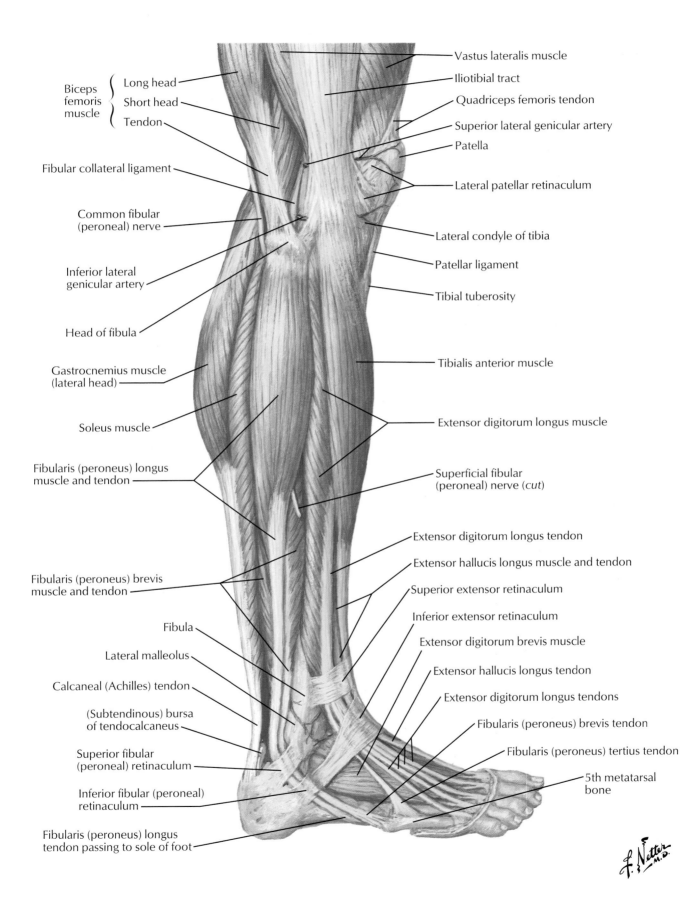

Biceps femoris muscle {
Long head
Short head
Tendon
}

Vastus lateralis muscle

Iliotibial tract

Quadriceps femoris tendon

Superior lateral genicular artery

Patella

Fibular collateral ligament

Lateral patellar retinaculum

Common fibular (peroneal) nerve

Lateral condyle of tibia

Patellar ligament

Inferior lateral genicular artery

Tibial tuberosity

Head of fibula

Tibialis anterior muscle

Gastrocnemius muscle (lateral head)

Soleus muscle

Extensor digitorum longus muscle

Fibularis (peroneus) longus muscle and tendon

Superficial fibular (peroneal) nerve (*cut*)

Extensor digitorum longus tendon

Extensor hallucis longus muscle and tendon

Fibularis (peroneus) brevis muscle and tendon

Superior extensor retinaculum

Inferior extensor retinaculum

Fibula

Extensor digitorum brevis muscle

Lateral malleolus

Extensor hallucis longus tendon

Calcaneal (Achilles) tendon

Extensor digitorum longus tendons

(Subtendinous) bursa of tendocalcaneus

Fibularis (peroneus) brevis tendon

Superior fibular (peroneal) retinaculum

Fibularis (peroneus) tertius tendon

5th metatarsal bone

Inferior fibular (peroneal) retinaculum

Fibularis (peroneus) longus tendon passing to sole of foot

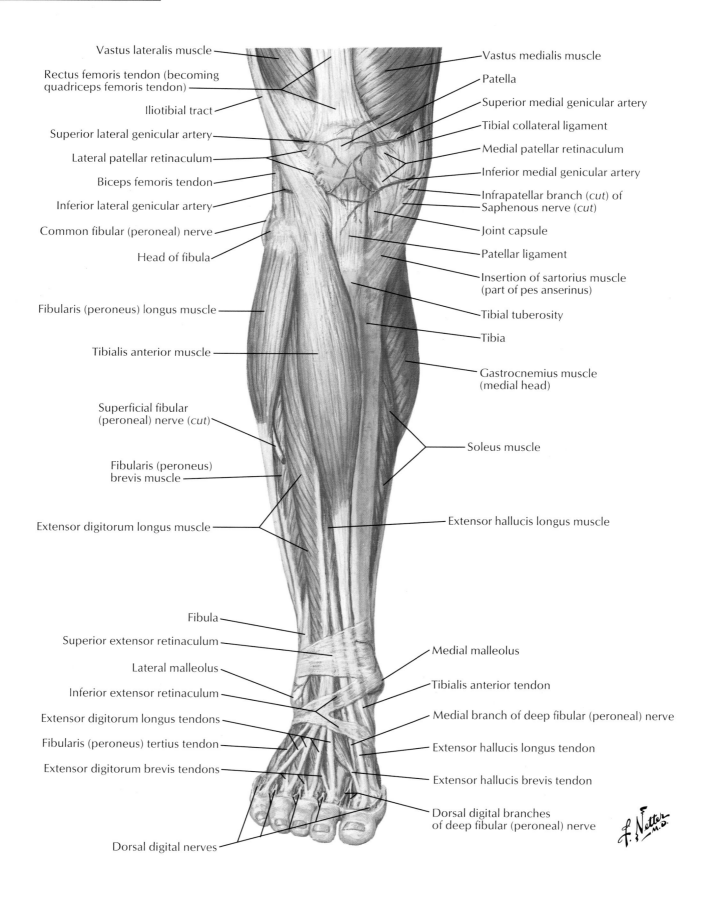

Vastus lateralis muscle

Rectus femoris tendon (becoming quadriceps femoris tendon)

Iliotibial tract

Superior lateral genicular artery

Lateral patellar retinaculum

Biceps femoris tendon

Inferior lateral genicular artery

Common fibular (peroneal) nerve

Head of fibula

Fibularis (peroneus) longus muscle

Tibialis anterior muscle

Superficial fibular (peroneal) nerve (*cut*)

Fibularis (peroneus) brevis muscle

Extensor digitorum longus muscle

Fibula

Superior extensor retinaculum

Lateral malleolus

Inferior extensor retinaculum

Extensor digitorum longus tendons

Fibularis (peroneus) tertius tendon

Extensor digitorum brevis tendons

Dorsal digital nerves

Vastus medialis muscle

Patella

Superior medial genicular artery

Tibial collateral ligament

Medial patellar retinaculum

Inferior medial genicular artery

Infrapatellar branch (*cut*) of Saphenous nerve (*cut*)

Joint capsule

Patellar ligament

Insertion of sartorius muscle (part of pes anserinus)

Tibial tuberosity

Tibia

Gastrocnemius muscle (medial head)

Soleus muscle

Extensor hallucis longus muscle

Medial malleolus

Tibialis anterior tendon

Medial branch of deep fibular (peroneal) nerve

Extensor hallucis longus tendon

Extensor hallucis brevis tendon

Dorsal digital branches of deep fibular (peroneal) nerve

**Plate 507**

**Leg**

Superior lateral genicular artery

Fibular collateral ligament

Lateral patellar retinaculum

Iliotibial tract (*cut*)

Biceps femoris tendon (*cut*)

Inferior lateral genicular artery

Common fibular (peroneal) nerve

Head of fibula

Fibularis (peroneus) longus muscle (*cut*)

Anterior tibial artery

Extensor digitorum longus muscle (*cut*)

Superficial fibular (peroneal) nerve

Deep fibular (peroneal) nerve

Fibularis (peroneus) longus muscle

Extensor digitorum longus muscle

Fibularis (peroneus)
brevis muscle and tendon

Fibularis (peroneus) longus tendon

Perforating branch of
fibular (peroneal) artery

Anterior lateral malleolar artery

Lateral malleolus and arterial network

Lateral tarsal artery and lateral
branch of deep fibular (peroneal) nerve

Extensor digitorum brevis and
extensor hallucis brevis muscles (*cut*)

Fibularis (peroneus) brevis tendon

Posterior perforating branches
from deep plantar arch

Extensor digitorum longus tendons (*cut*)

Extensor digitorum brevis tendons (*cut*)

Dorsal digital arteries

Branches of proper plantar
digital arteries and nerves

Superior medial genicular artery

Quadriceps femoris tendon

Tibial collateral ligament

Medial patellar retinaculum

Infrapatellar branch of saphenous nerve (*cut*)

Inferior medial genicular artery

Saphenous nerve (*cut*)

Patellar ligament

Insertion of sartorius tendon

Anterior tibial recurrent artery and
recurrent branch of deep fibular (peroneal) nerve

Interosseous membrane

Tibialis anterior muscle (*cut*)

Gastrocnemius muscle

Soleus muscle

Tibia

Superficial fibular (peroneal) nerve (*cut*)

Extensor hallucis longus muscle and tendon (*cut*)

Interosseous membrane

Anterior medial malleolar artery

Medial malleolus and arterial network

Anterior tibial artery

Tibialis anterior tendon

Medial tarsal artery

Dorsalis pedis artery

Medial branch of deep fibular (peroneal) nerve

Arcuate artery

Deep plantar artery

Dorsal metatarsal arteries

Extensor hallucis longus tendon (*cut*)

Extensor hallucis brevis tendon (*cut*)

Dorsal digital branches of
deep fibular (peroneal) nerve

F. Netter M.D.

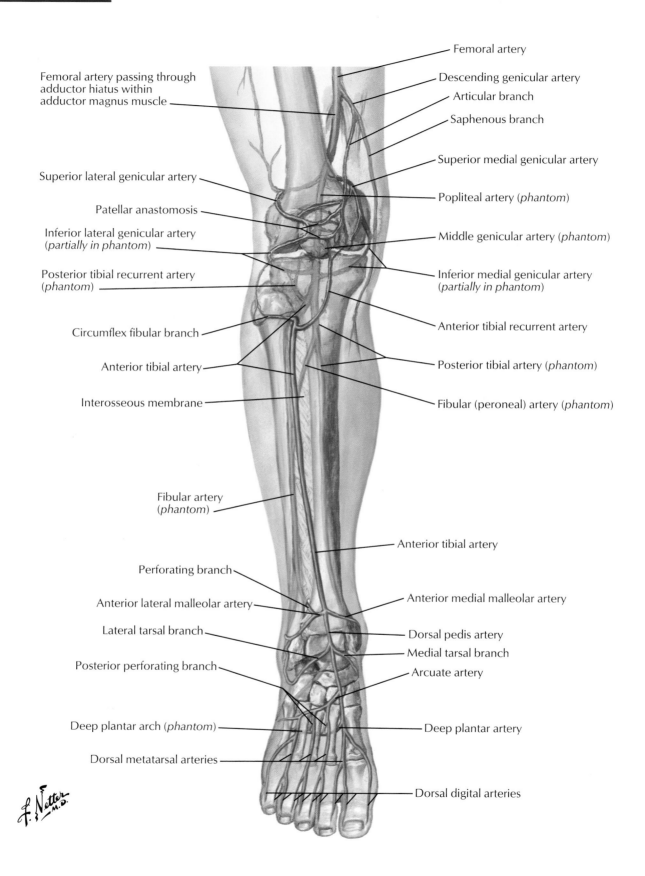

Femoral artery

Descending genicular artery

Articular branch

Saphenous branch

Femoral artery passing through adductor hiatus within adductor magnus muscle

Superior medial genicular artery

Superior lateral genicular artery

Popliteal artery (*phantom*)

Patellar anastomosis

Middle genicular artery (*phantom*)

Inferior lateral genicular artery (*partially in phantom*)

Inferior medial genicular artery (*partially in phantom*)

Posterior tibial recurrent artery (*phantom*)

Anterior tibial recurrent artery

Circumflex fibular branch

Anterior tibial artery

Posterior tibial artery (*phantom*)

Interosseous membrane

Fibular (peroneal) artery (*phantom*)

Fibular artery (*phantom*)

Anterior tibial artery

Perforating branch

Anterior lateral malleolar artery

Anterior medial malleolar artery

Lateral tarsal branch

Dorsal pedis artery

Medial tarsal branch

Posterior perforating branch

Arcuate artery

Deep plantar arch (*phantom*)

Deep plantar artery

Dorsal metatarsal arteries

Dorsal digital arteries

**Plate 509**

**Leg**

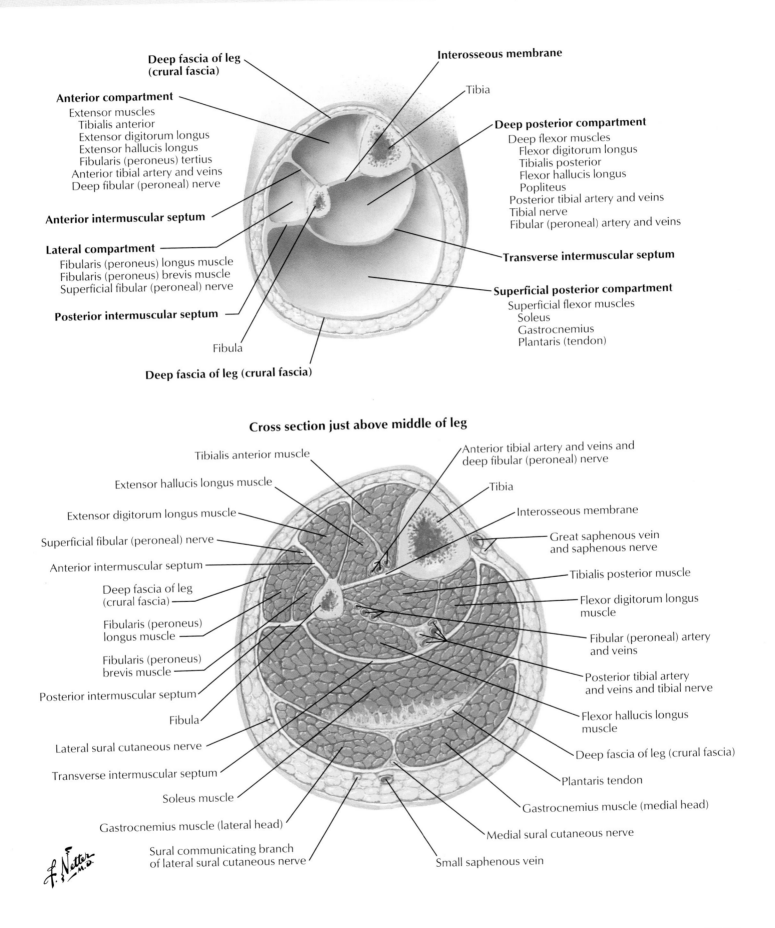

**Deep fascia of leg (crural fascia)**

**Interosseous membrane**

Tibia

**Anterior compartment**
Extensor muscles
Tibialis anterior
Extensor digitorum longus
Extensor hallucis longus
Fibularis (peroneus) tertius
Anterior tibial artery and veins
Deep fibular (peroneal) nerve

**Deep posterior compartment**
Deep flexor muscles
Flexor digitorum longus
Tibialis posterior
Flexor hallucis longus
Popliteus
Posterior tibial artery and veins
Tibial nerve
Fibular (peroneal) artery and veins

**Anterior intermuscular septum**

**Lateral compartment**
Fibularis (peroneus) longus muscle
Fibularis (peroneus) brevis muscle
Superficial fibular (peroneal) nerve

**Transverse intermuscular septum**

**Superficial posterior compartment**
Superficial flexor muscles
Soleus
Gastrocnemius
Plantaris (tendon)

**Posterior intermuscular septum**

Fibula

**Deep fascia of leg (crural fascia)**

**Cross section just above middle of leg**

Tibialis anterior muscle

Anterior tibial artery and veins and deep fibular (peroneal) nerve

Extensor hallucis longus muscle

Tibia

Extensor digitorum longus muscle

Interosseous membrane

Superficial fibular (peroneal) nerve

Great saphenous vein and saphenous nerve

Anterior intermuscular septum

Tibialis posterior muscle

Deep fascia of leg (crural fascia)

Flexor digitorum longus muscle

Fibularis (peroneus) longus muscle

Fibular (peroneal) artery and veins

Fibularis (peroneus) brevis muscle

Posterior tibial artery and veins and tibial nerve

Posterior intermuscular septum

Flexor hallucis longus muscle

Fibula

Deep fascia of leg (crural fascia)

Lateral sural cutaneous nerve

Plantaris tendon

Transverse intermuscular septum

Soleus muscle

Gastrocnemius muscle (medial head)

Gastrocnemius muscle (lateral head)

Medial sural cutaneous nerve

Sural communicating branch of lateral sural cutaneous nerve

Small saphenous vein

**Plate 510**

**Leg**

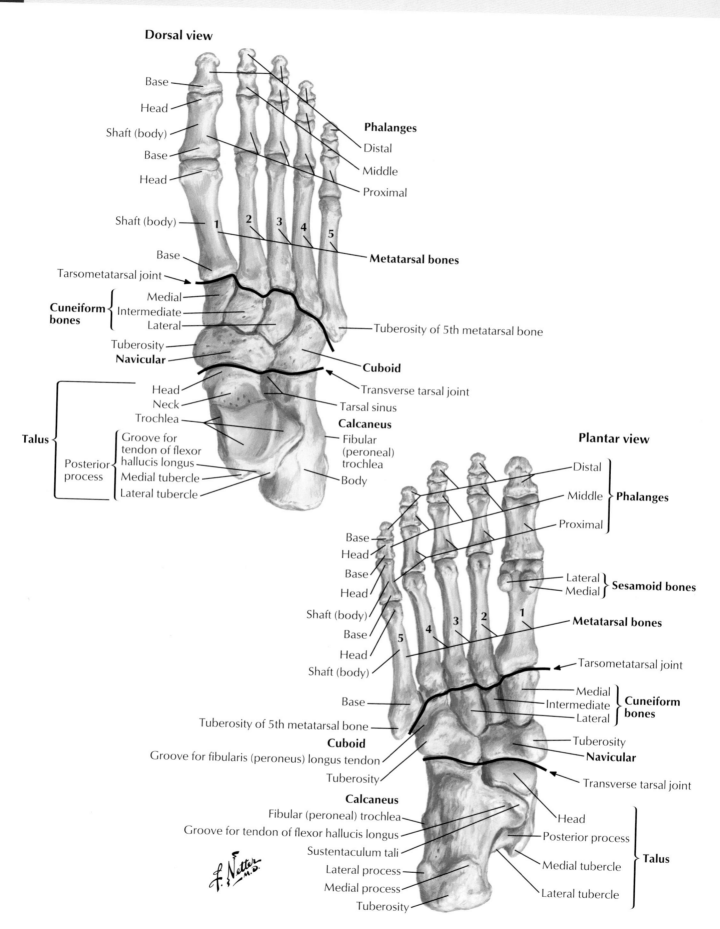

**Dorsal view**

Base
Head
Shaft (body)
Base
Head

**Phalanges**
Distal
Middle
Proximal

Shaft (body)
1  2  3  4  5

Base

**Metatarsal bones**

Tarsometatarsal joint

Medial
Intermediate
Lateral

**Cuneiform bones**

Tuberosity
**Navicular**

Tuberosity of 5th metatarsal bone

**Cuboid**

Transverse tarsal joint

Head
Neck
Trochlea

Tarsal sinus

**Calcaneus**

**Talus**

Groove for tendon of flexor hallucis longus
Posterior process
Medial tubercle
Lateral tubercle

Fibular (peroneal) trochlea

Body

**Plantar view**

Distal
Middle
Proximal

**Phalanges**

Base
Head
Base
Head

Lateral
Medial

**Sesamoid bones**

Shaft (body)
Base
Head
Shaft (body)

4  3  2  1

**Metatarsal bones**

Tarsometatarsal joint

Medial
Intermediate
Lateral

**Cuneiform bones**

Base

Tuberosity of 5th metatarsal bone

**Cuboid**

Groove for fibularis (peroneus) longus tendon

Tuberosity

Tuberosity
**Navicular**

Transverse tarsal joint

**Calcaneus**

Fibular (peroneal) trochlea
Groove for tendon of flexor hallucis longus
Sustentaculum tali
Lateral process
Medial process
Tuberosity

Head
Posterior process
Medial tubercle
Lateral tubercle

**Talus**

**Plate 511**

**Ankle and Foot**

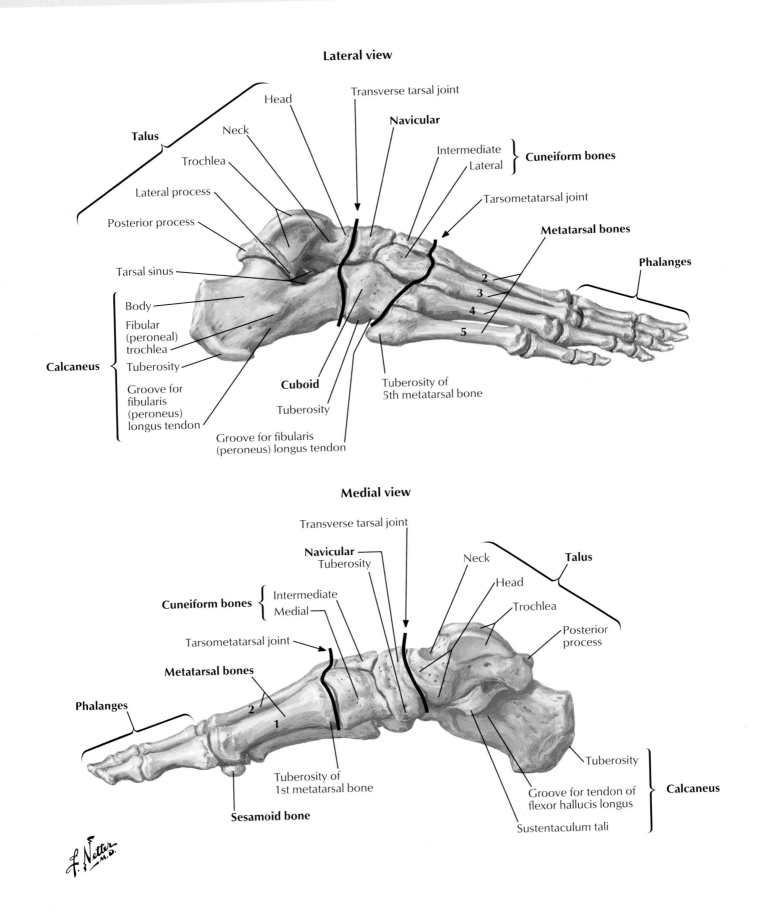

**Lateral view**

Transverse tarsal joint

Head

Neck

**Talus**

Trochlea

**Navicular**

Lateral process

Intermediate } **Cuneiform bones**
Lateral

Posterior process

Tarsometatarsal joint

Tarsal sinus

**Metatarsal bones**

Body

**Phalanges**

Fibular (peroneal) trochlea

2

3

**Calcaneus**

Tuberosity

4

5

Groove for fibularis (peroneus) longus tendon

**Cuboid**

Tuberosity of 5th metatarsal bone

Tuberosity

Groove for fibularis (peroneus) longus tendon

**Medial view**

Transverse tarsal joint

**Navicular**
Tuberosity

Neck

**Talus**

**Cuneiform bones** {
Intermediate

Head

Medial

Trochlea

Tarsometatarsal joint

Posterior process

**Metatarsal bones**

**Phalanges**

2

1

Tuberosity

Tuberosity of 1st metatarsal bone

Groove for tendon of flexor hallucis longus

**Calcaneus**

**Sesamoid bone**

Sustentaculum tali

**Right foot**

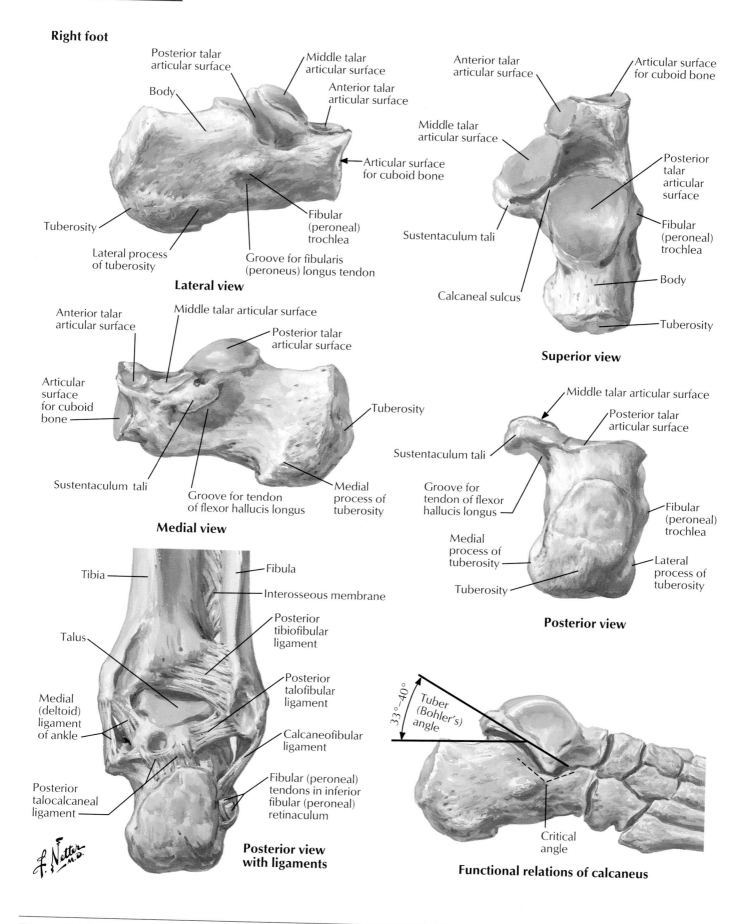

Posterior talar articular surface
Body
Middle talar articular surface
Anterior talar articular surface
Articular surface for cuboid bone
Tuberosity
Fibular (peroneal) trochlea
Lateral process of tuberosity
Groove for fibularis (peroneus) longus tendon

**Lateral view**

Anterior talar articular surface
Middle talar articular surface
Posterior talar articular surface
Articular surface for cuboid bone
Tuberosity
Sustentaculum tali
Groove for tendon of flexor hallucis longus
Medial process of tuberosity

**Medial view**

Anterior talar articular surface
Articular surface for cuboid bone
Middle talar articular surface
Posterior talar articular surface
Sustentaculum tali
Fibular (peroneal) trochlea
Calcaneal sulcus
Body
Tuberosity

**Superior view**

Middle talar articular surface
Posterior talar articular surface
Sustentaculum tali
Groove for tendon of flexor hallucis longus
Medial process of tuberosity
Tuberosity
Fibular (peroneal) trochlea
Lateral process of tuberosity

**Posterior view**

Tibia
Fibula
Interosseous membrane
Posterior tibiofibular ligament
Talus
Posterior talofibular ligament
Medial (deltoid) ligament of ankle
Calcaneofibular ligament
Posterior talocalcaneal ligament
Fibular (peroneal) tendons in inferior fibular (peroneal) retinaculum

**Posterior view with ligaments**

33°–40°
Tuber (Bohler's) angle
Critical angle

**Functional relations of calcaneus**

**Plate 513**

**Ankle and Foot**

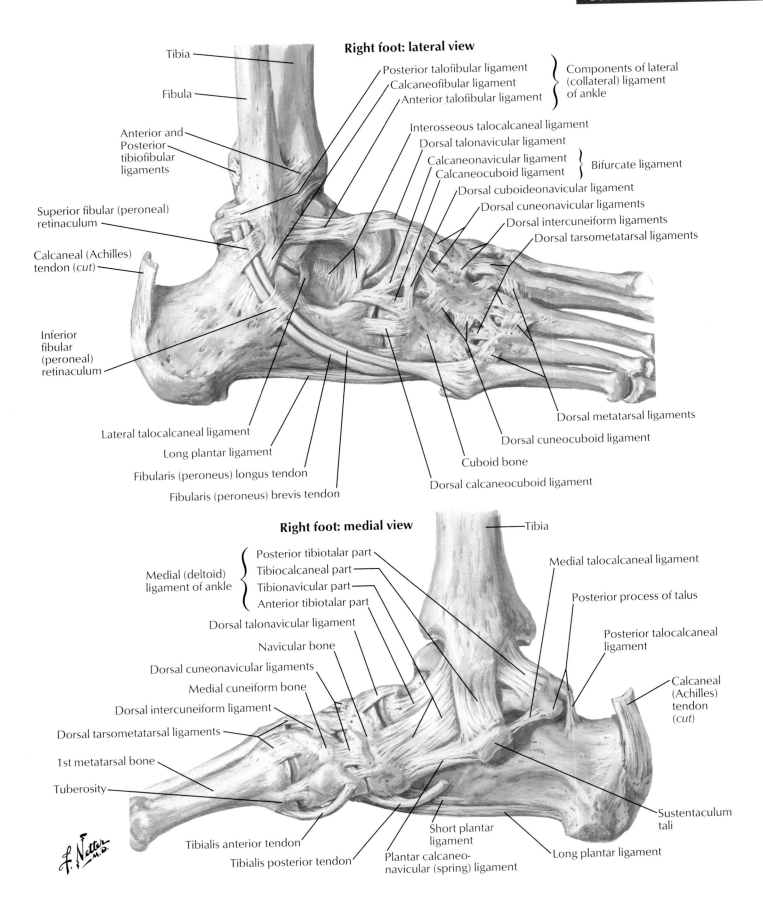

**Right foot: lateral view**

Tibia

Fibula

Anterior and Posterior tibiofibular ligaments

Superior fibular (peroneal) retinaculum

Calcaneal (Achilles) tendon (cut)

Inferior fibular (peroneal) retinaculum

Posterior talofibular ligament
Calcaneofibular ligament
Anterior talofibular ligament

Components of lateral (collateral) ligament of ankle

Interosseous talocalcaneal ligament
Dorsal talonavicular ligament
Calcaneonavicular ligament
Calcaneocuboid ligament

Bifurcate ligament

Dorsal cuboideonavicular ligament
Dorsal cuneonavicular ligaments
Dorsal intercuneiform ligaments
Dorsal tarsometatarsal ligaments

Dorsal metatarsal ligaments
Dorsal cuneocuboid ligament
Cuboid bone
Dorsal calcaneocuboid ligament

Lateral talocalcaneal ligament
Long plantar ligament
Fibularis (peroneus) longus tendon
Fibularis (peroneus) brevis tendon

**Right foot: medial view**

Tibia

Medial (deltoid) ligament of ankle

Posterior tibiotalar part
Tibiocalcaneal part
Tibionavicular part
Anterior tibiotalar part

Dorsal talonavicular ligament
Navicular bone
Dorsal cuneonavicular ligaments
Medial cuneiform bone
Dorsal intercuneiform ligament
Dorsal tarsometatarsal ligaments
1st metatarsal bone
Tuberosity

Medial talocalcaneal ligament
Posterior process of talus
Posterior talocalcaneal ligament
Calcaneal (Achilles) tendon (cut)
Sustentaculum tali

Tibialis anterior tendon
Tibialis posterior tendon
Short plantar ligament
Plantar calcaneonavicular (spring) ligament
Long plantar ligament

**Ankle and Foot**

**Plate 514**

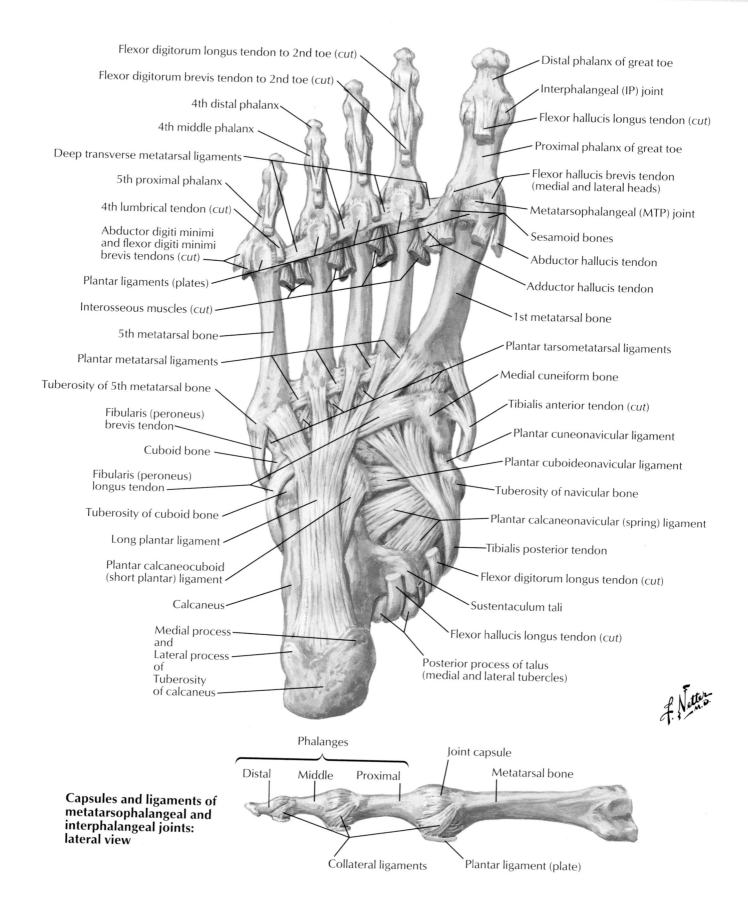

Flexor digitorum longus tendon to 2nd toe (*cut*)

Flexor digitorum brevis tendon to 2nd toe (*cut*)

4th distal phalanx

4th middle phalanx

Deep transverse metatarsal ligaments

5th proximal phalanx

4th lumbrical tendon (*cut*)

Abductor digiti minimi and flexor digiti minimi brevis tendons (*cut*)

Plantar ligaments (plates)

Interosseous muscles (*cut*)

5th metatarsal bone

Plantar metatarsal ligaments

Tuberosity of 5th metatarsal bone

Fibularis (peroneus) brevis tendon

Cuboid bone

Fibularis (peroneus) longus tendon

Tuberosity of cuboid bone

Long plantar ligament

Plantar calcaneocuboid (short plantar) ligament

Calcaneus

Medial process and Lateral process of Tuberosity of calcaneus

Distal phalanx of great toe

Interphalangeal (IP) joint

Flexor hallucis longus tendon (*cut*)

Proximal phalanx of great toe

Flexor hallucis brevis tendon (medial and lateral heads)

Metatarsophalangeal (MTP) joint

Sesamoid bones

Abductor hallucis tendon

Adductor hallucis tendon

1st metatarsal bone

Plantar tarsometatarsal ligaments

Medial cuneiform bone

Tibialis anterior tendon (*cut*)

Plantar cuneonavicular ligament

Plantar cuboideonavicular ligament

Tuberosity of navicular bone

Plantar calcaneonavicular (spring) ligament

Tibialis posterior tendon

Flexor digitorum longus tendon (*cut*)

Sustentaculum tali

Flexor hallucis longus tendon (*cut*)

Posterior process of talus (medial and lateral tubercles)

Phalanges

Distal    Middle    Proximal

Joint capsule

Metatarsal bone

**Capsules and ligaments of metatarsophalangeal and interphalangeal joints: lateral view**

Collateral ligaments

Plantar ligament (plate)

**Plate 515**

**Ankle and Foot**

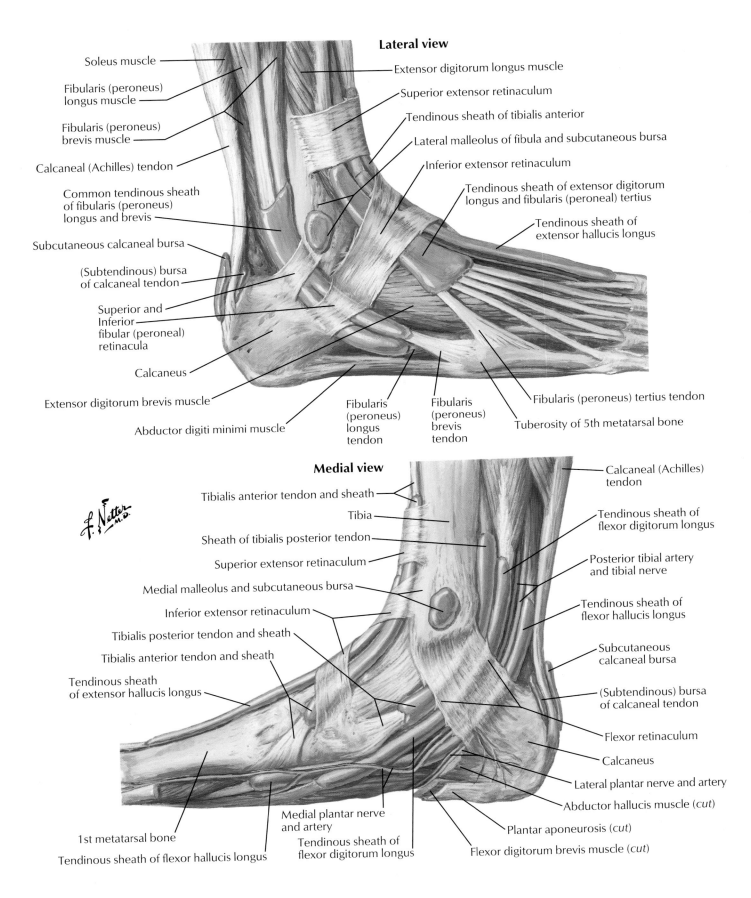

**Lateral view**

Soleus muscle

Fibularis (peroneus) longus muscle

Fibularis (peroneus) brevis muscle

Calcaneal (Achilles) tendon

Common tendinous sheath of fibularis (peroneus) longus and brevis

Subcutaneous calcaneal bursa

(Subtendinous) bursa of calcaneal tendon

Superior and Inferior fibular (peroneal) retinacula

Calcaneus

Extensor digitorum brevis muscle

Abductor digiti minimi muscle

Fibularis (peroneus) longus tendon

Fibularis (peroneus) brevis tendon

Extensor digitorum longus muscle

Superior extensor retinaculum

Tendinous sheath of tibialis anterior

Lateral malleolus of fibula and subcutaneous bursa

Inferior extensor retinaculum

Tendinous sheath of extensor digitorum longus and fibularis (peroneal) tertius

Tendinous sheath of extensor hallucis longus

Fibularis (peroneus) tertius tendon

Tuberosity of 5th metatarsal bone

**Medial view**

Tibialis anterior tendon and sheath

Tibia

Sheath of tibialis posterior tendon

Superior extensor retinaculum

Medial malleolus and subcutaneous bursa

Inferior extensor retinaculum

Tibialis posterior tendon and sheath

Tibialis anterior tendon and sheath

Tendinous sheath of extensor hallucis longus

1st metatarsal bone

Tendinous sheath of flexor hallucis longus

Medial plantar nerve and artery

Tendinous sheath of flexor digitorum longus

Calcaneal (Achilles) tendon

Tendinous sheath of flexor digitorum longus

Posterior tibial artery and tibial nerve

Tendinous sheath of flexor hallucis longus

Subcutaneous calcaneal bursa

(Subtendinous) bursa of calcaneal tendon

Flexor retinaculum

Calcaneus

Lateral plantar nerve and artery

Abductor hallucis muscle (cut)

Plantar aponeurosis (cut)

Flexor digitorum brevis muscle (cut)

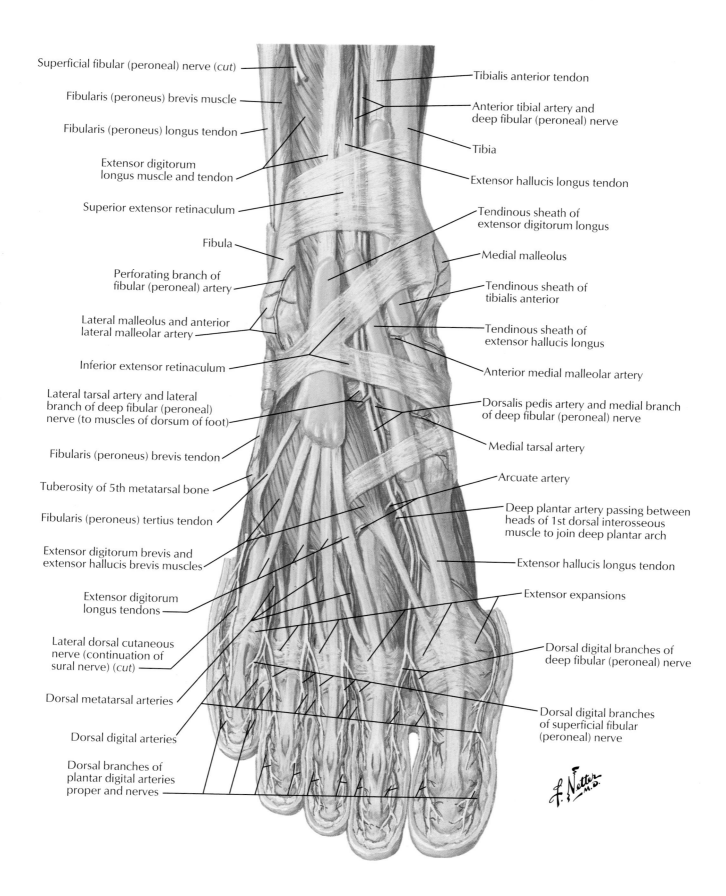

Superficial fibular (peroneal) nerve (cut)

Fibularis (peroneus) brevis muscle

Fibularis (peroneus) longus tendon

Extensor digitorum longus muscle and tendon

Superior extensor retinaculum

Fibula

Perforating branch of fibular (peroneal) artery

Lateral malleolus and anterior lateral malleolar artery

Inferior extensor retinaculum

Lateral tarsal artery and lateral branch of deep fibular (peroneal) nerve (to muscles of dorsum of foot)

Fibularis (peroneus) brevis tendon

Tuberosity of 5th metatarsal bone

Fibularis (peroneus) tertius tendon

Extensor digitorum brevis and extensor hallucis brevis muscles

Extensor digitorum longus tendons

Lateral dorsal cutaneous nerve (continuation of sural nerve) (cut)

Dorsal metatarsal arteries

Dorsal digital arteries

Dorsal branches of plantar digital arteries proper and nerves

Tibialis anterior tendon

Anterior tibial artery and deep fibular (peroneal) nerve

Tibia

Extensor hallucis longus tendon

Tendinous sheath of extensor digitorum longus

Medial malleolus

Tendinous sheath of tibialis anterior

Tendinous sheath of extensor hallucis longus

Anterior medial malleolar artery

Dorsalis pedis artery and medial branch of deep fibular (peroneal) nerve

Medial tarsal artery

Arcuate artery

Deep plantar artery passing between heads of 1st dorsal interosseous muscle to join deep plantar arch

Extensor hallucis longus tendon

Extensor expansions

Dorsal digital branches of deep fibular (peroneal) nerve

Dorsal digital branches of superficial fibular (peroneal) nerve

**Plate 517**

**Ankle and Foot**

Superficial fibular (peroneal) nerve (*cut*)

Fibularis (peroneus) longus tendon

Fibularis (peroneus) brevis muscle and tendon

Extensor digitorum longus muscle and tendon

Fibula

Perforating branch of fibular (peroneal) artery

Anterior lateral malleolar artery

Lateral malleolus

Lateral branch of deep fibular (peroneal) nerve (to muscles of dorsum of foot) and lateral tarsal artery

Fibularis (peroneus) longus tendon (*cut*)

Extensor digitorum brevis and extensor hallucis brevis muscles (*cut*)

Fibularis (peroneus) brevis tendon (*cut*)

Fibularis (peroneus) tertius tendon (*cut*)

Abductor digiti minimi muscle

Dorsal metatarsal arteries

Metatarsal bones

Dorsal interosseous muscles

Lateral dorsal cutaneous nerve (continuation of sural nerve) (*cut*)

Anterior perforating branches from plantar metatarsal arteries

Dorsal digital arteries

Dorsal branches of plantar digital arteries proper and nerves

Soleus muscle

Tibialis anterior muscle and tendon

Tibia

Anterior tibial artery and deep fibular (peroneal) nerve

Extensor hallucis longus muscle and tendon

Anterior medial malleolar artery

Medial malleolus

Medial branch of deep fibular (peroneal) nerve

Medial tarsal arteries

Tuberosity of navicular bone

Dorsalis pedis artery

Arcuate artery

Posterior perforating branches from deep plantar arch

Deep plantar artery to deep plantar arch

Abductor hallucis muscle

Extensor hallucis longus tendon

Extensor hallucis brevis tendon (*cut*)

Extensor digitorum brevis tendons (*cut*)

Extensor digitorum longus tendons (*cut*)

Extensor expansions

Dorsal digital branches of deep fibular (peroneal) nerve

Dorsal digital branches of superficial fibular (peroneal) nerve

*F. Netter, M.D.*

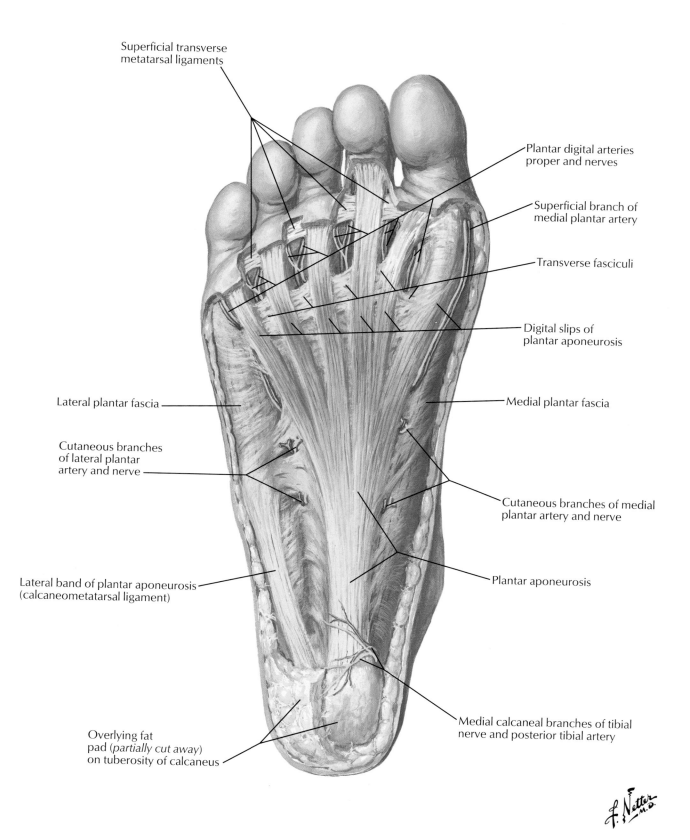

Superficial transverse
metatarsal ligaments

Plantar digital arteries
proper and nerves

Superficial branch of
medial plantar artery

Transverse fasciculi

Digital slips of
plantar aponeurosis

Lateral plantar fascia

Medial plantar fascia

Cutaneous branches
of lateral plantar
artery and nerve

Cutaneous branches of medial
plantar artery and nerve

Lateral band of plantar aponeurosis
(calcaneometatarsal ligament)

Plantar aponeurosis

Medial calcaneal branches of tibial
nerve and posterior tibial artery

Overlying fat
pad (*partially cut away*)
on tuberosity of calcaneus

**Plate 519**

**Ankle and Foot**

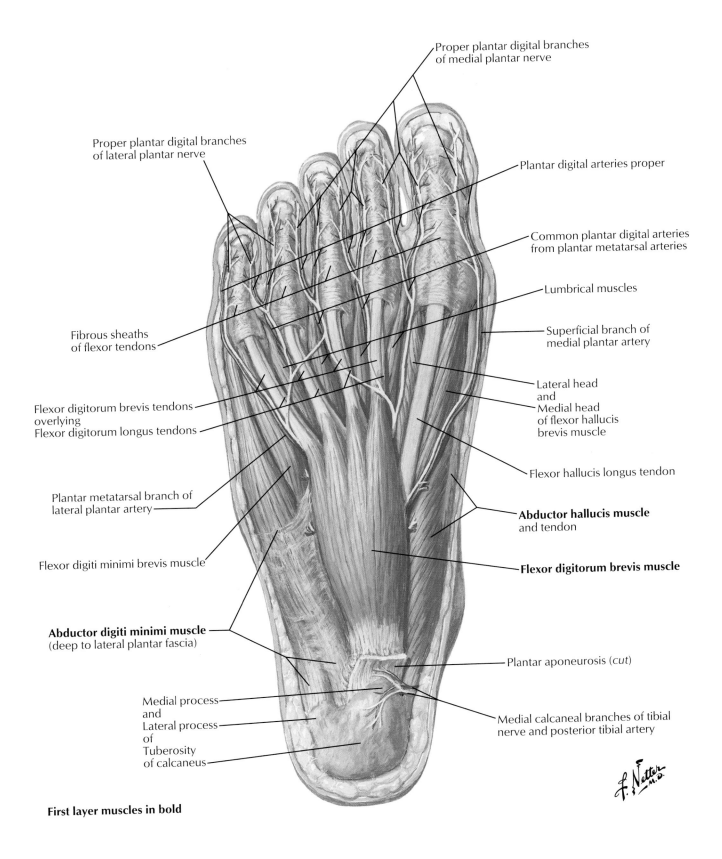

Proper plantar digital branches
of medial plantar nerve

Proper plantar digital branches
of lateral plantar nerve

Plantar digital arteries proper

Common plantar digital arteries
from plantar metatarsal arteries

Lumbrical muscles

Fibrous sheaths
of flexor tendons

Superficial branch of
medial plantar artery

Flexor digitorum brevis tendons
overlying
Flexor digitorum longus tendons

Lateral head
and
Medial head
of flexor hallucis
brevis muscle

Flexor hallucis longus tendon

Plantar metatarsal branch of
lateral plantar artery

**Abductor hallucis muscle**
and tendon

**Flexor digitorum brevis muscle**

Flexor digiti minimi brevis muscle

**Abductor digiti minimi muscle**
(deep to lateral plantar fascia)

Plantar aponeurosis (*cut*)

Medial process
and
Lateral process
of
Tuberosity
of calcaneus

Medial calcaneal branches of tibial
nerve and posterior tibial artery

**First layer muscles in bold**

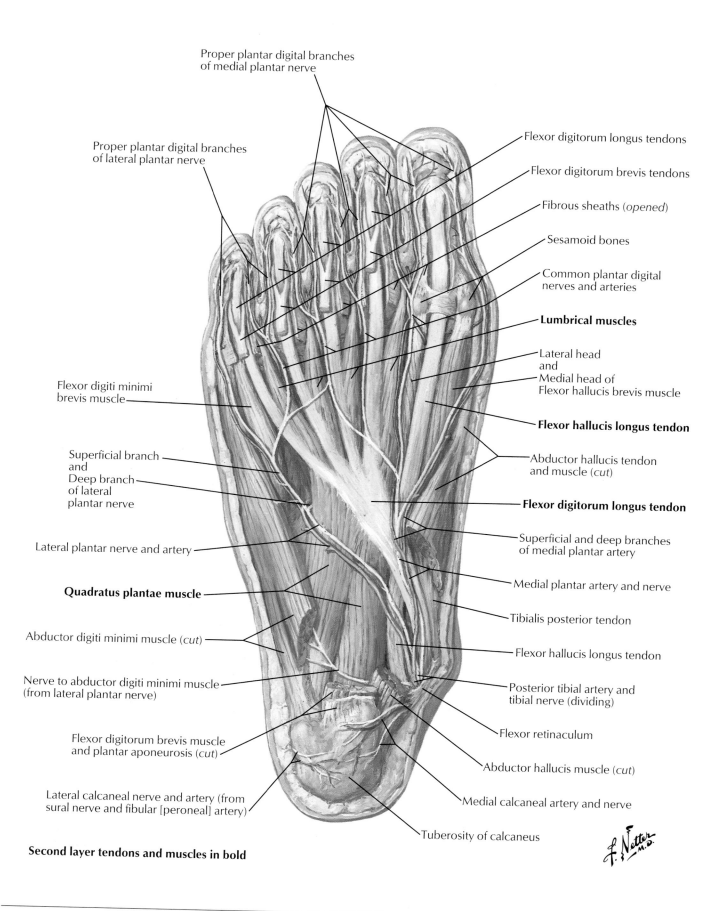

Proper plantar digital branches
of medial plantar nerve

Proper plantar digital branches
of lateral plantar nerve

Flexor digiti minimi
brevis muscle

Superficial branch
and
Deep branch
of lateral
plantar nerve

Lateral plantar nerve and artery

**Quadratus plantae muscle**

Abductor digiti minimi muscle (*cut*)

Nerve to abductor digiti minimi muscle
(from lateral plantar nerve)

Flexor digitorum brevis muscle
and plantar aponeurosis (*cut*)

Lateral calcaneal nerve and artery (from
sural nerve and fibular [peroneal] artery)

Flexor digitorum longus tendons

Flexor digitorum brevis tendons

Fibrous sheaths (*opened*)

Sesamoid bones

Common plantar digital
nerves and arteries

**Lumbrical muscles**

Lateral head
and
Medial head of
Flexor hallucis brevis muscle

**Flexor hallucis longus tendon**

Abductor hallucis tendon
and muscle (*cut*)

**Flexor digitorum longus tendon**

Superficial and deep branches
of medial plantar artery

Medial plantar artery and nerve

Tibialis posterior tendon

Flexor hallucis longus tendon

Posterior tibial artery and
tibial nerve (dividing)

Flexor retinaculum

Abductor hallucis muscle (*cut*)

Medial calcaneal artery and nerve

Tuberosity of calcaneus

**Second layer tendons and muscles in bold**

**Plate 521**

**Ankle and Foot**

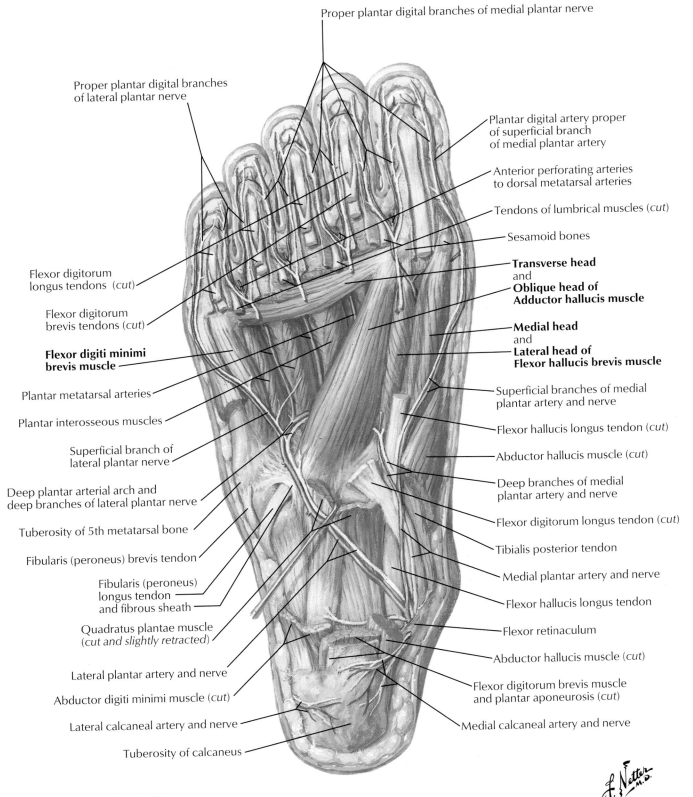

Proper plantar digital branches of medial plantar nerve

Proper plantar digital branches of lateral plantar nerve

Plantar digital artery proper of superficial branch of medial plantar artery

Anterior perforating arteries to dorsal metatarsal arteries

Tendons of lumbrical muscles (cut)

Sesamoid bones

**Transverse head** and **Oblique head of Adductor hallucis muscle**

Flexor digitorum longus tendons (cut)

Flexor digitorum brevis tendons (cut)

**Flexor digiti minimi brevis muscle**

**Medial head** and **Lateral head of Flexor hallucis brevis muscle**

Superficial branches of medial plantar artery and nerve

Plantar metatarsal arteries

Flexor hallucis longus tendon (cut)

Plantar interosseous muscles

Abductor hallucis muscle (cut)

Superficial branch of lateral plantar nerve

Deep branches of medial plantar artery and nerve

Deep plantar arterial arch and deep branches of lateral plantar nerve

Flexor digitorum longus tendon (cut)

Tuberosity of 5th metatarsal bone

Tibialis posterior tendon

Fibularis (peroneus) brevis tendon

Medial plantar artery and nerve

Fibularis (peroneus) longus tendon and fibrous sheath

Flexor hallucis longus tendon

Quadratus plantae muscle (cut and slightly retracted)

Flexor retinaculum

Lateral plantar artery and nerve

Abductor hallucis muscle (cut)

Abductor digiti minimi muscle (cut)

Flexor digitorum brevis muscle and plantar aponeurosis (cut)

Lateral calcaneal artery and nerve

Medial calcaneal artery and nerve

Tuberosity of calcaneus

**Third layer muscles in bold**

**Ankle and Foot**

**Plate 522**

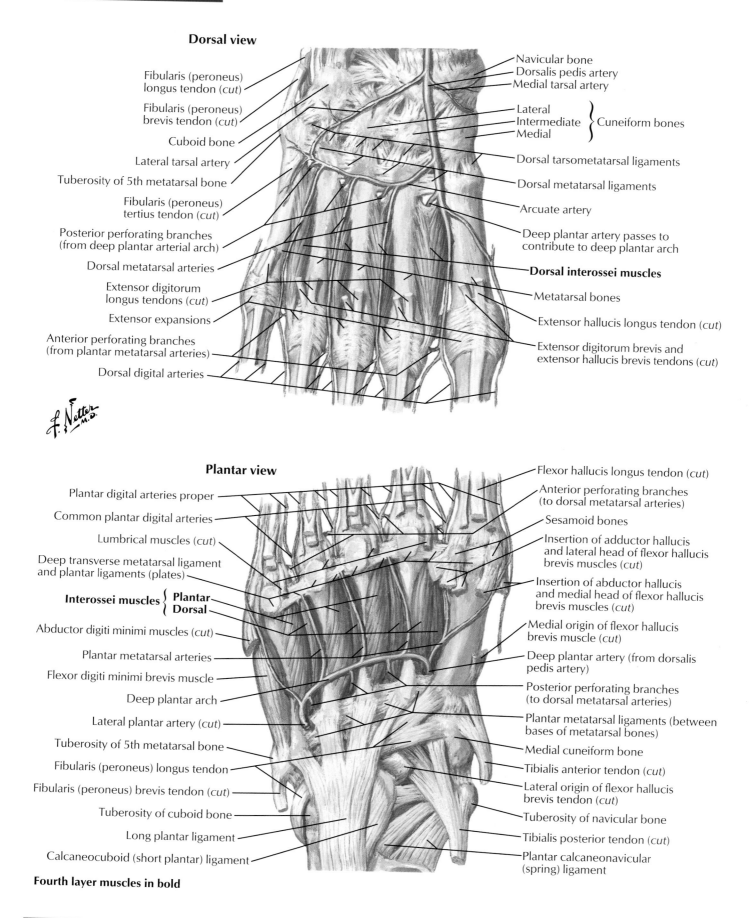

**Dorsal view**

Fibularis (peroneus) longus tendon (*cut*)

Fibularis (peroneus) brevis tendon (*cut*)

Cuboid bone

Lateral tarsal artery

Tuberosity of 5th metatarsal bone

Fibularis (peroneus) tertius tendon (*cut*)

Posterior perforating branches (from deep plantar arterial arch)

Dorsal metatarsal arteries

Extensor digitorum longus tendons (*cut*)

Extensor expansions

Anterior perforating branches (from plantar metatarsal arteries)

Dorsal digital arteries

Navicular bone

Dorsalis pedis artery

Medial tarsal artery

Lateral
Intermediate } Cuneiform bones
Medial

Dorsal tarsometatarsal ligaments

Dorsal metatarsal ligaments

Arcuate artery

Deep plantar artery passes to contribute to deep plantar arch

**Dorsal interossei muscles**

Metatarsal bones

Extensor hallucis longus tendon (*cut*)

Extensor digitorum brevis and extensor hallucis brevis tendons (*cut*)

**Plantar view**

Plantar digital arteries proper

Common plantar digital arteries

Lumbrical muscles (*cut*)

Deep transverse metatarsal ligament and plantar ligaments (plates)

**Interossei muscles** { **Plantar**
**Dorsal**

Abductor digiti minimi muscles (*cut*)

Plantar metatarsal arteries

Flexor digiti minimi brevis muscle

Deep plantar arch

Lateral plantar artery (*cut*)

Tuberosity of 5th metatarsal bone

Fibularis (peroneus) longus tendon

Fibularis (peroneus) brevis tendon (*cut*)

Tuberosity of cuboid bone

Long plantar ligament

Calcaneocuboid (short plantar) ligament

Flexor hallucis longus tendon (*cut*)

Anterior perforating branches (to dorsal metatarsal arteries)

Sesamoid bones

Insertion of adductor hallucis and lateral head of flexor hallucis brevis muscles (*cut*)

Insertion of abductor hallucis and medial head of flexor hallucis brevis muscles (*cut*)

Medial origin of flexor hallucis brevis muscle (*cut*)

Deep plantar artery (from dorsalis pedis artery)

Posterior perforating branches (to dorsal metatarsal arteries)

Plantar metatarsal ligaments (between bases of metatarsal bones)

Medial cuneiform bone

Tibialis anterior tendon (*cut*)

Lateral origin of flexor hallucis brevis tendon (*cut*)

Tuberosity of navicular bone

Tibialis posterior tendon (*cut*)

Plantar calcaneonavicular (spring) ligament

**Fourth layer muscles in bold**

**Plate 523**

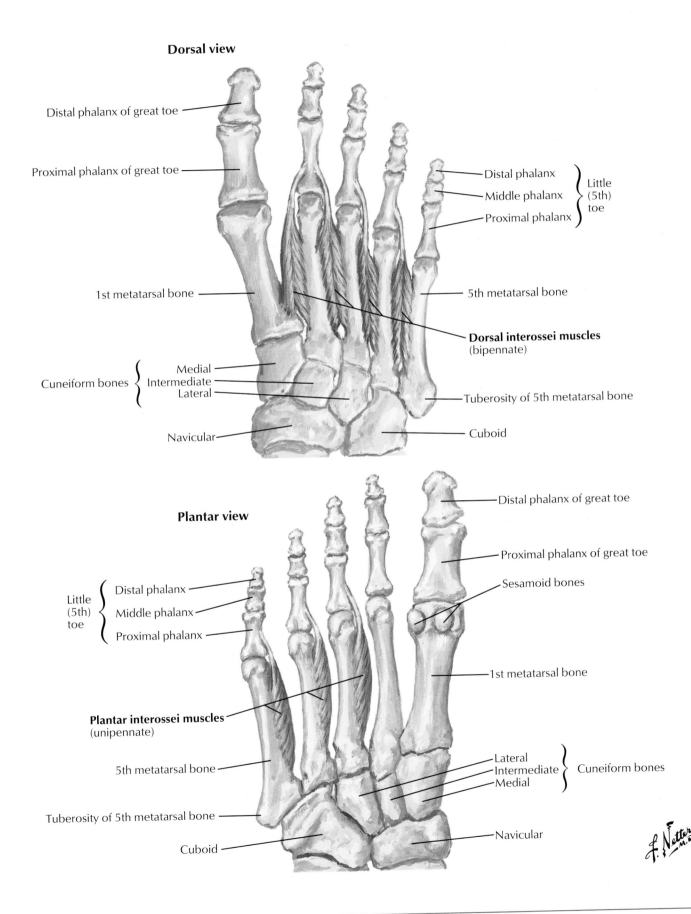

**Dorsal view**

Distal phalanx of great toe

Proximal phalanx of great toe

Distal phalanx
Middle phalanx
Proximal phalanx
} Little (5th) toe

1st metatarsal bone

5th metatarsal bone

**Dorsal interossei muscles** (bipennate)

Cuneiform bones {
Medial
Intermediate
Lateral

Tuberosity of 5th metatarsal bone

Navicular

Cuboid

**Plantar view**

Distal phalanx of great toe

Proximal phalanx of great toe

Sesamoid bones

Little (5th) toe {
Distal phalanx
Middle phalanx
Proximal phalanx

1st metatarsal bone

**Plantar interossei muscles** (unipennate)

5th metatarsal bone

Lateral
Intermediate
Medial
} Cuneiform bones

Tuberosity of 5th metatarsal bone

Navicular

Cuboid

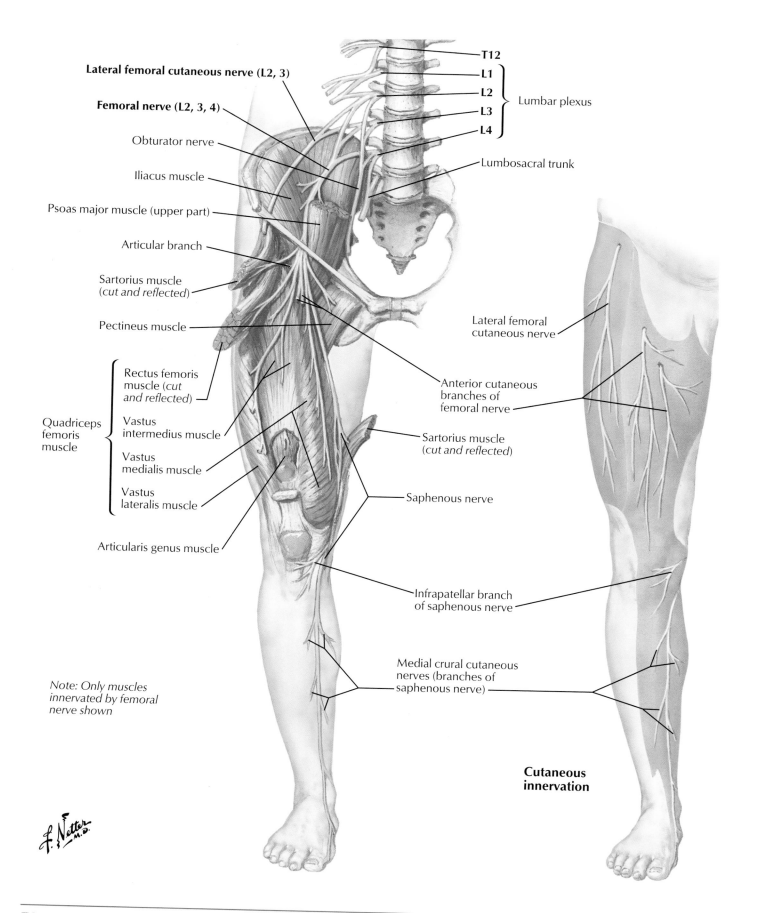

Lateral femoral cutaneous nerve (L2, 3)

Femoral nerve (L2, 3, 4)

Obturator nerve

Iliacus muscle

Psoas major muscle (upper part)

Articular branch

Sartorius muscle
(cut and reflected)

Pectineus muscle

Rectus femoris
muscle (cut
and reflected)

Quadriceps
femoris
muscle

Vastus
intermedius muscle

Vastus
medialis muscle

Vastus
lateralis muscle

Articularis genus muscle

Note: Only muscles
innervated by femoral
nerve shown

T12

L1

L2

L3

L4

Lumbar plexus

Lumbosacral trunk

Lateral femoral
cutaneous nerve

Anterior cutaneous
branches of
femoral nerve

Sartorius muscle
(cut and reflected)

Saphenous nerve

Infrapatellar branch
of saphenous nerve

Medial crural cutaneous
nerves (branches of
saphenous nerve)

**Cutaneous
innervation**

**Plate 525**

**Neurovasculature**

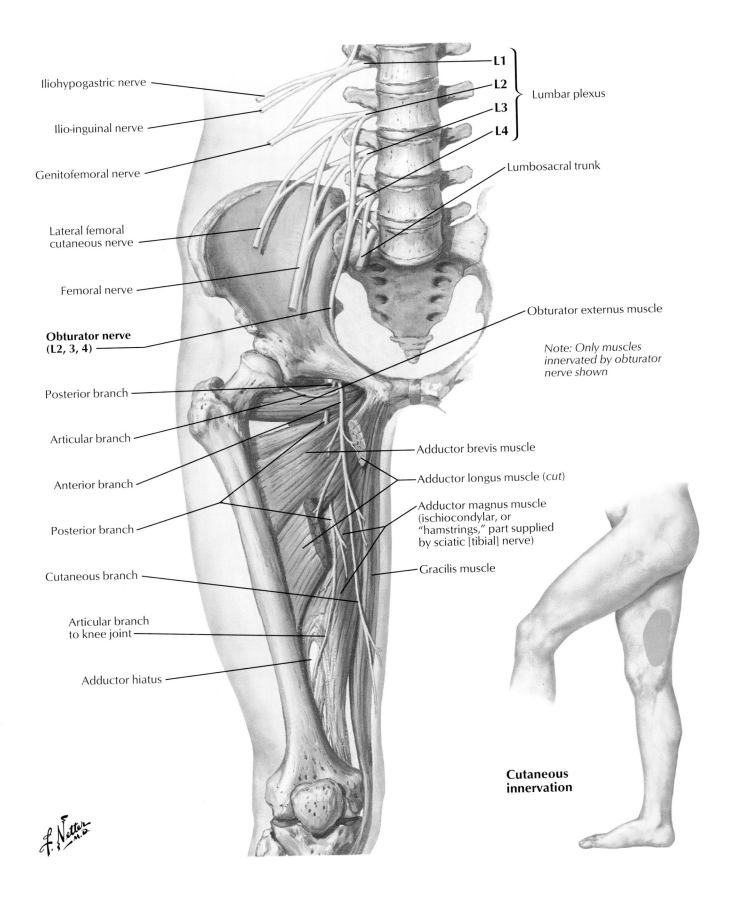

Iliohypogastric nerve

Ilio-inguinal nerve

Genitofemoral nerve

Lateral femoral cutaneous nerve

Femoral nerve

**Obturator nerve (L2, 3, 4)**

Posterior branch

Articular branch

Anterior branch

Posterior branch

Cutaneous branch

Articular branch to knee joint

Adductor hiatus

L1
L2
L3
L4

Lumbar plexus

Lumbosacral trunk

Obturator externus muscle

Note: Only muscles innervated by obturator nerve shown

Adductor brevis muscle

Adductor longus muscle (*cut*)

Adductor magnus muscle (ischiocondylar, or "hamstrings," part supplied by sciatic [tibial] nerve)

Gracilis muscle

**Cutaneous innervation**

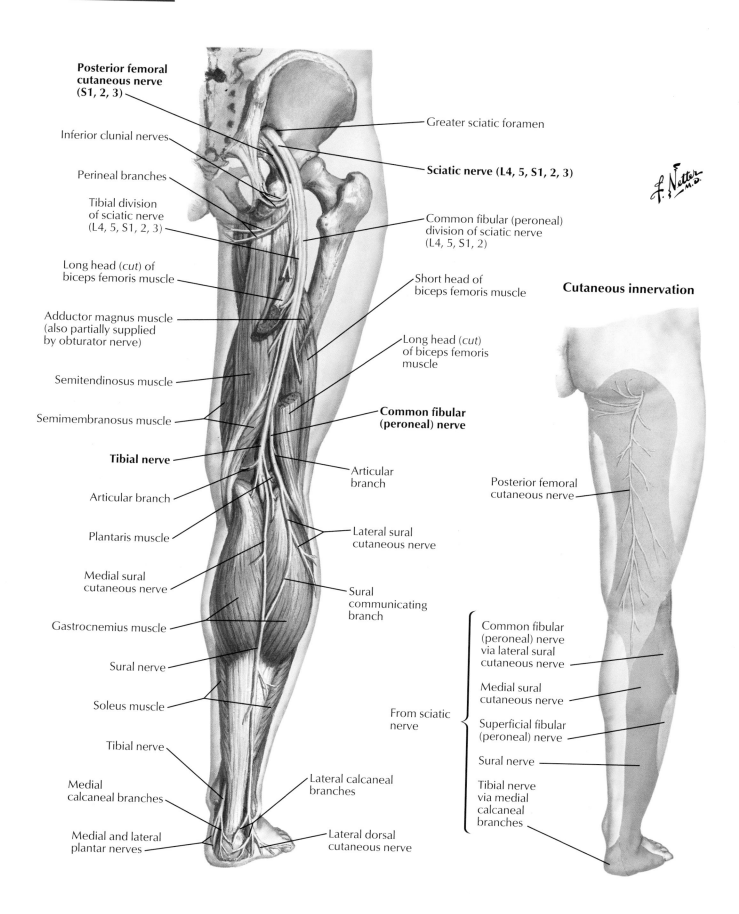

Posterior femoral
cutaneous nerve
(S1, 2, 3)

Inferior clunial nerves

Perineal branches

Tibial division
of sciatic nerve
(L4, 5, S1, 2, 3)

Long head (*cut*) of
biceps femoris muscle

Adductor magnus muscle
(also partially supplied
by obturator nerve)

Semitendinosus muscle

Semimembranosus muscle

**Tibial nerve**

Articular branch

Plantaris muscle

Medial sural
cutaneous nerve

Gastrocnemius muscle

Sural nerve

Soleus muscle

Tibial nerve

Medial
calcaneal branches

Medial and lateral
plantar nerves

Greater sciatic foramen

**Sciatic nerve (L4, 5, S1, 2, 3)**

Common fibular (peroneal)
division of sciatic nerve
(L4, 5, S1, 2)

Short head of
biceps femoris muscle

Long head (*cut*)
of biceps femoris
muscle

**Common fibular
(peroneal) nerve**

Articular
branch

Lateral sural
cutaneous nerve

Sural
communicating
branch

Lateral calcaneal
branches

Lateral dorsal
cutaneous nerve

**Cutaneous innervation**

Posterior femoral
cutaneous nerve

From sciatic
nerve

Common fibular
(peroneal) nerve
via lateral sural
cutaneous nerve

Medial sural
cutaneous nerve

Superficial fibular
(peroneal) nerve

Sural nerve

Tibial nerve
via medial
calcaneal
branches

**Plate 527**

**Neurovasculature**

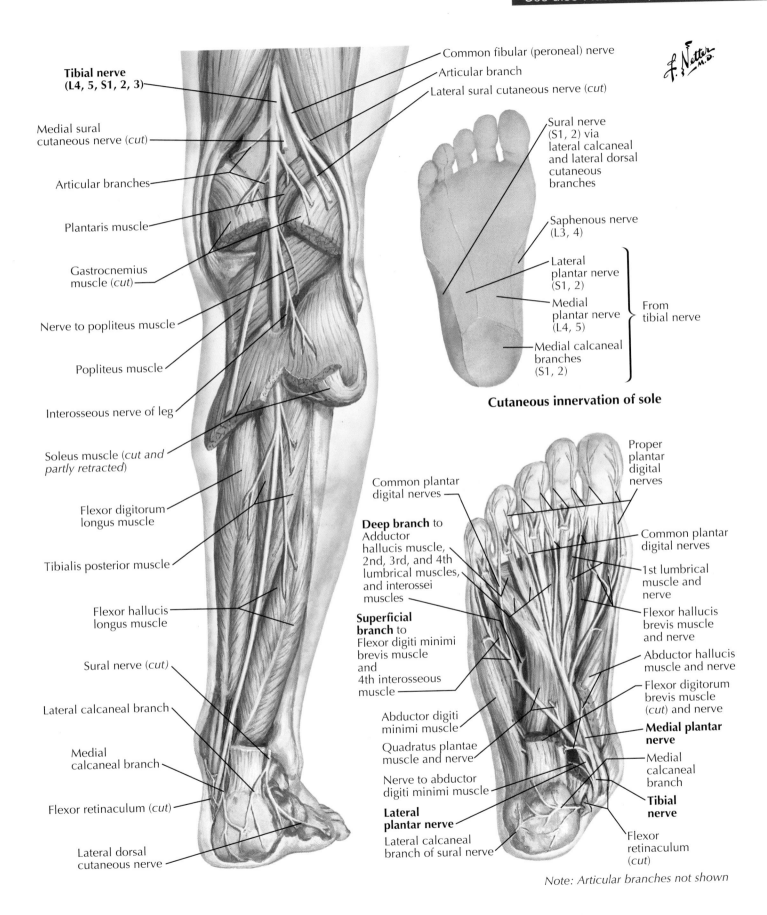

*f. Netter M.D.*

Tibial nerve
(L4, 5, S1, 2, 3)

Medial sural
cutaneous nerve (*cut*)

Articular branches

Plantaris muscle

Gastrocnemius
muscle (*cut*)

Nerve to popliteus muscle

Popliteus muscle

Interosseous nerve of leg

Soleus muscle (*cut and
partly retracted*)

Flexor digitorum
longus muscle

Tibialis posterior muscle

Flexor hallucis
longus muscle

Sural nerve (*cut*)

Lateral calcaneal branch

Medial
calcaneal branch

Flexor retinaculum (*cut*)

Lateral dorsal
cutaneous nerve

Common fibular (peroneal) nerve

Articular branch

Lateral sural cutaneous nerve (*cut*)

Sural nerve
(S1, 2) via
lateral calcaneal
and lateral dorsal
cutaneous
branches

Saphenous nerve
(L3, 4)

Lateral
plantar nerve
(S1, 2)

Medial
plantar nerve
(L4, 5)

Medial calcaneal
branches
(S1, 2)

From
tibial nerve

**Cutaneous innervation of sole**

Common plantar
digital nerves

**Deep branch** to
Adductor
hallucis muscle,
2nd, 3rd, and 4th
lumbrical muscles,
and interossei
muscles

**Superficial
branch** to
Flexor digiti minimi
brevis muscle
and
4th interosseous
muscle

Abductor digiti
minimi muscle

Quadratus plantae
muscle and nerve

Nerve to abductor
digiti minimi muscle

**Lateral
plantar nerve**

Lateral calcaneal
branch of sural nerve

Proper
plantar
digital
nerves

Common plantar
digital nerves

1st lumbrical
muscle and
nerve

Flexor hallucis
brevis muscle
and nerve

Abductor hallucis
muscle and nerve

Flexor digitorum
brevis muscle
(*cut*) and nerve

**Medial plantar
nerve**

Medial
calcaneal
branch

**Tibial
nerve**

Flexor
retinaculum
(*cut*)

*Note: Articular branches not shown*

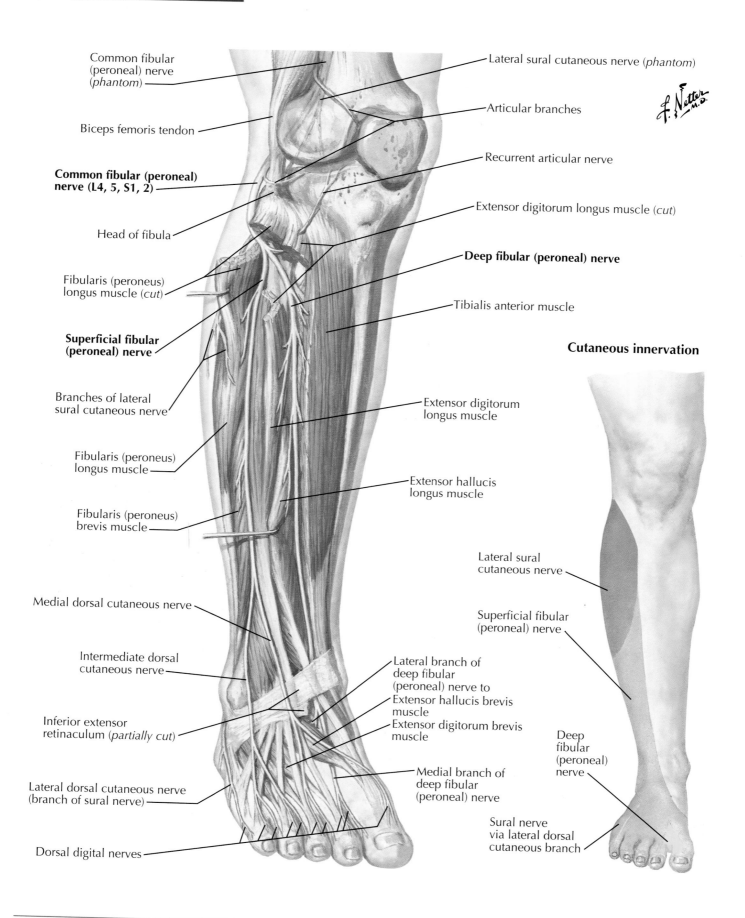

Common fibular
(peroneal) nerve
(*phantom*)

Biceps femoris tendon

**Common fibular (peroneal)
nerve (L4, 5, S1, 2)**

Head of fibula

Fibularis (peroneus)
longus muscle (*cut*)

**Superficial fibular
(peroneal) nerve**

Branches of lateral
sural cutaneous nerve

Fibularis (peroneus)
longus muscle

Fibularis (peroneus)
brevis muscle

Medial dorsal cutaneous nerve

Intermediate dorsal
cutaneous nerve

Inferior extensor
retinaculum (*partially cut*)

Lateral dorsal cutaneous nerve
(branch of sural nerve)

Dorsal digital nerves

Lateral sural cutaneous nerve (*phantom*)

Articular branches

Recurrent articular nerve

Extensor digitorum longus muscle (*cut*)

**Deep fibular (peroneal) nerve**

Tibialis anterior muscle

Extensor digitorum
longus muscle

Extensor hallucis
longus muscle

Lateral branch of
deep fibular
(peroneal) nerve to
Extensor hallucis brevis
muscle
Extensor digitorum brevis
muscle

Medial branch of
deep fibular
(peroneal) nerve

**Cutaneous innervation**

Lateral sural
cutaneous nerve

Superficial fibular
(peroneal) nerve

Deep
fibular
(peroneal)
nerve

Sural nerve
via lateral dorsal
cutaneous branch

**Plate 529**

**Neurovasculature**

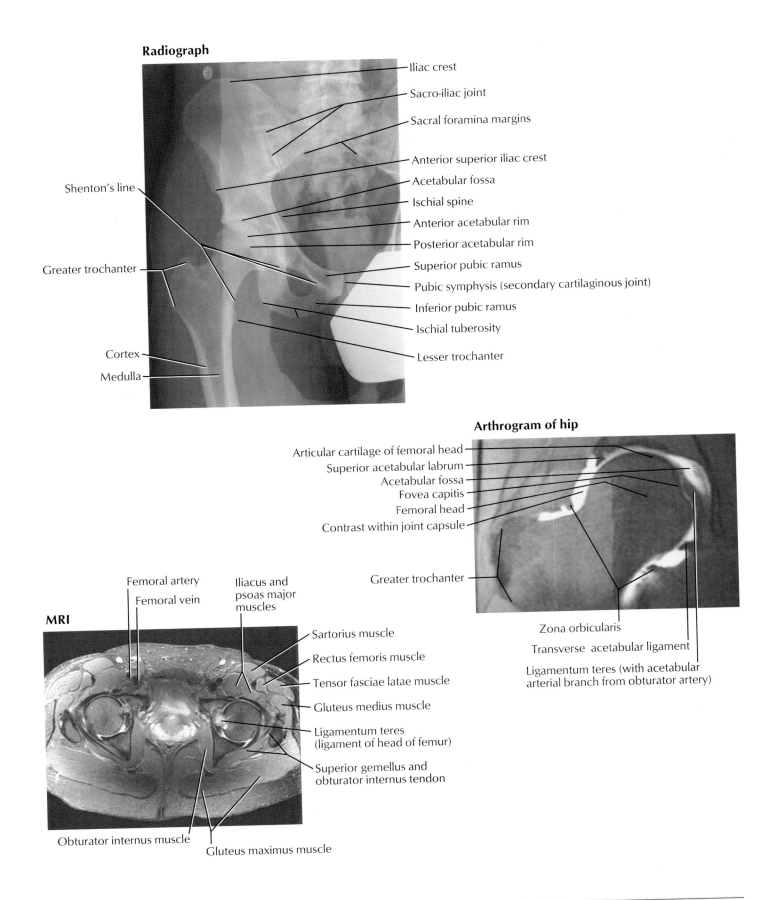

**Radiograph**

Iliac crest

Sacro-iliac joint

Sacral foramina margins

Anterior superior iliac crest

Acetabular fossa

Ischial spine

Anterior acetabular rim

Posterior acetabular rim

Superior pubic ramus

Pubic symphysis (secondary cartilaginous joint)

Inferior pubic ramus

Ischial tuberosity

Lesser trochanter

Shenton's line

Greater trochanter

Cortex

Medulla

**Arthrogram of hip**

Articular cartilage of femoral head

Superior acetabular labrum

Acetabular fossa

Fovea capitis

Femoral head

Contrast within joint capsule

Greater trochanter

Zona orbicularis

Transverse acetabular ligament

Ligamentum teres (with acetabular arterial branch from obturator artery)

Femoral artery

Femoral vein

Iliacus and psoas major muscles

**MRI**

Sartorius muscle

Rectus femoris muscle

Tensor fasciae latae muscle

Gluteus medius muscle

Ligamentum teres (ligament of head of femur)

Superior gemellus and obturator internus tendon

Obturator internus muscle

Gluteus maximus muscle

**Regional Scans**

**Plate 530**

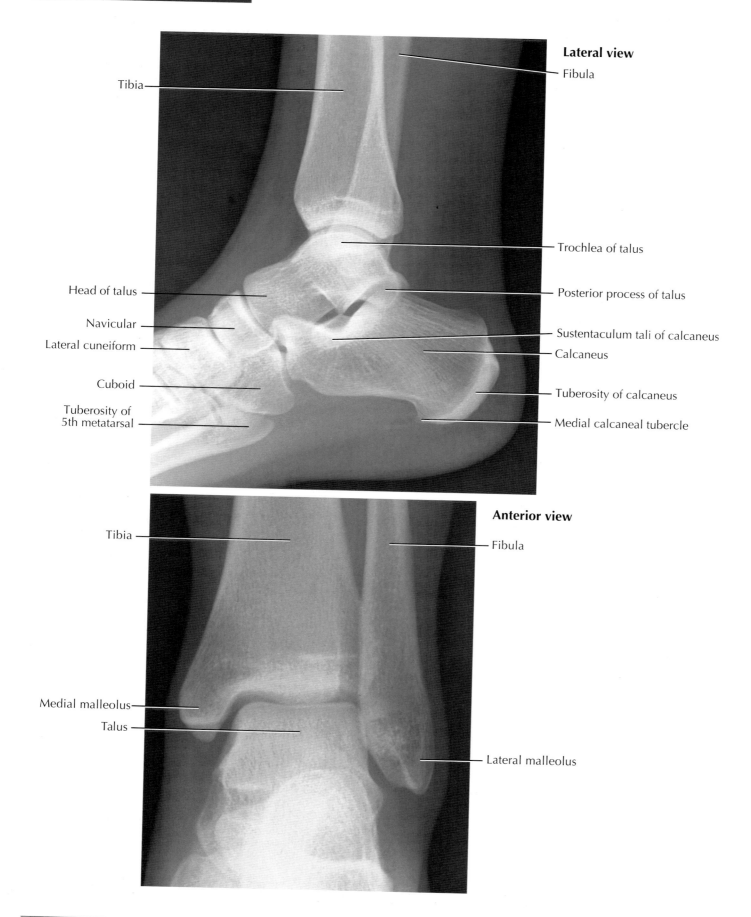

**Lateral view**

Fibula

Tibia

Trochlea of talus

Posterior process of talus

Head of talus

Navicular

Sustentaculum tali of calcaneus

Lateral cuneiform

Calcaneus

Cuboid

Tuberosity of calcaneus

Tuberosity of 5th metatarsal

Medial calcaneal tubercle

**Anterior view**

Tibia

Fibula

Medial malleolus

Talus

Lateral malleolus

**Plate 531**

**Regional Scans**

| MUSCLE | PROXIMAL ATTACHMENT (ORIGIN) | DISTAL ATTACHMENT (INSERTION) | INNERVATION | MAIN ACTIONS | BLOOD SUPPLY | MUSCLE GROUP |
|---|---|---|---|---|---|---|
| Abductor digiti minimi | Medial and lateral tubercles of tuberosity of calcaneus, plantar aponeurosis, and intermuscular septum | Lateral side of base of proximal phalanx of 5th digit | Lateral plantar nerve | Abducts and flexes 5th digit | Medial-lateral plantar artery, plantar metatarsal and plantar digital arteries to 5th digit | Foot |
| Abductor hallucis | Medial tubercle of tuberosity of calcaneus, flexor retinaculum, and plantar aponeurosis | Medial side of base of proximal phalanx of 1st digit | Medial plantar nerve | Abducts and flexes 1st digit | Medial plantar and 1st plantar metatarsal arteries | Foot |
| Adductor brevis | Body and inferior pubic ramus | Pectineal line and proximal part of linea aspera of femur | Obturator nerve | Adducts thigh at hip, weak hip flexor | Profunda femoris, medial circumflex femoral, and obturator arteries | Medial thigh |
| Adductor hallucis | *Oblique head:* bases of 2nd through 4th metatarsals<br><br>*Transverse head:* ligaments of metatarsophalangeal joints of digits 3-5 | Tendons of both heads lateral to side of base of proximal phalanx of 1st digit | Deep branch of lateral plantar nerve | Adducts 1st digit, maintains transverse arch of foot | Medial and lateral plantar arteries and plantar arch, plantar metatarsal arteries | Foot |
| Adductor longus | Body of pubis inferior to pubic crest | Middle third of linea aspera of femur | Obturator nerve (anterior division) | Adducts thigh at hip | Profunda femoris and medial circumflex femoral arteries | Medial thigh |
| Adductor magnus | Inferior pubic ramus, ramus of ischium<br><br>*Hamstring part:* ischial tuberosity | Gluteal tuberosity, linea aspera, medial supracondylar line<br><br>*Hamstring part:* adductor tubercle of femur | *Adductor part:* obturator nerve<br><br>*Hamstring part:* sciatic nerve (tibial division) | *Adductor part:* adducts and flexes thigh<br><br>*Hamstring part:* extends thigh | Femoral, profunda femoris, and obturator arteries | Medial thigh |
| Articularis genus | Distal femur on anterior surface | Suprapatellar bursa | Femoral nerve | Pulls suprapatellar bursa superiorly with extension of knee | Femoral artery | Anterior thigh |
| Biceps femoris | *Long head:* ischial tuberosity<br><br>*Short head:* Linea aspera and lateral supracondylar line of femur | Lateral side of head of fibula | *Long head:* sciatic nerve (tibial division) (L5–S2)<br><br>*Short head:* sciatic nerve (common fibular division) | Flexes and laterally rotates leg, extends thigh at hip | Perforating branches of profunda femoris, inferior gluteal, and medial circumflex femoral arteries | Posterior thigh |
| Dorsal interossei (four muscles) | Adjacent sides of 1st through 5th metatarsals | *1st:* medial side of proximal phalanx of 2nd digit<br><br>*2nd through 4th:* lateral sides of digits 2–4 | Lateral plantar nerve | Abduct 2nd through 4th toes, flex metatarsophalangeal joints, and extend phalanges | Arcuate artery, dorsal and plantar metatarsal arteries | Foot |
| Extensor digitorum brevis and extensor hallucis brevis | Superolateral surface of calcaneus, lateral talocalcaneal ligament, cruciate crural ligament | First tendon into dorsal surface of base of proximal phalanx of great toe; other 3 tendons into lateral sides of tendons of extensor digitorum longus to digits 2-4 | Deep fibular nerve | Aids the extensor digitorum longus in extending of 4 medial digits at the metatarsophalangeal and interphalangeal joints | Dorsalis pedis, lateral tarsal, arcuate, and fibular arteries | Foot |

Variations in spinal nerve contributions to the innervation of muscles, their arterial supply, their attachments, and their actions are common themes in human anatomy. Therefore, expect differences between texts and realize that anatomical variation is normal.

# Muscle Tables

| MUSCLE | PROXIMAL ATTACHMENT (ORIGIN) | DISTAL ATTACHMENT (INSERTION) | INNERVATION | MAIN ACTIONS | BLOOD SUPPLY | MUSCLE GROUP |
|---|---|---|---|---|---|---|
| Extensor digitorum longus | Lateral condyle of tibia, proximal 3/4 of anterior surface of interosseous membrane and fibula | Middle and distal phalanges of lateral four digits | Deep fibular nerve | Extends lateral four digits and dorsiflexes foot at ankle | Anterior tibial artery | Anterior leg |
| Extensor hallucis longus | Middle part of anterior surface of fibula and interosseous membrane | Dorsal aspect of base of distal phalanx of great toe | Deep fibular nerve | Extends great toe, dorsiflexes foot at ankle | Anterior tibial artery | Anterior leg |
| Fibularis peroneus brevis | Distal 2/3 of lateral surface of fibula | Dorsal surface of tuberosity on lateral side of 5th metatarsal | Superficial fibular nerve | Everts foot and weakly plantarflexes foot at ankle | Anterior tibial and fibular arteries | Lateral leg |
| Fibularis peroneus longus | Head and proximal 2/3 of lateral fibula | Plantar base of 1st metatarsal and medial cuneiform | Superficial fibular nerve | Everts foot and weakly plantarflexes foot at ankle | Anterior tibial and fibular arteries | Lateral leg |
| Fibularis peroneus tertius | Distal third of anterior surface of fibula and interosseous membrane | Dorsum of base of 5th metatarsal | Deep fibular nerve | Dorsiflexes foot at ankle and aids in eversion of foot | Anterior tibial artery | Anterior leg |
| Flexor digiti minimi brevis | Base of 5th metatarsal | Lateral base of proximal phalanx of 5th digit | Superficial branch of lateral plantar nerve | Flexes proximal phalanx of 5th digit | Lateral plantar artery, plantar digital artery to 5th digit, arcuate artery | Foot |
| Flexor digitorum brevis | Medial tubercle of tuberosity of calcaneus, plantar aponeurosis, and intermuscular septum | Both sides of middle phalanges of lateral four digits | Medial plantar nerve | Flexes 2nd through 5th digits | Medial and lateral plantar arteries and plantar arch, plantar metatarsal and plantar digital arteries | Foot |
| Flexor digitorum longus | Medial part of posterior tibia inferior to soleal line | Plantar bases of distal phalanges of lateral four digits | Tibial nerve | Flexes lateral four digits and plantarflexes foot at ankle; supports longitudinal arches of foot | Posterior tibial artery | Posterior leg |
| Flexor hallucis brevis | Plantar surfaces of cuboid and lateral cuneiform | Both sides of base of proximal phalanx of 1st digit | Medial plantar nerve | Flexes proximal phalanx of 1st digit | Medial plantar artery, first plantar metatarsal artery | Foot |
| Flexor hallucis longus | Distal 2/3 of posterior fibula and interosseous membrane | Base of distal phalanx of great toe (hallux) | Tibial nerve | Flexes all joints of great toe, weakly plantarflexes foot at ankle | Fibular artery | Posterior leg |
| Gastrocnemius | *Lateral head:* lateral aspect of lateral condyle of femur<br><br>*Medial head:* popliteal surface above medial condyle of femur | Posterior aspect of calcaneus via calcaneal tendon | Tibial nerve | Plantarflexes foot at ankle joint, assists in flexion of knee joint, raises heel during walking | Popliteal and posterior tibial arteries | Posterior leg |
| Gluteus maximus | Ilium posterior to posterior gluteal line, dorsal surface of sacrum and coccyx, sacrotuberous ligament | Most fibers end in iliotibial tract that inserts into lateral condyle of tibia; some fibers insert into gluteal tuberosity of femur | Inferior gluteal nerve | Extends flexed thigh, assists in lateral rotation, and abducts thigh | Inferior gluteal arteries mainly, and superior gluteal arteries occasionally | Gluteal region |

**Table 7-2**

**Muscle Tables**

| MUSCLE | PROXIMAL ATTACHMENT (ORIGIN) | DISTAL ATTACHMENT (INSERTION) | INNERVATION | MAIN ACTIONS | BLOOD SUPPLY | MUSCLE GROUP |
|---|---|---|---|---|---|---|
| Gluteus medius | Lateral surface of ilium between anterior and posterior gluteal lines | Lateral surface of greater trochanter of femur | Superior gluteal nerve | Abducts and medially rotates thigh at hips; steadies pelvis on leg when opposite leg is raised | Superior gluteal artery | Gluteal region |
| Gluteus minimus | Lateral surface of ilium between anterior and inferior gluteal lines | Anterior surface of greater trochanter of femur | Superior gluteal nerve | Abducts and medially rotates thigh at hips; steadies pelvis on leg when opposite leg is raised | Main trunk and deep branch of superior gluteal artery | Gluteal region |
| Gracilis | Body and inferior ramus of pubis | Superior part of medial surface of tibia | Obturator nerve | Adducts thigh, flexes and medially rotates leg | Profunda femoris artery, medial circumflex femoral artery | Medial thigh |
| Iliacus (Iliopsoas) | Superior 2/3 of iliac fossa, iliac crest, ala of sacrum, anterior sacro-iliac ligaments | Lesser trochanter of femur and shaft inferior to it, to psoas major tendon | Femoral nerve | Flexes thigh at hips and stabilizes hip joint, acts with psoas major | Iliac branches of iliolumbar artery | Anterior thigh |
| Inferior gamellus | Ischial tuberosity | Medial surface of greater trochanter of femur | Nerve to quadratus femoris | Laterally rotates extended thigh at the hip | Medial circumflex femoral artery | Gluteal region |
| Lumbricals | Tendons of flexor digitorum longus | Medial side of dorsal digital expansions of lateral 4 digits | *Medial one:* medial plantar nerve  *Lateral three:* lateral plantar nerve | Flexes proximal phalanges at MTP joint, extends phalanges at PIP and DIP joints | Lateral plantar artery and plantar metatarsal arteries | Foot |
| Obturator externus | Margins of obturator foramen, obturator membrane | Trochanteric fossa of femur | Obturator nerve | Laterally rotates thigh, stabilizes head of femur in acetabulum | Medial circumflex femoral artery, obturator artery | Medial thigh |
| Obturator internus | Pelvic surface of obturator membrane and surrounding bone | Medial surface of greater trochanter of femur | Nerve to obturator internus | Laterally rotates extended thigh, abducts flexed thigh at hip | Internal pudendal and obturator arteries | Gluteal region |
| Pectineus | Superior ramus of pubis | Pectineal line of femur | Femoral nerve and sometimes obturator nerve | Adducts and flexes thigh at hip | Medial circumflex femoral artery, obturator artery | Medial thigh |
| Piriformis | Anterior surface of sacral segments 2–4, sacrotuberous ligament | Superior border of greater trochanter of femur | Ventral rami of L5, S1, S2 | Laterally rotates extended thigh, abducts flexed thigh at hip | Superior and inferior gluteal arteries, internal pudendal artery | Gluteal region |
| Plantar interossei (three muscles) | Bases and medial sides of 3rd through 5th metatarsals | Medial sides of bases of proximal phalanges of 3rd through 5th digits | Lateral plantar nerve | Adduct digits (3-5) and flex metatarsophalangeal joint and extend phalanges | Lateral plantar artery and plantar arch, plantar metatarsal and plantar digital arteries | Foot |
| Plantaris | Inferior end of lateral supracondylar line of femur and oblique popliteal ligament | Posterior aspect of calcaneus via calcaneal tendon | Tibial nerve | Weakly assists gastrocnemius | Popliteal artery | Posterior leg |
| Popliteus | Lateral aspect of lateral condyle of femur, lateral meniscus | Posterior tibia superior to soleal line | Tibial nerve (L4–S1) | Weakly flexes knee and unlocks it by rotating femur on fixed tibia | Inferior medial and lateral genicular arteries | Posterior leg |
| Psoas major (Iliopsoas) | Transverse processes of lumbar vertebrae, sides of bodies of T12–L5 vertebrae, intervening intervertebral discs | Lesser trochanter of femur | Ventral rami of first lumbar nerve | Acting superiorly with iliacus, flexes hip; acting inferiorly, flexes vertebral column laterally; used to balance trunk in sitting position; acting inferiorly with iliacus, flexes trunk | Lumbar branches of iliolumbar artery | Anterior thigh |
| Quadratus femoris | Lateral margin of ischial tuberosity | Quadrate tubercle on intertrochanteric crest of femur | Nerve to quadratus femoris | Laterally rotates thigh at hip | Medial circumflex femoral artery | Gluteal region |

# Muscle Tables

| MUSCLE | PROXIMAL ATTACHMENT (ORIGIN) | DISTAL ATTACHMENT (INSERTION) | INNERVATION | MAIN ACTIONS | BLOOD SUPPLY | MUSCLE GROUP |
|---|---|---|---|---|---|---|
| Quadratus plantae | Medial and lateral sides of plantar surface of calcaneus | Posterolateral edge of flexor digitorum longus tendon | Lateral plantar nerve | Corrects for oblique pull of flexor digitorum longus tendon, thus assists in flexion of toes | Medial and lateral plantar arteries and deep plantar arterial arch | Foot |
| Rectus femoris (quadriceps) | Anterior inferior iliac spine and ilium superior to acetabulum | Base of patella and to tibial tuberosity via patellar ligament | Femoral nerve | Extends leg at knee joint and flexes thigh at hip joint | Profunda femoris and lateral circumflex femoral arteries | Anterior thigh |
| Sartorius | Anterior superior iliac spine and superior part of notch below it | Superior part of medial surface of tibia | Femoral nerve | Abducts, laterally rotates, and flexes thigh; flexes knee joint | Femoral artery | Anterior thigh |
| Semimembranosus | Ischial tuberosity | Posterior part of medial condyle of tibia | Sciatic nerve (tibial division) | Flexes leg, extends thigh | Perforating branch of profunda femoris and medial circumflex femoral arteries | Posterior thigh |
| Semitendinosus | Ischial tuberosity | Superior part of medial surface of tibia | Sciatic nerve (tibial division) | Flexes leg, extends thigh | Perforating branch of profunda femoris and medial circumflex femoral arteries | Posterior thigh |
| Soleus | Posterior aspect of head of fibula, proximal 1/4 of posterior surface of fibula, soleal line of tibia | Posterior aspect of calcaneus via calcaneal tendon | Tibial nerve | Plantarflexes foot at ankle, stabilizes leg over foot | Popliteal, posterior tibial, and fibular arteries | Posterior leg |
| Superior gemellus | Outer surface of ischial spine | Medial surface of greater trochanter of femur | Nerve to obturator internus | Laterally rotates extended thigh at the hip | Inferior gluteal and internal pudendal arteries | Gluteal region |
| Tensor fasciae latae | Anterior superior iliac spine and anterior part of iliac crest | Iliotibial tract that attaches to lateral condyle of tibia | Superior gluteal nerve | Abducts, medially rotates, and flexes thigh at hip; helps to keep knee extended | Ascending branch of lateral circumflex femoral artery | Gluteal region |
| Tibialis anterior | Lateral condyle, proximal half of lateral tibia, interosseous membrane | Medial plantar surfaces of medial cuneiform and base of 1st metatarsal | Deep fibular nerve | Dorsiflexes foot at ankle and inverts foot | Anterior tibial artery | Anterior leg |
| Tibialis posterior | Posterior tibia below soleal line, interosseous membrane, proximal half of posterior fibula | Tuberosity of navicular bone, all cuneiforms, cuboid, and bases of 2nd through 4th metatarsals | Tibial nerve | Plantarflexes foot at ankle and inverts foot | Fibular artery | Posterior leg |
| Vastus intermedius (quadriceps) | Anterior and lateral surfaces of body of femur | Base of patella and to tibial tuberosity via patellar ligament | Femoral nerve | Extends leg at knee joint | Lateral circumflex femoral and profunda femoris arteries | Anterior thigh |
| Vastus lateralis (quadriceps) | Greater trochanter, lateral lip of linea aspera of femur | Base of patella and to tibial tuberosity via patellar ligament | Femoral nerve | Extends leg at knee joint | Lateral circumflex femoral and profunda femoris arteries | Anterior thigh |
| Vastus medialis (quadriceps) | Intertrochanteric line, medial lip of linea aspera of femur | Base of patella and to tibial tuberosity via patellar ligament | Femoral nerve | Extends leg at knee joint | Femoral and profunda femoris arteries | Anterior thigh |

Table 7-4

# References

**Plates 8, 36-38, 43-45**
Lang J. Clinical Anatomy of the Nose, Nasal Cavity, and Paranasal Sinuses. Thieme Medical Publishers, New York, 1989.

**Plates 19-21**
Baccetti T, Franchi L, McNamara J Jr. The cervical vertebral maturation (CVM) method for the assessment of optimal treatment timing in dentofacial orthopedics. Semin Orthod 2005;11:119-29.

Roman PS. Skeletal maturation determined by cervical vertebrae development. Eur J Orthod 2002;24:303-11.

**Plate 23**
Tubbs RS, Kelly DR, Humphrey ER, et al. The tectorial membrane: anatomical, biomechanical, and histological analysis. Clin Anat 2007;20:382-6.

**Plates 25, 27-29, 48, 49, 58, 67, 70**
Noden DM, Francis-West P. The differentiation and morphogenesis of craniofacial muscles. Dev Dyn 2006;235: 1194-218.

**Plates 32, 34, 126-132**
Tubbs RS, Salter EG, Oakes WJ. Anatomic landmarks for nerves of the neck: a vade mecum for neurosurgeons. Neurosurgery 2005;56:256-60.

**Plate 48**
Benninger B, Lee BI. Clinical importance of morphology and nomenclature of distal attachment of temporalis tendon. J Maxillofac Surg 2012;70:557-61.

**Plates 50, 58**
Benninger B, Kloenne J, Horn JL. Clinical anatomy of the lingual nerve and identification with ultrasonography. Br J Oral Maxillofac Surg 2013;51:541-4.

**Plates 57, 62**
Benninger B, Andrew K, Carter B. Clinical measurements of hard palate and implications for subepithelial connective tissue grafts with suggestions for palatal nomenclature. J Oral Maxillofac Surg 2012;70:149-53.

**Plates 65, 95, 96**
Kierner AC, Mayer R, v Kirschlhofer K. Do the tensor tympani and tensor veli palatini muscles of man form a functional unit? A histochemical investigation of their putative connections. Hear Res 2002;165:48-52.

**Plates 74, 75**
Benninger B, Barrett R. A head and neck lymph node classification using an anatomical grid system while maintaining clinical relevance. J Oral Maxillofac Surg 2011;69: 2670-3.

**Plates 80-82**
Ludlow CL. Central nervous system control of the laryngeal muscles in humans. Respir Physiol Neurobiol 2005;147: 205-22.

**Plates 102-116**
Rhoton AL. Cranial Anatomy and Surgical Approaches. Congress of Neurological Surgeons, Schaumburg, IL, 2003.

**Plates 105, 141**
Tubbs RS, Hansasuta A, Loukas M, et al. Branches of the petrous and cavernous segments of the internal carotid artery. Clin Anat 2007;20:596-601.

**Plates 117-119, 125**
Schrott-Fischer A, Kammen-Jolly K, Scholtz AW, et al. Patterns of GABA-like immunoreactivity in efferent fibers of the human cochlea. Hear Res 2002;174:75-85.

**Plates 160, 175**
Tubbs RS, Loukas M, Slappy JB, et al. Clinical anatomy of the C1 dorsal root, ganglion, and ramus: a review and anatomical study. Clin Anat 2007;20:624-7.

**Plate 162**
Lee MWL, McPhee RW, Stringer MD. An evidence-based approach to human dermatomes. Clin Anat 2008;21: 363-73.

**Plates 162, 399, 469, 513**
Forester O. The dermatomes in man. Brain 1933; 56:1-39.

Garrett FD. The segmental distribution of the cutaneous nerves in the limbs of man. Anat Rec 1948;102:409-37.

Keegan JJ. Dermatome hypalgesia with posterolateral herniation of lower cervical intervertebral disc. J Neurosurg 1947;4:115-39.

**Plate 168**
Turnball IM. Bloody supply of the spinal cord. In Vinken PJ, Bruyn GW (eds). Handbook of Clinical Neurology, XII. Amsterdam, 1972, pp 478-91.

**Plate 169**
Stringer MD, Restieaux M, Fisher AL, Crosado B. The vertebral venous plexuses: the internal veins are muscular and external veins have valves. Clin Anat 2012;25:609-18.

**Plates 174, 175**
Tubbs RS, Mortazavi MM, Loukas M, et al. Anatomical study of the third occipital nerve and its potential role in occipital headache/neck pain following midline dissections of the craniocervical junction. J Neurosurg Spine 2011; 15:71-5.

**Plates 179-181**
Hassiotou F, Geddes D. Anatomy of the human mammary gland: current status of knowledge. Clin Anat 2013;26: 29-48.

**Plates 197, 198**
Jackson CL, Huber JF. Correlated applied anatomy of the bronchial tree and lungs with a system of nomenclature. Dis Chest 1943;9:319-26.

**Plate 200**
Ikeda S, Ono Y, Miyazawa S, et al. Flexible broncho-fiberscope. Otolaryngology (Tokyo) 1970;42:855.

**Plate 215**
Angelini, P, Velasco JA, Flamm S. Coronary anomalies: incidence, pathophysiology, and clinical relevance. Circulation 2002;105:2449-54.

**Plates 215, 216**
Chiu IS, Anderson RH. Can we better understand the known variations in coronary arterial anatomy? Ann Thorac Surg 2012;94:1751-60.

**Plate 222**
James TN. The internodal pathways of the human heart. Prog Cardiovasc Dis 2001;43:495-535.

**Plates 222-224**
Hildreth V, Anderson RH, Henderson DJ. Autonomic innervation of the developing heart: origins and function. Clin Anat 2009;22:36-46.

**Plate 236**
Ang HJ, Gill YC, Lee WJ, et al. Anatomy of thoracic splanchnic nerves for surgical resection. Clin Anat 2008;21:171-7.

**Plate 279**
Elias H. Morphology of the Liver. New York, Academic Press, 1969.

MacSween RNM, Anthony PP, Scheuer PJ, et al (eds). Pathology of the Liver. London, Churchill Livingstone, 2002.

Robinson PJ. MRI of the Liver: A Practical Guide. New York, Taylor & Francis, 2006.

**Plates 283, 284**
Odze RD. Surgical Pathology of the GI Tract, Liver, Biliary Tract, and Pancreas. Philadelphia, Saunders, 2004.

**Plate 305**
Thomas MD. In The Ciba Collection of Medical Illustrations, vol 3, part II. Summit, NJ, CIBA, p 78.

**Plates 321, 344, 362, 374, 392**
Stormont TJ, Cahill DR, King BF, Myers RP. Fascias of the male external genitalia and perineum. Clin Anat 1994;7:115-24.

**Plates 335, 340, 346, 350, 355, 356**
Oelrich TM. The striated urogenital sphincter muscle in the female. Anat Rec 1983;205:223-32.

**Plates 339, 344**
Myers RP, Goellner JR, Cahill DR. Prostate shape, external striated urethral sphincter, and radical prostatectomy: the apical dissection. J Urol 1987;138:543-50.

**Plates 339, 344, 361, 362**
Oelrich TM. The urethral sphincter muscle in the male. Am J Anat 1980;158:229-46.

**Plate 381**
Flocks RH, Kerr HD, Elkins HB, et al. Treatment of carcinoma of the prostate by interstitial radiation with radio-active gold (Au 198): A preliminary report. J Urol 1952;68:510-22.

**Plate 399**
Keegan JJ, Garrett FD. The segmental distribution of the cutaneous nerves in the limbs of man. Anat Rec 1948;102:409.

**Plate 469**
Keegan JJ. Neurological interpretation of dermatome hypalgesia with herniation of the lumbar intervertebral disc. J Bone Joint Surg Am 1944;26:238-48.

Last RJ. Innervation of the limbs. J Bone Joint Surg Br 1949;31:452.

Anal canal, 371
  arteries of, male, 376
  longitudinal muscle of, 338–339
  muscularis mucosae of, 371–372
  veins of, female, 377
Anal columns, 371
Anal crypt, 371
Anal glands, 371
Anal (rectal) nerves
  branch of, 357
  inferior, 388–389, 391–392, 484, 490
Anal pit, 366
Anal sinus, 371
Anal sphincter muscle
  external, 276, 303, 321, 335, 340, 346,
    355–356, 359–360, 370, 376, 382,
    397
    attachment of, 337
    deep, 344, 369, 371–374
    perineal views of, 373
    subcutaneous, 344, 369, 371–374
    superficial, 344, 369, 371–374
  internal, 370–372
Anal triangle, 358
Anal tubercle, 366
Anal valve, 371
Anal verge, 371
Anastomosis
  in arteries to brain, 139
  internal to external carotid artery, 138
  paravertebral, 168
  prevertebral, 168
Anastomotic loops, 287, 290
  to anterior spinal artery, 167
  of ileal arteries, 272
  of jejunal arteries, 272
  to posterior spinal artery, 167
Anastomotic vein
  inferior (of Labbé), 103, 146
  superior (of Trolard), 103
Anatomical snuffbox, 398, 430, 454,
  456–457
Anconeus muscle, 406, 418, 430–431, 436,
  438, 465–467
  nerve to, 418
Angle of mandible, 1, 15, 17, 66
Angular artery, 3, 35, 51, 72, 87, 139
Angular gyrus, 106
  branch to, 142–143
Angular notch, 269
Angular vein, 3, 73, 87
Ankle
  dorsiflexion of, 469
  ligaments of, 514
  medial ligament of, 501
  plantarflexion of, 469
  radiographs of, 531
  tendon sheaths of, 516
  tendons of, 514
Anococcygeal body (ligament), 337,
  355–356, 360, 373–374
Anococcygeal nerve, 389, 391, 484,
  486
Anocutaneous line, 370–372
Anoderm, 371
Anorectal hiatus, 338
Anorectal junction
  circular muscle layer of, 339
  conjoined longitudinal muscle of, 339
Anorectal line, 371
Anorectal musculature, 372
Ansa cervicalis, 31, 129–130
  inferior root of, 32, 34, 71, 76, 129–130
  superior root of, 32, 34, 71, 76, 129–130
Ansa of Galen, 82
Ansa pectoralis, 415
Ansa subclavia, 131, 206, 223–224, 236
Anserine bursa, 493–494

Antebrachial cutaneous nerves
  lateral, 400–401
    branches of, 401
  medial, 400
    branches of, 401
  posterior, 400–401
Antebrachial fascia, 436
  deep, 441
Antebrachial vein, median, 401–402, 436
Anterior chamber of eye, 83, 89–92
  endothelium of, 90
Anterolateral central (lenticulostriate)
  arteries, 138, 140–142, 144
Anteromedial central (perforating)
  arteries, 141
Antihelix, 1, 95
  crura of, 95
Antitragus, 1, 95
Anular ligament of radius, 424
Anular (intercartilaginous) ligaments, 199
Anulus fibrosus, 21, 155, 159
  collagen lamellae of, 159
Anus, 337, 340, 354, 358, 360, 366, 373
Aorta, 26, 204, 216–217, 226, 258, 306, 309,
  320
  abdominal, 176, 192, 229, 259, 264,
    267–268, 271, 283–284, 303, 308, 310,
    314–315, 320–321, 341–342, 345, 376,
    378–381, 390
    arteriogram of, 285
    axial CT images of, 323
    transverse section of, 326–328
  ascending, 139, 212, 214, 217, 220–222, 237,
    240
    coronal section of, 214
  axial CT images of, 322
  thoracic (descending), 139, 168, 188, 191,
    213, 228–229, 233, 237, 240–241
    lung groove for, 196
    transverse section of, 324–325
  ureteric branch from, 314
Aortic arch, 76–77, 139, 193, 203, 207–212,
  218, 222, 228–230, 233, 239
  lung groove for, 196
Aortic arch lymph node of ligamentum
  arteriosum, 205
Aortic heart valve, 210, 214, 218–222
  left semilunar cusp of, 218–222
  posterior semilunar cusp of, 218–222
  right semilunar cusp of, 218–222
Aortic hiatus, 192
Aortic lymph nodes, lateral, 261, 316, 384
Aortic plexus, 300
Aortic sinus, 210, 220
Aorticorenal ganglion, 163, 262, 297,
  299–303, 317–319, 387, 392–393, 395
  left, 388, 394
Apical collecting vessels, 75
Apical foramina, 63
Apical ligament, of dens, 23, 64–65
Appendicular artery, 273, 287–288, 301–302
Appendicular lymph nodes, 296
Appendicular plexus, 301–302
Appendicular vein, 291–292
Appendix, 127, 275
  of epididymis, 365, 367
  fibrous, of liver, 277
  omental (epiploic), 265
  of testis, 365, 367
  vermiform, 265, 273–276
    orifice of, 274
  vesicular, 352, 367
Arachnoid, 101, 103, 110
  dura mater interface with, 103
  superior cerebral veins penetrating, 103
Arachnoid granulations, 101–103, 110
  granular foveolae for, 9
Arachnoid mater, 165–166

Arcuate arteries, 312, 517–518, 523
  lymph vessels along, 316
Arcuate eminence, 11, 94
Arcuate ligament
  dorsal radial metaphyseal, 442
  lateral, 192, 258
  medial, 192, 258
  median, 192, 258
Arcuate line, 243, 247, 249, 251, 255, 330,
  334–335, 338, 473
  of ilium, 336
Arcuate (infundibular) nucleus, 148
Arcus tendineus fasciae pelvis, 351
Areola, 179
Areolar glands (of Montgomery),
  179
Areolar tissue, 245, 344
  loose, 103
Areolar venous plexus, 252
Arm
  arteries of, 420
  cutaneous nerves of, 401
  muscles of
    anterior view of, 417
    posterior view of, 418
  radial nerve in, 465
  serial cross sections of, 421
  superficial veins of, 401
Arrector pili muscles, innervation to,
  163
Arteriae rectae, 288, 305
Arterial arch, deep plantar, 522
Arterial circle of iris
  major, 90, 92–93
  minor, 90, 92–93
Arterial rete, marginal, 96
Arteries. See also specific arteries
  of abdominal wall
    anterior, 251
    posterior, 259
  of anal canal, male, 376
  of arm, 420
  of brain, 137
    frontal section of, 142
    frontal view of, 142
    inferior view of, 140
    lateral view, 143
    medial view, 143
    schema of, 139
  of duodenum, 284, 286
  of esophagus, 233
  of eye, intrinsic, 92
  of face, 3
  of femoral head and neck, 491
  of foot, 509
    deep, 523
  of forearm, 435
  of hand, 453
  of head of pancreas, 286
  of hypothalamus and hypophysis,
    149
  intrarenal, 312
  of iris, 93
  of knee, 499, 509
  of large intestine, 288
  of leg, 509
  of liver, 283–284
  of mallear stria, 96
  of mammary gland, 180
  to meninges, 137
  of nasal cavity, 40
  of oral and pharyngeal regions, 72
  of orbit and eyelids, 87
  of pancreas, 284
  of pelvic organs, female, 378
  of pelvis
    female, 380
    male, 381

**Atlas of Human Anatomy**

**Colles' fascia**, 344, 348, 350, 355–361, 369, 373–374, 382–383, 389
  superficial, 359
**Colliculus**
  facial, 116
  inferior, 107, 112, 115–116
    brachia of, 115
    brachium of, 112
    left, 145
  seminal, 348
  superior, 107–108, 112, 115–117, 133, 144
    brachia of, 115
    brachium of, 112
    left, 145
**Colon**
  ascending, 127, 265, 268, 271, 276, 309, 341, 345
    transverse section of, 326–328
  circular muscle of, 274
  descending, 265, 271, 276, 302, 315, 341, 345
    axial CT images of, 322–323
    innervation of, 163–164
    transverse section of, 325–328
  innervation of, 163
  radiography of, 156
  sigmoid, 263, 265, 276, 302, 341–342, 345, 369–372, 390
    innervation of, 163–164
  transverse, 263–265, 267, 271, 276, 281–282, 290, 321
    axial CT images of, 322–323
    transverse section of, 325–328
  tributary from, 291
**Commissure**
  anterior, 107, 116, 120, 147–148
  of fornix, 113
  habenular, 107, 112, 116
  of labia majora
    anterior, 354
    posterior, 354
  of lips, 1
  posterior, 107, 112, 116, 366
**Common bony limbs**, 97–98
**Common membranous limbs**, 97–98
**Common tendinous ring (of Zinn)**, 85–86, 88, 122
**Common trunk**, 46, 73
**Common-extensor tendon**, 406
**Communicating artery**
  anterior, 137–143
    imaging of, 150
  posterior, 105, 137–144
    imaging of, 150
**Communicating nerve, sural**, 471
**Communicating vein**, 31, 170
**Compressor urethrae muscle**, 335, 350, 356–357, 382, 397
  growth of, 347
**Concha**
  of auricle, 95
  inferior, 16
**Conducting system, of heart**, 222
**Condylar canal**, 10, 13
**Condylar fossa**, 10
**Condylar process, of mandible**, 15, 17
  head of, 6
**Condyles**
  of femur
    lateral, 476, 494–497
    medial, 476, 494–497
  of mandible, 7
  occipital, 8, 10–11, 16
  of tibia
    lateral, 481, 497, 500–501, 506
    medial, 494, 496–497, 500–501
**Cone of light**, 95

**Cones**, 121
**Conjoined longitudinal muscle**, 370–372
**Conjoint tendon**, 246, 249, 255–256
**Conjunctiva**, 93
**Conjunctival artery, posterior**, 93
**Conjunctival fornix**
  inferior, 83
  superior, 83
**Conjunctival vein, posterior**, 93
**Conjunctival vessels**, 92
**Connective tissue**
  of skull, 103
  subserous, 305
**Conoid ligament**, 404, 408, 411
**Conoid tubercle**, 404
**Conus arteriosus**, 209, 217–219
**Conus elasticus**, 80, 82
**Conus medullaris**, 156, 160–161
  transverse section of, 327
**Cooper's ligament**, 179, 246–247, 249, 255, 257–258
**Coraco-acromial ligament**, 408, 411, 413, 417
**Coracobrachialis muscle**, 239–240, 405, 410, 412–413, 415, 417, 419, 421, 460, 462, 467
**Coracobrachialis tendon**, 410, 413
**Coracoclavicular ligament**, 408, 411
**Coracohumeral ligament**, 408
**Coracoid process**, 185–186, 405–408, 410–415, 417, 419
  of scapula, 183
**Cornea**, 83, 85, 89–90, 92–93
**Corneal limbus**, 83
**Corneoscleral junction**, 83
**Corniculate cartilage**, 79
**Corniculate tubercle**, 66–67, 80
**Coronal sulcus**, 366
**Coronal suture**, 4–9, 14
**Coronary arteries**, 215, 221
  imaging of, 216
  left, 215–216, 220
    anterior interventricular branch of (left anterior descending artery), 215–216
    circumflex branch of, 215–216, 219
    interventricular branch of, 209
    interventricular septal branches of, 215–216
    left (obtuse) marginal branch of, 215–216
    posterior left ventricular branch of, 215
    posterolateral branches of, 216
  right, 209, 211, 215–216, 219–220
    atrial branch of, 215
    AV nodal branch of, 216, 219
    interventricular septal branches of, 215
    posterior interventricular branch of (posterior descending artery), 211, 215–216, 219
    right (acute) marginal branch of, 215–216
    SA nodal branch of, 215–216
**Coronary ligament**, 277, 321
  hepatorenal portion of, 277
  of liver, 268
**Coronary sinus**, 211–213, 215, 218, 241
  opening of, 214, 217, 220
  valve (thebesian) of, 217
**Coronary sulcus**, 209, 211
**Coronoid fossa**, 405, 422
**Coronoid process**
  of mandible, 6–7, 15, 17, 42
  temporalis muscle insertion to, 6
  of ulna, 422, 425, 429
    radiographs of, 423
**Corpora cavernosa, of penis**, 360
**Corpora quadrigemina**, 108
**Corpus albicans**, 352

**Corpus callosum**, 107, 109, 112, 142, 144
  cistern of, 110
  dorsal vein of, 145, 147
  genu of, 107–108, 111, 113, 147
    imaging of, 151
  imaging of, 151
  posterior cerebral artery to, 143
  rostrum of, 107, 142, 146
  splenium of, 107–108, 111, 113, 116, 144–147
    imaging of, 151
  sulcus of, 107
  trunk of, 107, 142
**Corpus cavernosum**, 344, 359, 361, 363
  tunica albuginea of, 359, 363
**Corpus luteum**, 352
**Corpus spongiosum**, 344, 348, 359–361, 363
  tunica albuginea of, 359, 363
**Corpus striatum**, 111, 142
**Corrugator cutis ani muscle**, 371–372
**Corrugator supercilii muscle**, 25, 124, 151
**Corti**
  spiral ganglion of, 98
  spiral organ of, 94, 98
**Cortical lymph vessels**, 316
**Cortical radiate (interlobular) arteries**, 312
  lymph vessels along, 316
**Costal cartilages**, 183–184, 243, 404
  fifth, 191, 213
  first, 193, 238
  second, 240
  seventh, 195
  sixth, 409
  transverse section of, 324
**Costal facet**, 154
  inferior, 154, 184
  superior, 154, 184
  transverse, 154, 184
**Costal groove**, 184
**Costal impressions**, 277
**Costal lamella**, 20
**Costocervical trunk**, 33, 137, 139, 170
**Costochondral joints**, 184
**Costoclavicular ligament**, 184, 404, 412
  impression for, 404
**Costocoracoid ligament**, 412
**Costocoracoid membrane**, 412
**Costodiaphragmatic recess**, 193–195, 210, 214, 227–228, 309, 315
  transverse section of, 324
**Costomediastinal space**, 195
**Costotransverse joint**, 238
**Costotransverse ligament**, 184
  lateral, 184
  superior, 184
**Costoxiphoid ligament**, 184
**Cough receptors**, 207
**Cowper's gland**, 249, 321, 344, 348, 361–363, 367
  duct of, 361
  primordium of, 367
**Cranial base**
  foramina and canals of
    inferior view of, 12
    superior view of, 13
  inferior view of, 10
  nerves of, 55
  superior view of, 11
  vessels of, 55
**Cranial fossa**
  anterior, 11
  middle, 11
  posterior, 11
    arteries of, 144
    veins of, 145
**Cranial imaging**, 150–151

**Digastric muscle** (*Continued*)
  phantom, 34
  posterior belly of, 27–29, 34, 46–47, 50–51, 58–59, 67, 70, 75, 124
    innervation of, 119
    nerve to, 24
**Digastric tendon, intermediate**, 47, 59
  fibrous loop for, 27–28, 58–59
**Digital artery**
  dorsal, 456, 458, 508–509, 517, 523
  palmar, 435
    common, 435
    proper, 435
  proper, 453
**Digital fibrous sheaths**, 445
**Digital nerves, dorsal**, 402, 458, 466, 470, 507, 529
**Digital veins, dorsal**, 402, 470
**Digits**
  extensors of, 427
  flexors of, 429
**Dilator pupillae muscle**, 90, 122, 133, 151
**Diploë**, 9
**Diploic veins**, 101, 103
  frontal, 101
  occipital, 101
  temporal
    anterior, 101
    posterior, 101
**Direct vein, lateral**, 146–147
**Distal interphalangeal (DIP) joint**, 398, 445
**Distributing vein**, 279
**Dome of pleura, parietal**, 193–194, 227–228
**Dorsal artery**
  of clitoris, 357, 382
  of penis, 359, 361, 383
    deep, 379, 383
**Dorsal nerve**
  of clitoris, 357, 391–392, 484
  of penis, 359, 361, 383, 387–389, 394, 484, 490
**Dorsal nucleus, of vagus nerve**, 117
  posterior, 118
**Dorsal rami**, 254
  of cervical spinal nerves, 2, 22–24
  of lumbar spinal nerves, 158, 174
  of sacral spinal nerves, 174
  of spinal nerves, 165–166
  of thoracic spinal nerves, 174, 177, 250
**Dorsal root ganglion**, 129, 133, 166, 177, 188, 254, 300, 303–304, 306–307, 318, 395
**Dorsal rootlets, of spinal nerves**, 160
**Dorsal vein**
  of clitoris, deep, 335–337, 340, 343, 346, 357
  of corpus callosum, 145, 147
  of penis
    deep, 245, 339, 344, 359, 361, 379, 381
    superficial, 245, 252, 329, 359, 381
**Dorsal venous network**, 402, 455
**Dorsiflexion, of ankle**, 469
**Dorsum of foot**, 518
**Douglas, recto-uterine pouch of**, 340, 342, 352, 369
**Duct system, of liver**, 278
**Ductus arteriosus**, 226
**Ductus (vas) deferens**, 249, 255–257, 259, 313, 344–345, 348, 362, 364–365, 367–369, 387, 394, 472
  ampulla of, 362
  artery to, 251, 259, 365, 376, 379, 381
  inferior, 381
**Ductus reuniens**, 98
**Ductus venosus**, 226
**Duodenal flexure**
  inferior, 272
  superior, 272

**Duodenal fold**
  inferior, 264, 271
  superior, 264
**Duodenal fossa**
  inferior, 264, 271
  superior, 264
**Duodenal impression**, 277
**Duodenal muscle fibers**, 280
**Duodenal papilla**
  major (of Vater), 272, 280
  minor, 272, 280
**Duodenojejunal flexure**, 264, 271–272, 281, 315, 320
**Duodenojejunal junction**, 176
**Duodenum**, 127, 267–269, 271, 277–278, 281, 308, 313, 315, 320
  arteries of, 284, 286
  ascending part of, 264, 271–272
  autonomic nerves of, 298–300
  descending part of, 176, 264, 266, 271–272, 280
    transverse section of, 326
  inferior part of, 264, 271–272, 321
  mucosa and musculature of, 272
  in situ, 271
  superior part of, 270–272
    transverse section of, 325
  suspensory muscle of, 264
  transverse section of, 327
  veins of, 289
**Dura mater**, 38, 95, 98, 102–103, 110, 120
  arachnoid interface with, 103
  endosteal layer, 103
  meningeal layer, 101, 103
  periosteal layer, 101
  skull interface with, 101, 103
  spinal, 160, 165–166, 170, 176
    posterior intercostal artery branch to, 168
  superior cerebral veins penetrating, 103
**Dural sac, termination of**, 160–161
**Dural venous sinuses**
  sagittal section of, 104
  superior view of, 105

## E

**Ear**
  ampulla of, 94, 98
  bony and membranous labyrinths of, 97–98
    orientation of, 99
  external, 95
  innervation of, 119
  tympanic cavity of, 96
  vestibule of, 94, 97–98
**Edinger-Westphal nucleus**, 117–118, 122, 133
**Efferent ductules**, 367–368
**Efferent fibers**, 117–118, 122–124, 126, 128–130
  of autonomic reflex pathways, 304
  to olfactory bulb, 120
**Ejaculatory duct**
  beginning of, 362
  opening of, 362–363, 367, 396
**Elbow**
  bones of, 422
  ligaments of, 424
  radiographs of, 423
**Elliptical recess**, 97
**Emissary vein**, 13, 73, 101, 103
  condylar, 170
  mastoid, 3, 101, 170
    in mastoid foramen, 12
  occipital, 101
  parietal, 3, 101
    parietal foramen for, 9
  to superior sagittal sinus, 13
**Enamel of teeth**, 63

**Endolymphatic duct**, 13, 97–99
**Endolymphatic sac**, 98
**Endometrium**, 352
**Endopelvic fascia, female**, 343
**Enteric plexus**, 304
**Ependyma**, 109
**Epicolic lymph nodes**, 296
**Epicondyles**
  of femur
    lateral, 476, 480, 497
    medial, 476, 488–489, 493–494, 496–497
  of humerus
    lateral, 405–406, 417–418, 422–424, 426, 428–429, 431, 434, 466
    medial, 405–406, 417–419, 422–424, 426–434, 464–465
**Epicranial aponeurosis**, 3, 25, 103, 175
**Epicranius muscle, occipital belly of**, 151
**Epididymal duct**, 368
**Epididymis**, 364, 368, 394
  appendix of, 365, 367
  body of, 365, 368
  head of, 365, 368
  sinus of, 368
  tail of, 368
**Epidural hematoma, site of**, 101, 103
**Epidural space, fat in**, 166
**Epigastric artery**
  inferior, 245, 247, 249, 251, 255–257, 259, 268, 314, 341, 343, 345, 376, 378–379, 381, 499
    cremasteric branch of, 247, 249, 259
    pubic branch of, 247, 249, 255, 259, 343, 345
    transverse section of, 328
  superficial, 186, 208, 245, 247, 251, 259, 487, 499
  superior, 185, 187–188, 247, 251
**Epigastric lymph nodes, inferior**, 261
**Epigastric region**, 244
**Epigastric veins**
  inferior, 245, 247, 249, 252, 255–257, 260, 268, 341, 345, 378–379, 381
    pubic branch of, 255
    transverse section of, 328
  superficial, 186, 242, 245, 252, 260, 329, 470, 487
  superior, 187, 189, 247, 252
**Epiglottis**, 15, 60, 64, 66–69, 78–80, 82, 136, 230
**Epiphysis**, 458
  nutrient branches to, 458
**Episcleral artery**, 92
**Episcleral space**, 85, 89
**Episcleral vein**, 92–93
  segment of, 93
**Epithelial tag**, 366
**Epithelium, gingival**, 63
**Epitympanic recess**, 94–95
**Eponychium**, 458
**Epoöphoron**, 352, 367
**Erector spinae muscles**, 152, 171–173, 176–177, 188, 238, 254, 309
  transverse section of, 324, 328
**Esophageal artery**, 204
**Esophageal hiatus**, 192, 264
**Esophageal impression**, 277
**Esophageal mucosa**, 69, 232
**Esophageal muscles**, 64, 199
  circular, 65, 67, 69
    in V-shaped area of Laimer, 69, 77
  longitudinal, 65, 67, 69, 77
    attachment of, 69
    cricoid attachment of, 65, 67
**Esophageal plexus**, 127, 203, 206, 213, 227–229, 234, 236, 300
  nerve branches to, 236
  sympathetic branch to, 206

**Flexor pollicis longus muscle**, 405, 429, 433–434, 436–437, 447, 460, 463, 467
 tendinous sheath of, 448, 450
**Flexor pollicis longus tendon**, 434, 436, 441, 449–450
**Flexor retinaculum**, 433, 441, 447, 449–450, 452–453, 460, 503–505, 516, 521–522, 528
**Flexor sheath, common**, 447–450, 453
**Flexor tendon**, 450, 453
 common, 405–406, 428–429, 432, 437–438
 fibrous sheaths of, 520
 in fingers, 451
 at wrist, 449
**Flexor tendon sheath**, 447
**Floating ribs**, 183
**Flocculonodular lobe**, 114
**Flocculus**, 114–115
**Folds of iris**, 90
**Foliate papillae**, 60, 136
**Folium**, 114, 116
**Follicle (graafian)**, 352
**Fontanelle**
 anterior, 14
 posterior, 14
**Foot**
 arteries of, 509
 bones of, 511–512
 deep arteries, 523
 dorsum of, 518
  muscles of, 517
 eversion of, 469
 interosseous muscles of, 523–524
 inversion of, 469
 ligaments of, 515
 muscles of sole of
  first layer, 520
  second layer, 521
  third layer, 522
 plantar surface of, 468
 sole of, 519
 tendons of, 515
**Foramen**
 interventricular (of Monro), 107, 109–110, 112, 116, 146–147
 of Luschka, 109–110
 of Magendie, 109–110, 116, 118
**Foramen cecum**, 11, 13, 60, 64
**Foramen lacerum**, 10, 13, 100
 recurrent artery of, 138
**Foramen magnum**, 8, 10, 12–13, 100, 128
**Foramen ovale**, 6, 10, 12–13, 16, 49–50, 100, 226
 branch to, 138
 valve of, 218
**Foramen rotundum**, 5, 13, 52
 branch to, 138
 maxillary nerve entering, 53
**Foramen spinosum**, 10, 13, 16, 50, 100
 accessory, 12
 branch to, 138
**Foramen transversarium**, 20–21
 bony spicule dividing, 20
 septated, 20
**Forearm**
 arteries of, 435
 bones of, 425
 cutaneous nerves of, 402, 461–462
 muscles of
  attachments of, 437–438
  deep layer, 431, 434
  extensors of wrist and digits, 427
  flexors of digits, 429
  flexors of wrist, 428
  intermediate layer, 433
  rotators of radius, 426
  superficial layer, 430, 432

**Forearm** *(Continued)*
 proximal, arteries of, 420
 radial nerve in, 466
 serial cross sections of, 436
 superficial veins of, 402
**Fornix**, 107, 113, 148
 anterior, 351
 body of, 107, 109, 113, 116
 columns of, 107, 111–113, 146
 commissure of, 113
 conjunctival
  inferior, 83
  superior, 83
 crus of, 107, 111, 113, 144
 imaging of, 151
 vaginal, 352
  anterior, 340
  posterior, 340
**Fossa ovalis**, 214, 217, 226, 470
 limbus of, 217
**Fovea, inferior**, 116
**Fovea capitis**, 530
**Fovea centralis in macula**, 89, 92
**Free taenia**, 265, 273–274, 276, 369, 372
**Frenulum**, 274
 artery to, 59
 of clitoris, 354
 of labia minora, 354
 of lower lip, 56
 of penis, 360
 of tongue, 46, 56
 of upper lip, 56
**Frontal artery**, 3
 polar, 142–143
**Frontal bone**, 1, 4, 6, 8–11, 35, 37, 83–84
 foramen cecum of, 11
 frontal crest of, 11
 glabella of, 4, 6
 groove for anterior meningeal vessels, 11
 groove for superior sagittal sinus of, 11
 growth of, 45
 lateral view of, 14
 nasal spine of, 37–38
 of newborn, 14
 orbital surface, 4
 sinus of, 8, 37–38
 squamous part of, 14, 37–38
 superior surface of orbital part, 11
 superior view of, 14
 supra-orbital notch of, 4, 6
**Frontal crest**, 9, 11
**Frontal gyrus**
 inferior
  opercular part of, 106
  orbital part of, 106
  triangular part of, 106
 medial, 107
 middle, 106
 superior, 106
**Frontal (anterior) horn**, 109
**Frontal lobe**, 106
**Frontal nerve**, 13, 52, 85, 88, 122–123, 132
**Frontal operculum**, 106
**Frontal pole**, 106, 108
**Frontal sinus**, 7, 36–38, 43–44, 64
 growth of, 45
**Frontal sulcus**
 inferior, 106
 superior, 106
**Frontal (metopic) suture**, 14
**Frontal vein**, 3
**Frontobasal artery**
 lateral, 140, 142–143
 medial, 138, 140, 142–143
**Frontonasal canal**
 infundibulum leading to, 37
 opening of, 37

**Frontonasal duct**, 36
 opening of, 44
**Fundiform ligament**, 245, 255, 344
**Fundus**
 of gallbladder, axial CT images of, 323
 of stomach, 230, 232, 269–270
  transverse section of, 324
 of urinary bladder, 344, 346, 348
 of uterus, 340, 342, 346, 352
  sagittal CT images of, 375
**Fungiform papilla**, 60, 136
**Funiculus, lateral**, 116

### G

**Galen, great cerebral veins of**, 104–105, 107, 116, 145–147
 imaging of, 150
**Gallaudet's fascia**, 344, 348, 350, 355–356, 359–361, 369
**Gallbladder**, 127, 193, 263, 266, 269, 277–278, 280–281, 284
 axial CT images of, 322
 fundus of, axial CT images of, 323
 innervation of, 163–164
 transverse section of, 325
**Ganglion, of trigeminal nerve**, 117–118, 132
**Ganglion cells**, 121
**Gartner's duct**, 367
**Gasserian ganglion**, 105, 117–118
**Gastric artery**
 left, 233, 259, 266, 268, 283–284, 297–300, 388
  arteriogram of, 285
  esophageal branch of, 233, 236, 283
 right, 272, 280, 283–284, 298–300
  arteriogram of, 285
 short, 268, 282–284, 300
**Gastric canal, longitudinal folds of**, 270
**Gastric folds (rugae)**, 232, 270
 transverse section of, 324
**Gastric impression**, 277, 282
**Gastric lymph nodes**, 235, 293–294
**Gastric plexus**, 388
 left, 297–299
 right, 298–299
**Gastric veins**
 left, 234, 289–292
  esophageal tributary of, 289
 right, 234, 289–290, 292
 short, 234, 268, 282, 289, 292
**Gastrocnemius muscle**, 478, 481, 489, 493–494, 502–508, 510, 527–528, 531
 lateral head of, 468, 482, 497–498, 503
 lateral subtendinous bursa of, 498
 medial head of, 468, 482, 497–498, 503
**Gastrocolic ligament**, 266
 anterior layers of, 266
 posterior layers of, 266
**Gastroduodenal artery**, 272, 280, 283–284, 286–287, 300–301, 306
 arteriogram of, 285
 plexus on, 299
**Gastroduodenal plexus**, 301, 306
**Gastro-omental (gastro-epiploic) artery**, 268, 282
 anastomosis of, 266
 left, 283–284, 289, 292, 300
 plexus on, 298–299
 right, 266, 283–284, 286–287, 289, 292, 300
**Gastro-omental (gastro-epiploic) lymph nodes**, 293
**Gastro-omental (gastro-epiploic) vein**, 268, 282
 left, 234
 right, 234, 289, 291
**Gastropancreatic fold**, 266

**Gastrophrenic ligament**, 266, 268, 308
**Gastrosplenic (gastrolienal) ligament**, 266–267, 282
**Gemellus muscle**, 530
  inferior, 396–397, 477–478, 482, 489–490, 531
    nerve to, 490
  superior, 477–478, 482, 489–490, 531
    nerve to, 484, 489
**Genial tubercle**, 58
**Genicular artery**
  descending, 487–488, 492, 499, 509
  inferior
    lateral, 499, 504–509
    medial, 488, 499, 504–505, 507–509
  middle, 499, 509
  superior
    lateral, 489, 499, 503–509
    medial, 487–489, 499, 503–505, 507–509
**Geniculate body**
  lateral, 108, 111–112, 115–117, 121, 133, 140, 144–146
  medial, 108, 111–112, 115–116, 140, 144–146
**Geniculate ganglion**, 50, 53, 96, 99, 117, 124–126, 132, 136
**Geniculate nucleus, dorsal lateral**
  left, 121
  right, 121
**Geniculum, of facial nerve**, 50, 53, 99, 117, 125–126, 132
**Genioglossus muscle**, 43, 47, 59, 64, 129, 151
  superior mental spine for origin of, 58
**Geniohyoid fascia**, 26
**Geniohyoid muscle**, 26, 43, 58–59, 64, 129–130, 151
  communication with cervical plexus, 33
**Genital cord**, 367
**Genital tubercle**
  anal pit of, 366
  anal tubercle of, 366
  epithelial tag of, 366
  glans area of, 366
  lateral part of, 366
  urogenital fold of, 366
**Genitalia**
  external
    female, 354
    homologues of, 366
    innervation of, 163–164
    male, 358–359
  internal, homologues of, 367
  lymph vessels and nodes of
    female, 384
    male, 386
  nerves of
    female, 391
    male, 387
**Genitofemoral nerve**, 257, 262, 308, 313, 387, 483, 485, 526
  femoral branches of, 253, 257, 262, 387, 470, 484–485
  genital branch of, 253, 255–257, 262, 365, 387, 470, 484–485
  nerves to, 484
  transverse section of, 328
**Genu**
  of corpus callosum, 107–108, 111, 113, 147
    imaging of, 151
  internal, of facial nerve, 118
  of internal capsule, 111
**Gerdy's tubercle**, 481, 494, 496, 500–501
**Gerota's fascia.** *See* Renal (Gerota's) fascia
**GI tract, innervation of**, 119
**Gimbernat's (lacunar) ligament**, 246–247, 249, 255, 257–258, 472
**Gingiva, lamina propria of**, 63
**Gingival epithelium**, 63

**Gingival groove**, 63
**Glabella**, 1, 4, 6
**Gland lobules**, 179
**Gland orifices**, 280
**Glans, of clitoris**, 354, 366
**Glans penis**, 329, 344, 360, 363, 366
  corona of, 360
  neck of, 360
**Glenohumeral joint**, 408, 467
  capsule of, 418
**Glenohumeral ligament**
  inferior, 408
  middle, 408
  superior, 408
**Glenoid cavity, of scapula**, 183, 405, 407–408, 467
**Glenoid labrum**, 408, 467
**Globus pallidus**, 109, 111
**Glomerulus**, 120
**Glossoepiglottic fold**
  lateral, 60
  median, 60
**Glossoepiglottic ligament, median**, 80
**Glossopharyngeal nerve (IX)**, 34, 42, 55, 61, 71–72, 105, 115, 117–118, 124, 126–127, 131–132, 134–136, 207
  branch of, 164
  carotid branch of, 34, 127, 132
  in carotid sheath, 47
  carotid sinus branch (of Hering), 71, 126, 131
  distribution of, 119
  inferior, 13
  inferior (petrosal) ganglion of, 55, 96, 126, 135–136, 207
  in jugular fossa, 12
  lesser petrosal nerve from, 123
  lingual branches of, 61, 126
  pharyngeal branches of, 126
  schema of, 126
  superior ganglion of, 126
  tonsillar branches of, 61, 68, 71, 126
  tympanic branch of, 12
**Gluteal aponeurosis**, 309, 481–482, 489
  over gluteus medius muscle, 250
**Gluteal artery**
  inferior, 259, 314, 376, 380–381, 486, 489
  superior, 259, 314, 376, 380–381, 486, 489
**Gluteal fold**, 152, 468
**Gluteal lines**
  anterior, 334, 473
  inferior, 334, 473
  posterior, 334, 473
**Gluteal nerves**
  inferior, 160, 484, 486, 489–490
  superior, 160, 484, 486, 489–490
**Gluteal vein, superior**, 260, 291
**Gluteus maximus muscle**, 152, 171, 174, 250, 309, 339, 356, 359–360, 373–374, 388–389, 391, 396, 468, 478, 481–482, 489–490, 492, 530–531
**Gluteus medius muscle**, 152, 309, 396–397, 468, 478–479, 482–483, 487–490, 530–531
  gluteal aponeurosis over, 250
**Gluteus minimus muscle**, 477, 482–483, 487–490, 531
**Gluteus minimus tendon**, 396
**Gonads**, 364, 367
**Graafian follicle**, 352
**Gracile fasciculus**, 115–116
**Gracile tubercle**, 115–116
**Gracilis muscle**, 477, 480, 482, 487–489, 492–493, 497, 502–503, 526, 531
**Gracilis tendon**, 468, 477, 479–480, 493–494
**Granular foveolae**, 9, 101, 103
**Granule cell**, 120

**Gray matter**
  imaging of, 151
  intermediolateral nucleus of, preganglionic sympathetic cell bodies in, 53, 133–135
  lateral horn of, 165–166, 319
  of spinal nerves, 165
**Gray rami communicantes**, 131, 133–135, 163, 166, 177, 188, 206, 224–225, 227–228, 236, 254, 262, 297, 300, 303–304, 317–318, 388, 390, 393–395, 485–486
  of spinal nerves, 165
  to and from sympathetic trunk, 165
**Great auricular nerve**, 2
**Great cardiac vein**, 215
**Great cerebral veins (of Galen)**, 104–105, 107, 116, 145–147
  imaging of, 150
**Great toe**
  dorsal digital nerve and vein of, 470
  phalanx of, 515, 524
**Great vessels**
  pericardium at site of reflection from, 209
  of superior mediastinum, 203
**Greater occipital nerve**, 2
**Groin**
  left, 244
  right, 244
**Gubernaculum**, 364, 367
**Gyrus**
  angular, 106
    branch to, 142–143
  cingulate, 107
    isthmus of, 107
  dentate, 107, 109, 113, 120
  frontal
    inferior, 106
    medial, 107
    middle, 106
    superior, 106
  lingual, 107
  long, 106
  occipitotemporal
    lateral, 107–108
    medial, 107–108
  orbital, 108
  parahippocampal, 107–109, 120
  postcentral, 106
  precentral, 106
  straight, 108
  subcallosal, 107
  supramarginal, 106
  temporal
    inferior, 106, 108
    middle, 106
    superior, 106

## H

**Habenula**, 111
**Habenular commissure**, 107, 112, 116
**Habenular trigone**, 112, 116
**Hair cells**
  inner, 98
  outer, 98
**Hamate**, 440, 442–443, 449
  hook of, 428, 434, 439, 441, 443–445, 453
  radiographs of, 444
**Hand**
  arteries of, 453
  bones of, 443
  bursae of, 450
  cutaneous nerves of, 459, 463–464
  deep dorsal dissection of, 456
  dorsum of, lymph vessels passing to, 403
  fascia of, 450
  intrinsic muscles of, 452
  nerves of, 453

**J**

**Jacobson, tympanic nerve of**, 124, 126, 135
**Jejunal arteries**, 287–288, 290
  anastomotic loops of, 272
**Jejunal vein**, 290–291
**Jejunum**, 263–265, 271–272, 281, 290, 295
  axial CT images of, 323
  transverse section of, 325–328
**Joint capsule**
  of femur, 491
  of foot, 515
  of hand and fingers, 424, 445
  of knee, 493, 495, 507
    attachment of, 498
  of shoulder, 413
**Jugular foramen**, 8, 10, 13, 104–105, 126–128
**Jugular fossa**, 10, 12
**Jugular lymph nodes**
  anterior, 74
  external, 74
  internal, 74–75
**Jugular nerve**, 131
**Jugular notch**, 1, 27, 178, 193
  of sternum, 183
**Jugular trunk**, 74
  right, 295
**Jugular vein**
  anterior, 31, 73, 76
  external, 3, 31–32, 46, 73, 76, 195, 203, 208, 214, 234
  internal, 3, 26–28, 30–31, 33–34, 42, 46–47, 55, 59, 73, 75–78, 94, 96, 99, 129, 182, 186–187, 195, 208, 229, 234
    imaging of, 150
    inferior bulb of, 77, 170
    in jugular fossa, 12
    left, 209, 214
    right, 203
    superior bulb of, 170
**Jugulodigastric lymph nodes**, 74–75
**Jugulo-omohyoid lymph nodes**, 74–75
**Jugum**, 11

**K**

**Keratinized tip, of papilla**, 60
**Kidneys**, 176, 226, 266, 271, 278, 364, 378
  autonomic nerves of, 317–318
  cortex of, 311
    transverse section of, 326
  fibrous capsule of, 315
  gross structure of, 311
  hilum of, 311
  inferior pole of, 311
  innervation of, 163–164
  lateral border of, 311
  left, 194, 267, 281–282, 308, 313, 315, 320
    axial CT images of, 322
    transverse section of, 326–327
  lymph vessels and nodes of, 316
  major calyces of, 311
    transverse section of, 327
  medial border of, 311
  medulla (pyramids) of, 311
    transverse section of, 326
  minor calyces of, 311
  renal capsule of, 311
  renal papilla of, 311
  renal pelvis of, 311
    transverse section of, 327
  renal sinus of, 311
  right, 194, 267–269, 277, 281, 308–309, 313, 315, 320
    axial CT images of, 322
    transverse section of, 327

**Kidneys** (Continued)
  in situ
    anterior view of, 308
    posterior view of, 309
  superior pole of, 311
    transverse section of, 325–326
  vascular renal segments of, 312
**Knee**
  anterior view of, 494
  arteries of, 499, 509
  bursa of, 495
  cruciate and collateral ligaments, 496
  extension of, 469, 494
  flexion of, 469, 494
  interior of, 495
  lateral view of, 493
  medial view of, 493
  posterior view of, 497–498
  radiograph of, 497
  sagittal view of, 498
  transverse ligament of, 496

**L**

**Labbé, inferior anastomotic vein of**, 103, 146
**Labia majora**
  anterior commissure of, 354
  posterior commissure of, 354
**Labia majus**, 340
**Labia minora, frenulum of**, 354
**Labia minus**, 340
**Labial arteries**
  inferior, 35, 72
  posterior, 357, 382
  superior, 35, 72
    nasal septal branch of, 40
**Labial nerve**
  anterior, 391
  posterior, 391–392
**Labial vein**
  inferior, 73
  superior, 73
**Labioscrotal swelling**, 366
**Labium majus**, 340, 346, 350, 354, 366
**Labium minus**, 340, 346, 350, 354, 357, 366
**Labyrinthine artery**, 13, 96, 140–142, 144
  left, 137
**Labyrinths**
  bony, 97
  membranous, 97
  orientation of, 99
**Lacrimal apparatus**, 84
**Lacrimal artery**, 87, 139
  recurrent meningeal branch of, 102
**Lacrimal bone**, 4, 6, 8, 37
  of newborn, 14, 45
**Lacrimal canaliculi**, 84
**Lacrimal caruncle**, 83–84
**Lacrimal gland**, 85, 87–88, 134
  excretory ducts of, 84
  innervation of, 119, 163–164
  orbital part of, 84
  palpebral part of, 84
**Lacrimal lake**, 83–84
**Lacrimal nerve (V₁)**, 13, 52, 54, 85, 88, 122–123, 132
  communicating branch of, 52
  cutaneous branch of, 52
  palpebral branch of, 2
**Lacrimal papilla**
  inferior, 83–84
  superior, 83–84
**Lacrimal punctum**
  inferior, 83–84
  superior, 83–84
**Lacrimal sac**, 83–84
  fossa for, 4, 6

**Lactiferous duct**, 179
**Lactiferous sinus**, 179
**Lacuna, lateral (venous) of Trolard**, 101–102
**Lacuna magna**, 363
**Lacunar (Gimbernat's) ligament**, 246–247, 249, 255, 257–258, 472
**Lacus lacrimalis**, 83
**Lambda**, 9
**Lambdoid suture**, 5–9, 14
**Lamina**
  cervical, 20
  lumbar, 155–156, 158–159
  of mesovarium, 353
  thoracic, 154
**Lamina affixa**, 112
**Lamina cribrosa of sclera**, 89
**Lamina propria, of gingiva**, 63
**Lamina terminalis**, 107–108, 116, 148
**Large intestine**
  arteries of, 288
  autonomic nerves of, 302–303
  innervation of, 163–164
  lymph vessels and nodes of, 296
  mucosa and musculature of, 276
  veins of, 291
**Laryngeal artery**
  inferior, 82
  superior, 34, 72, 76–78, 137
    foramen for, 80
    internal branch of, 69
**Laryngeal inlet (aditus)**, 64, 66, 69
**Laryngeal nerve**
  inferior, 82
    anterior branches of, 82
    posterior branches of, 82
  recurrent, 26, 33, 69, 71, 82, 131, 229, 236
    left, 76–78, 127, 190, 203, 206–209, 223, 228–229, 236, 238–239
    right, 76–78, 82, 127, 209, 223, 236
  superior, 76, 82, 131–132, 136, 207, 236
    external branch of, 71, 76–78, 82, 127
    fold over internal branch of, 66
    internal branch of, 61, 65, 67, 69, 71, 76–78, 80, 82, 127
**Laryngeal prominence**, 79
**Laryngeal vein, superior**, 73
  foramen for, 80
  internal branch of, 69
**Laryngopharyngeal sympathetic branch**, 131
**Laryngopharynx**, 64, 66
**Larynx**, 136, 207
  cartilages of, 79
  infraglottic region of, 82
  innervation of, 119, 163–164
  muscles of, 80
    action of intrinsic, 81
  nerves of, 82
  sensory branches to, 82
  vestibule of, 82
**Lateral aperture**, 110
  of fourth ventricle, 147
  left, 109
**Lateral direct vein**, 146–147
**Lateral funiculus**, 116
**Lateral ligament**
  of ankle, 514
  of bladder, 343
**Lateral process**
  of malleus, 95
  of nasal septal cartilage, 35, 37–38
  of talus, 512
**Lateral recess**, 116
  left, 109
  vein of, 145

**Atlas of Human Anatomy**

Atlas of Human Anatomy

**Pudendum**, 354
**Pulmonary arteries**, 202
  left, 196, 203, 210–211, 218, 226, 228, 240
  right, 196, 203, 209, 211, 217–218, 226–227, 240
**Pulmonary heart valve**, 217, 219, 222
  anterior semilunar cusp of, 217, 219
  left semilunar cusp of, 217, 219
  right semilunar cusp of, 217, 219
**Pulmonary ligament**, 195–196, 205, 227–228
**Pulmonary (intrapulmonary) lymph nodes**, 205
**Pulmonary plexus**, 127, 207, 236
  anterior, 206
  branches to, 206
  posterior, 206
**Pulmonary trunk**, 203, 209–210, 212, 217, 221–222, 226, 237, 240
  bifurcation of, 214
**Pulmonary veins**, 202
  inferior
    left, 196, 211, 213
    right, 196, 211, 213, 217, 241
  left, 203, 212, 218, 221, 226, 228
  right, 203, 212, 218, 222, 226–227
  septum of, 202
  superior
    left, 196, 209, 211, 218
    right, 196, 209, 211, 217, 221
**Pulmonic heart valve**, 210
**Pulvinar**, 111–112
  left, 145
  right, 145
  of thalamus, 108, 112, 115–116, 140, 146
**Pupil**, 83
**Purkinje fibers**
  of left bundle, 222
  of right bundle, 222
**Putamen**, 109, 111
**Pyloric antrum**, 269
**Pyloric canal**, 269
  transverse section of, 325
**Pyloric lymph nodes**, 294
**Pyloric orifice**, 272
**Pyloric sphincter**, 270
**Pyloric zone**, 270
**Pylorus**, 269–271
  transverse section of, 325
**Pyramid, cerebellar**, 115
  decussation of, 115–116
  of inferior vermis, 114, 116
**Pyramidal eminence**, 96
**Pyramidal lobe, of thyroid gland**, 76
**Pyramidal process**, 10, 14, 16
**Pyramidalis muscle**, 246, 256, 328

## Q

**Quadrangular lobule**, 114
**Quadrangular space**, 413–414
**Quadrate ligament**, 424
**Quadrate tubercle**, 476
**Quadratus femoris muscle**, 477–478, 480, 482, 488–490, 531
  nerve to, 484, 486, 490
**Quadratus lumborum fascia**, 176, 192, 258–260, 262, 308, 315, 328, 341, 345
  transverse section of, 328
**Quadratus lumborum muscle**, 173, 176, 309, 483, 485
**Quadratus plantae muscle**, 521–522, 528, 531
**Quadratus plantae nerve**, 528
**Quadriceps femoris muscle**, 502, 525
**Quadriceps femoris tendon**, 468, 477, 488, 493–494, 498, 506–508
**Quadrigeminal cistern**, 110
  imaging of, 151

## R

**Radial artery**, 419–420, 431–436, 441, 447, 449, 452–454, 456–457, 460
  dorsal carpal branch of, 454
  palmar branch of, 433, 453
    superficial, 434–435, 441, 447, 452–453
  palmar carpal branches of, 434, 452
**Radial collateral artery**, 418, 420–421
**Radial collateral ligament**, 424
**Radial fossa**, 405, 422
**Radial groove**, 406
**Radial longitudinal crease**, 398
**Radial metaphyseal arcuate ligament, dorsal**, 442
**Radial nerve**, 400, 410, 413, 415–416, 418, 421, 433–434, 454, 459–463, 465
  in arm, 465
  communicating branches of, 455
  deep branch of, 433, 436, 460, 466
  dorsal digital branches, 400, 454, 459, 466
  in forearm, 466
  inferior lateral brachial cutaneous nerve from, 400–401
  lateral branch of, 454
  medial branch of, 454
  posterior antebrachial cutaneous nerve from, 400–401, 459
  posterior brachial cutaneous nerve from, 400–401
  superficial branch of, 400, 402, 430, 433, 436, 454–456, 459–460, 466
**Radial notch, of ulna**, 422, 425
**Radial recurrent artery**, 419–420, 433–435
**Radial tuberosity**, 417, 422, 425
  radiograph of, 423
**Radialis indicis artery**, 435, 453
**Radiate ligament, of head of rib**, 184
**Radiate sternocostal ligament**, 184, 404
**Radicular artery**
  anterior, 167–168
  posterior, 168
**Radicular vein, segmental**, 169
  anterior, 169
  posterior, 169
**Radiocarpal joint**, 439, 442
  articular disc of, 439, 442
**Radiocarpal ligament, dorsal**, 442
**Radiology, of heart**, 210
**Radiolunate ligament**
  long, 441
  palmar, 441
  short, 441
**Radioscaphocapitate ligament**, 441
**Radio-ulnar joint, distal**, 442
**Radio-ulnar ligament, dorsal**, 442
**Radius**, 422, 426–429, 431, 434, 436–439, 441–442, 452
  anterior border of, 425
  anterior surface of, 425
  dorsal (Lister's) tubercle of, 425
  head of, 417, 422–423, 425
  interosseous border of, 425
  interosseous membrane of, 425, 429
  neck of, 422–423, 425
  posterior border of, 425
  posterior surface of, 425
  radiograph of, 423
  rotators of, 426
  styloid process of, 425, 439
    radiographs of, 444
**Rathke's pouch**, 45
**Rectal artery**
  inferior, 288, 376, 380–383
  middle, 259, 288, 302, 313, 343, 376, 378, 380–381

**Rectal artery** *(Continued)*
  superior, 259, 268, 288, 297, 302–303, 313, 376, 378
    branch of, 288
**Rectal fascia**, 342–343, 355, 362, 369–372, 374
**Rectal lymph nodes**
  middle, 296
  superior, 296
**Rectal nerves**
  inferior, 303, 388–389, 391–392, 484, 490
  superior, 303
**Rectal plexus**, 302–303, 317, 388, 390
  communication between, 377
  external, 377
  internal, 377
  middle, 302
  superior, 297, 302
**Rectal vein**
  inferior, 292, 377
    right, 291
  middle, 260, 291–292, 377
    right, 291
  superior, 268, 291–292, 377
**Rectal venous plexus**, 260
  external, 291, 371–372
  internal, 371–372
  perimuscular, 291
**Rectocervical spaces**, 342
**Rectococcygeus muscle**, 258
**Rectoprostatic (Denonvilliers') fascia**, 321, 339, 344, 362, 369, 374
**Rectosigmoid arteries**, 376
**Rectosigmoid junction**, 276, 369, 371–372
**Recto-urethralis superior muscle**, 339
**Recto-uterine fold**, 342
**Recto-uterine ligament**, 342
**Recto-uterine pouch (of Douglas)**, 340, 342, 352, 369
**Rectovaginal spaces**, 342–343
**Rectovesical fascia**, 362, 374
**Rectovesical pouch**, 321, 344–345, 369
**Rectovesical space**, 374
**Rectum**, 258, 265, 268, 276, 308, 321, 335–337, 340–341, 343–346, 362, 371, 378, 390
  ampulla of, 346
  arteries of, male, 376
  circular muscle layer of, 371–372
  innervation of, 163–164
  longitudinal muscle layer of, 371–372
  muscularis mucosae of, 372
  radiography of, 156
  sagittal CT images of, 375
  in situ, 369
  transverse folds of, 371
  transverse section of, 397
  veins of, female, 377
**Rectus abdominis muscle**, 7, 178, 185–186, 188, 242, 246–247, 249, 251, 253–256, 321, 328–329, 341, 343–345, 355
  axial CT images of, 322
  sagittal CT images of, 375
  transverse section of, 324, 328
**Rectus capitis muscle**
  anterior, 30, 42, 75, 151
    communication with cervical plexus, 33
    nerves to, 130
  lateral, 30, 151
    communication with cervical plexus, 33
    nerves to, 130
  posterior
    major, 172–173, 175, 177
    minor, 172–173, 175, 177
**Rectus femoris muscle**, 396–397, 468, 477, 479, 481, 487–488, 492, 525, 530–531
**Rectus femoris tendon**, 468, 479–480, 494, 507

**Atlas of Human Anatomy**

**Tongue**, 38, 46–47, 59–60, 68
apex of, 60
body of, 43, 60, 64
dorsum of, 60
frenulum of, 46, 56
inferior longitudinal muscle of, 59
innervation of, 119
intrinsic muscles of, 60, 129
inferior longitudinal, 129
superior longitudinal, 129
transverse, 129
vertical, 129
lingual glands of, 60
longitudinal muscle of
inferior, 47, 151
superior, 47, 151
lymph follicles of, 60
lymph vessels and nodes of, 75
mucous glands of, 60
root of, 60, 64, 66–67, 69, 80
taste buds of, 60
transverse muscle of, 151
vertical muscle of, 151
**Tonsil**
of cerebellum, 114, 116
lingual, 60, 64, 68, 80
palatine, 47, 56–57, 60, 64, 66, 68
pharyngeal, 64, 66–68
imaging of, 151
**Tonsillar artery**, 51, 72
**Torus levatorius**, 66
**Torus tubarius**, 36, 38, 66, 68
posterior, opening of, 36
**Trabecula**, 149
artery of, 149
**Trabeculae carneae**, 217
**Trabecular meshwork and spaces of
iridocorneal angle**, 90
**Trachea**, 15, 26, 28, 64, 70, 76–80, 127, 193,
195, 199–200, 203–204, 208, 210, 214, 227,
229–231, 233, 237–239
connective tissue sheath of, 199
cross section through, 199
elastic fibers of, 199
epithelium of, 199
glands of, 199
innervation of, 119, 163–164
lung area for
left, 196
right, 196
lymph vessels of, 199
nerves of, 199
small arteries of, 199
**Tracheal cartilages**, 199
**Tracheal wall**
anterior, 199
posterior, 199
mucosa of, 199
**Trachealis muscle**, 199
**Tracheobronchial lymph nodes**, 261
inferior, 235, 240
superior, 235, 239
left, 205
right, 205
**Tracheobronchial (carinal) lymph nodes,
inferior**, 205
**Tracheobronchial tree, innervation of,
schema of**, 207
**Tracheo-esophageal groove**, 70
**Tragus**, 1, 95
**Transpyloric plane**, 244
**Transversalis fascia**, 7, 176, 245, 249,
255–257, 259, 315, 321, 341, 343–344, 346,
355
within inguinal triangle, 255
transverse section of, 328
**Transverse fasciculi**, 446, 519
**Transverse foramen**, 19

**Transverse ligament**
of atlas, 23
of knee, 496
**Transverse pericardial sinus**, 209, 212,
217–218
**Transverse process**, 176, 184
cervical, 19, 22, 30, 173
anterior tubercle of, 20, 30
C6, 137
posterior tubercle of, 20, 30
of coccyx, 157
lumbar, 155–156, 158–159, 243, 330
lumbosacral, L1, 192
thoracic, 154
of vertebral body, articular facet for,
184
**Transverse ridges**, 157
**Transverse sinus**, 99, 104–105, 146
groove for, 8, 11
imaging of, 150
sigmoid sinus continuation of, 105
**Transversospinalis muscle**, 238
**Transversus abdominis muscle**, 7,
172–173, 176, 186–187, 245, 247, 249, 251,
253–256, 258, 262, 308–309, 328, 341,
345
aponeurosis of, 7, 251, 309
tendon of origin of, 172–173, 176,
250
transverse section of, 328
**Transversus muscle**, 151
**Transversus thoracis muscle**, 177,
186–188, 213, 241
**Trapeziocapitate ligament**, 441–442
**Trapeziotrapezoid ligament**, 441–442
**Trapezium**, 439, 442–443, 445, 449, 454
radiographs of, 444
tubercle of, 439, 441, 443
**Trapezium bone**, 439
**Trapezius muscle**, 1, 26–29, 31, 128, 130,
152, 171, 174–175, 177, 185–186, 188,
238–241, 250, 398, 404–406, 409–410, 412,
415, 467
accessory nerve to, 128
innervation of, 119
**Trapezoid bone**, 439, 442–443, 449
radiographs of, 444
**Trapezoid ligament**, 404, 408, 411
**Treitz, ligament of**, 264
**Triangle**
anal, 358
of auscultation, 241, 409
auscultatory, 152, 250
cystohepatic (Calot's), 280, 284
deltopectoral, 409
inguinal (Hesselbach's), 249, 255
transversalis fascia within, 255
lumbar (of Petit), 152, 250
internal oblique muscle in, 171
lumbocostal, 192
of neck, 175
posterior, 171, 185
sternocostal, 187
suboccipital, 175
urogenital, 358
**Triangular aponeurosis**, 451
**Triangular fold**, 68
**Triangular fossa**, 95
**Triangular ligament**
left, 268, 277
right, 268, 277
**Triangular space**, 413
**Triceps brachii muscle**, 152, 178, 405–406,
409–410, 413–415, 418–419, 421, 438, 465,
467
lateral head of, 152, 239–240, 398
long head of, 152, 238–240, 398
tendon of, 152, 398

**Triceps brachii tendon**, 424, 430–431, 465
**Tricuspid heart valve**, 210, 213–214,
219–221, 241
anterior cusp of, 213, 217, 219–221
posterior cusp of, 213, 217, 219–221
right fibrous ring of, 219, 222
septal cusp of, 213, 217, 219–221
**Trigeminal (semilunar) ganglion**, 50, 52,
88, 105, 133–136
**Trigeminal impression**, 11
**Trigeminal nerve (V)**, 52, 55, 61, 99, 115,
123, 134–135, 145, 207
distribution of, 119
ganglion of, 117–118, 123, 132
mandibular division of, 2, 61
maxillary division of, 2, 61
mesencephalic nucleus of, 117–118, 123,
136
motor nucleus of, 117–118, 123, 132,
136
nuclei of, 123
ophthalmic division of, 2
schema of, 123
sensory root of, 115, 117–118, 123, 132
spinal nucleus of, 117–118, 123, 126–127
spinal tract of, 117–118, 123, 126–127
**Trigeminal tubercle**, 116
**Trigonal ring**, 347
**Trigone**
collateral, 112
habenular, 112, 116
hypoglossal, 116
olfactory, 120
of urinary bladder, 344, 346, 348,
362–363
vagal, 116
**Triquetrocapitate ligament**, 441
**Triquetrohamate ligament**, 441–442
**Triquetrum bone**, 439–440, 442–443
radiographs of, 444
**Triticeal cartilage**, 79
**Trochanter of femur**
greater, 152, 243, 330, 396–397, 468,
474–476, 479–480, 483, 489–490, 530
radiograph of, 331
lesser, 243, 258, 330, 474–476, 530
radiograph of, 331
**Trochanteric fossa**, 476
**Trochlea**, 86, 405–406, 422
fibular, 512–513
radiographs of, 423
of talus, 512, 531
**Trochlear nerve (IV)**, 55, 85–86, 88, 105,
115–118, 122, 145
distribution of, 119
schema of, 122
superior, 13
**Trochlear notch, of ulna**, 425
**Trochlear nucleus**, 117–118, 122
**Trolard**
lateral lacuna of, 101–102
superior anastomotic vein of, 103
**True cords**. *See* Vocal fold
**True pelvis**, 334
**True ribs**, 183
**Tubal artery**, 96, 382
**Tuber, of inferior vermis**, 114, 116
**Tuber (Bohler's) angle**, 513
**Tuber cinereum**, 107–108, 115
median eminence of, 148
**Tuberohypophyseal tract**, 148
**Tufted cell**, 120
**Tunica albuginea**, 359, 363, 368
**Tunica vaginalis**
cavity of, 364
parietal layer of, 365, 368
testis, 321
visceral layer of, 365, 368

**Turbinate**, 36, 44
**Tympanic artery**
anterior, 51, 72, 96, 139
inferior, 55, 96
superior, 96
**Tympanic canaliculus**, 10, 12
**Tympanic cavity**, 53, 94–96, 98,
125–126
**Tympanic membrane**, 94–96, 98
**Tympanic nerve**, 55, 95
inferior, 96
of Jacobson, 124, 126, 135
**Tympanic plexus**, 96, 124, 126, 133,
135
promontory with, 95
tubal branch of, 126
**Tyson's gland, opening of**, 360

# U

**Ulna**, 422, 426–429, 431, 436–439,
441–442, 452
anterior border of, 425
anterior surface of, 425
coronoid process of, 422, 425, 429
radiographs of, 423
interosseous border of, 425
interosseous membrane of, 425,
429
oblique cord of, 425
olecranon of, 398, 418, 422, 425, 427,
430–431, 465
radiographs of, 423
radial notch of, 422, 425
radiographs of, 423
styloid process of, 425, 439
radiographs of, 444
trochlear notch of, 425
**Ulna fascia**, 436
**Ulnar artery**, 419–420, 432–436, 441,
446–447, 449, 452–453, 460
carpal branch of, 456
deep palmar branch of, 433–435, 441,
446–447, 452–453, 460
palmar branch of, 453
palmar carpal branches of, 434,
452
**Ulnar bursa**, 449–450, 453
**Ulnar collateral artery**
inferior, 419–420, 431, 435
superior, 419–421, 430–431, 435
**Ulnar collateral ligament**, 424
**Ulnar nerve**, 400, 415–416, 418–419, 421,
430–434, 436, 441, 447, 449, 452–453,
459–464
articular branch of, 464
communicating branches of, 455
deep branch of, 434, 441, 446–447, 452–453,
460, 464
deep palmar branch of, 453
dorsal branch of, 400, 402, 430, 433–434,
436, 455–456, 459–460, 464
dorsal digital branch of, 400, 459
groove for, 406, 422
palmar branch of, 400, 402, 433, 446, 459,
464
palmar digital branch of, 400, 456,
459–460
superficial branch of, 433, 446–447, 453,
460, 464
superficial palmar arch of, 460
**Ulnar recurrent artery**
anterior, 420, 433–435
posterior, 420, 431, 434–435
**Ulnar tuberosity**, 417, 422, 425
**Ulnocapitate ligament**, 441
**Ulnolunate ligament**, 441
**Ulnotriquetral ligament**, 441–442

**Umbilical artery**, 226, 249, 259, 313, 376,
381
left, 249
occluded part of, 245, 257, 259, 268, 313,
343, 345, 378, 380–381
patent part of, 314, 378, 380–381
**Umbilical fold**
lateral, 249, 268, 341, 345
medial, 268, 341, 345, 378
median, 249, 268, 341, 345
right medial, 249
**Umbilical ligament**
medial, 226, 245, 249, 255–257, 259,
313–314, 341, 343, 345, 378, 380–381
left, 249
median, 256–257, 321, 341, 343, 345–346,
378, 381
**Umbilical prevesical fascia**, 249, 256,
343–344, 346
**Umbilical region**, 244
**Umbilical vein**, 226, 269
**Umbilicus**, 242, 249, 292, 329
sagittal CT images of, 375
**Umbo**, 95, 98
**Uncal vein**, 146
**Uncinate process**
cervical, 20
of ethmoidal bone, 36–37, 44
of newborn, 45
of pancreas, 281
transverse section of, 327
**Uncovertebral joints**, 21
**Uncus**, 107–108, 120
**Unerupted teeth**, 5
**Upper limb**
arteries of, 460
cutaneous innervation of, 400
dermatomes of, 399
lymph vessels and nodes of, 403
nerves of, 460–461
surface anatomy of, 398
**Urachus**, 249, 256–257, 268, 321, 341,
343–344, 346, 355, 378
median, 346
**Ureteric fold**, 341–342, 345
**Ureteric orifice**, 362
left, 348
right, 348
**Ureteric plexus**, 388
**Ureteropelvic junction, transverse
section of**, 327
**Ureters**, 249, 257, 260, 265, 268, 297, 308,
311, 313–314, 340–346, 350, 352, 362,
369–370, 378–382, 388, 390, 395
in abdomen and pelvis, 313
arteries of, 314
autonomic nerves of, 317–318
in female, 313
innervation of, 395
left, 313
transverse section of, 328
in male, 313
retroperitoneal, 313
right, 313, 353
**Urethra**, 258, 335–337, 339–340, 346, 348,
351, 356, 359, 361–363, 367, 396
bulbous portion of, 363
floor of, 363
growth of, 347
hiatus for, 338
intermediate part of, 363
musculofascial extensions to, 337
pendulous portion of, 363
prostatic, 348, 363
roof of, 363
spongy, 363
bulbous portion of, 348
transverse section of, 397

**Urethrae muscle**
compressor, 335, 350, 356–357, 382, 397
growth of, 347
sphincter, 335, 339, 356, 374, 395, 397
growth of, 347
**Urethral artery**, 361, 383
**Urethral crest**, 362–363
**Urethral fold**, 366
**Urethral glands (of Littré)**, 363
**Urethral lacunae, of Morgagni**,
363
**Urethral meatus, external**, 344
**Urethral orifice, external**, 329, 340, 354,
357, 360, 363, 366, 373
**Urethral sphincter muscle**
external, 249, 344, 361–363, 381
internal, 348, 362–363
**Urethrovaginal sphincter muscle**,
335
growth of, 347
**Urinary bladder**, 249, 256–257, 263, 268,
302, 308, 313, 321, 340, 342, 361–362, 364,
369, 378, 390, 395–396
apex of, 344, 346
arteries of, 314
autonomic nerves of, 317
body of, 344, 346
fascia of, 344
female, 341, 343, 348
growth of, 347
fundus of, 344, 346, 348
innervation of, 163–164, 395
lateral ligament of, 343
loop of Heiss, 347
lymph vessels and nodes of, 316
male, 344–345, 348
neck of, 344, 346, 348
orientation and supports of, 346
posterior loop of, 347
sagittal CT images of, 375
trigonal ring of, 347
trigone of, 344, 346, 348, 362–363
ureteric orifice of, 346
uvula of, 348, 362–363
**Urinary bladder-prostate junction**,
396
**Urogenital fold**, 366
**Urogenital groove**, 366
**Urogenital hiatus, growth of**, 347
**Urogenital sinus**, 367
**Urogenital triangle**, 358
**Uterine artery**, 313–314, 342, 350, 352–353,
378, 380, 382
branches of, 382
ovarian branches of, 353
vaginal branches of, 382
**Uterine fascia**, 343
**Uterine ostium**, 352
**Uterine (fallopian) tube**, 340–342, 350–352,
367, 378, 390, 393
abdominal ostium of, 352
ampulla of, 352–353
fimbriae of, 352–353
folds of, 352
infection of, 353
infundibulum of, 352–353
isthmus of, 352
uterine part of, 352
**Uterine vein**, 260, 342, 350, 352, 382
ovarian branches of, 353
superior, 377
**Uterosacral fold**, 313, 341, 370
**Uterosacral ligament**, 340, 343, 351–352
**Uterovaginal fascia**, 342, 350, 355
**Uterovaginal plexus**, 390, 392–393
**Uterovaginal venous plexus**, 260
**Uterovesical pouch.** *See* Vesico-uterine
pouch

**Uterus**, 341, 346, 350, 367, 369, 378, 390, 393
  adnexa and, 352
  arteries of, 382
  body of, 340, 342, 352
  cervix of, 340, 342–343, 350, 352
  fascial ligaments of, 351
  fundus of, 340, 342, 346, 352
    sagittal CT images of, 375
  growth of, 349
  hysterosalpingogram of, 353
  isthmus of, 352
  round ligament of, 260, 340–342, 350–351, 353, 355, 367, 378, 382
    terminal part of, 350
  supporting structures of, 350
  veins of, 382
**Utricle**, 94, 97–98, 125
  prostatic, 362
**Uvula**, 56, 66–68
  of bladder, 348
  of inferior vermis, 114, 116
  of urinary bladder, 362–363
**Uvular muscle**, 57, 151

## V

**Vagal cardiac nerves**, 131
**Vagal fibers**, 127
**Vagal trigone**, 116
**Vagal trunk**, 258, 297
  anterior, 127, 206, 229, 236, 298–302, 306–307, 317, 319, 388
    celiac branch of, 127, 298–299, 301
    gastric branches of, 127, 298
    hepatic branch of, 127, 298–299, 302, 306
  posterior, 236, 299–302, 306–307, 317, 319, 388
    celiac branch of, 127, 298–301, 388
    gastric branch of, 299
**Vagina**, 335–337, 340, 346, 350, 352, 356, 367, 369, 373, 378, 393
  growth of, 347
  horizontal portion of, 351
  musculofascial extensions to, 337
  sagittal CT images of, 375
  supporting structures of, 350
  transverse section of, 397
  vertical portion of, 351
  vestibule of, 350, 354, 367
**Vaginal artery**, 313, 350, 353, 378, 380, 382
  inferior, 343, 346
**Vaginal fascia**, 369
**Vaginal fornix**, 352
  anterior, 340
  posterior, 340
**Vaginal orifice**, 340, 354, 357, 366
**Vaginal vein**, 377
**Vaginal venous plexus**, 377, 397
**Vaginal wall**, 350–351
**Vaginorectal fascial fibers**, 343
**Vagus nerve (X)**, 26, 32–34, 42, 55, 61, 71–72, 76–78, 105, 115, 117–118, 126–128, 131–132, 136, 164, 203, 206–208, 224, 229, 236, 303–304, 318
  auricular branch of, 2, 12, 127
    communication to, 126
  in carotid sheath, 47
  celiac branch of, 300
  cervical cardiac branch of
    inferior, 127
    superior, 71–72, 127, 131–132
  communicating branch of, 127
  communication with cervical plexus, 33
  cranial root of, 127
  distribution of, 119

**Vagus nerve (X)** *(Continued)*
  dorsal nucleus of, 117, 127, 303
    posterior, 118
  ganglion of
    inferior, 55, 127–129, 236
    superior, 127–128, 236
  inferior, 13
  inferior (nodose) ganglion of, 136, 207
  in jugular fossa, 12
  left, 77, 190, 203, 209, 223, 228, 238–239
  meningeal branch of, 127
  pharyngeal branch of, 126–127, 131–132, 236
  posterior (dorsal) nucleus of, 224, 318
  right, 77, 190, 203, 209, 223, 227, 238
  schema of, 127
  sympathetic trunk and, 73, 126
  thoracic cardiac branch of, 127, 206, 223–224
  vagal branches of, 236
**Vallate papillae**, 60, 136
**Vallecula**, 60, 68
**Valves.** *See* Heart valves
**Valves of Houston**, 371
**Valves of Kerckring**, 272, 280
**Vas deferens**, 249
**Vascular fold, of cecum**, 273
**Vascular smooth muscle, innervation to**, 163
**Vascular system, of liver**, 278
**Vastus intermedius muscle**, 477–480, 488, 492, 494, 525, 531
**Vastus lateralis muscle**, 397, 468, 477–481, 487, 489, 492–494, 506–507, 525, 531
**Vastus medialis muscle**, 468, 477–478, 480, 487–488, 492–494, 507, 525, 531
  nerve to, 487, 492
**Vater**
  hepatopancreatic ampulla of, 280
  major duodenal papilla of, 272, 280
**Veins.** *See also specific veins*
  of abdominal wall
    anterior, 252
    posterior, 260
  of anal canal, female, 377
  of brain
    deep, 146
    subependymal, 147
  of duodenum, 289
  of esophagus, 234
  of eye, intrinsic, 92
  of face, 3
  of hypothalamus and hypophysis, 149
  of internal thoracic wall, 189
  of iris, 93
  of large intestine, 291
  of oral and pharyngeal regions, 73
  of orbit and eyelids, 87
  of pancreas, 289
  of pelvic organs, female, 378
  of pelvis, male, 381
  of perineum, 382
    male, 383
  of posterior cranial fossa, 145
  of rectum, female, 377
  of scalp, 3
  of small intestine, 290
  of spinal cord, 169
  of spleen, 289
  of stomach, 289
  of suprarenal glands, 320
  of testis, 379
  of uterus, 382
  of vertebral column, 169–170

**Vena cava**, 380
  inferior, 176, 203, 206, 211–212, 214, 217–218, 220, 222, 226–227, 229, 234, 237, 260, 266–268, 271, 277, 281, 286, 289, 308–310, 315, 320, 341, 345, 376, 378–379, 381, 390
    axial CT images of, 322–323
    groove for, 277
    lung groove for, 196
    transverse section of, 324–328
    valve (eustachian) of, 217
  superior, 76–77, 190, 203, 208–214, 217, 221–222, 226–227, 234, 237, 239–241
    lung groove for, 196
**Vena comitans, of hypoglossal nerve**, 47, 59, 73
**Venae comitantes**, 59, 447
**Venae rectae**, 290
**Venous arch, dorsal**, 470
**Venous plexus**, 353
  basilar, 104–105
  external, 370
    communication with, 377
  in foramen magnum, 12
  internal, 370
    communication with, 377
  of internal carotid artery, 55
  pampiniform, 252, 365, 379, 381
  prostatic, 344, 381
  rectal, 260
    external, 291
    perimuscular, 291
  vaginal, 377, 397
  vertebral (of Batson), 104
    internal, 166
  around vertebral artery, 170
  vesical, 381
**Venous sinuses, dural**
  sagittal section of, 104
  superior view of, 105
**Ventral posteromedial nucleus, of thalamus**, 136
**Ventral rami**
  of cervical spinal nerves, 32, 71, 129, 174, 190
  of lumbar spinal nerves, 158, 174, 388, 393, 485
  of sacral spinal nerves, 388, 392
  in situ, 160
  of spinal nerves, 165–166
  of thoracic spinal nerve, 174, 177, 388, 392
**Ventricles (cardiac)**, 221
  left, 209–214, 216, 218, 221, 237, 241
    posterior vein of, 215
    right coronary artery branches to back of, 216
  right, 209, 211–214, 217, 221, 237, 241
**Ventricles (cerebral)**, 109
  fourth, 109, 116, 144, 147
    cerebellum and, 114, 116
    choroid plexus of, 107, 110, 115–116, 145
    choroidal branch to, 144
    imaging of, 151
    lateral apertures of, 147
    left lateral aperture of, 109
    left lateral recess of, 109, 116
    median apertures of, 109, 147
    rhomboid fossa of, 115
    taenia of, 116
    vein of lateral recess of, 145
  interventricular foramen (of Monro), 109–110
  lateral, 109, 111, 113, 140, 147
    central part of, 109
    choroid plexus of, 101, 109–111, 140, 144, 146
    frontal (anterior) horn of, 109
    imaging of, 151

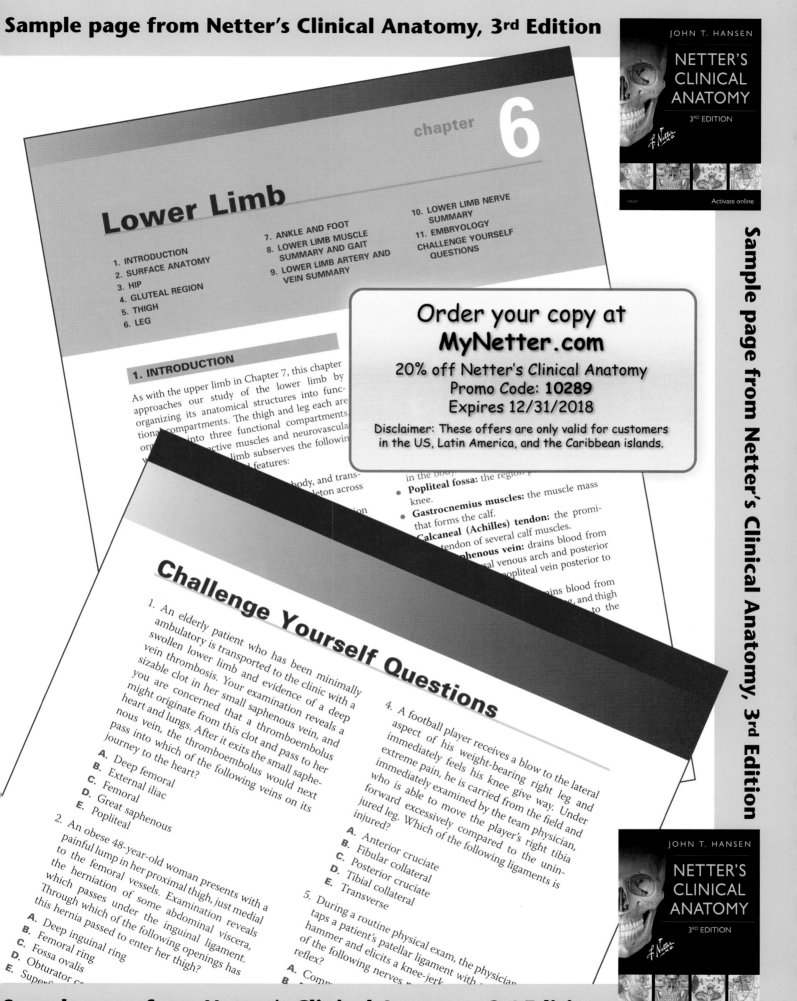

chapter **6**

# Lower Limb

## 1. INTRODUCTION

As with the upper limb in Chapter 7, this chapter approaches our study of the lower limb by organizing its anatomical structures into functional compartments. The thigh and leg each are organized into three functional compartments, with protective muscles and neurovascular... limb subserves the following... ...features:

...body, and trans-...leton across

...in the body.

- **Popliteal fossa:** the region...knee.
- **Gastrocnemius muscles:** the muscle mass that forms the calf.
- **Calcaneal (Achilles) tendon:** the prominent tendon of several calf muscles.
- ...**phenous vein:** drains blood from ...sal venous arch and posterior to ...popliteal vein posterior to
- ...ains blood from ...g, and thigh ...to the

# Challenge Yourself Questions

1. An elderly patient who has been minimally ambulatory is transported to the clinic with a swollen lower limb and evidence of a deep vein thrombosis. Your examination reveals a sizable clot in her small saphenous vein, and you are concerned that a thromboembolus might originate from this clot and pass to her heart and lungs. After it exits the small saphenous vein, the thromboembolus would next pass into which of the following veins on its journey to the heart?

   A. Deep femoral
   B. External iliac
   C. Femoral
   D. Great saphenous
   E. Popliteal

2. An obese 48-year-old woman presents with a painful lump in her proximal thigh, just medial to the femoral vessels. Examination reveals the herniation of some abdominal viscera, which passes under the inguinal ligament. Through which of the following openings has this hernia passed to enter her thigh?

   A. Deep inguinal ring
   B. Femoral ring
   C. Fossa ovalis
   D. Obturator ca...
   E. Superc...

4. A football player receives a blow to the lateral aspect of his weight-bearing right leg and immediately feels his knee give way. Under extreme pain, he is carried from the field and immediately examined by the team physician, who is able to move the player's right tibia forward excessively compared to the uninjured leg. Which of the following ligaments is injured?

   A. Anterior cruciate
   B. Fibular collateral
   C. Posterior cruciate
   D. Tibial collateral
   E. Transverse

5. During a routine physical exam, the physician taps a patient's patellar ligament with a hammer and elicits a knee-jerk with... of the following nerves... reflex?

   A. Comm...
   B. ...

# Intervertebral Disc Herniation—cont'd

The most common sites for disc herniation in the cervical region are the C5-C6 and C6-C7 levels, resulting in shoulder and upper limb pain. In the lumbar region the primary sites are the L4-L5 and L5-S1 levels. Lumbar disc herniation is much more common than cervical herniation and results in pain over the sacro-iliac joint, hip, posterior thigh, and leg.

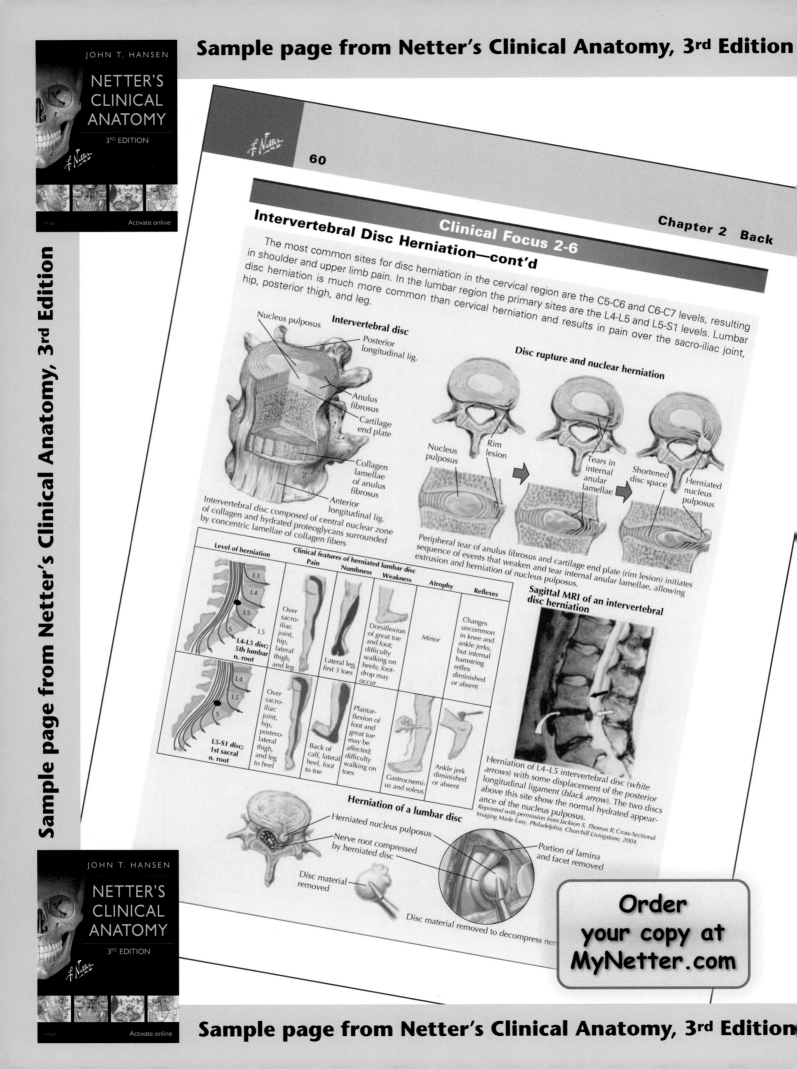

Intervertebral disc composed of central nuclear zone of collagen and hydrated proteoglycans surrounded by concentric lamellae of collagen fibers

**Nucleus pulposus**
**Intervertebral disc**
Posterior longitudinal lig.
Anulus fibrosus
Cartilage end plate
Collagen lamellae of anulus fibrosus
Anterior longitudinal lig.

**Disc rupture and nuclear herniation**

Nucleus pulposus
Rim lesion
Tears in internal anular lamellae
Shortened disc space
Herniated nucleus pulposus

Peripheral tear of anulus fibrosus and cartilage end plate (rim lesion) initiates sequence of events that weaken and tear internal anular lamellae, allowing extrusion and herniation of nucleus pulposus.

**Sagittal MRI of an intervertebral disc herniation**

Herniation of L4–L5 intervertebral disc (*white arrows*) with some displacement of the posterior longitudinal ligament (*black arrow*). The two discs above this site show the normal hydrated appearance of the nucleus pulposus.
*Reprinted with permission from Jackson S, Thomas R: Cross-Sectional Imaging Made Easy. Philadelphia, Churchill Livingstone, 2004.*

## Clinical features of herniated lumbar disc

| Level of herniation | Pain | Numbness | Weakness | Atrophy | Reflexes |
|---|---|---|---|---|---|
| **L4-L5 disc; 5th lumbar n. root** | Over sacro-iliac joint, hip, lateral thigh, and leg | Lateral leg, first 3 toes | Dorsiflexion of great toe and foot; difficulty walking on heels; foot-drop may occur | Minor | Changes uncommon in knee and ankle jerks, but internal hamstring reflex diminished or absent |
| **L5-S1 disc; 1st sacral n. root** | Over sacro-iliac joint, hip, postero-lateral thigh, and leg to heel | Back of calf, lateral heel, foot to toe | Plantar-flexion of foot and great toe may be affected; difficulty walking on toes | Gastrocnemius and soleus | Ankle jerk diminished or absent |

**Herniation of a lumbar disc**

Herniated nucleus pulposus
Nerve root compressed by herniated disc
Disc material removed
Portion of lamina and facet removed
Disc material removed to decompress ner...

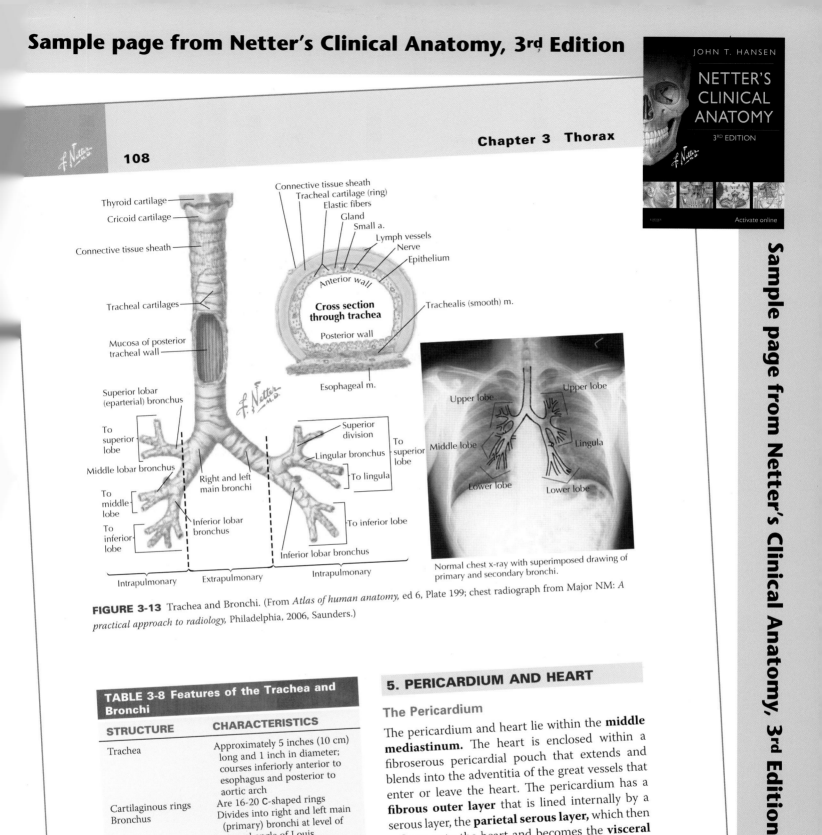

Thyroid cartilage
Cricoid cartilage
Connective tissue sheath
Tracheal cartilages
Mucosa of posterior tracheal wall
Superior lobar (eparterial) bronchus
To superior lobe
Middle lobar bronchus
To middle lobe
To inferior lobe
Inferior lobar bronchus
Intrapulmonary
Extrapulmonary
Intrapulmonary

Connective tissue sheath
Tracheal cartilage (ring)
Elastic fibers
Gland
Small a.
Lymph vessels
Nerve
Epithelium
Anterior wall
**Cross section through trachea**
Posterior wall
Trachealis (smooth) m.
Esophageal m.

Right and left main bronchi
Superior division
Lingular bronchus
To superior lobe
To lingula
Inferior lobar bronchus
To inferior lobe

Upper lobe
Upper lobe
Middle lobe
Lingula
Lower lobe
Lower lobe

Normal chest x-ray with superimposed drawing of primary and secondary bronchi.

**FIGURE 3-13** Trachea and Bronchi. (From *Atlas of human anatomy*, ed 6, Plate 199; chest radiograph from Major NM: *A practical approach to radiology*, Philadelphia, 2006, Saunders.)

**TABLE 3-8 Features of the Trachea and Bronchi**

| STRUCTURE | CHARACTERISTICS |
|---|---|
| Trachea | Approximately 5 inches (10 cm) long and 1 inch in diameter; courses inferiorly anterior to esophagus and posterior to aortic arch |
| Cartilaginous rings Bronchus | Are 16-20 **C**-shaped rings Divides into right and left main (primary) bronchi at level of sternal angle of Louis |
| Right bronchus | Shorter, wider, and more vertical than left bronchus; aspirated foreign objects more likely to [enter] into right bronchus [Sharp], keel-like cartilage at [biforcation] of trachea [To] lobes of each lung (three [on right], two on left) [To] bronchopulmonary [segm]ents (10 for each lung) |

## 5. PERICARDIUM AND HEART

### The Pericardium

The pericardium and heart lie within the **middle mediastinum.** The heart is enclosed within a fibroserous pericardial pouch that extends and blends into the adventitia of the great vessels that enter or leave the heart. The pericardium has a **fibrous outer layer** that is lined internally by a serous layer, the **parietal serous layer,** which then reflects onto the heart and becomes the **visceral serous layer,** which is the outer covering of the heart itself, also known as the **epicardium** (Fi[g] 3-14 and Table 3-9). These two serous layers for[m] a potential space known as the **pericardial s**[pace] **(cavity).**

### The Heart

The heart is essentially two muscular pumps [in] series. The two atria contract in unison, follow[ed]

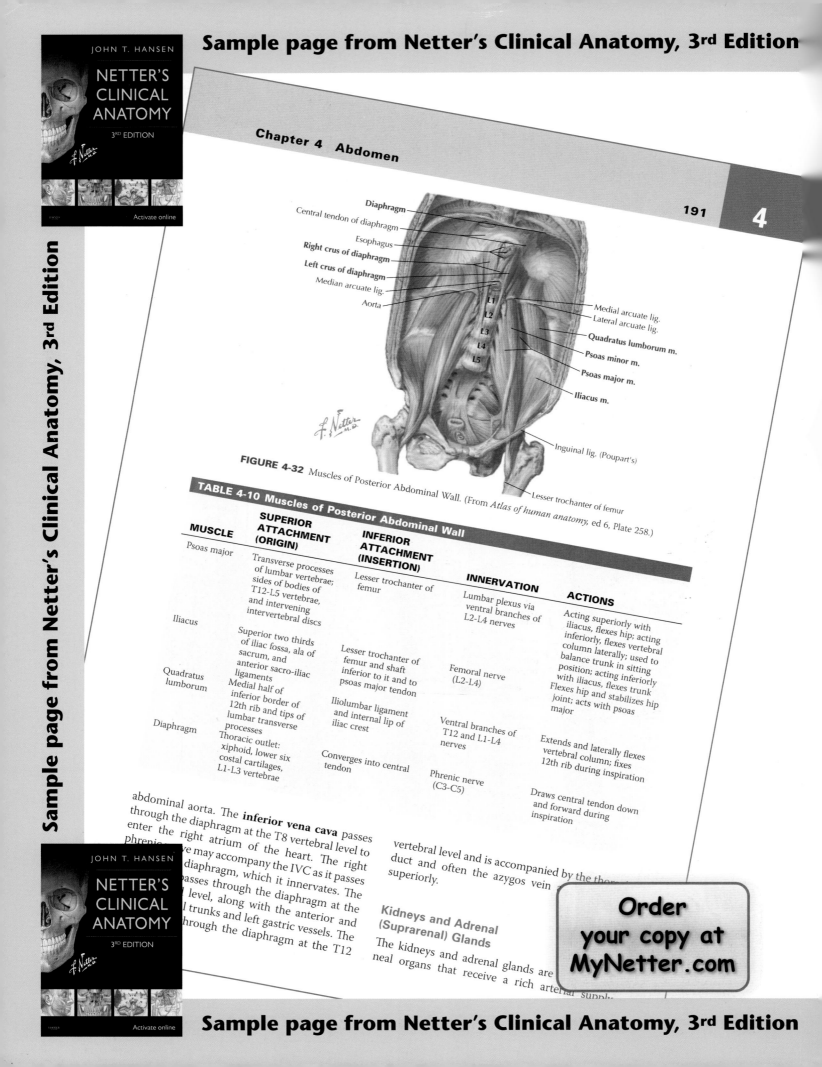

**FIGURE 4-32** Muscles of Posterior Abdominal Wall. (From *Atlas of human anatomy*, ed 6, Plate 258.)

**TABLE 4-10 Muscles of Posterior Abdominal Wall**

| MUSCLE | SUPERIOR ATTACHMENT (ORIGIN) | INFERIOR ATTACHMENT (INSERTION) | INNERVATION | ACTIONS |
|---|---|---|---|---|
| Psoas major | Transverse processes of lumbar vertebrae; sides of bodies of T12-L5 vertebrae, and intervening intervertebral discs | Lesser trochanter of femur | Lumbar plexus via ventral branches of L2-L4 nerves | Acting superiorly with iliacus, flexes hip; acting inferiorly, flexes vertebral column laterally; used to balance trunk in sitting position; acting inferiorly with iliacus, flexes trunk |
| Iliacus | Superior two thirds of iliac fossa, ala of sacrum, and anterior sacro-iliac ligaments | Lesser trochanter of femur and shaft inferior to it and to psoas major tendon | Femoral nerve (L2-L4) | Flexes hip and stabilizes hip joint; acts with psoas major |
| Quadratus lumborum | Medial half of inferior border of 12th rib and tips of lumbar transverse processes | Iliolumbar ligament and internal lip of iliac crest | Ventral branches of T12 and L1-L4 nerves | Extends and laterally flexes vertebral column; fixes 12th rib during inspiration |
| Diaphragm | Thoracic outlet: xiphoid, lower six costal cartilages, L1-L3 vertebrae | Converges into central tendon | Phrenic nerve (C3-C5) | Draws central tendon down and forward during inspiration |

abdominal aorta. The **inferior vena cava** passes through the diaphragm at the T8 vertebral level to enter the right atrium of the heart. The right phrenic [nerve] may accompany the IVC as it passes [through the] diaphragm, which it innervates. The [esophagus] passes through the diaphragm at the [T10] level, along with the anterior and [posterior vaga]l trunks and left gastric vessels. The [aorta passes] through the diaphragm at the T12

vertebral level and is accompanied by the thor[acic] duct and often the azygos vein [and] superiorly.

## Kidneys and Adrenal (Suprarenal) Glands

The kidneys and adrenal glands are [retroperito]neal organs that receive a rich arterial supply.

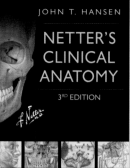

inguinal region, rectus sheath, and lateral thoracic wall. Most of its connections ultimately drain into the **axillary vein (4)** and then into the **subclavian vein**, **brachiocephalic veins**, which form the **superior vena cava**, and then into the **heart (6)**. The inferior epigastric veins (from the external iliac veins) enter the posterior rectus sheath and course cranially above the umbilicus as the superior epigastric veins and then anastomose with the internal thoracic veins that drain into the subclavian veins (Fig. 4-3).

The superficial veins can become enlarged during portal hypertension, when the venous flow through the liver is compromised. Important **portosystemic anastomoses** between the portal system and caval system can allow venous blood to gain access to the caval veins (both deep and

superficial veins) to assist in returning blood to the heart.

Variations in the venous pattern and in the number of veins and their size are common, so it is best to understand the major venous channels and realize that smaller veins often are more variable.

### Hepatic Portal System of Veins

The hepatic portal system of veins drains the abdominal GI tract and two of its accessory organs (pancreas and gallbladder) and the spleen (immune system organ) (Fig. 4-40). This blood then collects largely in the liver, where processing of absorbed GI contents takes place. (However, most fats are absorbed by the lymphatics and returned via the thoracic duct to the venous system in the neck, at the junction of the left internal jugular and left

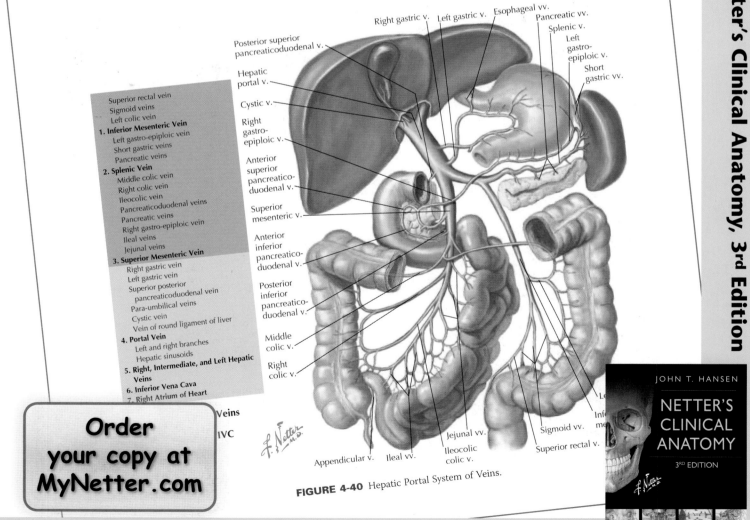

Superior rectal vein
Sigmoid veins
Left colic vein
**1. Inferior Mesenteric Vein**
    Left gastro-epiploic vein
    Short gastric veins
    Pancreatic veins
**2. Splenic Vein**
    Middle colic vein
    Right colic vein
    Ileocolic vein
    Pancreaticoduodenal veins
    Pancreatic veins
    Right gastro-epiploic vein
    Ileal veins
    Jejunal veins
**3. Superior Mesenteric Vein**
    Right gastric vein
    Left gastric vein
    Superior posterior
        pancreaticoduodenal vein
    Para-umbilical veins
    Cystic vein
    Vein of round ligament of liver
**4. Portal Vein**
    Left and right branches
    Hepatic sinusoids
**5. Right, Intermediate, and Left Hepatic Veins**
**6. Inferior Vena Cava**
**7. Right Atrium of Heart**

**FIGURE 4-40** Hepatic Portal System of Veins.

### Nosebleed

A nosebleed, or **epistaxis,** is a common occurrence and often involves the richly vascularized region of the vestibule and the anteroinferior aspect of the nasal septum (Kiesselbach's area). Nosebleeds usually result from trauma to the septal branch of the superior labial artery from the facial artery.

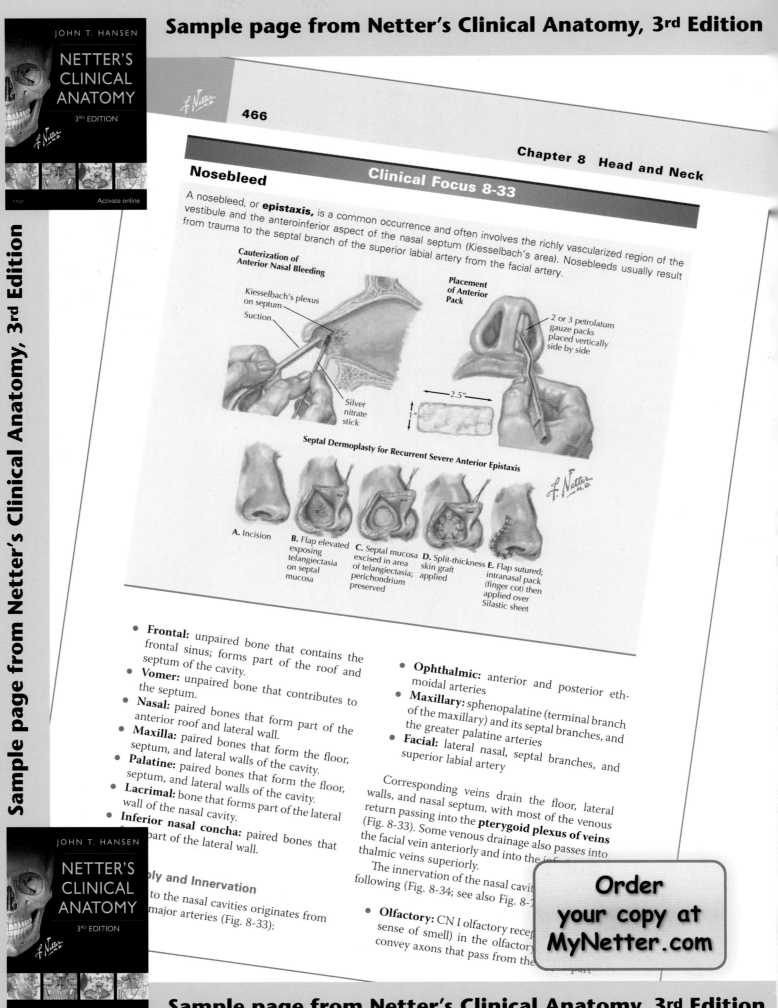

Cauterization of Anterior Nasal Bleeding

Kiesselbach's plexus on septum

Suction

Silver nitrate stick

Placement of Anterior Pack

2 or 3 petrolatum gauze packs placed vertically side by side

2.5"

1"

Septal Dermoplasty for Recurrent Severe Anterior Epistaxis

A. Incision

B. Flap elevated exposing telangiectasia on septal mucosa

C. Septal mucosa excised in area of telangiectasia; perichondrium preserved

D. Split-thickness skin graft applied

E. Flap sutured; intranasal pack (finger cot) then applied over Silastic sheet

- **Frontal:** unpaired bone that contains the frontal sinus; forms part of the roof and septum of the cavity.
- **Vomer:** unpaired bone that contributes to the septum.
- **Nasal:** paired bones that form part of the anterior roof and lateral wall.
- **Maxilla:** paired bones that form the floor, septum, and lateral walls of the cavity.
- **Palatine:** paired bones that form the floor, septum, and lateral walls of the cavity.
- **Lacrimal:** bone that forms part of the lateral wall of the nasal cavity.
- **Inferior nasal concha:** paired bones that ... part of the lateral wall.

...ly and Innervation

...to the nasal cavities originates from ...major arteries (Fig. 8-33):

- **Ophthalmic:** anterior and posterior ethmoidal arteries
- **Maxillary:** sphenopalatine (terminal branch of the maxillary) and its septal branches, and the greater palatine arteries
- **Facial:** lateral nasal, septal branches, and superior labial artery

Corresponding veins drain the floor, lateral walls, and nasal septum, with most of the venous return passing into the **pterygoid plexus of veins** (Fig. 8-33). Some venous drainage also passes into the facial vein anteriorly and into the inf... thalmic veins superiorly.

The innervation of the nasal cavi... following (Fig. 8-34; see also Fig. 8-7...

- **Olfactory:** CN I olfactory recep... sense of smell) in the olfactory... convey axons that pass from the... part

*Netter's Online Dissection Modules by UNC*

### Head & Neck

| UNC 1. | Posterior Neck and Suboccipital Region: Step 5. Suboccipital triangle |
| UNC 2. | Posterior Neck and Suboccipital Region: Step 6. Exposure of the posterior arch of C1 and related structures |
| UNC 3. | Posterior Neck and Suboccipital Region: Step 7. Vertebral artery and suboccipital nerve |
| UNC 4. | Anterior Neck: Step 6. Infrahyoid and digastric muscles; submandibular gland |
| UNC 5. | Anterior Neck: Step 7. Subdivisions of the anterior triangle |
| UNC 6. | Brain: Step 1. Cerebral hemispheres, lobes, fissures, gyri and sulci |
| UNC 7. | Brain: Step 2. Diencephalon: mammillary bodies, pituitary gland, tuber cinereum, optic nerves, and pineal gland |
| UNC 8. | Brain: Step 3. Mesencephalon: cerebral peduncles, interpeduncular fossa, oculomotor nerve, trochlear nerve, and corpora quadrigemini |
| UNC 9. | Brain: Step 4. Metencephalon: pons and cerebellum and associated cranial nerves |
| UNC 10. | Brain: Step 5. Medulla oblongata: olive, pyramids, apertures, and choroid plexus of the fourth ventricle |
| UNC 11. | Brain: Step 6. Cerebral arterial circle (of Willis) |
| UNC 12. | Brain: Step 7. Middle, anterior and posterior cerebral arteries |
| UNC 13. | Brain: Step 8. Midsagittal section of the brain |
| UNC 14. | Brain: Step 9. CN III, V, and VI in the floor of the cranial cavity; trigeminal cave and ganglion; mandibular division of CN V |
| UNC 15. | Cranial Cavity and Dural Venous Sinuses: Step 10. Reflection of the tentorium cerebelli and removal of the brain |
| UNC 16. | Cranial Cavity and Dural Venous Sinuses: Step 11. Dural venous sinuses |
| UNC 17. | Eye and Orbit I: Step 2. Frontal nerve |
| UNC 18. | Eye and Orbit I: Step 3. Superior oblique muscle; trochlear and lacrimal nerves |
| UNC 19. | Osteology of the Head and Neck: Step 7. Cranial sutures |
| UNC 20. | Osteology of the Head and Neck: Step 19. Foramina in the base of the skull |

### Back & Spinal Cord

| UNC 21. | Vertebral Column and Its Contents: Step 2. Epidural space and dura mater |
| UNC 22. | Vertebral Column and Its Contents: Step 3. Spinal cord, conus medullaris, internal filum terminale, arachnoid membrane |

### Thorax

| UNC 23. | Coronary Circulation and Internal Structure of the Heart: Step 4. Internal anatomy of the right atrium |

UNC 24.    Coronary Circulation and Internal Structure of the Heart: Step 5. Internal anatomy of the right ventricle

UNC 25.    Posterior Mediastinum, Azygos System: Step 1. Vagus and recurrent laryngeal nerves

UNC 26.    Posterior Mediastinum, Azygos System: Step 2. Relationship of the esophagus to the tracheal bifurcation and thoracic vertebrae

### Abdomen

UNC 27.    Anterior Abdominal Wall and Abdominal Viscera in situ: Step 11. Ligaments of the liver

UNC 28.    Anterior Abdominal Wall and Abdominal Viscera in situ: Step 12. Abdominal viscera in situ

UNC 29.    Stomach, Duodenum, Portal System, and Inferior Mesenteric Artery: Step 8. Internal anatomy of the duodenum

UNC 30.    Stomach, Duodenum, Portal System, and Inferior Mesenteric Artery: Step 9. Duct system within the pancreas

### Pelvis & Perineum

UNC 31.    Female Pelvic Viscera: Step 1. Pelvic viscera in situ

UNC 32.    Female Pelvic Viscera: Step 5. Pelvic ligaments and uterine tube

UNC 33.    Somatic Nerves of the Greater and Lesser Pelvis; Pelvic Diaphragm: Step 6. Lumbosacral trunk and sacral plexus

UNC 34.    Somatic Nerves of the Greater and Lesser Pelvis; Pelvic Diaphragm: Step 7. Obturator internus fascia and the arcus tendineus

### Upper Limb

UNC 35.    Posterior Shoulder: Step 2. Rhomboid major, rhomboid minor, and levator scapulae muscles; accessory nerve

UNC 36.    Posterior Shoulder: Step 3. Innervation of the rhomboid and latissimus dorsi muscles; the dorsal scapular and thoracodorsal nerves

UNC 37.    Flexor Surface of the Forearm: Step 4. Pronator teres and muscular branches of the median nerve

UNC 38.    Flexor Surface of the Forearm: Step 5. Sectioning of first layer of flexor muscles

### Lower Limb

UNC 39.    Medial and Anterior Thigh: Step 4. Sartorius muscle; medial and lateral inter muscular septa

UNC 40.    Medial and Anterior Thigh: Step 5. Quadriceps femoris muscle

UNC 41.    Popliteal Fossa, Knee Joint, and Posterior Compartment of the Leg: Step 5. Triceps surae and its innervation

UNC 42.    Popliteal Fossa, Knee Joint, and Posterior Compartment of the Leg: Step 6. Contents of the deep posterior compartment of the leg